Inborn Errors of Metabolism

OXFORD MONOGRAPHS ON MEDICAL GENETICS
General Editors
Judith G. Hall
Peter S. Harper
Louanne Hudgkins
Evan Eichler

1. R.B. McConnell: *The genetics of gastrointestinal disorders*
2. A.C. Kopéc: *The distribution of the blood groups in the United Kingdom*
3. E. Slater and V.A. Cowie: *The genetics of mental disorders*
4. C.O. Carter and T.J. Fairbank: *The genetics of locomotor disorders*
5. A.E. Mourant, A.C. Kopéc, and K. Domaniewska-Sobezak: *The distribution of the human blood groups and other polymorphisms*
6. A.E. Mourant, A.C. Kopéc, and K. Domaniewska-Sobezak: *Blood groups and diseases*
7. A.G. Steinbert and C.E. Cook: *The distribution of the human immunoglobulin allotypes*
8. D. Tills, A.C. Kopéc, and R.E. Tills *The distribution of the human blood groups and other polymorphisms: Supplement I*
10. D.Z. Loesch: *Quantitative dermatoglyphics: classification, genetics, and pathology*
11. D.J. Bond and A.C. Chandley: *Aneuploidy*
12. P.F. Benson and A.H. Fensom: *Genetic biochemical disorders*
13. G.R. Sutherland and F. Hecht: *Fragile sites on human chromosomes*
14. M. d'A. Crawfurd: *The genetics of renal tract disorders*
16. C.R. Scriver and B. Child: *Garrod's inborn factors in disease*
18. M. Baraitser: *The genetics of neurological disorders*
19. R.J. Gorlin, M.M. Cohen, Jr., and L.S. Levin: *Syndromes of the head and neck, third edition*
21. D. Warburton, J. Byrne, and N. Canki: *Chromosome anomalies and prenatal development: an atlas*
22. J.J. Nora, K. Berg, and A.H. Nora: *Cardiovascular disease: genetics, epidemiology, and prevention*
24. A.E.H. Emery: *Duchenne muscular dystrophy, second edition*
25. E.G.D. Tuddenham and D.N. Cooper: *The molecular genetics of haemostasis and its inherited disorders*
26. A. Boué: *Foetal medicine*
27. R.E. Stevenson, J.G. Hall, and R.M. Goodman: *Human malformations*
28. R.J. Gorlin, H.V. Toriello, and M.M. Cohen, Jr.: *Hereditary hearing loss and its syndromes*
29. R.J.M. Gardner and G.R. Sutherland: *Chromosomes abnormalities and genetic counseling, second edition*
30. A.S. Teebi and T.I. Farag: *Genetic disorders among Arab populations*
31. M.M. Cohen, Jr.: *The child with multiple birth defects*
32. W.W. Weber: *Pharmacogenetics*
33. V.P. Sybert: *Genetic skin disorders*
34. M. Baraitser: *Genetics of neurological disorders, third edition*
35. H. Ostrer: *Non-Mendelian genetics in humans*
36. E. Traboulsi: *Genetic factors in human disease*
37. G.L. Semenza: *Transcription factors and human disease*
38. L. Pinsky, R.P. Erickson, and R.N. Schimke: *Genetic disorders of human sexual development*
39. R.E. Stevenson, C.E. Schwartz, and R.J. Schroer: *X-linked mental retardation*
40. M.J. Khoury, W. Burke, and E. Thomson: *Genetics and public health in the 21st century*
41. J. Weil: *Psychosocial genetic counseling*
42. R.J. Gorlin, M.M. Cohen, Jr., and R.C.M. Hennekam: *Syndromes of the head and neck, fourth edition*
43. M.M. Cohen, Jr., G. Neri, and R. Weksberg: *Overgrowth syndromes*
44. R.A. King, J.I. Rotter, and A.G. Motulsky: *The genetic basis of common diseases, second edition*
45. G.P. Bates, P.S. Harper, and L. Jones: *Huntington's disease, third edition*
46. R.J.M. Gardner and G.R. Sutherland: *Chromosome abnormalities and genetic counseling, third edition*
47. I.J. Holt: *Genetics of mitochondrial disease*
48. F. Flinter, E. Maher, and A. Saggar-Malik: *The genetics of renal disease*
49. C.J. Epstein, R.P. Erickson, and A. Wynshaw-Boris: *Inborn errors of development: the molecular basis of clinical disorders of morphogenesis*
50. H.V. Toriello, W. Reardon, and R.J. Gorlin: *Hereditary hearing loss and its syndromes, second edition*
51. P.S. Harper: *Landmarks in medical genetics*
52. R.E. Stevenson and J.G. Hall: *Human malformations and related anomalies, second edition*
53. D. Kumar and S.D. Weatherall: *Genomics and clinical medicine*
54. C.J. Epstein, R.P. Erickson, and A. Wynshaw-Boris: *Inborn errors of development: the molecular basis of clinical disorders of morphogenesis, second edition*
55. W. Weber: *Pharmacogenetics, second edition*
56. P.L. Beales, I.S. Farooqi, and S. O'Rahilly: *The genetics of obesity syndromes*
57. P.S. Harper: *A short history of medical genetics*
58. R.C.M. Hennekam, I.D. Krantz, and J.E. Allanson: *Gorlin's syndromes of the head and neck, fifth edition*
59. D. Kumar and P. Elliot: *Principles and practices of cardiovascular genetics*
60. V.P. Sybert: *Genetic skin disorders, second edition*
61. R.J.M. Gardner, G.R. Sutherland, and L.C. Shaffer: *Chromosome abnormalities and genetic counseling, fourth edition*
62. D. Kumar: *Genomics and health in the developing world*
63. G. Bates, S. Tabrizi, and L. Jones: *Huntington's disease, fourth edition*
64. B. Lee and F. Scaglia: *Inborn errors of metabolism: from neonatal screening to metabolic pathways*

Inborn Errors of Metabolism

From Neonatal Screening to Metabolic Pathways

EDITED BY
Brendan Lee
AND
Fernando Scaglia

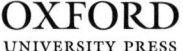

OXFORD
UNIVERSITY PRESS

Oxford University Press is a department of the University of
Oxford. It furthers the University's objective of excellence in research,
scholarship, and education by publishing worldwide.

Oxford   New York
Auckland   Cape Town   Dar es Salaam   Hong Kong   Karachi
Kuala Lumpur   Madrid   Melbourne   Mexico City   Nairobi
New Delhi   Shanghai   Taipei   Toronto

With offices in
Argentina   Austria   Brazil   Chile   Czech Republic   France   Greece
Guatemala   Hungary   Italy   Japan   Poland   Portugal   Singapore
South Korea   Switzerland   Thailand   Turkey   Ukraine   Vietnam

Oxford is a registered trademark of Oxford University Press
in the UK and certain other countries.

Published in the United States of America by
Oxford University Press
198 Madison Avenue, New York, NY 10016

© Oxford University Press 2015

All rights reserved. No part of this publication may be reproduced, stored in
a retrieval system, or transmitted, in any form or by any means, without the prior
permission in writing of Oxford University Press, or as expressly permitted by law,
by license, or under terms agreed with the appropriate reproduction rights organization.
Inquiries concerning reproduction outside the scope of the above should be sent to the
Rights Department, Oxford University Press, at the address above.

You must not circulate this work in any other form
and you must impose this same condition on any acquirer.

Library of Congress Cataloging-in-Publication Data
Inborn errors of metabolism (Lee)
Inborn errors of metabolism : from neonatal screening to metabolic pathways / edited by
Brendan Lee and Fernando Scaglia.
p. ; cm.
Includes bibliographical references.
ISBN 978–0–19–979758–5 (alk. paper)
I. Lee, Brendan, editor.   II. Scaglia, Fernando, editor.   III. Title.
[DNLM: 1. Metabolism, Inborn Errors. WD 205]
RC627.8
616.3'9042—dc23
2014010620

This material is not intended to be, and should not be considered, a substitute for medical or other professional
advice. Treatment for the conditions described in this material is highly dependent on the individual circumstances.
And, while this material is designed to offer accurate information with respect to the subject matter covered and
to be current as of the time it was written, research and knowledge about medical and health issues is constantly
evolving and dose schedules for medications are being revised continually, with new side effects recognized and
accounted for regularly. Readers must therefore always check the product information and clinical procedures with
the most up-to-date published product information and data sheets provided by the manufacturers and the most
recent codes of conduct and safety regulation. The publisher and the authors make no representations or warranties
to readers, express or implied, as to the accuracy or completeness of this material. Without limiting the foregoing,
the publisher and the authors make no representations or warranties as to the accuracy or efficacy of the drug dosages
mentioned in the material. The authors and the publisher do not accept, and expressly disclaim, any responsibility for
any liability, loss or risk that may be claimed or incurred as a consequence of the use and/or application of any of the
contents of this material.

1 3 5 7 9 8 6 4 2
Printed in the United States of America
on acid-free paper

Contents

Contributors vii
About the Editors xi
Introduction xiii

SECTION 1 Newborn Screening

1. Newborn Screening for Inborn Errors of Metabolism: Introduction and Approaches for Confirmation — 3
   V. Reid Sutton and Brett H. Graham

SECTION 2 Pathways

2. Human Glycosylation Disorders: Many Faces, Many Pathways — 37
   Hudson H. Freeze, Erik A. Eklund, and Donna M. Krasnewich
3. Gluconeogenesis — 68
   Erin M. Coffee and Dean R. Tolan
4. Branched Chain Amino Acid Disorders — 92
   Irini Manoli and Charles P. Venditti
5. Glycolysis — 119
   Areeg El-Gharbawy and Dwight Koeberl
6. Urea Cycle: Ureagenesis and Non-Ureagenic Functions — 134
   Oleg A. Shchelochkov, Sandesh C.S. Nagamani, Philippe M. Campeau, Ayelet Erez, and Brendan Lee
7. Fatty Acid Metabolism and Defects — 152
   Marwan S. Shinawi and Lutfi A. Abu-Elheiga
8. Mitochondrial Disorders — 180
   Ayman W. El-Hattab and Fernando Scaglia
9. Cholesterol, Sterols, and Isoprenoids — 203
   Yasemen Eroglu, Jean-Baptiste Roullet, and Robert D. Steiner

10. Disorders of One-Carbon Metabolism   225
Luis Umaña and William J. Craigen
11. Neurotransmission and Neurotoxicity (Phenylketonuria and Dopamine)   241
Uta Lichter-Konecki

SECTION 3   Therapeutic Approaches

12. Cell and Organ Transplantation for Inborn Errors of Metabolism   271
Alberto Burlina, Andrea Bordugo, Georg F. Hoffmann, and Jochen Meyburg
13. Gene Replacement Therapy for Inborn Errors of Metabolism   280
Nicola Brunetti-Pierri
14. Enzyme Replacement and Other Therapies for the Lysosomal Storage Disorders   303
Gregory M. Pastores and Christine M. Eng
15. Chaperone Therapy for the Lysosomal Storage Disorders   328
Alexander J. Choi, Robert Burnett, Ehud Goldin, Wei Zheng, and Ellen Sidransky
16. Substrate Deprivation Therapy   346
Marc C. Patterson

Index   357

Contributors

Lutfi A. Abu-Elheiga, Ph.D.
Verna and Marrs McLean Department of
 Biochemistry and Molecular Biology
Baylor College of Medicine
Houston, Texas

Andrea Bordugo, M.D.
Division of Inherited Metabolic Disorders
Department of Pediatrics
University Hospital
Padova, Italy

Nicola Brunetti-Pierri, M.D., F.A.C.M.G.
Telethon Institute of Genetics and
 Medicine; and
Department of Translational Medical
 Sciences
Federico II University of Naples
Naples, Italy

Alberto Burlina, M.D.
Division of Inherited Metabolic Disorders
Department of Pediatrics
University Hospital
Padova, Italy

Robert Burnett, B.S.
Medical Genetics Branch
National Human Genome Research
 Institute
Bethesda, Maryland

Philippe M. Campeau, M.D.
Department of Pediatrics
University of Montreal
Montreal, Quebec

Alexander J. Choi, B.S.
Medical Genetics Branch
National Human Genome Research
 Institute
Bethesda, Maryland

Erin M. Coffee, Ph.D.
Biology Department
Boston University
Boston, Massachusetts

William J. Craigen, M.D., Ph.D.
Department of Molecular and Human
 Genetics
Baylor College of Medicine
Houston, Texas

Contributors

Erik A. Eklund, M.D., Ph.D.
Department of Clinical Sciences
Lund University
Lund, Sweden

Ayman W. El-Hattab, M.D.
Division of Medical Genetics
Department of Pediatrics
The Children's Hospital
King Fahad Medical City
Riyadh, Saudi Arabia
Faculty of Medicine
King Saud bin Abdulaziz University for Health Sciences
Riyadh, Saudi Arabia

Christine M. Eng, M.D.
Professor of Molecular and Human Genetics
Director
DNA Diagnostic Laboratory
Baylor College of Medicine
Houston, TX

Ayelet Erez, M.D., Ph.D.
Incumbent of the Leah Omenn Career Development Chair
Senior Scientist
Department of Biological Regulation
Weizmann Institute of Science
Rehovot, Israel

Yasemen Eroglu, M.D.
Pediatric Gastroenterology and Hepatology
Oregon Health & Science University
Portland, Oregon

Hudson H. Freeze, Ph.D.
Human Genetics Program
Sanford-Burnham Medical Research Institute
La Jolla, California

Areeg El-Gharbawy, M.D.
Division of Medical Genetics, Department of Pediatrics
Children's hospital of Pittsburgh of UPMC-University of Pittsburgh School of Medicine
Durham, North Carolina

Ehud Goldin, Ph.D.
Medical Genetics Branch
National Human Genome Research Institute
Bethesda, Maryland

Brett H. Graham, M.D., Ph.D.
Department of Molecular and Human Genetics
Baylor College of Medicine
Houston, Texas

Georg F. Hoffmann, M.D.
Department of General Pediatrics
University Children's Hospital
Heidelberg, Germany

Dwight Koeberl, M.D., Ph.D.
Division of Medical Genetics, Department of Pediatrics
Duke University Medical Center
Durham, North Carolina

Donna M. Krasnewich, M.D., Ph.D.
National Institute of General Medical Sciences
National Institutes of Health
Bethesda, Maryland

Brendan Lee, M.D., Ph.D.
Robert and Janice Endowed Chair in Molecular and Human Genetics
Department of Molecular and Human Genetics
Baylor College of Medicine
Houston, Texas

Uta Lichter-Konecki, M.D., Ph.D.
Columbia University
Department of Pediatrics
Division of Clinical Genetics
New York, New York

Irini Manoli, M.D., Ph.D.
Organic Acid Research Section
National Human Genome Research
 Institute
National Institutes of Health
Bethesda, Maryland

Jochen Meyburg, M.D.
Department of General Pediatrics
University Children's Hospital
Heidelberg, Germany

Sandesh C.S. Nagamani, M.D.
Department of Molecular and Human
 Genetics
Baylor College of Medicine
Houston, Texas

Gregory M. Pastores, M.D.
Consultant
Department of Medicine/National Centre
 for Inherited Metabolic Disorders
Mater Misericordiae University Hospital
Dublin, Ireland
and
Visiting Professor
Department of Medicine
Yale University School of Medicine
New Haven, CT

Marc C. Patterson, M.D., F.R.A.C.P.
Pediatrics and Medical Genetics
Mayo Clinic College of Medicine
Chair, Division of Child and Adolescent
 Neurology
Mayo Clinic
Rochester, Minnesota

Jean-Baptiste Roullet, Ph.D.
Department of Pediatrics
Oregon Health & Science University
Portland, Oregon

Fernando Scaglia, M.D.
Department of Molecular and Human
 Genetics
Baylor College of Medicine
Houston, Texas
Texas Children's Hospital
Houston, Texas

Oleg A. Shchelochkov, M.D., F.A.A.P.
Division of Genetics
Department of Pediatrics
University of Iowa Hospitals and Clinics
Iowa City, Iowa

Marwan S. Shinawi, M.D.
Division of Genetics and Genomic
 Medicine
Department of Pediatrics
Washington University School of
 Medicine
St. Louis, Missouri

Ellen Sidransky, M.D.
Medical Genetics Branch
National Human Genome Research
 Institute
Bethesda, Maryland

Robert D. Steiner, M.D.
Marshfield Clinic Research Foundation
Department of Pediatrics
University of Wisconsin
Madison and Marshfield, Wisconsin

V. Reid Sutton, M.D.
Department of Molecular and Human
 Genetics
Baylor College of Medicine
Houston, Texas

Dean R. Tolan, Ph.D.
Biology Department
Boston University
Boston, Massachusetts

Luis A. Umaña, M.D.
Department of Molecular and Human Genetics
Baylor College of Medicine
Houston, Texas

Charles P. Venditti, M.D., Ph.D.
Organic Acid Research Section
National Human Genome Research Institute
National Institutes of Health
Bethesda, Maryland

Wei Zheng, M.D., Ph.D.
Therapeutics for Rare and Neglected Disease Program
National Center for Advancing Translational Sciences
National Institutes of Health
Bethesda, Maryland

About the Editors

Brendan Lee, MD, PhD, is Professor and Chair in the Department of Molecular and Human Genetics at Baylor College of Medicine. As a pediatrician and geneticist, Dr. Lee studies structural birth defects and inborn errors of metabolism. In the area of metabolic disease, he is developing new treatments for maple syrup urine disease and urea cycle disorders.

Fernando Scaglia, MD, is a Professor in the Department of Molecular and Human Genetics at Baylor College of Medicine. His primary research interests include the natural history and molecular characterization of mitochondrial cytopathies, clinical trials for Leigh syndrome, and the study of nitric oxide and glucose metabolism in patients with MELAS syndrome.

Introduction

Typically, textbooks on inborn errors of metabolism have focused on presenting the classical biochemical defects, correlating them with different clinical presentations and describing the current therapeutic approaches. However, with the advent of comprehensive newborn screening and improvement in diagnostic methodologies, we are beginning to appreciate the complex natural histories of these disorders. They together underscore that the increasingly diverse disease phenotypes that arise from Mendelian disorders reflect not only the primary effect of the metabolic disturbance, that is, accumulation of toxic metabolites upstream of a biochemical block and deficiency of the product downstream. We and others now appreciate secondary effects of the block as well as new "moonlighting" functions of components of the pathway. Hence, the aim of this textbook focuses on a pathways approach to presenting the phenotypes of inborn errors of metabolism. This textbook covers a myriad of topics from the principles of newborn screening, to presenting the basic underlying biochemical and molecular alterations, to explaining how these basic alterations in pathways may in fact lead to complex secondary and tertiary effects in metabolism that contribute to the complex natural histories of these disorders. The boundaries between Mendelian and complex disorders have become increasingly blurred as we recognize that Mendelian inborn errors of metabolism are indeed complex disorders. An evolving paradigm shift now supported by robust evidence points to complex signaling pathways and networks in inborn errors of metabolism. Thus a new focus on understanding these diseases should be based on studying how their natural histories can inform us about the secondary and tertiary consequences of the primary metabolic defects. The focus on the broad pathway effects of specific metabolic derangements will lead us to a deeper understanding of the mechanisms of pathogenesis. Hence, we hope to extend beyond basic descriptions of the classical biochemistry to prepare future generations of students, clinicians, and scientists in the study of these disorders. We hope that this approach will stimulate new ideas for therapeutic strategies and management.

SECTION 1

Newborn Screening

1

Newborn Screening for Inborn Errors of Metabolism

Introduction and Approaches for Confirmation

V. REID SUTTON AND BRETT H. GRAHAM

History of Newborn Screening

In the early 1960s, Robert Guthrie and Ada Susi published a method for the detection of phenylketonuria (PKU) in newborns.[1] A small punch from a blood or urine spot on a filter paper card was applied to an agar plate. Elevated phenylalanine (Phe) levels impaired the growth of *Bacillus subtilis* ATCC 6051, and the diameter of clearing of bacterial growth could be correlated with Phe levels in the blood spot. Screening programs were rapidly developed in the industrialized world, and the early detection and treatment of PKU has led to dramatically improved, and sometimes normal, outcomes. This method for screening, known as a bacterial inhibition assay, was employed to detect other inborn errors of metabolism such as galactosemia, maple syrup urine disease (MSUD), homocystinuria, and others, though they were not as widely adopted as screening for PKU. Enzyme assays were subsequently developed for newborn screening (NBS) bloodspots for detection of disorders, including galactosemia in 1964[2] and biotinidase in 1984.[3] In 1975, an immunoassay procedure was published for the detection of neonatal hypothyroidism,[4] and over the next few decades immunoassays were developed for congenital adrenal hyperplasia (21-hydroxylase deficiency) and other disorders. In the 1980s and 1990s, fluorimetric assays replaced bacterial inhibition assays for analyte analysis. In 1990, tandem mass spectroscopy (MS/MS), which had been used clinically to measure urine acylcarnitines, was demonstrated to be amenable to the detection of analytes in NBS bloodspots.[5] The adoption of this methodology by NBS programs in North America and in most industrialized nations rapidly expanded the number of disorders included in NBS programs. This rapid expansion reflected the large number of analytes that could be detected with a single assay; the high level of automation; and the speed of the sample preparation, assay, and analysis. In 2006, the American College of Medical Genetics (ACMG) proposed a uniform NBS panel[6] that was endorsed by the March of Dimes and has now been widely adopted by NBS programs.

Principles Underlying NBS

The original tenets for NBS were based upon the idea that there is an individual and separate test for every disease screened for. Those original tenets are

- the disorder occurs with significant frequency.
- an inexpensive and reliable method of testing exists.
- an effective treatment/intervention exists.
- if untreated, the baby may die or develop severe mental retardation.
- the affected baby may appear normal at birth.

The advent of MS/MS for NBS has allowed for the interrogation for multiple disorders using a single, multianalyte assay. This has led to a shift in the aforementioned tenets, since adding a test using the same method adds very little expense. For example, even if a disorder were extremely rare, if it could be detected and there were an effective intervention, the minimal cost of adding it to a MS/MS panel might be cost effective. Similarly, if one could add a disorder for which there was no accepted effective treatment, it might be cost effective to add it based upon minimizing diagnostic testing to determine the cause of the phenotype and being able to counsel parents about their reproductive options. The minimum criteria for diseases considered for inclusion in NBS as proposed by the ACMG are

- The disorder can be identified at a phase (24 to 48 hours after birth) at which it would not ordinarily be clinically detected.
- A test with the appropriate sensitivity and specificity is available.
- There are demonstrated benefits of early detection, timely intervention, and efficacious treatment of the condition being tested.[6]

Current Technologies

NBS programs currently employ a variety of methods for initial detection of targeted disorders.

Fluoroimmunoassay

Also known as fluorescence spectroscopy, this method utilizes light (often ultraviolet) to excite the electrons of a particular analyte/antibody interaction that is the product of an enzyme reaction. Readings of sample fluorescence at a specific wavelength or set of wavelengths can be used to determine the concentration of a particular analyte. This method is commonly employed in the measurement of congenital adrenal hypoplasia, congenital hypothyroidism, cystic fibrosis, biotinidase, and galactose-1-phosphate uridyltransferase enzyme activities. It was also used commonly in the past for PKU but has been widely replaced in the United States by MS/MS.

Radioimmunoassay

In radioimmunoassay, a known quantity of an antigen is made radioactive. This radiolabeled (or "hot") antigen is then mixed with a known amount of antibody for that antigen, and, as a result, the two chemically bind to one another. Then a soluabilized NBS bloodspot punch sample is added that contains natural, unlabled ("cold") antigen. This causes the unlabeled (cold) antigen from the bloodspot sample to compete with the radiolabeled antigen (hot) for antibody binding sites. The higher the concentration of cold antigen in the NBS sample, the more it binds to the antibody, displacing the radiolabeled antigen and thus reducing the ratio of *antibody-bound* radiolabeled antigen to *free* radiolabeled antigen. The bound antigens are then separated from the unbound ones, and the radioactivity of the free antigen remaining in the supernatant is measured using a gamma counter. Using known standards, a binding curve can then be generated that allows the amount of antigen in the patient's serum to be determined. This method has been used for the detection of congenital hypothyroidism, congenital adrenal hyperplasia (21-hydroxylase deficiency), and cystic fibrosis; however, it has been widely replaced by enzyme-linked immunosorbent assay or fluoroimmunoassay to avoid the use of radioactive substrates.

Enzyme-Linked Immunosorbent Assay

Enzyme-linked immunosorbent assay is another method that may be used for congenital hypothyroidism and congenital adrenal hyperplasia. It uses an antibody linked to an enzyme. When the NBS specimen containing the antigen of interest (e.g., T4) is mixed with the antibody-enzyme complex, it binds to the antibody. A substrate is then added that the enzyme metabolized and produces a signal, such as fluorescence at a particular wavelength, or other signal that can be detected.

Electrophoresis

The use of an electrical current to separate proteins by mass and charge is known as electrophoresis. This is typically performed in a gel-based medium but can also be done on paper. Electrophoresis has been used by NBS programs to separate different hemoglobin chains in the detection of sickle cell disease and other hemoglobinopathies, but this has widely been replaced by isoelectric focusing or high-performance liquid chromatography as these methods better resolve the types and quantities of hemoglobins.

Isoelectric Focusing

Employment of a gel-based medium to separate molecules by charge and pH is used by NBS to test for hemoglobinopathies. It is the most common method currently employed by NBS programs in the United States. High-performance liquid chromatograph is significantly more expensive but is generally viewed to be a superior method as it is more automated and more quantitative.

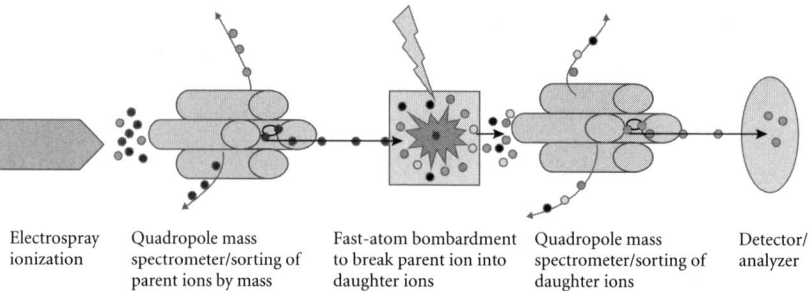

FIGURE 1.1 Tandem mass spectrometry. The specimen is injected into the machine and undergoes electrospray ionization. The first quadrupole uses an electromagnetic field to sort and select the ions of interest (that the scientist has programmed the machine to look for). The ions of interest then undergo fast-atom bombardment to break the parent ion into a host of daughter ions. The daughter ions then enter a second quadrupole that sorts out and selects the daughter ions of interest and the detector then measures the quantity.

Tandem Mass Spectroscopy

MS/MS is presently used in the detection of multiple analytes for the detection of amino acid disorders, organic acidemias, and fatty acid oxidation disorders by NBS. A soluabilized bloodspot sample may be either derivatized (e.g., butylated) or underivatized. In certain cases, derivatization may be more sensitive; underivatized methods may be quicker and allow for the detection of analytes (such as succinylacetone) that cannot be detected using a derivatized method. Most methods employ electrospray technology to ionize the sample and separate the parent ions by mass (this is the first mass spectrometry in MS/MS). The parent ion is then subjected to a force that breaks it into daughter ions, and a second mass spectrometer searches for the mass of a specific daughter ion associated with the analyte of interest (Figure 1.1). For example, propionyl(C3)carnitine is used to detect both methylmalonic and propionic acidemias, and the butylated mass transition is 274; the most commonly used daughter ion in this case is carnitine, which has a mass transition of 85. When the first mass spectrometer detects a mass transition of 274 and the second mass spectrometer detects a mass transition of 85, then the quantity of the parent ion is measured to determine the amount of propionylcarnitine. One problem with this method is that if there is another compound in the specimen that has the same parent ion mass transition and daughter ion mass, it will be assumed to be the analyte of interest, even if it is not. This occurs with pentanoyl(C5)carnitine; pivalic acid, which is a metabolite of ampicillin, has the same mass transition as pentanoylcarnitine and also has a daughter ion that has the same mass as that commonly used by NBS programs.

Selection of Primary and Secondary Analytes

Selection of primary and secondary analytes is dependent on the preference of the individual NBS program. Secondary analytes are typically utilized to improve sensitivity and reduce the false positive rate and tend to vary more from program to program. Commonly accepted primary analytes and the diseases they are able to detect are found in Table 1.1.

Certain NBS programs may reflex to a second-tier test based on an abnormal primary screen result. This is commonly done for cystic fibrosis, whereby individuals with an elevated

TABLE 1.1 Screening Metabolites and Confirmatory Testing for Inborn Errors of Metabolism Detected by Tandem Mass Spectrometry.

Disease Category	Screening Analyte [Secondary Analytes]	Primary Metabolic Confirmatory Test(s)	Disorder	Other Metabolic Markers	Additional Confirmatory Test(s)[¶]
Disorders of amino acid catabolism and transport.	Arginine	PAA[1]	Argininemia (Arginase Deficiency)	Orotic acid	Arginase enzyme activity in RBC[2]'s or liver; *ARG1* gene sequencing
	Citrulline	PAA	Argininosuccinic Aciduria (Argininosuccinate Lyase or ASL Deficiency)	Argininosuccinic Acid Orotic acid	ASL enzyme activity in RBCs, SFC[3] or liver; *ASL* gene sequencing
			Citrullinemia, type I (Argininosuccinate Synthetase or ASS Deficiency)	Low Arginine	ASS enzyme activity in SFC or liver; *ASS1* gene sequencing
			Citrullinemia, type II (Citrin Deficiency)	Arginine; Methionine; Threonine; Tyrosine; ↑Threonine/Serine ratio	*SLC25A13* gene sequencing
	Leucine [Valine]	PAA & UOA[4]	Maple Syrup Urine Disease (Branched-Chain Ketoacid Dehydrogenase Deficiency)	Isoleucine; Alloisoleucine	BCKD[5] enzyme activity in LB[6], SFC; *BCKDHA, BCKDHB, DBT* gene sequencing
	Methionine	PAA & total plasma homocysteine	Homocystinuria (CBS Deficiency)	Homocysteine	*CBS* gene sequencing
			Hypermethionemia (MAT[7] I/III, GNMT[8], or S-AdoHcy[9] hydrolase deficiencies)	S-AdoMet[10] (↑ in GNMT or S-AdoHcy hydrolase deficiencies); S-AdoHcy (↑ in S-AdoHcy hydrolase deficiency)	plasma S-AdoMet & S-AdoHcy; *MAT1A* gene sequencing for MAT I/III def.
	Phenylalanine [↑Phe/Tyr ratio]	Plasma Phe	PKU or hyperphenylalaninemia (PAH or Phe hydroxylase deficiency)	Increased urine hydroxyphenylacetic acid, phenylpyruvic acid, phenylacetic acid and phenylacetylglutamine	*PAH* gene sequencing
			Disorders of biopterin metabolism (GTPCH[11], PTPS[12], PCD[13], or DHPR[14] deficiencies)	Biopterin (↓ in all); neopterin (↓ in GTPCH, ↑ or N in others); 5HIAA[15] & HVA[16] in CSF[17] (↓ in all)	urine pterins; CSF neurotransmitters; RBC DHPR enzyme assay; *GCH1, PTS,* or *QDPR* gene sequencing

(continued)

TABLE 1.1 (Continued)

Disease Category	Screening Analyte [Secondary Analytes]	Primary Metabolic Confirmatory Test(s)	Disorder	Other Metabolic Markers	Additional Confirmatory Test(s)¶
	Succinylacetone	PAA; succinylacetone in blood or urine	Tyrosinemia, type I (Fumarylacetoacetate Hydrolase Deficiency)	Tyrosine; 4-hydroxyphenylpyruvate, 4-hydroxyphenyllactate, and 4-hydroxyphenylacetate in urine; 5-aminolevulinic acid in urine	*FAH* gene sequencing
	Tyrosine	PAA	Tyrosinemia, type II (Tyrosine Aminotransferase Deficiency)	4-hydroxyphenylpyruvate, 4-hydroxyphenyllactate, and 4-hydroxyphenylacetate in urine	
			Tyrosinemia, type III (4-Hydroxy-phenylpyruvate Dioxygenase Deficiency)	4-hydroxyphenylpyruvate, 4-hydroxyphenyllactate, and 4-hydroxyphenylacetate in urine	
Disorders of Fatty Acid Oxidation	C0 (↓) (Free carnitine)	Total & free plasma carnitine	Carnitine Uptake Defect		carnitine transport assay in SFC; *OCTN2* gene sequencing
	C0/[C16+C18] [↑C0]	Total & free plasma carnitine, ACP[17]	Carnitine Palmitoyl Transferase I (CPT1) Deficiency		CPT assay in SFC; *CPT1A* gene sequencing
	C4 (Butyrylcarnitine)	ACP, UAG[19], UOA	Short-Chain Acyl-CoA Deficiency (SCAD)	Ethylmalonic Acid; Butyrylglycine	*ACADS* gene sequencing
			Ethylmalonic Encephalopathy	C5; Ethylmalonic Acid; Isovalerylglycine	*ETHE1* gene sequencing
			Glutaric Aciduria, Type II or Multiple Acyl-CoA Dehydrogenase Deficiency (MADD)	↑ C6-C18; ethylmalonic acid, isovaleric acid, glutaric acid; isovalerylglycine and hexanoylglycine	ETF/ETF:QO enzyme assays on SFC; *ETFA, ETFB, ETFDH* gene sequencing
	C4-OH (3-Hydroxybutyrylcarnitine)	ACP, UOA	Medium/Short-Chain Hydroxy Acyl-CoA Deficiency (M/SCHAD)	↑ Hydroxy-dicarboxylic acids; elevated insulin	*HADH* gene sequencing
	C8 (Octanoylcarnitine) [C6; C10; C10:1; C8/C10; C8/C2]	ACP, UOA, UAG	Medium Chain Acyl-CoA Dehydrogenase Deficiency (MCAD)	↑ medium chain dicarboxylic acids; hexanoyl-, suberyl-, and 3-phenylpropionylglycines	*ACADM* gene sequencing
	C14:1 (Tetradecenoylcarnitine) [C14; C14:2; C16; C18:1; C14:1/C2]	ACP	Very Long Chain Acyl-CoA Dehydrogenase Deficiency (VLCAD)	↑ medium/long chain dicarboxylic acids	*ACADVL* gene sequencing

Analyte	Codes	Disorder	Metabolites	Testing
C16 (Hexadecanoylcarnitine) [C18; C18:1; C18:2]	ACP	Carnitine Palmitoyl Transferase II Deficiency (CPT2)		$CPT2$ gene sequencing
		Carnitine/Acylcarnitine Translocase Deficiency (CACT)		$SLC25A20$ gene sequencing
C16-OH (Hydroxyhexadecanoyl-carnitine) [C16:1-OH; C18:1-OH; C18-OH]	ACP	Long-Chain 3-Hydroxyacyl-CoA Dehydrogenase Deficiency (LCHAD)	↑ 3-hydroxy long chain dicarboxylic acids	$HADHA$ gene sequencing
		Trifunctional Protein Deficiency		$HADHA$, $HADHB$ gene sequencing

Organic Acidemias

Analyte	Codes	Disorder	Metabolites	Testing
C3 (Propionylcarnitine) [C3/C2]	ACP, UOA, UAG	Methylmalonic Acidemia (Methylmalonyl-CoA Mutase Deficiency)	Methylmalonic acid, 3-OH propionic acid, methylcitric acid, and tiglylglycine	plasma methylmalonic acid; enzyme assay in SFC; MUT gene sequencing
		Propionic Acidemia (Propionyl-CoA Carboxylase Deficiency)	Propionic acid, 3-OH propionic acid, methylcitric acid, and tiglylglycine	enzyme assay in SFC, WBC[20]; $PCCA$, $PCCB$ gene sequencing
		Disorders of Cobalamin Metabolism (Cbl A, B, C, D)	Methylmalonic acid; homocysteine (normal with Cbl A, B; ↑ with Cbl C, D)	plasma methylmalonic acid, plasma homocysteine; Cbl complementation studies in SFC; $MMAA$, $MMAB$, or $MMACHC$ gene sequencing
C3-DC (Malonylcarnitine)	ACP, UOA	Malonic Aciduria (Malonyl-CoA Decarboxylase Deficiency)	Malonic acid; Methylmalonic acid	$MLYCD$ gene sequencing
C4 (Isobutyrylcarnitine)	ACP, UAG	Isobutyryl-CoA Dehydrogenase Deficiency (Isobutyric Aciduria)	Isobutyrylglycine	$ACAD8$ gene sequencing
C5 (Isovalerylcarnitine or Methylbutyrylcarnitine)	ACP, UOA, UAG	Isovaleric Acidemia (Isovaleryl-CoA Dehydrogenase Deficiency)	Isovalerylglycine; 3-OH-isovaleric acid	IVD gene sequencing
		2-Methylbutyrylglycinuria (Short/Branched-Chain Acyl-CoA Dehydrogenase Deficiency)	2-Methylbutyrylglycine	$ACADSB$ gene sequencing
C5-DC (Glutarylcarnitine)	ACP, UOA	Glutaric Aciduria, Type I (Glutaryl-CoA Dehydrogenase Deficiency)	3-Hydroxyglutaric acid; Glutaric acid	enzyme assay in SFC; $GDCH$ gene sequencing

(continued)

TABLE 1.1 (Continued)

Disease Category	Screening Analyte [Secondary Analytes]	Primary Metabolic Confirmatory Test(s)	Disorder	Other Metabolic Markers	Additional Confirmatory Test(s)[1]
	C5-OH (3-Hydroxyisovaleryl-carnitine)	ACP, UOA, UAG (Biotinidase enzyme assay should be done if not part of the NBS panel)	Biotinidase Deficiency[21]	3-Hydroxyisovaleric acid; 3-methylcrotonylglycine; propionic acid; lactate	Biotinidase enzyme assay in serum; *BTD* gene sequencing
			Holocarboxylase Deficiency[21]	3-Hydroxyisovaleric acid; 3-methylcrotonylglycine; propionic acid; lactate	multiple carboxylases enzyme testing in SFC, WBC; *HLCS* gene sequencing
			3-Methylcrotonyl Carboxylase Deficiency (3-MCC Deficiency)	3-Hydroxyisovaleric acid; 3-Methylcrotonylglycine	enzyme testing in SFC, WBC; *MCCC1*, *MCCC2* gene sequencing
			3-Hydroxy-3-Methylglutaryl-CoA Lyase Deficiency (HMG-CoA Lyase Deficiency)	3-Hydroxyisovaleric acid; 3-Hydroxy-3-methylglutaric acid; 3-Methylglutaconic acid; 3-Methylglutaric acid; 3-Methylcrotonylglycine	*HMGCL* gene sequencing
			3-Methylglutaconic Aciduria, Type I (3-Methylglutaconyl-CoA Hydratase Deficiency)	3-Hydroxyisovaleric acid; 3-Methylglutaconic acid; 3-methylglutaric acid	enzyme testing in SFC; *AUH* gene sequencing
	C5-OH (2-methyl-3-hydroxybutyrylcarnitine)	ACP, UOA	Beta-Ketothiolase Deficiency (Methylacetoacetyl-CoA Thiolase Deficiency)	2-Methyl-3-hydroxbutyric acid; 2-Methylacetoacidic acid; Tiglylglycine	enzyme testing in SFC; *ACAT1* gene sequencing
			2-Methyl-3-Hydroxybutyric Acidemia (2-Methyl-3-Hydroxybutyryl-CoA Dehydrogenase Deficiency)	2-Methyl-3-hydroxbutyric acid; Tiglylglycine	enzyme testing in SFC; *HSD17B10* (*MHBD*) gene sequencing

[1]Additional tests to complement metabolic confirmation and/or to provide molecular and/or biochemical confirmation. [2]PAA = plasma amino acids, [3]RBC = red blood cell, [4]SFC = skin fibroblast cell culture, [5]UOA = urine organic acids, [6]BCKD = branch chain α-keto acid dehydrogenase, [7]LB = transformed lymphoblasts, [8]MAT = methionine S-adenosyltransferase, [9]GNMT = glycine N-methyltransferase deficiency, [10]S-AdoHcy = S-adenosylhomocysteine, [11]S-AdoMet = S-adenosylmethionine, [12]GTPCH = guanosine triphosphate cyclohydrolase I, [13]PTPS = 6-pyruvoyl-tetrahydropterin synthase, [14]PCD = pterin-4α-carbinolamine dehydratase, [15]DHPR = dihydropteridine reductase, [16]5HAA = 5-hydroxyindole acetic acid, [17]HVA = homovanilic acid, [18]CSF = cerebrospinal fluid, [19]ACP = acylcarnitine profile, [20]UAG = urine acylglycines, [21]Multiple Carboxylase Deficiency (MCD) can be caused by either biotinidase or holocarboxylase deficiencies.

immunoreactive trypsinogen receive reflex deoxyribonucleic acid (DNA) testing for cystic fibrosis. Such second-tier reflex testing may use another analyte or another method, or it may be done by targeted DNA mutation analysis or DNA sequencing.

Determination of Analyte Cut-Offs

Each screening program determines where to set cut-off values for each analyte or test, based on their population, the assay, and consideration of the positive predictive value and false negative rate. Programs typically set the cut-off range between the 99th percentile for the normal population and the 5th percentile for affected individuals. When there is overlap between normal and affected individuals, programs typically elect for a higher false positive rate to ensure that false negatives are minimized. Separate cut-off values may be used for low-birthweight infants, for infants receiving parenteral nutrition, and for second or follow-up screens. When secondary analytes are measured, an algorithm may be developed so that, rather than or in addition to a single analyte cut-off, all the data is considered in the determination of whether the screen is positive. Fatty acid oxidation disorders are particularly amenable to such an analysis. In the United States, the Health Resources and Services Administration division of the Department of Health and Human Services funds the Region 4 Genetics Collaborative, which collects data from NBS programs and provides assistance and advice regarding altering cut-offs to maximize sensitivity and specificity.[7,8] Definitions commonly used in discussing NBS cut-off values include

- **True Positives (TP):** The number of individuals who both test positive and actually have the disease.
- **True Negatives (TN):** The number of individuals who both test negative and do not have the disease.
- **False Positives (FP):** The number of individuals who test positive but do *not* have the disease.
- **False Negatives (FN):** The number of individuals who have the disease but have a normal newborn screen result.
- **Sensitivity:** The proportion of individuals with the disorder who have a positive (abnormal) newborn screen = TP ÷ (TP + FN).
- **Specificity:** The proportion of individuals without the disorder who have a normal newborn screen = TN ÷ (FP + TN).
- **False Positive Rate (FPR):** The percentage of healthy (normal) subjects who test positive. FPR = FP ÷ (FP + TN) = 1 − specificity.
- **False Negative Rate (FNR):** The percentage of affected subjects not detected by the newborn screen. FNR = FN ÷ (FN + TP) = 1 − sensitivity.
- **Presumptive Positive Rate:** The percentage of all screened who test positive. TP ÷ (TP + TN + FP + FN).
- **Positive Predictive Value (PPV):** The probability that the patient has the disease when restricted to those patients who test positive. PPV = TP ÷ (TP + FP).

Quality Control for Newborn Screening Programs

Each NBS laboratory and program is responsible for quality control and quality assurance that should monitor preanalytical, analytical, and postanalytical procedures. Assistance with quality assurance is also available through the U.S. Centers for Disease Control and Prevention Newborn Screening Quality Assurance Program. Founded in 1978 to provide assistance with the testing for congenital hypothyroidism, the program now offers quality assurance testing for 44 analytes (and 48 disorders). Nearly 500 NBS laboratories in more than 60 countries participate in this quality assurance program.[9] Accreditation of NBS labs in the United States is through the College of American Pathology program for laboratory accreditation and improvement.

Incidental Detection of Nontargeted Disorders

As discussed previously, MS/MS measures in parallel multiple amino acid and acylcarnitine species from a single sample, allowing for expanded NBS of the ACMG-defined core and secondary metabolic disorders.[6] It is important to realize that there are disorders not included in the ACMG uniform panel that can also present in the newborn period with alterations of amino acid or acylcarnitine markers that are screened by NBS programs and therefore should be considered in the differential diagnosis when confronted with a positive NBS result. Prominent examples include pyruvate carboxylase deficiency, succinyl-CoA ligase deficiency, and hydroxyprolinemia.[10] Pyruvate carboxylase deficiency can be detected through NBS through the presence of elevated citrulline, which results from secondary mitochondrial relative deficiency of oxaloacetate and aspartate. Succinyl-CoA ligase deficiency can be detected through NBS through the presence of mildly elevated methylmalonic acid, which results from the accumulation of succinyl-CoA. Hydroxyprolinemia, a clinically benign biochemical disorder caused by a deficiency of hydroxy-L-proline oxidase, can be detected through NBS because hydroxyproline is indistinguishable from leucine/isoleucine by MS/MS.

Confirmation of Individual Inborn Errors of Metabolism Detected by Tandem Mass Spectroscopy

In this section, individual inborn errors of metabolism targeted for NBS by MS/MS are presented with brief clinical descriptions and the various approaches for biochemical and molecular confirmation. The screening and confirmatory testing for each disorder is summarized in Table 1.1.

Biochemical Versus Molecular Confirmation

When an infant presents with a positive result on the newborn screen, the NBS program typically refers the patient to the local primary care provider or metabolic specialist for confirmation. The initial step usually consists of confirmation of abnormal metabolite pattern(s) through analysis of plasma amino acids (PAAs), urine organic acids (UOAs), and/or acylcarnitine profile (ACP) analyses to rule out false positives cases from further evaluations. Historically, the next step has been to obtain biochemical confirmation through demonstration of enzymatic deficiency in the appropriate cell or tissue. With the sequencing of the human genome and the dramatic advancement of relatively economical DNA sequencing technologies, the utilization of DNA testing for molecular diagnostic confirmation in lieu of enzymatic confirmation has become an attractive option in many cases. Enzymatic testing can be technically difficult, often requiring invasive tissue biopsies and, given the particular enzymatic test, may be limited to only a few or even a single diagnostic laboratory worldwide. In contrast, testing for pathological mutations in the gene of interest requires only a single blood sample for DNA, which can be obtained in essentially any medical setting. For the more common disorders, these tests are offered by numerous clinical diagnostic laboratories. In addition, molecular confirmation provides an opportunity for prenatal diagnosis in future pregnancies if the parents are so inclined. As with any diagnostic test, DNA sequencing is not 100% specific, with noncoding mutations (except for invariant splice site mutations) typically not detectable or identifiable with current diagnostic approaches. In addition, the detection of novel, unclassified variants can provide interpretive challenges to the physician. In our experience, the combination of metabolic analyses and DNA testing often provides convincing diagnostic confirmation. Also, in the current "postgenomic" age, the ability to recognize rare benign polymorphisms will continue to improve as the number of publicly available sequenced genomes or whole exomes grows from dozens to tens of thousands and beyond in the very near future. In cases where metabolite and/or DNA analyses are equivocal, enzymatic testing for confirmation of a diagnosis should be pursued. Of course, there are examples where enzymatic testing is the preferred option for confirmation, or even screening, as is the case for biotinidase deficiency and galactosemia due to deficiency of galactose-1-phosphate uridyltransferase.

Disorders of Amino Acid Catabolism and Transport
Argininemia (Arginase Deficiency)

Primary Screening Analyte: Arginine
Secondary Screening Analyte(s): None
Other Metabolic Markers: Elevated urine orotic acid

Clinical Summary: Argininemia is a urea cycle disorder due to deficiency of the liver isoform of arginase (ARG1). Argininemia is an autosomal recessive disorder (*ARG1* is encoded on 6q23) with a U.S. incidence of 1:363,000.[11] Arginase deficiency classically presents as spastic diplegia and developmental delay. Rarely, it can present as an infantile acute encephalopathy with mild to moderate hyperammonemia.

Confirmatory Testing: Analysis of PAAs will demonstrate significantly elevated arginine levels (usually greater than 200 µM) and is pathognomonic for arginase deficiency. Enzyme deficiency can be confirmed by measuring arginase enzyme activity in red blood cells (RBCs) or liver tissue. Molecular confirmation is obtained by *ARG1* gene sequencing and identifying known or suspected pathogenic mutations in the homozygous or compound heterozygous state.

Argininosuccinic Aciduria (Argininosuccinate Lyase Deficiency)

Primary Screening Analyte: Citrulline
Secondary Screening Analyte(s): None
Other Metabolic Markers: Elevated serum argininosuccinic aciduria (ASA), elevated urine orotic acid

Clinical Summary: ASA is a urea cycle disorder due to deficiency of argininosuccinate lyase (ASL). ASA is an autosomal recessive disorder (*ASL* is encoded on 7q11.21) with a U.S. incidence of 1:70,000.[11] ASL deficiency can present as an infantile acute encephalopathy with mild to moderate hyperammonemia or as a chronic encephalopathy with developmental delay/intellectual disability as the predominant feature. Progressive cirrhosis may also be seen.

Confirmatory Testing: Analysis of PAAs will demonstrate mild to moderate elevations of citrulline. In addition, detectable levels of argininosuccinic acid will be present and is pathognomonic for arginase deficiency. Enzyme deficiency can be confirmed by measuring ASL enzyme activity in RBCs, fibroblasts (skin fibroblast cell culture [SFC]), or liver tissue. Molecular confirmation is obtained by *ASL* gene sequencing and identifying known or suspected pathogenic mutations in the homozygous or compound heterozygous state.

Citrullinemia, Type I (Argininosuccinate Synthetase Deficiency)

Primary Screening Analyte: Citrulline
Secondary Screening Analyte(s): None
Other Metabolic Markers: Low serum arginine, elevated urine orotic acid

Clinical Summary: Citrullinemia, type I is a urea cycle disorder due to deficiency of argininosuccinate synthetase (ASS). Citrullinemia, type I is an autosomal recessive disorder (*ASS1* is encoded on 9q34.11) with a U.S. incidence of 1:57,000.[11] ASS deficiency can present as an infantile acute encephalopathy with hyperammonemia or as later onset progressive cirrhosis.

Confirmatory Testing: Analysis of PAAs will demonstrate significant elevations of citrulline (1 to 3 mM is typical). In addition, low levels of plasma arginine will be observed in the untreated state. Enzyme deficiency can be confirmed by measuring ASS enzyme activity in fibroblasts or liver tissue. Molecular confirmation is obtained by *ASS1* gene sequencing and identifying known or suspected pathogenic mutations in the homozygous or compound heterozygous state.

Citrullinemia, Type II (Citrin Deficiency)

Primary Screening Analyte: Citrulline
Secondary Screening Analyte(s): None
Other Metabolic Markers: Elevated arginine, methionine, threonine, and tyrosine (Tyr). Increased threonine/serine ratio

Clinical Summary: Citrullinemia, type II is a metabolic disorder due to deficiency of the mitochondrial aspartate-glutamate solute carrier (CITRIN or SLC25A13). Citrullinemia, type II is an autosomal recessive disorder (*SLC25A13* is encoded on 7q21.3) with incidences in East Asian populations estimated to range between 1:17,000 and 1:50,000[12] but has been observed worldwide at much lower frequencies.[13] ASS deficiency can present as an infantile hepatitis with intrahepatic cholestasis or as an adult encephalopathy with hyperammonemia.

Confirmatory Testing: Analysis of PAAs will demonstrate mild to moderate elevations of citrulline (100 to 600 μM is typical). In addition, plasma arginine, methionine, threonine, and Tyr are typically elevated with the threonine/serine ratio usually elevated (1.5 to 3.0). Molecular confirmation is obtained by *SLC25A13* gene sequencing and identifying known or suspected pathogenic mutations in the homozygous or compound heterozygous state.

Maple Syrup Urine Disease (Branched-Chain Ketoacid Dehydrogenase Deficiency)

Primary Screening Analyte: Leucine + isoleucine
Secondary Screening Analyte(s): Valine
Other Metabolic Markers: Alloisoleucine

Clinical Summary: MSUD is a metabolic disorder due to deficiency of the branched-chain ketoacid dehydrogenase deficiency (BCKD) complex. MSUD has a worldwide incidence of 1:250,000 but can be as high as 1:150 in certain reproductively isolated populations, such as Old Order Mennonite communities.[14] The BCKD complex consists of three catalytic subcomplexes: E1, a branched chain α-ketoacid decarboxylase that exists as a heterotetrameric subcomplex, composed of two α (E1α) and two β (E1β) subunits; E2, a homo-24-meric dihydrolipoyl transacylase; and E3, a homodimeric dihydrolipoamide dehydrogenase. MSUD can present along a spectrum of disease severity, including a classic severe acute infantile toxic encephalopathy, an intermediate later-onset form with developmental delay, and an intermittent form with acute episodes of encephalopathy often precipitated by illness or other forms of catabolic stress. MSUD is an autosomal recessive disorder that can be caused by mutations in the genes encoding E1α (*BCKDHA* on 19q13.2), E1β (*BCKDHB* on 6q14.1), or E2 (*DBT* on 1p21.2). Since E3 is also a component of the pyruvate dehydrogenase and the α-ketoglutarate dehydrogenase complexes, mutations in the gene encoding E3 (*DLD* on 7q31.1) causing dihydrolipoamide dehydrogenase deficiency presents as multiple dehydrogenase deficiencies with combined features of MSUD and lactic acidemia.

Confirmatory Testing: Analysis of PAAs will demonstrate significantly elevations of branch chain amino acids leucine, valine, and isoleucine, with perturbation of the normal 1:2:3 ratio of isoleucine:leucine:valine. In addition, detection of plasma alloisoleucine is pathognomonic. UOA analysis will demonstrate 2-keto-methylvalerate (which results in the maple syrup smell) as well as other 2-oxo and 2-hydroxy analytes. Enzyme deficiency can be confirmed by measuring BCKD activity from liver biopsy or SFC. Sequencing *BCKDHA*, *BCKDHB*, or *DBT* and identifying known or suspected pathogenic mutations in the homozygous or compound heterozygous state will provide molecular confirmation.

Homocystinuria (Cystathionine β-Synthase Deficiency)

Primary Screening Analyte: Methionine
Secondary Screening Analyte(s): None
Other Metabolic Markers: Homocysteine

Clinical Summary: Homocystinuria is a disorder of sulfur metabolism and has a worldwide estimated prevalence of 1:344,000 based on NBS for elevated blood methionine levels.[15] Homocystinuria is caused be deficiency of cystathionine β-synthase (CBS), which is a pyridoxine-dependent enzyme, and there are both pyridoxine-responsive and pyridoxine-unresponsive forms of the disease. Homocystinuria classically presents in the first or second decade of life with marfanoid habitus, ectopia lentis, myopia, mental retardation, and increased risk for thromboembolic events. Homocystinuria is an autosomal recessive disorder caused by mutations in the gene encoding CBS (*CBS* on 21q22.3).

Confirmatory Testing: Analysis of PAAs will demonstrate elevated methionine and possibly elevated free homocysteine (although total plasma homocysteine level and urine homocysteine should be measured separately to definitively demonstrate elevations). Sequencing *CBS* and identifying known or suspected pathogenic mutations in the homozygous or compound heterozygous state will provide molecular confirmation.

Hypermethioninemia (Methionine S-Adenosyltransferase, Glycine N-Methyltransferase, or S-Adenosylhomocysteine Hydrolase Deficiencies)

Primary Screening Analyte: Methionine
Secondary Screening Analyte(s): None
Other Metabolic Markers: Elevated plasma S-adenosylmethionine (S-AdoMet) (increased in glycine N-methyltransferase [GNMT] or S-adenosylhomocysteine [S-AdoHcy] hydrolase deficiencies); elevated plasma S-AdoHcy (increased in S-AdoHcy hydrolase deficiency).

Clinical Summary: Hypermethioninemia in the absence of significantly elevated homocysteine (isolated hypermethioninemia) can be caused by a deficiency in any of the three enzymatic steps of conversion of methionine to homocysteine in the transsulfuration pathway. Methionine is adenosylated to S-AdoMet by methionine S-adenosyltransferase (MAT I/III). S-AdoMet is converted to S-AdoHcy by GNMT, and S-AdoHcy is converted to homocysteine by S-adenosylhomocysteine hydrolase (AHCY). The true incidence of MAT I/III deficiency is unknown but may be between 1:30,000 and 1:100,000.[16] MAT I/III deficiency has identified mostly from NBS, and most individuals are asymptomatic, with only a small subset of patients with neurological findings.[16] The other two deficiencies are quite rare with only a handful of patients described to date demonstrating hepatomegaly and/or neurodevelopmental defects.[17] These disorders are predominantly autosomal recessive and caused by mutations in the genes encoding MAT I/III (*MAT1A* on 10q23.1), GNMT (*GNMT* on 6p21.1), or AHCY (*AHCY* on 20q11.22).

Confirmatory Testing: Analysis of PAAs will demonstrate elevated methionine in all instances. Plasma S-AdoMet will be elevated in both GNMT and AHCY deficiencies, while S-AdoHcy will be elevated in AHCY deficiency. No enzymatic testing is clinically available at this time. Sequencing *MAT1A, GNMT,* or *AHCY* and identifying known or

Phenylalanine Hydroxylase Deficiency

Primary Screening Analyte: Phe

Secondary Screening Analyte(s): Phe/Tyr ratio

Other Metabolic Markers: Increased urine phenyl ketoacids (hydroxyphenylacetic acid, phenylpyruvic acid, phenylacetic acid, and phenylacetylglutamine)

Clinical Summary: PKU is caused by deficiency of Phe hydroxylase (PAH). PKU is an autosomal recessive disorder (*PAH* is encoded on 12q23.2) with incidences in Caucasian populations estimated at 1:10,000 but much less frequent in Asian and African populations.[18] Untreated, PAH deficiency will present as developmental delay and intellectual disability.

Confirmatory Testing: Analysis of plasma Phe and Tyr will demonstrate significantly elevated Phe levels (typically between 10 and 30 mg/dL for classical PKU and less for milder forms) and elevated Phe/Tyr ratio (typically greater than 2.5). Analysis of UOA will demonstrate elevations of hydroxyphenylacetic acid, phenylpyruvic acid, phenylacetic acid, and phenylacetylglutamine. Sequencing of *PAH* and identifying known or suspected pathogenic mutations in the homozygous or compound heterozygous state will provide molecular confirmation.

Disorders of Biopterin Metabolism (Guanosine Triphosphate Cyclohydrolase I, 6-Pyruvoyl-Tetrahydropterin Synthase, Pterin-4α-Carbinolamine Dehydratase, or Dihydropterin Reductase Deficiencies)

Primary Screening Analyte: Phe

Secondary Screening Analyte(s): Phe/Tyr ratio

Other Metabolic Markers: Biopterin (↓ in all); neopterin (↓ in guanosine triphosphate cyclohydrolase I [GTPCH], ↑ or *N* in others); 5-hydroxyindole acetic acid, and homovanelic acid in cerebral spinal fluid (↓ in all)

Clinical Summary: Approximately 1% to 2% of cases of hyperphenylalanemia are caused by disorders of biopterin metabolism disrupting synthesis or recycling of tetrahydrobiopterin (a cofactor for PAH).[18] Deficiencies of GTPCH, 6-pyruvoyl-tetrahydropterin synthase, pterin-4α-carbinolamine dehydratase, or dihydropterin reductase can result in secondary PAH deficiency and hyperphenalanemia. These disorders are autosomal recessive and due to mutations in genes encoding GTPCH (*GCH1* on 14q22.2), 6-pyruvoyl-tetrahydropterin synthase (*PTS* on 11q23.1), pterin-4α-carbinolamine dehydratase (*PCBD1* on 10q22.1), or dihydropterin reductase (*QDPR* on 4q15.32).

Confirmatory Testing: Analysis of plasma Phe and Tyr will demonstrate significantly elevated Phe levels (typically between 10 and 30 mg/dL) and elevated Phe/Tyr ratio (typically greater than 2.5). Analysis of UOA will demonstrate elevations of hydroxyphenylacetic acid, phenylpyruvic acid, phenylacetic acid, and phenylacetylglutamine. Analysis of urine pterins will demonstrate reduced biopterin in all deficiencies.

Urine neopterin may be elevated in 6-pyruvoyl-tetrahydropterin synthase deficiency and low in GTPCH deficiency. Measurement of neurotransmitters in cerebral spinal fluid will demonstrate reduced levels of 5-hydroxyindolacetic acid and homovanelic acid. Deficiency of dihydropterin reductase can be demonstrated by enzyme assay in RBCs. Sequencing of *GCH1*, *PTS*, *PCBD1*, or *QDPR* and identifying known or suspected pathogenic mutations in the homozygous or compound heterozygous state will provide molecular confirmation.

Tyrosinemia, Type I (Fumarylacetoacetate Hydrolase Deficiency)

Primary Screening Analyte: Succinylacetone and/or Tyr
Secondary Screening Analyte(s): None
Other Metabolic Markers: Elevated Tyr, Phe, methionine; elevated Tyr metabolites in urine (4-hydroxyphenylpyruvate, 4-hydroxyphenyllactate, and 4-hydroxyphenylacetate); elevated 5-aminolevulinic acid in urine

Clinical Summary: Tyrosinemia type I is an inborn error of Tyr metabolism caused by deficiency of fumarylacetoacetate hydrolase (FAH). FAH deficiency is an autosomal recessive disorder with an overall estimated incidence of 1:100,000 to 1:120,000.[19] Tyrosinemia type I can present as a severe infantile progressive hepatopathy or later in infancy as a renal tubulopathy with rickets, failure to thrive, and hepatopathy. Untreated individuals can display porphyria-like intermittent episodes of acute neurological crises and progress to fatal hepatic failure and/or hepatocellular carcinoma. Tyrosinemia type I is caused by mutations in the gene encoding FAH (*FAH* on 15q25.1).

Confirmatory Testing: Detection of succinylacetone in blood or urine is pathognomonic for FAH deficiency. Analysis of PAAs may reveal normal or modest elevations of Tyr (typically less than 300 µM), Phe, and methionine. The use of Tyr as the primary screening analyte for tyrosinemia type I has generally been abandoned due to unacceptable high false positive rates given that the modest elevations of Tyr as observed in tyrosinemia type I can also be seen in other conditions with relatively high frequency, including hepatic immaturity, transient hypertyrosinemia of the newborn, and other extrinsic causes of hepatic dysfunction (TPN cholestasis, etc). Analysis of UOA will demonstrate elevations of Tyr metabolites (4-hydroxyphenylpyruvate, 4-hydroxyphenyllactate, and 4-hydroxyphenylacetate). Elevations in urine 5-aminolevulinic acid will be present secondary to inhibition of 5-aminolevulinic acid dehydratase (porphobilinogen synthase) in the liver and RBCs by elevated succinylacetone. Sequencing of *FAH* and identifying known or suspected pathogenic mutations in the homozygous or compound heterozygous state will provide molecular confirmation.

Tyrosinemia, Type II (Tyr Aminotransferase Deficiency) and Type III (4-Hydroxy-Phenylpyruvate Dioxygenase Deficiency)

Primary Screening Analyte: Tyr
Secondary Screening Analyte(s): None

Other Metabolic Markers: Elevated Tyr metabolites in urine (4-hydroxyphenylpyruvate, 4-hydroxyphenyllactate, and 4-hydroxyphenylacetate)

Clinical Summary: Tyrosinemia type II is an inborn error of Tyr metabolism caused by deficiency of the hepatic cytosolic isoform of Tyr aminotransferase (TAT). It is a rare autosomal recessive disorder also known as oculocutaneous tyrosinemia or Richner-Hanhart Syndrome. Ophthalmologic features include recalcitrant pseudodendritic keratitis and corneal ulcerations, while dermatologic manifestations consist of painful palmoplan`tar keratodermatitis.[20] Tyrosinemia type II is caused by mutations in the gene encoding TAT (*TAT* on 16q22.2). Tyrosinemia type III is an inborn error of Tyr metabolism caused by deficiency of 4-hydroxy-phenylpyruvate dioxygenase. It is a very rare autosomal recessive disorder with only a handful of affected individuals reported; therefore, the phenotype remains poorly defined. Like TAT deficiency, the few patients described with HPD deficiency do not have liver involvement but may have skin, eye, and neurological effects.[21] Tyrosinemia type III is caused by mutations in the gene encoding HPD (*HPD* on 12q24.31).

Confirmatory Testing: Analysis of PAAs will demonstrate elevated Tyr for both conditions. TAT deficiency typically presents with a plasma Tyr greater than 1000 μM while HPD deficiency typically presents with a plasma Tyr between 350 and 650 μM. Analysis of UOA will demonstrate elevations of Tyr metabolites (4-hydroxyphenylpyruvate, 4-hydroxyphenyllactate, and 4-hydroxyphenylacetate). In theory, enzyme deficiency for either condition could be demonstrated on liver biopsy; however, this is not readily available clinically. Sequencing of *TAT* or *HPD* and identifying known or suspected pathogenic mutations in the homozygous or compound heterozygous state will provide molecular confirmation for tyrosinemia types II and III, respectively.

Disorders of Fatty Acid Oxidation

Carnitine Uptake Defect (Primary Carnitine Deficiency)

Primary Screening Analyte: Low C0 (free carnitine)
Secondary Screening Analyte(s): None
Other Metabolic Markers: Low total plasma carnitine

Clinical Summary: Primary carnitine deficiency is a defect of the cellular uptake of carnitine due to deficiency of the carnitine transporter OCTN2. OCTN2 deficiency is an autosomal recessive disorder with an estimated incidence of 1:30,000 to 1:60,000.[22,23] Primary carnitine deficiency exhibits prominent variable expressivity, ranging from classic presentations of cardiomyopathy, hepatoencephalopathy, or episodic hypoketotic hypoglycemia to asymptomatic deficient mothers identified through detection of low carnitine via NBS of their unaffected children. Primary carnitine deficiency is caused by mutations in the gene encoding OCTN2 (*SLC22A5* on 5q31.1).

Confirmatory Testing: Analysis of free and total plasma carnitine will demonstrate deficiency. It is important to measure the mother's free and total plasma carnitine levels as well, because newborns of affected mothers will have transient secondary carnitine deficiency. Enzyme deficiency can be shown by carnitine transport assay in SFC. Sequencing of

OCTN2 and identifying known or suspected pathogenic mutations in the homozygous or compound heterozygous state will provide molecular confirmation.

Carnitine Palmitoyl Transferase I Deficiency

Primary Screening Analyte: C0/(C16+C18) ratio
Secondary Screening Analyte(s): C0
Other Metabolic Markers: Generalized decrease of acylcarnitines

Clinical Summary: Carnitine palmitoyl transferase 1 deficiency is a disorder of long-chain fatty acid oxidation that is caused by deficiency of the hepatic isoform of carnitine palmitoyl transferase (CPT1A). It is a rare autosomal recessive disorder with an estimated incidence of 1:750,000 to 1:2,000,000.[24] CPT1A deficiency presents predominantly as episodic hypoketotic hypoglycemia often triggered by catabolic stress. CPT1A deficiency is caused by mutations in the gene encoding CPT1A (*CPT1A* on 11q13.3).

Confirmatory Testing: Analysis of total and free plasma carnitine will demonstrate increased free carnitine. An ACP will exhibit a generalized decrease of acylcarnitines. Enzyme deficiency can be inferred by radiolabeled fatty acid in SFC. Sequencing of *CPT1A* and identifying known or suspected pathogenic mutations in the homozygous or compound heterozygous state will provide molecular confirmation.

Short-Chain Acyl-CoA Dehydrogenase Deficiency

Primary Screening Analyte: C4
Secondary Screening Analyte(s): None
Other Metabolic Markers: Ethylmalonic acid and butyrylglycine

Clinical Summary: Short-chain acyl-CoA dehydrogenase (SCAD) deficiency is an inborn error of short-chain fatty acid oxidation. SCAD deficiency is autosomal recessive with an estimated incidence of 1:95,000.[24] While initially thought to be a clinically severe disorder, the identification of numerous asymptomatic individuals through expanded NBS over the past decade has shifted the general consensus toward SCAD deficiency being a biochemical abnormality without clear clinical significance.[25] SCAD deficiency is caused by mutations in the gene encoding SCAD (*ACADS* on 12q24.31).

Confirmatory Testing: Analysis of ACP will demonstrate elevated butyrylcarnitine (C4). Analysis of urine acylglycines (UAG) will demonstrate elevated butyrylglycine. Analysis or UOA will demonstrate elevations of ethylmalonic acid. Sequencing of *ACADS* and identifying known or suspected pathogenic mutations in the homozygous or compound heterozygous state will provide molecular confirmation.

Ethylmalonic Encephalopathy

Primary Screening Analyte: C4
Secondary Screening Analyte(s): C5
Other Metabolic Markers: Ethylmalonic acid, isovalerylglycine, lactic acid

Clinical Summary: Ethylmalonic encephalopathy is a rare autosomal recessive disorder due to deficiency of ETHE1, a mitochondrial matrix sulfur dioxygenase. This disorder presents with encephalopathy, chronic diarrhea, and orthostatic acrocyanosis. A mouse model suggests that the metabolic abnormalities, including elevations of ethylmalonic acid, butyrylcarnitine, and lactic acid, are caused by secondary inhibition of SCAD and cytochrome c oxidase by increased cellular sulfides.[26] Ethylmalonic encephalopathy is caused by mutations in the gene encoding ETHE1 (*ETHE1* on 19q31.13).

Confirmatory Testing: Analysis of ACP will demonstrate elevations in butyrylcarnitine (C4) and isovalerylcarnitine (C5). Evaluation of UOA will show elevations of ethylmalonic acid, isovalerylglycine, and lactic acid. Sequencing of *ETHE1* and identifying known or suspected pathogenic mutations in the homozygous or compound heterozygous state will provide molecular confirmation.

Glutaric Aciduria, Type II or Multiple Acyl-CoA Dehydrogenase Deficiency

Primary Screening Analyte: C4
Secondary Screening Analyte(s): C5
Other Metabolic Markers: ↑ C6-C18; ethylmalonic acid, isovaleric acid, glutaric acid; isovalerylglycine and hexanoylglycine

Clinical Summary: Glutaric aciduria, type II (GA II) is a disorder of fatty acid oxidation caused by deficiencies of components of the system that transfers electrons released from β-oxidation to the electron transport chain. This includes the electron-transfer flavoprotein (ETF) and the ETF dehydrogenase (ETF-DH). Because this system is required for proper β-oxidation of all fatty acids, this disorder effectively presents as a deficiency of multiple acyl-CoA dehydrogenases. In addition, this system is required for oxidation of branched chain amino acids, sarcosine, and lysine. GA II is autosomal recessive and genetically heterogeneous with an estimated incidence that ranges from 1:15,000 in Turkey to 1:750,000 to 1:2,000,000 in North America and Europe.[24] In its most severe form, GA II clinically presents as neonatal cardiomyopathy, hypoglycemia, and encephalopathy, while milder forms can present with episodic hypoglycemia induced by catabolic stress. GA II is caused by mutations in the genes encoding components of the electron transfer system, including *ETFA* (15q24.2), *ETFB* (19q13.41), and *ETFDH* (4q32.1).

Confirmatory Testing: Analysis ACP will reveal a generalized elevation of acylcarnitines (C4-C18). Examination of UOA will reveal presence of ethylmalonic acid, isovaleric acid, and glutaric acid and 2-hydroxyglutaric acid. Analysis of UAG will demonstrate presence of isovalerylglycine and hexanoylglycine. Enzyme deficiency can be demonstrated by EFT/EFT:ubiquinone oxidoreductase enzyme assay on SFC. Sequencing of *ETFA, ETFB*, or *ETFDH* and identifying known or suspected pathogenic mutations in the homozygous or compound heterozygous state will provide molecular confirmation.

Medium/Short-Chain Hydroxy Acyl-CoA Deficiency

Primary Screening Analyte: C4-OH
Secondary Screening Analyte(s): None
Other Metabolic Markers: ↑ Hydroxydicarboxylic acids; elevated insulin

Clinical Summary: Medium/short-chain hydroxy acyl-CoA (M/SCHAD) deficiency is a rare autosomal recessive disorder involving deficiency of the penultimate step of β-oxidation. While M/SCHAD deficiency causes a biochemical abnormality (elevated 3-hydroxybutyrylcarnitine), its clinical significance is uncertain, although there are reports of mutations associated with hyperinsulinemic hypoglycemia.[27,28] M/SCHAD deficiency is caused by mutations in the gene encoding M/SCHAD (*HADH* on 4q25).

Confirmatory Testing: Analysis of ACP will demonstrate elevated 3-hydroxybutyrylcarnitine (C4-OH), while analysis of UOA will show elevations of hydroxydicarboxylic acids. Hyperinsulinism in the presence of hypoglycemia may also be present. Sequencing of *HADH* and identifying known or suspected pathogenic mutations in the homozygous or compound heterozygous state will provide molecular confirmation.

Medium-Chain Acyl-CoA Dehydrogenase Deficiency

Primary Screening Analyte: C8
Secondary Screening Analyte(s): C6; C10; C10:1; C8/C10; C8/C2
Other Metabolic Markers: ↑ medium-chain dicarboxylic acids; hexanoyl-, suberyl-, and 3-phenylpropionylglycines

Clinical Summary: Medium-chain acyl-CoA dehydrogenase (MCAD) deficiency is an autosomal recessive inborn error of β-oxidation. MCAD deficiency has an incidence of 1:15,000 in Caucasian populations.[24] MCAD deficiency presents as a potentially fatal fasting hypoglycemia often induced by catabolic stress. MCAD deficiency is caused by mutations in the gene encoding MCAD (*ACADM* on 1p31.1).

Confirmatory Testing: Analysis ACP will demonstrate elevations in hexanoylcarnitine (C6), octanoylcarnitine (C8), decenoylcarnitine (C10:1), and, to a lesser extent, decanoylcarnitine (C10). Evaluation of UOA will show elevations of medium-chain dicarboxylic acids. Analysis of UAG will demonstrate the presence of hexanoylglycine, suberylglycine, and 3-phenylpropionylglycine. Sequencing of *ACADM* and identifying known or suspected pathogenic mutations in the homozygous or compound heterozygous state will provide molecular confirmation.

Very Long-Chain Acyl-CoA Dehydrogenase Deficiency

Primary Screening Analyte: C14:1
Secondary Screening Analyte(s): C14; C14:2; C16; C18:1; C14:1/C2
Other Metabolic Markers: ↑ medium/long-chain dicarboxylic acids

Clinical Summary: Very long-chain acyl-CoA dehydrogenase (VLCAD) deficiency is an autosomal recessive inborn error of β-oxidation. VLCAD deficiency has an incidence of 1:85,000 in Caucasian populations.[24] VLCAD deficiency can present along a spectrum of severity that includes neonatal hypoketotic hypoglycemia, cardiomyopathy, or exercise-induced rhabdomyolysis. VLCAD deficiency is caused by mutations in the gene encoding VLCAD (*ACADVL* on 17p13.1).

Confirmatory Testing: Analysis of ACP will demonstrate elevations of long-chain acylcarnitines, with tetradecenoylcarnitine (C14:1) typically most prominent. Evaluation of UOA will reveal elevations of medium- and long-chain dicarboxylic acids. Sequencing of *ACADVL* and identifying known or suspected pathogenic mutations in the homozygous or compound heterozygous state will provide molecular confirmation.

Carnitine Palmitoyl Transferase II Deficiency

Primary Screening Analyte: C16
Secondary Screening Analyte(s): C18; C18:1; C18:2
Other Metabolic Markers: None

 Clinical Summary: Carnitine palmitoyl transferase II (CPT2) deficiency is a disorder of long-chain fatty acid oxidation that is caused by deficiency of CPT2. It is a rare autosomal recessive disorder with an estimated incidence of 1:750,000 to 1:2,000,000.[24] CPT2 deficiency presents predominantly as episodic hypoketotic hypoglycemia often triggered by catabolic stress. CPT2 deficiency can present along a spectrum of severity that includes neonatal hypoketotic hypoglycemia, cardiomyopathy, or exercise-induced rhabdomyolysis. CPT2 deficiency is caused by mutations in the gene encoding CPT2 (*CPT2* on 1p32.3).

 Confirmatory Testing: Analysis of ACP will reveal elevations of long-chain acylcarnitines, in particular hexadecanoylcarnitine (C16). Sequencing of *CPT2* and identifying known or suspected pathogenic mutations in the homozygous or compound heterozygous state will provide molecular confirmation.

Carnitine/Acylcarnitine Translocase Deficiency

Primary Screening Analyte: C16
Secondary Screening Analyte(s): C18; C18:1; C18:2
Other Metabolic Markers: None

 Clinical Summary: Carnitine/acylcarnitine translocase (CACT) deficiency is a disorder of long-chain fatty acid oxidation that is caused by deficiency of the CACT. It is a rare autosomal recessive disorder with an estimated incidence of 1:750,000 to 1:2,000,000.[24] CACT deficiency presents predominantly as infantile episodic hypoketotic hypoglycemia triggered by fating/catabolic stress with encephalopathy and cardiomyopathy/ventricular arrhythmias. CACT deficiency is caused by mutations in the gene encoding CACT (*SLC25A20* on 3p21.31).

 Confirmatory Testing: Analysis of ACP will reveal elevations of long-chain acylcarnitines, in particular hexadecanoylcarnitine (C16). Sequencing of *SLC25A20* and identifying known or suspected pathogenic mutations in the homozygous or compound heterozygous state will provide molecular confirmation.

Long-Chain 3-Hydroxyacyl-CoA Dehydrogenase Deficiency and Trifunctional Protein Deficiency

Primary Screening Analyte: C16-OH
Secondary Screening Analyte(s): C16:1-OH; C18:1-OH; C18-OH
Other Metabolic Markers: ↑ 3-hydroxy long-chain dicarboxylic acids

 Clinical Summary: The mitochondrial trifunctional protein complex, an octamer composed of four α- and four β-subunits, contains three enzymatic activities important for long-chain fatty acid oxidation: a long-chain 3-hydroxyacyl-CoA dehydrogenase (LCHAD) (α), long-chain enoyl-CoA hydratase (α), and 3-ketoacyl-CoA thiolase (β) activities. LCHAD deficiency is a disorder of long-chain fatty acid oxidation that is caused by isolated deficiency of the α-subunit LCHAD activity of the mitochondrial trifunctional protein complex. It is an autosomal recessive disorder with an overall incidence of 1:250,000.[24] Complete trifunctional protein (TFP) deficiency is caused by deficiency of either the α- or β-subunits leading to deficiencies of all three activities. It is a more rare autosomal recessive disorder with an overall incidence of 1:750,000.[24] These disorders have similar and overlapping clinical features that can present along a spectrum of severity that includes neonatal hypoketotic hypoglycemia, cardiomyopathy, and/or acute rhabdomyolysis. Peripheral neuropathy and retinopathy are long-term complications of these disorders, and a subset of women who present with maternal hemolysis, liver dysfunction, and low platelets (hemolysis, elevated liver enzymes, and low platelets syndrome) or acute fatty liver of pregnancy are carriers with an affected fetus.[29] LCHAD deficiency is caused by mutations in the gene encoding the α-subunit of TFP (*HADHA* on 2p23.3), with homozygosity for the highly prevalent c.1528G>C (p.E510Q) common mutation being the most common genotype. TFP deficiency can be caused by mutations in either the α-subunit of TFP (*HADHA*) or the β-subunit of TFP (*HADHB* on 2p23.3).

Confirmatory Testing: Analysis of ACP will reveal elevations of long-chain hydroxylated acylcarnitines, in particular hydroxyhexadecanoylcarnitine (C16-OH). Evaluation of UOA will reveal elevations of 3-hydroxy long-chain dicarboxylic acids (*C6-C14*).[30,31] Sequencing of *HADHA* (LCHAD or TFP) or *HADHB* (TFP) and identifying known or suspected pathogenic mutations in the homozygous or compound heterozygous state will provide molecular confirmation.

Organic Acidemias
Methylmalonic Acidemia (Methylmalonyl-CoA Mutase Deficiency)
Primary Screening Analyte: C3
Secondary Screening Analyte(s): C3/C2 ratio
Other Metabolic Markers: Methylmalonic acidemia (MMA), 3-OH propionic acid, methylcitric acid, and tiglylglycine

Clinical Summary: Primary MMA is a disorder of amino acid metabolism caused by the deficiency of methylmalonyl-CoA mutase (MUT) affecting the catabolism of isoleucine, valine, methionine, and threonine. It is an autosomal recessive disorder with an estimated incidence of 1:50,000 to 1:100,000.[32] MMA classically presents as an infantile toxic encephalopathy with a prominent acute metabolic anion gap acidosis. MUT deficiency is caused by mutations in the gene encoding methylmalonyl-CoA mutase (*MUT* on 6p12.3).

Confirmatory Testing: Analysis of ACP will reveal elevations in propionylcarnitine (C3) and the ratio of propionylcarnitine to acetylcarnitine (C3/C2). Measurement of plasma methylmalonic acid levels will show significant elevations (typically 10 to 1000 μM). Analysis of UOA and UAG will demonstrate the presence of 3-methylmalonic acid, methylcitric acid, and tiglylglycine. Biochemical confirmation can be obtained by demonstration of enzyme deficiency in SFC. Sequencing of *MUT* and identifying known or suspected pathogenic mutations in the homozygous or compound heterozygous state will provide molecular confirmation.

Propionic Acidemia (Propionyl-CoA Carboxylase Deficiency)

Primary Screening Analyte: C3
Secondary Screening Analyte(s): C3/C2 ratio
Other Metabolic Markers: Propionic acid, 3-OH propionic acid, methylcitric acid, and tiglylglycine

Clinical Summary: Propionic acidemia is a disorder of amino acid metabolism caused by the deficiency of propionyl-CoA carboxylase affecting the catabolism of isoleucine, valine, methionine, and threonine. It is an autosomal recessive disorder with an estimated incidence of 1:75,000 to 1:300,000.[33,34] Propionic acidemia classically presents as an infantile toxic encephalopathy with a prominent acute metabolic anion gap acidosis, mild hyperammonemia, and neutropenia. Propionic acidemia is caused by mutations in either the gene encoding the α-subunit (*PCCA* on 13q32.3) or β-subunit (*PCCB* on 3q22.3) of propionyl-CoA carboxylase.

Confirmatory Testing: Analysis of ACP will reveal elevations in propionylcarnitine (C3) and the ratio of propionylcarnitine to acetylcarnitine (C3/C2). Measurement of PAA will typically show elevations of glycine and alanine. Analysis of UOA and UAG will demonstrate the presence of propionic acid, 3-hydroxy-propionic acid, methylcitric acid, and tiglylglycine. Biochemical confirmation can be obtained by demonstration of enzyme deficiency in SFC or leukocytes. Sequencing of *PCCA* or *PCCB* and identifying known or suspected pathogenic mutations in the homozygous or compound heterozygous state will provide molecular confirmation.

Disorders of Cobalamin Metabolism (CblA, B, C, D, F)

Primary Screening Analyte: C3
Secondary Screening Analyte(s): C3/C2 ratio
Other Metabolic Markers: Methylmalonic acid, homocysteine (normal with Cbl A, B; ↑ with Cbl C, D, F)

Clinical Summary: Cobalamin (Vitamin B_{12}) is a cobalt-containing water-soluble vitamin that is converted into two distinct bioactive forms intracellularly. Adenosyl cobalamin (AdoCbl) is a required cofactor for the mitochondrial methylmalonyl-CoA mutase, and methylcobalamin (MeCbl) is a required cofactor for the cytoplasmic methionine synthase. Inherited disorders affecting the intracellular metabolism of cobalamin, which result in deficiency of AdoCbl, will present with MMA. Biochemical complementation studies of fibroblasts from patients with defects of intracellular metabolism of cobalamin defined seven genetically distinct complementation groups, CblA-G.[35] Of these, CblA and CblB present as isolated MMA similar to MUT deficiency, while CblC, CblD, and CblF (which are involved in intracellular processing of cobalamin prior to conversion to either AdoCbl or MeCbl) present with combined MMA and hyperhomocysteinemia that can include megaloblastic anemia and neurological abnormalities. These disorders are rare autosomal recessive conditions for which true incidences are currently unknown. However, in our experience, CblC is by far the most common of these disorders. CblA is caused by mutations in the MMAA gene (*MMAA* on 4q31.21); CblB is caused by mutations in the MMAB gene (*MMAB* on 12q24.11); CblC is caused by mutations in the MMACHC gene (*MMACHC* on 1p34.1); CblD is caused by mutations in the MMADHC gene (*MMADHC* on 2q23.2); and CblF is caused by mutations in the LMBRD1 gene (*LMBRD1* on 6q13).

Confirmatory Testing: Analysis of ACP will reveal elevations in propionylcarnitine (C3) and the ratio of propionylcarnitine to acetylcarnitine (C3/C2). Measurement of plasma methylmalonic acid levels will show elevations (typically 10 to 100 μM). For CblC, D, and F, measurement of total plasma homocysteine will show elevations (typically 30 to 100 μM) in the context of normal or low plasma methionine. Analysis of UOA and UAG may demonstrate the presence of 3-hydroxy-propionic acid, methylcitric acid, and tiglylglycine. Genetic complementation studies in SFC can establish the specific affected biochemical step. Sequencing of *MMAA, MMAB, MMACHC, MMADHC,* or *LMBRD1* and identifying known or suspected pathogenic mutations in the homozygous or compound heterozygous state will provide molecular confirmation.

Malonic Aciduria (Malonyl-CoA Decarboxylase Deficiency)
Primary Screening Analyte: C3-DC
Secondary Screening Analyte(s): None
Other Metabolic Markers: Malonic acid, methylmalonic acid

Clinical Summary: Malonic aciduria is a defect of branch-chain amino acid catabolism caused by a deficiency of malonyl-CoA decarboxylase. It is a very rare autosomal recessive disorder of unknown incidence that may present as an acute metabolic acidosis with hypoglycemia or as a progressive developmental delay. Malonic aciduria is caused by mutations in the gene encoding malonyl-CoA decarboxylase (*MLYCD* on 16q23.3).

Confirmatory Testing: Analysis of ACP demonstrates significant elevation of malonylcarnitine (C3-DC). Evaluation of UOA will show elevations of both malonic acid and methylmalonic acid. Sequencing of *MLYCD* and identifying known or suspected pathogenic mutations in the homozygous or compound heterozygous state will provide molecular confirmation.

Isobutyryl-CoA Dehydrogenase Deficiency (Isobutyric Aciduria)
Primary Screening Analyte: C4
Secondary Screening Analyte(s): None
Other Metabolic Markers: Isobutyrylglycine

Clinical Summary: Isobutyric aciduria is a rare autosomal disorder of valine metabolism due to deficiency of isobutyryl-CoA dehydrogenase (IBD). While IBD deficiency causes a biochemical abnormality (isobutyric aciduria), the detection of multiple asymptomatic individuals through NBS raises doubts regarding its clinical significance.[36] IBD deficiency is caused by mutations in the gene encoding IBD (*ACAD8* on 11q25).

Confirmatory Testing: Analysis of ACP will demonstrate elevations of isobutyrylcarnitine (C4), while analysis of UAG will show elevated isobutyrylglycine. Isobutyrylcarnitine and butyrylcarnitine (also elevated in SCAD deficiency and ethylmalonic encephalopathy) are C4 acylcarnitine isomers and cannot be distinguished by routine MS/MS, but can be differentiated by using ultra-pressure liquid chromatography followed by MS/MS.[37]

Sequencing of *ACAD8* and identifying known or suspected pathogenic mutations in the homozygous or compound heterozygous state will provide molecular confirmation.

Isovaleric Acidemia (Isovaleryl-CoA Dehydrogenase Deficiency)
Primary Screening Analyte: C5
Secondary Screening Analyte(s): None
Other Metabolic Markers: Isovalerylglycine, 3-OH-isovaleric acid

Clinical Summary: Isovaleric acidemia is a disorder of leucine catabolism caused by deficiency of isovaleryl-CoA dehydrogenase (IVD). IVD deficiency is an autosomal recessive disorder with an estimated incidence of 1:60,000 to 1:250,000.[38] Similar to MSUD, isovaleric acidemia can present along a spectrum of disease severity, including a classic severe acute infantile toxic encephalopathy, an intermediate later-onset form with developmental delay, and an intermittent form with acute episodes of encephalopathy often precipitated by illness or other forms of catabolic stress. Isovaleric acidemia is caused by mutations in the gene encoding IVD (*IVD* on 15q15.1). Individuals that harbor the hypomorphic *IVD* c.932C>T (p.A282V) mutation either in the homozygous or compound heterozygous state are likely to be clinically asymptomatic.[38]

Confirmatory Testing: Analysis of ACP will reveal elevations of isovalerylcarnitine (C5). Examination of UOA and UAG will demonstrate elevated 3-hydroxyisovaleric acid and isovalerylglycine, respectively. Sequencing of *IVD* and identifying known or suspected pathogenic mutations in the homozygous or compound heterozygous state will provide molecular confirmation.

2-Methylbutyrylglycinuria (Short/Branched-Chain Acyl-CoA Dehydrogenase Deficiency)
Primary Screening Analyte: C5
Secondary Screening Analyte(s): None
Other Metabolic Markers: 2-methylbutyrylglycine

Clinical Summary: 2-methylbutyrylglycinuria is a rare autosomal recessive disorder of isoleucine catabolism caused by deficiency of 2-methylbutyryl-CoA dehydrogenase or short/branched-chain acyl-CoA dehydrogenase (SBCAD). SBCAD deficiency was first reported among the Hmong Chinese population secondary to a founder population, but it has recently been reported in non-Hmong individuals as well.[39] While detectable as a biochemical abnormality through NBS, the majority of individuals described to date are asymptomatic.[39] 2-methylbutyrylglycinuria is caused by mutations in the gene encoding SBCAD (*ACADSB* on 10q26.13).

Confirmatory Testing: Analysis of ACP will demonstrate elevation of methylbutyrylcarnitine (C5). Methylbutyrylcarnitine and isovalerylcarnitine are C5 acylcarnitine isomers and cannot be distinguished by routine MS/MS but can be differentiated by using ultra-pressure liquid chromatography followed by MS/MS.[37] Examination of UAG will show presence of 2-methylbutyrylglycine. Sequencing of *ACADSB* and identifying known or suspected pathogenic mutations in the homozygous or compound heterozygous state will provide molecular confirmation.

Glutaric Aciduria, Type I (Glutaryl-CoA Dehydrogenase Deficiency)

Primary Screening Analyte: C5-DC
Secondary Screening Analyte(s): None
Other Metabolic Markers: 3-hydroxyglutaric acid, glutaric acid

Clinical Summary: Glutaric aciduria, type I (GA1) is a disorder of lysine and tryptophan catabolism caused by deficiency of glutaryl-CoA dehydrogenase. GA1 is an autosomal recessive disorder with an overall estimated incidence of 1:50,000 to 1:100,000 but can be as high as 1:300 in some reproductively isolated populations such as Old Order Amish.[40-42] Untreated, GA1 classically presents with macrocephaly and frontotemporal atrophy, followed by acute metabolic-encephalopathic crises precipitated by catabolic stress, which results in irreversible injury to the striatum and a subsequent dystonia-dyskinesia movement disorder. GA1 is caused by mutations in the gene encoding glutaryl-CoA dehydrogenase (*GCDH* on 19p13.2).

Confirmatory Testing: Analysis of ACP will demonstrate elevated glutarylcarnitine (C5-DC). Examination of UOA will show elevated 3-hydroxyglutaric (essentially pathognomonic) and glutaric acids. Demonstration of GCDH deficiency in SFC by enzyme assay will provide biochemical confirmation. Sequencing of *GDCH* and identifying known or suspected pathogenic mutations in the homozygous or compound heterozygous state will provide molecular confirmation.

Multiple Carboxylase Deficiency

Primary Screening Analyte: C5-OH (Note: Many NBS programs screen for biotinidase deficiency directly in addition to the potential detection of C5-OH by MS/MS.)
Secondary Screening Analyte(s): None
Other Metabolic Markers: 3-hydroxyisovaleric acid; 3-methylcrotonylglycine; propionic acid; lactate

Clinical Summary: Multiple carboxylase deficiency (MCD) is a disorder of biotin metabolism resulting from a deficiency of either biotinidase or holocarboxylase synthetase (HCS). Biotin is a required cofactor for acetyl-CoA, 3-methylcrotonyl-CoA, propionyl-CoA, and pyruvate carboxylases. With both deficiencies being autosomal recessive, biotinidase deficiency has an estimated worldwide incidence of 1:50,000 to 1:75,000[43], while HCS deficiency is much rarer. MCD classically presents with neurological dysfunction including seizures and developmental delay, metabolic acidosis, and an eczematous skin rash with alopecia. MCD is caused by mutations in either the gene encoding biotinidase (*BTD* on 3p25.1) or the gene encoding HCS (*HLCS* on 21q22.13).

Confirmatory Testing: Analysis of ACP will demonstrate elevated 3-hydroxyisovalericcarnitine (C5-OH). UOA and UAG analysis will show elevated 3-hydroxyisovaleric acid and 3-methylcrotonylglycine, respectively. Biotinidase enzyme assay in serum will show profound or partial deficiency for biotinidase deficiency but will be normal for HCS deficiency. Demonstration of deficiency of multiple carboxylase activities by enzyme testing in SFC or leukocytes will provide a biochemical diagnosis. Sequencing of

BTD or *HLCS* and identifying known or suspected pathogenic mutations in the homozygous or compound heterozygous state will provide molecular confirmation.

3-Methylcrotonyl-CoA Carboxylase Deficiency

Primary Screening Analyte: C5-OH
Secondary Screening Analyte(s): None
Other Metabolic Markers: 3-hydroxyisovaleric acid, 3-methylcrotonylglycine

Clinical Summary: 3-methylcrotonylglycinuria is a disorder of leucine catabolism resulting from the isolated deficiency of methylcrotonyl-CoA carboxylase (3-MCC). It is an autosomal recessive disease with an estimated incidence of at least 1:35,000 to 1:40,000, making it one of the more frequent deficiencies detected by NBS.[33,42] Initially described in some individuals with severe neurological deficits and developmental delay, the majority of 3-MCC deficient individuals detected by NBS, including mothers detected through secondary elevation in their newborns, are asymptomatic.[44] 3-MCC deficiency is caused by mutations in either the gene encoding the α–subunit (*MCCC1* on 3q27.1) or the gene encoding the β–subunit (*MCCC2* on 5q13.2).

Confirmatory Testing: Analysis of ACP will demonstrate elevations of 3-hydroxyisovalerylcarnitine (C5-OH). UOA and UAG testing will show increased 3-hydroxyisovaleric acid and 3-methylcrotonylglycine, respectively. 3-MCC deficiency can be directly demonstrated by enzyme testing in SFC or leukocytes. Sequencing of *MCCC1* or *MCCC2* and identifying known or suspected pathogenic mutations in the homozygous or compound heterozygous state will provide molecular confirmation.

3-Hydroxy-3-Methylglutaryl-CoA Lyase Deficiency

Primary Screening Analyte: C5-OH
Secondary Screening Analyte(s): C6DC
Other Metabolic Markers: 3-hydroxyisovaleric acid; 3-hydroxy-3-methylglutaric acid; 3-methylglutaconic acid; 3-methylglutaric acid

Clinical Summary: 3-hydroxy-3-methylglutaryl-CoA (HMG-CoA) lyase deficiency is a disorder of ketogenesis and leucine catabolism. It is a rare autosomal recessive condition overall[45], but has higher incidence in some reproductively isolated populations, such as the Saudi.[46] HMG-CoA lyase deficiency classically presents as neonatal hypoketotic hypoglycemia with relatively short fasting tolerance; however, some individuals present later in infancy with episodic hypoketotic hypoglycemia triggered by catabolic stress. This disorder is caused by mutations in the gene encoding HMG-CoA lyase (*HMGCL* on 1p36.11).

Confirmatory Testing: Analysis of ACP will demonstrate elevations of 3-hydroxyisovalerylcarnitine (C5-OH) and 3-methylglutarylcarnitine (C6DC). UOA testing will show increased levels of 3-hydroxyisovaleric, 3-hydroxy-3-methylglutaric, 3-methylglutaconic, and 3-methylglutaric acids. Sequencing of *HMGCL* and identifying known or suspected pathogenic mutations in the homozygous or compound heterozygous state will provide molecular confirmation.

3-Methylglutaconic Aciduria, Type I (3-Methylglutaconyl-CoA Hydratase Deficiency)

Primary Screening Analyte: C5-OH

Secondary Screening Analyte(s): None

Other Metabolic Markers: 3-hydroxyisovaleric acid; 3-methylglutaconic aciduria (MGA); 3-methylglutaric acid

Clinical Summary: MGA type I is a disorder of leucine catabolism resulting from the deficiency of 3-methylglutaconyl-CoA hydratase (AUH). It is a rare autosomal recessive condition with an unknown incidence. AUH deficiency exhibits an apparently wide clinical spectrum, ranging from severe childhood-onset encephalopathy to an adult-onset slowly progressive leukoencephalopathy.[47] MGA type I is caused by mutations in the gene encoding AUH (*AUH* on 9q22.31).

Confirmatory Testing: Analysis of ACP will demonstrate elevations of 3-hydroxyisovalerylcarnitine (C5-OH). UOA testing will show increased levels of 3-hydroxyisovaleric, 3-methylglutaconic, and 3-methylglutaric acids. Biochemical confirmation can be obtained by enzyme testing in SFC. Sequencing of *AUH* and identifying known or suspected pathogenic mutations in the homozygous or compound heterozygous state will provide molecular confirmation.

Beta-Ketothiolase Deficiency (Methyl-acetoacetyl-CoA Thiolase Deficiency)

Primary Screening Analyte: C5-OH

Secondary Screening Analyte(s): C5:1

Other Metabolic Markers: 2-methyl-3-hydroxbutyric acid; 2-methylacetoacidic acid; tiglylglycine

Clinical Summary: Beta-ketothiolase (BKT) deficiency (methyl-acetoacetyl-CoA thiolase deficiency) is a disorder of isoleucine catabolism and ketolysis. It is a rare autosomal recessive condition, and the true incidence is currently unknown. The phenotypic severity of BKT deficiency varies from severe to asymptomatic but classically presents during infancy with episodic ketoacidosis and metabolic decompensation. BKT deficiency is caused by mutations in the gene encoding methyl-acetoacetyl-CoA thiolase (*ACAT1* on 11q22.3).

Confirmatory Testing: Analysis of ACP will demonstrate elevated 2-methyl-3-hydroxybutyrylcarnitine (C5-OH) and tiglylcarnitine (C5:1). Evaluation of UOA and UAG will show elevated 2-methyl-3-hydroxybutyric acid, 2-methylacetoacidic acid, and tiglylglycine. BKT deficiency can be directly demonstrated by enzyme testing in SFC. Sequencing of *ACAT1* and identifying known or suspected pathogenic mutations in the homozygous or compound heterozygous state will provide molecular confirmation.

2-Methyl-3-Hydroxybutyric Acidemia (2-Methyl-3-Hydroxybutyryl-CoA Dehydrogenase Deficiency)

Primary Screening Analyte: C5-OH

Secondary Screening Analyte(s): None

Other Metabolic Markers: 2-methyl-3-hydroxybutyric acid; tiglylglycine

Clinical Summary: 2-methyl-3-hydroxybutyric acidemia is a disorder of isoleucine catabolism resulting from the deficiency of 2-methyl-3-hydroxybutyryl-CoA dehydrogenase (MHBD). MHBD deficiency is a very rare X-linked disorder with only a small number of patients described to date.[48] The affected males have presented with infantile developmental delay followed by progressive neurodegeneration with female carriers having a milder phenotype.[48] 2-methyl-3-hydroxybutyric acidemia is caused by mutations in the gene encoding MHBD (*HSD17B10* on Xp11.22).

Confirmatory Testing: Analysis of ACP will demonstrate elevated 2-methyl-3-hydroxybutyrylcarnitine (C5-OH). Evaluation of UOA will show elevated 2-methyl-3-hydroxybutyric acid and tiglylglycine. MHBD deficiency can be directly demonstrated by enzyme testing in SFC. Sequencing of *HSD17B10* and identifying a known or suspected pathogenic mutation in the hemizygous or heterozygous state will provide molecular confirmation.

Disorders of Galactose Metabolism

Galactose-1-Phosphate Uridyltransferase Deficiency

Primary Screening: Galactose-1-phosphate uridyltransferase (GALT) activity
Secondary Screening Analyte(s): Galactose
Other Metabolic Markers: Galactose-1-phosphate, galactitol

Clinical Summary: GALT deficiency is a disorder of galactose metabolism that classically presents as neonatal hepatic failure with feeding intolerance and high risk of Gram-negative sepsis. It is an autosomal recessive disorder with an estimated incidence in Caucasians of 1:47,000.[49] This form of galactosemia is caused by mutations in the gene that encodes GALT (*GALT* on 9p13.3). When the common hypomorphic Duarte allele (N314D) is present in a compound heterozygote, there is only a partial GALT deficiency with no apparent significant clinical consequences.

Confirmatory Testing: Currently the vast majority of NBS programs screen for GALT deficiency directly by enzyme assay, but some also screen for elevated galactose by fluorimetry, allowing for the possible detection of other rare forms of galactosemia (see below). In addition, some NBS programs also secondarily reflexively screen GALT deficient newborns for common mutations in order to distinguish classic and Duarte galactosemia. Confirmatory GALT activity testing on RBCs will demonstrate severe GALT deficiency for classic galactosemia and partial GALT deficiency for Duarte galactosemia (typically approximately 25% of normal activity for a Duarte/classic compound heterozygote). Galactose-1-phosphate in RBCs and urine galactitol will be elevated. If the *GALT* genotype is not determined or tested by the NBS program, sequencing of *GALT* and detecting known or suspected pathogenic mutations in the homozygous or compound heterozygous state will provide molecular confirmation.

Galactokinase Deficiency or UDP-Galactose 4-Epimerase Deficiency

Primary Screening Analyte: Galactose
Secondary Screening Analyte(s): None

Other Metabolic Markers: Galactose-1-phosphate, galactitol

Clinical Summary: Galactokinase (GALK) deficiency is a disorder of galactose metabolism that presents with rapid, progressive central cataracts. UDP-galactose 4-epimerase (GALE) deficiency is a disorder of galactose metabolism that presents with neonatal hepatopathy and cataracts. GALK and GALE deficiencies are very rare autosomal recessive disorders with worldwide incidences of less than 1:200,000. GALK and GALE deficiencies are caused by mutations in the genes encoding the respective enzymes (*GALK1* on 17q25.1; and *GALE* on 1p36.11).

Confirmatory Testing: NBS programs that screen for elevated galactose by fluorimetry will potentially detect individuals with GALK or GALE deficiencies. Testing GALK or GALE activity on RBCs to demonstrate deficiency will provide biochemical confirmation. Galactose-1-phosphate in RBCs will be elevated in GALE deficiency but low in GALK deficiency. Urine galactitol will be elevated in both disorders. Sequencing of *GALK* or *GALE* and detecting known or suspected pathogenic mutations in the homozygous or compound heterozygous state will provide molecular confirmation.

Future Directions

Given the rapid improvement and reducing costs of many high throughput technologies, the expansion of disorders included in NBS programs worldwide is highly likely. Over the past few years, many conditions have been under active investigation for the feasibility and validation of high throughput population screening. The list includes disorders of creatine metabolism, glucose-6-phasphate dehydrogenase deficiency, various lysosomal storage disorders, severe combined immunodeficiency, disorders of sterol metabolism (particularly Smith-Lemli-Optiz syndrome), Wilson disease, X-linked adrenoleukodystrophy, familial hypercholesterolemia, Fragile X syndrome, Duchene muscular dystrophy, and spinal muscular atrophy.[10] In addition to feasibility, the principles described in Section II of this chapter should be applied in the decision regarding whether to add a particular disorder to NBS programs. Finally, especially as the cost of next-generation sequencing technologies continues to plummet and as our ability to accumulate and analyze large DNA sequence data sets continues to improve, it is intriguing to consider the future possibility of whole genome or whole exome sequencing as an additional or even replacement technology for NBS.

References

1. Guthrie R, Susi A. A simple phenylalanine method for detecting phenylketonuria in large populations of newborn infants. *Pediatrics.* 1963; 32(3): 338–343.
2. Beutler E, Baluda M, Donnell GN. A new method for the detection of galactosemia and its carrier state. *J Lab Clin Med.* 1964; 64: 694–705.
3. Heard GS, McVoy SJ, Wolf B. A screening method for biotinidase deficiency in newborns. *Clin Chem.* 1984; 30(1): 125–127.
4. Dussault JH, Coulombe P, Laberge C, Letarte J, Guyda H, Khoury K. Perliminary report on a mass screening program for neonatal hypothyroidism. *J Pediatr.* 1975; 86(5): 670–674.
5. Millington DS, Kodo N, Norwood DL, Roe CR. Tandem mass spectroscopy: a new method for acylcarnitine profiling with potential for neonatal screening for inborn errors of metabolism. *J Inher Metab Dis.* 1990; 13: 321–324.

6. Watson MS, Lloyd-Puryear MA, Mann MY, Rinaldo P, Howell RR. Newborn screening: toward a uniform screening panel and system. *Genet in Med*. 2006; 8(5S): 12S-252S.
7. Region 4 Genetics Collaborative. http://region4genetics.org.
8. Rinaldo P, Zafari S, Tortorelli S, Matern D. Making the case for objective performance metrics in newborn screening by tandem mass spectroscopy. *Ment Retard Dev Disabil Res Rev*. 2006; 12(4): 255–261.
9. U.S. Centers for Disease Control and Prevention. Newborn Screening Quality Assurance Program. Atlanta, GA: Author. http://www.cdc.gov/labstandards/nsqap.html
10. Rinaldo P, Lim JS, Tortorelli S, Gavrilov D, Matern D. Newborn screening of metabolic disorders: recent progress and future developments. *Nestle Nutr Workshop Ser Pediatr Program*. 2008; 62: 81–93; discussion 93–96.
11. Brusilow SW, Maestri NE. Urea cycle disorders: Diagnosis, pathophysiology, and therapy. *Adv Pediatr*. 1996; 43: 127–170.
12. Lu YB, Kobayashi, K, Ushikai M, et al. Frequency and distribution in East Asia of 12 mutations identified in the SLC25A13 gene of Japanese patients with citrin deficiency. *J Hum Genet*. 2005; 50(7): 338–346.
13. Song YZ, Li BX, Chen FP, et al. Neonatal intrahepatic cholestasis caused by citrin deficiency: clinical and laboratory investigation of 13 subjects in mainland of China. *Dig Liver Dis*. 2009; 41(9): 683–689.
14. Carleton SM, Peck DS, Grasela J, Dietiker KL, Phillips CL. DNA carrier testing and newborn screening for maple syrup urine disease in Old Order Mennonite communities. *Genet Test Mol Biomarkers*. 2010; 14(2): 205–208.
15. Skovby F, Gaustadnes M, Mudd SH. A revisit to the natural history of homocystinuria due to cystathionine beta-synthase deficiency. *Mol Genet Metab*. 2010; 99(1): 1–3.
16. Couce ML, Boveda MD, Castineiras DE, et al. Hypermethioninaemia due to methionine adenosyltransferase I/III (MAT I/III) deficiency: diagnosis in an expanded neonatal screening programme. *J Inherit Metab Dis*. 2008; 31: 233–239.
17. Baric, I. Inherited disorders in the conversion of methionine to homocysteine. *J Inherit Metab Dis*. 2009; 32(4): 459–471.
18. Donlon J, Levy H, Scriver CR. Donlon J,Levy H, Scriver C.R. Hyperphenylalaninemia: Phenylalanine Hydroxylase Deficiency. In: Valle D, Beaudet AL, Vogelstein B, et al. eds. *OMMBID - The Online Metabolic and Molecular Bases of Inherited Diseases*. New York, NY: McGraw-Hill; 2013. http://ommbid.mhmedical.com.ezproxyhost.library.tmc.edu/content.aspx?bookid=474&Sectionid=45374059. Accessed May 19, 2014.
19. Mitchell GA, Grompe M, Lambert M, Tanguay RM. Hypertyrosinemia. In: Valle D, Beaudet AL, Vogelstein B, et al., eds. *OMMBID - The Online Metabolic and Molecular Bases of Inherited Diseases*. New York, NY: McGraw-Hill; 2013. http://ommbid.mhmedical.com.ezproxyhost.library.tmc.edu/content.aspx?bookid=474&Sectionid=45374064. Accessed May 19, 2014.
20. Macsai MS, Schwartz TL, Hinkle D, Hummel MB, Mulhern MG, Rootman D. Tyrosinemia type II: nine cases of ocular signs and symptoms. *Am J Ophthalmol*. 2001; 132(4): 522–527.
21. Ellaway CJ, Holme E, Standing S, et al. Outcome of tyrosinaemia type III. *J Inherit Metab Dis*. 2001; 24(8): 824–832.
22. Koizumi A, Nozaki J, Ohura T, et al. Genetic epidemiology of the carnitine transporter OCTN2 gene in a Japanese population and phenotypic characterization in Japanese pedigrees with primary systemic carnitine deficiency. *Hum Mol Genet*. 1999; 8(12): 2247–2254.
23. Lee NC, Tang NL, Chien YH, et al. Diagnoses of newborns and mothers with carnitine uptake defects through newborn screening. *Mol Genet Metab*. 2010; 100(1): 46–50.
24. Lindner M, Hoffmann GF, Matern D. Newborn screening for disorders of fatty-acid oxidation: experience and recommendations from an expert meeting. *J Inherit Metab Dis*. 2010; 33(5): 521–526.
25. van Maldegem BT, Wanders RJ, Wijburg FA. Clinical aspects of short-chain acyl-CoA dehydrogenase deficiency. *J Inherit Metab Dis*. 2010; 33(5): 507–511.
26. Viscomi C, Burlina AB, Dweikat I, et al. Combined treatment with oral metronidazole and N-acetylcysteine is effective in ethylmalonic encephalopathy. *Nat Med*. 2010; 16(8): 869–871.
27. Clayton PT, Eaton S, Aynsley-Green A, et al. Hyperinsulinism in short-chain L-3-hydroxyacyl-CoA dehydrogenase deficiency reveals the importance of beta-oxidation in insulin secretion. *J Clin Invest*. 2001; 108(3): 457–465.
28. Molven A, Matre GE, Duran M, et al. Familial hyperinsulinemic hypoglycemia caused by a defect in the SCHAD enzyme of mitochondrial fatty acid oxidation. *Diabetes*. 2004; 53(1): 221–227.

29. Spiekerkoetter, U. Mitochondrial fatty acid oxidation disorders: clinical presentation of long-chain fatty acid oxidation defects before and after newborn screening. *J Inherit Metab Dis.* 2010; 33(5): 527–532.
30. Hagenfeldt L, von Dobeln U, Holme E, et al. 3-Hydroxydicarboxylic aciduria—a fatty acid oxidation defect with severe prognosis. *J Pediatr.* 1990; 116(3): 387–392.
31. Rocchiccioli F, Wanders RJ, Aubourg P, et al. Deficiency of long-chain 3-hydroxyacyl-CoA dehydrogenase: a cause of lethal myopathy and cardiomyopathy in early childhood. *Pediatr Res.* 1990; 28(6): 657–662.
32. Manoli I, Venditti CP. Methylmalonic acidemia. In: Pagon, R.A., ed. *GeneReviews.* Seattle: University of Washington, 2010.
33. Frazier DM, Millington DS, McCandless SE, et al. The tandem mass spectrometry newborn screening experience in North Carolina: 1997–2005. *J Inherit Metab Dis.* 2006; 29(1): 76–85.
34. Kasper DC, Ratschmann R, Metz TF, et al. The National Austrian Newborn Screening Program—eight years experience with mass spectrometry: Past, present, and future goals. *Wien Klin Wochenschr.* 2010; 122(21–22): 607–613.
35. Rosenblatt DS, Fenton, WA. Inherited Disorders of folate and cobalamin transport and metabolism. In: Scriver, C.R., et al., eds. *The Metabolic and Molecular Bases of Inherited Disease.* New York: McGraw-Hill, 2001.
36. Oglesbee D, He M, Majumder N, et al. Development of a newborn screening follow-up algorithm for the diagnosis of isobutyryl-CoA dehydrogenase deficiency. *Genet Med.* 2007; 9(2): 108–116.
37. Forni S, Fu X, Palmer SE, Sweetman, L. Rapid determination of C4-acylcarnitine and C5-acylcarnitine isomers in plasma and dried blood spots by UPLC-MS/MS as a second tier test following flow-injection MS/MS acylcarnitine profile analysis. *Mol Genet Metab.* 2010; 101(1): 25–32.
38. Ensenauer R, Vockley J, Willard JM, et al. A common mutation is associated with a mild, potentially asymptomatic phenotype in patients with isovaleric acidemia diagnosed by newborn screening. *Am J Hum Genet.* 2004; 75(6): 1136–1142.
39. Alfardan J, Mohsen AW, Copeland S, et al. Characterization of new ACADSB gene sequence mutations and clinical implications in patients with 2-methylbutyrylglycinuria identified by newborn screening. *Mol Genet Metab.* 2010; 100(4): 333–338.
40. Boneh A, Beauchamp M, Humphrey M, Watkins J, Peters H, Yaplito-Lee J. Newborn screening for glutaric aciduria type I in Victoria: treatment and outcome. *Mol Genet Metab.* 2008; 94(3): 287–291.
41. Hedlund GL, Longo N, Pasquali M. Glutaric acidemia type 1. *Am J Med Genet C, Semin Med Genet.* 2006; 142C(2): 86–94.
42. Niu DM, Chien YH, Chiang CC, et al. Nationwide survey of extended newborn screening by tandem mass spectrometry in Taiwan. *J Inherit Metab Dis.* 2010; 33(Suppl 2): S295–S305.
43. Wolf, B. Worldwide survey of neonatal screening for biotinidase deficiency. *J Inherit Metab Dis.* 1991; 14(6): 923–927.
44. Stadler SC, Polanetz R, Maier EM, et al. Newborn screening for 3-methylcrotonyl-CoA carboxylase deficiency: population heterogeneity of MCCA and MCCB mutations and impact on risk assessment. *Hum Mutat.* 2006; 27(8): 748–759.
45. Chace DH, Kalas TA, Naylor EW. Use of tandem mass spectrometry for multianalyte screening of dried blood specimens from newborns. *Clin Chem.* 2003; 49(11): 1797–1817.
46. Al-Sayed M, Imtiaz F, Alsmadi OA, Rashed MS, Meyer BF. Mutations underlying 3-hydroxy-3-methylglutaryl CoA lyase deficiency in the Saudi population. *BMC Med Genet.* 2006; 7: 86.
47. Wortmann SB, Kluijtmans LA, Engelke UF, Wevers RA, Morava E. The 3-methylglutaconic acidurias: what's new? *J Inherit Metab Dis.* 2010; 35(1): 13–22.
48. Korman, SH. Inborn errors of isoleucine degradation: a review. *Mol Genet Metab.* 2006; 89(4): 289–299.
49. Suzuki M, West C, Beutler E. Large-scale molecular screening for galactosemia alleles in a pan-ethnic population. *Human Genetics.* 2001; 109: 210–215.

SECTION 2

Pathways

2

Human Glycosylation Disorders

Many Faces, Many Pathways

HUDSON H. FREEZE, ERIK A. EKLUND,
AND DONNA M. KRASNEWICH

Introduction

An explosive discovery of rare human glycosylation disorders began in 1984 thanks to a simple serum test that queried the structures of N-linked oligosaccharides. Since that time, the analysis of this glycoprotein, transferrin, has become a diagnostic test specifically for individuals with congenital disorders of glycosylation (CDG), with indications for other glycosylation pathways as well. In addition, researchers have developed biochemical assays for the steps in the N-linked oligosaccharide synthetic pathway, cloned genes encoding these enzymes, and described many different types of human glycosylation disorders. The emergence of the group of human disorders resulting from defects in steps within glycosylation pathways has dramatically underscored the importance of educating clinicians in their identification and treatment.

Currently, over 100 distinct disorders, each with a known genetic basis, have been described and encompass several different glycosylation pathways as well as common substrate biosynthetic steps. *These disorders collectively define the CDGs.* In this chapter we describe the clinical presentation of these disorders as well as their classifications, diagnostic strategies, and the basic metabolic pathways underlying their pathology. However, this is only the beginning. With the advances in genome sequencing and the fact that at least 2% of the translated genome is needed for optimal glycosylation, it is inevitable that new disorders will be defined. Partnerships between medical specialists and basic scientists will be needed to advance our understanding of the impact of glycosylation on human biology and disease.

This chapter discusses the clinical findings and metabolic features of human disorders resulting from defects in the synthesis of (a) N-linked glycans or multiple glycosylation pathways including N-linked glycans, (b) O-linked glycans, (c) glycosphingolipids, and (d) glycosylphosphatidylinositol (GPI-anchors). Figure 2.1 shows the types and representative

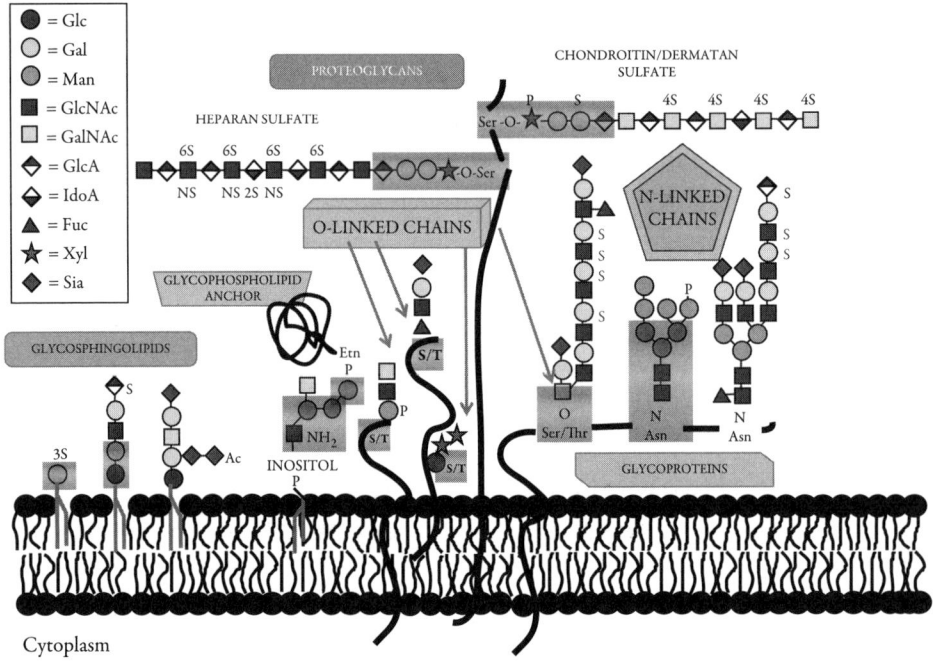

FIGURE 2.1 Major types of ER-Golgi formed glycans.

structures of these glycans. Figure 2.2 indicates the general biosynthetic pathways in the endoplasmic reticulum (ER) and Golgi.

Clinical Disorders Resulting from Defective Synthesis of N-Linked Oligosaccharides or Multiple Glycosylation Pathways

PMM2-CDG (CDG-Ia): The Most Common Type of CDG

The first children with CDG, initially termed "carbohydrate deficient glycoprotein syndrome," were described by Dr. Jaak Jaeken in 1980. A study on the underlying metabolic defect, phosphomannomutase (PMM) deficiency, was published almost 15 years later.[1] Since that time, 56 different genes coding for distinct enzymes, transporters, or structural proteins, only or partly involved in the synthesis of N-linked oligosaccharides, have been described and constitute the majority of the subtypes of the CDGs. Each of these genes defines a distinct subtype of CDG. Historically, the types were denoted as types I and II (e.g., CDG-Ia [PMM2-deficiency] and CDG-IIa [MGAT2-deficiency]) based on the pattern of underglycosylation of transferrin and order of publication.[2] A new nomenclature is now used with the gene name CDG (e.g., PMM2-CDG and MGAT-CDG), where some authors prefer to add the old denotation in parenthesis—that is, PMM2-CDG (CDG-Ia)—when available. It is notable that OMIM has kept annotating newly discovered disorders by the old nomenclature.[3] With more than 800 cases identified worldwide in both adults and

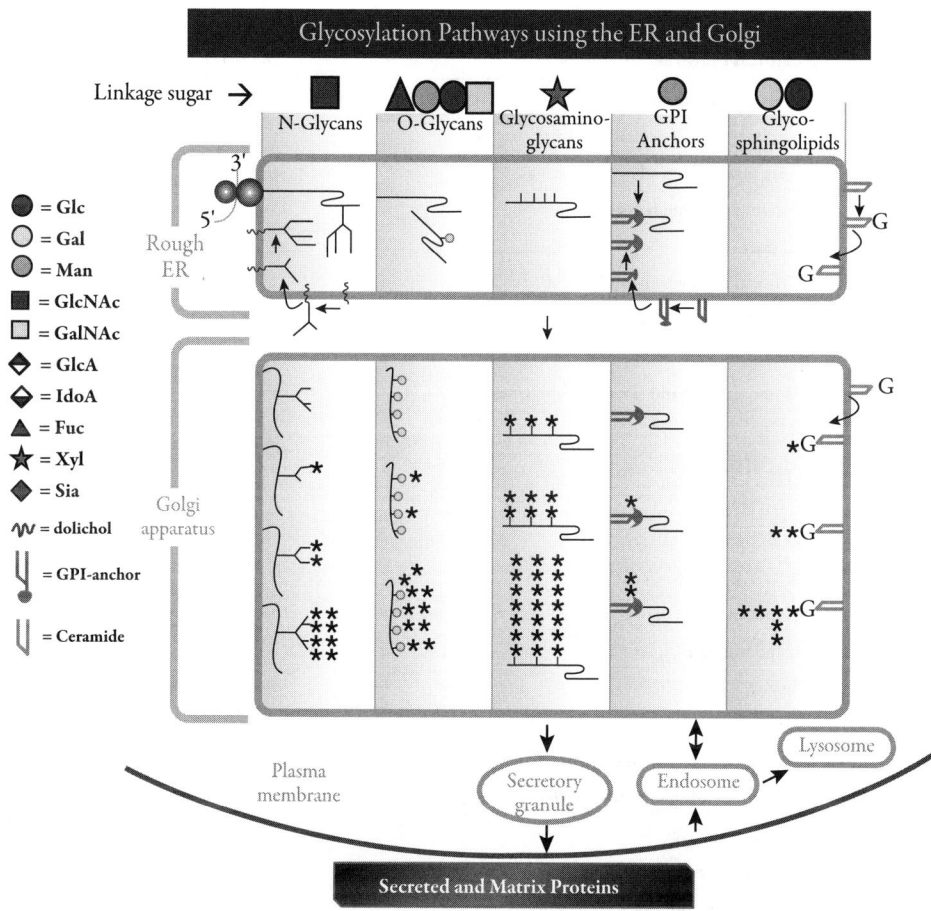

FIGURE 2.2 Major glycosylation pathways in ER-Golgi.

children, there is an increasing need to understand the common pathology and management and to devise novel therapeutic strategies.

The clinical spectrum of CDGs is very broad. It ranges from severe neurologic involvement and complications in multiple organ systems to normal development with only significant gastrointestinal symptoms. The clinical manifestations are variable both between and within subtypes. With almost 700 cases of PMM2-CDG patients identified, it is the most common type. More than 20 cases of PMI-CDG, ALG6-CDG, ALG1-CDG, and PGM1-CDG are known with other types having only one or a few documented cases. As is true with most rare metabolic disorders, the clinical spectrum of each of these CDG types is much broader than reported. This suggests that clinical knowledge of the most common presentations is important; however, clinicians must remember that many organ systems are known to be affected in disorders of N-linked glycosylation. This will open the door to identifying both unusual presentations of known CDG types as well as new types of CDG.

The range of clinical phenotypes of the most common type of CDG (PMM2-CDG) presents a lesson in the breadth of human embryologic and physiologic processes dependent on normal N-linked glycosylation for full function (Table 2.1).[4] Infants with PMM2-CDG

TABLE 2.1 **Clinical Features of PMM2-CDG Patients**

Clinical Features	Occurrence
Presentation in infancy	
Normal pregnancy, delivery, birthweight	+++
Failure to thrive and hypotonia	+++
Ascites, multiorgan system failure	+
Hydrops fetalis	+
Clinical features in adulthood	
Variable intellectual impairment	+++
Ataxia, dysarthria, dysmetria	+++
Kyphoscoliosis and skeletal involvement	+++
Range of functional life skills	+++
Risk of thrombosis	++
Neurology	
Developmental delay	+++
Ataxia, dysarthria, dysmetria	+++
Hypotonia	+++
Hyporeflexia	+++
Seizures	++
Stroke-like episodes	++
Progressive peripheral neuropathy with muscle wasting	++
Gastroentrology/Hepatopathy	
Failure to thrive	+++
Gastroesophogeal reflux	+++
Liver dysfunction/elevated liver function tests	+++
Hematology	
Risk of thrombosis	++
Decreased levels of procoagulation cascade	+++
Decreased levels of protein C, protein S, antithrombin III	+++
Nephrology	
Microcystic kidneys	+++
Proteinuria	++
Nephrotic syndrome	+
Cardiology	
Pericardial effusion	+++
Hypertrophic cardiomyopathy	+
Ophthalmology	
Esotropia	+++
Retinitis pigmentosa	+++
Myopia	+++
Orthopedics	
Osteopenia	+++
Kyphosis/kyphoscoliosis	+++

(continued)

TABLE 2.1 **Continued**

Clinical Features	Occurrence
Chest deformaties	+++
Contractures	++
Dermatologic	
Atypical fat distribution	+++
Inverted nipples	++
Endocrinologic	
Hypergonadotropic hypogonadism	+++
Hyperinsulinemic hypoglycemia	+
Growth dysregulation	+++

Note. (+) = rare; (++) = occasional; (+++) = common.

typically present after an uneventful pregnancy and delivery with normal birthweight. Pediatricians may note failure to thrive, hypotonia, developmental delay, inverted nipples, abnormal fat distribution, hepatopathy, and, in some cases, a small cerebellum on an MRI at four to six months of age. Most affected children continue to gain skills and advance to adulthood, are never hospitalized, and have variable involvement of different organ systems. However, about 20% of children may die in infancy from multiorgan system failure. Typically, these more severely affected infants have difficult newborn courses with multiple hospitalizations for failure to thrive and more severe courses of common childhood diseases. Complications of hypoalbuminemia with catastrophic fluid imbalance and anasarca lead to increased morbidity and mortality.[5] Each affected child has a different collection of developmental skills and medical issues reflecting the many factors that modulate the clinical effects of the basic glycobiologic defect.

Neurologic, hepatic, skeletal, cardiac, coagulation, and endocrine manifestations are typically recognized after the diagnosis and may pose important management issues in infants and children with PMM2-CDG. The diagnosis of PMM2-CDG in both infants with hydrops fetalis as well as adults with ataxia and normal cognition document the phenotypic spectrum of this disorder.[6,7]

Central and Peripheral Nervous System

Hypotonia and developmental delay are typically the first recognized neurologic signs in infants with PMM2-CDG. Affected children continue to make slow developmental progress without regression throughout their lives. A combination of ataxia, dysarthria, and dysmetria, due to documented cerebellar hypoplasia, is recognized in early childhood.[4,8] The cerebellum may appear normal sized in infancy; however, serial imaging has consistently shown a mismatch between cerebellar growth and growth in other parts of the brain. Cognition varies greatly; most children have intellectual disabilities while a few adults have been reported to have normal intelligence.[7,9] It is critical to note that cognitive function is difficult to test because of speech involvement and slow processing time. Seizures are common, typically first occurring in childhood, and are responsive to anticonvulsants.

Progressive peripheral neuropathy with muscle wasting is seen variably in teens and adults. Stroke-like episodes, sudden hemiplegia, or obtunded consciousness are other complications that have been reported in early childhood through the teen years. These stroke-like episodes typically do not result in permanent neurologic changes; instead, affected individuals show gradual improvement with a return to normal after weeks or months.[4] The etiology is not well understood.

Gastrointestinal Tract and Liver

Children with PMM2-CDG commonly present with failure to thrive. Oral motor dysfunction, as well as gastroesophogeal reflux, compound the feeding issues, especially in the first two years of life. Elevated transaminases and decreased serum levels of both pro- and anticoagulation factors reflect the typical episodic hepatopathy. Although most affected children show this hepatic dysfunction, the elevation of liver function tests rarely reach a level causing clinical concern, and there are no reports of liver failure in individuals with PMM2-CDG. Liver biopsies have been performed on children prior to diagnosis and show steatosis, fibrosis, and involvement of the portal tracts. The elevated liver function tests typically decrease by age five; however, the coagulopathy continues to require vigilance throughout life.[10]

Renal

Renal involvement is typically limited in individuals affected with PMM2-CDG, with echogenic kidneys being the most common finding. There are rare reports of affected children with nephrotic syndrome, which typically resolves. Renal function is preserved throughout the life of the affected individuals.[11]

Cardiac

The most frequent cardiac finding in infants with PMM2-CDG is a small pericardial effusion that disappears over time. There are also reports of hypertrophic cardiomyopathy and pericardial effusions requiring pericardial windows; however, this is rare.[12]

Ophthalmologic

Infants with PMM2-CDG have esotropia typically with progressive myopia. Appropriate management by a pediatric ophthalmologist leads to minimal visual deficits in older children. Progressive retinitis pigmentosa, has been reported in affected children with variable age of onset and becomes more symptomatic in affected adults.[13]

Orthopedic

Both children and adults with PMM2-CDG show radiologic evidence of osteopenia without significantly increased risk of fracture. As children grow, they may develop contractures of the extremities especially if hypotonia is profound and physical therapy does not address range of motion. The onset of scoliosis and progressive kyphosis in childhood with truncal shortening and chest deformity may lead to functional limitation in adulthood.[14]

Dermatologic

One of the cardinal features of PMM2-CDG is the unusual fat pads seen in early childhood, including suprapubital fat pads with asymmetric fat accumulation and distinctive lipodystrophy of the buttocks. These disappear with age and thus are an age-dependent diagnostic finding.[4]

Endocrinologic

Endocrine issues in individuals with PMM2-CDG are present in many of the hormone pathways. Affected individuals may present with hypergonadotropic hypogonadism, with minimal pubertal development in females. Males undergo normal pubertal changes followed by hypogonadism in adulthood with low testosterone levels and small testes. Some individuals have low cortisol or transcortin, and most have failure to thrive, suggesting growth dysregulation. Each of these hormonal cascades include glycosylated receptors and agonist/peptides with the exact nature of how defective N-linked oligosaccharide structures change endocrine function an area of active research.[15] In some children, there is also a hyperinsulinemic hypoglycemia that requires clinical attention.[16]

Adulthood

Adults with PMM2-CDG continue to gain skills and thrive into adulthood with the oldest known patient in her sixties. Their cheerful, interactive personalities highlight their function despite, in most cases, both cognitive and physical disabilities. Affected adults live in assisted-living settings with cognitive impairment and ataxia causing limitations in their functional life skills and independence. Otherwise, affected adults are relatively healthy and social members of the community. The generation of children diagnosed in the past few decades will teach us more about the spectrum of phenotypes of affected adults.[7,17,18]

Clinical Disorders From Defects in Other Steps in N-Linked Oligosaccharide Synthesis or Multiple Glycosylation Pathways

Once the first cases of CDG were recognized, clinicians slowly began looking for N-linked glycosylation disorders among their patients without diagnoses. Any child or adult with multiorgan system involvement should be considered for serum transferrin analysis, the clinical diagnostic test, especially individuals with central nervous system and multisystemic, hepatic, or gastrointestinal involvement. However, the spectrum of clinical stories that have emerged from cases identified by astute clinicians performing transferrin analysis on their patients has led to a stunning expansion of the phenotypes now recognized to be due to defects in N-linked oligosaccharide synthesis.

There are now 98 recognized types of human glycosylation diseases, with a type delineated when causative mutations in a novel gene have been identified.[2,19] Of these, 56 are known to disrupt the N-linked pathway or multiple pathways including the N-linked pathway. The N-linked pathway subtypes have been broadly classified into type I and II based on whether the defect is in the pathway where the growing oligosaccharide is linked to dolichol, type I, or to protein, type II. Most types have only a few described individuals, leaving much of the phenotypic variability to be documented in future cases. Being able to pick the type by knowing the phenotype is not possible, since there is significant overlap both in organ involvement and in clinical severity.

Some types of CDG have a phenotypic feature not typically seen in other CDGs. These include: normal development with severe protein losing enteropathy and hepatic involvement in MPI-CDG and ALG8-CDG[20–22]; icthyosis in SRD5A3-CDG,[23] MPDU1-CDG,[24,25] and DOLK-CDG[26]; and *cutis laxa* in ATP6VOA2-CDG.[24,27] Developmental eye anomalies, including coloboma and optic atrophy, occur in ALG3-CDG,[28] ALG2-CDG,[29] and SRD5A3-CDG.[30,31] Other hematologic anomalies can be seen, including increased risk of infections in ALG12-CDG[32] and COG4-CDG,[33] increased peripheral lymphocytes in SLC35C1-CDG,[34,35] and thrombocytopenia in SLC35A1-CDG.[36] One of the most recently discovered type, DHDDS-CDG, caused by a mutation in the Ashkenazi Jewish population, causes only *retinitis pigmentosa*.[37] Other mutations in DHDDS could have additional pathologies.

PMI-CDG is notable in that it is treatable with alimentary mannose supplementation. The clinical manifestations include failure to thrive, hypoglycemia, and protein losing enteropathy with normal development. Children treated for several years with oral mannose may develop severe progressive hepatic fibrosis and cirrhosis. Further experience is needed to determine whether this is the natural course of the disorder or whether oral mannose exacerbates the hepatic manifestations.[38]

Diagnosis

For many years, the analysis of the serum glycoprotein transferrin has been used as a diagnostic tool in individuals with clinical features of CDG. This is usually done using isoelectric focusing, high-performance liquid chromatography, or mass spectrometry. Serum transferrin glycoprotein analysis assesses whether a complete N-linked oligosaccharide is attached to transferrin. An abnormal serum transferrin glycoform analysis implies that there is a problem with N-linked glycan synthesis, thus a CDG. However, the test can have both false positives and false negatives. False positives are seen in individuals with galactosemia, fructosemia, alcohol abuse, hemolytic uremic syndrome, and transferrin protein polymorphisms. Affected infants younger than one month may have a normal serum transferrin analysis, which eventually becomes abnormal by six weeks to two months of age. Conversely, abnormal patterns can be seen with normal neonates giving a false positive that normalize by the third month of life. In those cases, another glycoprotein marker, α1-antitrypsin, can be used since it provides greater reliability.[39] There have been reports that older affected individuals, with proven mutations in CDG genes, develop normal transferrin glycosylation without a corresponding improvement in their clinical features. Defects uniquely disrupting glycosylation pathways other than N-linked do not show abnormal transferrin glycosylation.

If the serum transferrin glycoform analysis on an individual shows abnormal N-linked glycosylation, the diagnosis of CDG is made. This analysis will reveal either a type I or type II pattern. A type I pattern suggests that the defective step is in the cytosol or ER and involves a step early in the pathway before the sugar chains are transferred to protein. A type II pattern highlights defects later in the synthetic pathway, in the ER or the Golgi, after the N-linked glycan is attached to the protein. If an individual has an abnormal transferrin glycan analysis but no molecular defect is found, they are given the diagnosis of CDG-X or, if applicable, CDG-Ix, where the analysis shows a type I pattern, or CDG-IIx, where the analysis shows a type II pattern. In some cases, transferrin will have a "mixed pattern" with the absence of entire glycan chains *and* loss of several individual sugars,[40] as is the case of PGM1-CDG.

The research laboratory approach to defining the CDG type is guided by the serum transferrin glycan analysis pattern, type I or type II. Since the defect in CDG-Ix individuals is likely in the early part of the pathway, an analysis of dolichol-linked oligosaccharides in fibroblasts may reveal an increase in the oligosaccharide that is the substrate for the defective enzyme, so lipid-linked oligosaccharide analysis is useful.[41] If the transferrin analysis shows a type II pattern, then C-III isoelectric focusing has been used to look for specific mucin-type glycosylation defects.[42] Other studies such as O-linked and N-linked serum glycan profiling in plasma are also available to give direction to which step may be defective in these glycosylation pathways.[43,44]

At present, enzyme assays are rarely used to find the CDG type; however, in some instances a PMM2 assay can precede genetic testing. Full sequencing of candidate genes is clinically available for the most common CDG types, PMM-CDG, MPI-CDG, and ALG6-CDG. However, unless the indicated mutations have been proven to be pathologic, introduce early stop signals, or severely disrupt protein structure, they may require further confirmation before being designated a causative mutation. Testing of some genes is available on a research basis. Plasma and serum oligosaccharides are also being examined on a clinical basis by GC-Mass Spec looking for glycans that may indicate the type of CDG.[45]

While disorders of N-linked glycan synthesis are detectable with the serum transferrin glycan analysis, disorders of other glycosylation pathways may not be detected by this blood test. Other laboratory tests that are being used currently include muscle biopsy with alpha-dystroglycan glycosylation analysis by immunofluorescence for the diagnosis of the congenital muscular dystrophies, a type of O-linked glycan synthetic disorder. The molecular diagnostics, on either a clinical or a research basis, are available for many of the disorders where the genetic basis has been defined. The caveat that changes in the DNA sequence of candidate genes must be proven to be causative is critical in the context of clinical care and genetic counseling.

Whole exome and genome sequencing are becoming increasingly more available in the clinical setting as well, and both will greatly facilitate diagnosis of CDG in known genes and find disorders in hitherto unknown ones. One must, however, stress caution when reading the results of these massive approaches and the great importance of using second-tier biochemical analyses of any unclear genetic result from these screenings before assigning a mutation as causative.

It is clear that there are many undiscovered types of CDG considering that there are approximately 200 steps in the pathway, with only ~100 known types. It is important clinicians consider glycosylation disorders in individuals who have suggested features, including multisystemic involvement; stroke-like episodes or unexpected deep venous thrombosis, retinal pigmentary changes, or congenital eye anomalies; cerebellar atrophy or cortical abnormalities; osteopenia or scoliosis; hepatic fibrosis or recurrent generalized edema/ascites; coagulopathy; or recurrent infections.

N-Linked Glycosylation: The Metabolic Pathway

N-linked glycosylation is the attachment of a sugar chain to a protein via the terminal amino group (N) of the side chain of the amino acid asparagine. The synthesis of N-linked oligosaccharides involves a dynamic, complex pathway beginning with the formation of a 14 sugar oligosaccharide. It is constructed on the lipid, dolichol, by glycosyltransferases, which add simple sugars, monosaccharides, one at a time in a sequential, defined order. This process is structure rather than template driven, and each transfer of a monosaccharide to the growing structure is catalyzed by a specific transferase. This dolichol-linked structure, consisting of 2 GlcNAc, 9 mannose, and 3 glucose units, is then transferred en bloc to selected asparagines in nascent proteins entering the ER. These structures are then trimmed, with 3 glucoses and up to 6 mannoses removed by glycosidases. A diverse range of hundreds of N-glycan structures can be built at this point with different branching patterns and monosaccharide modifications. Both the complexity of this pathway and the dynamic nature of the N-linked oligosaccharide structure itself imply the existence of many more steps that, when perturbed, may lead to human pathology or fetal lethality.[2]

Defects have been found in affected individuals in both the reactions leading to the addition of the chains and in their modification after they are added, including the trimming reactions. The order of many modifications requires a preceding step, while others compete with each other in the Golgi. The outcome can be a diverse assembly of different related structures at a specific glycosylation site. It depends on many factors, such as the supply of donor substrates, abundance of each of the complementing and competing transferases, their catalytic efficiency, proper location within the dynamic Golgi, and time the proteins coreside with the modifying enzymes. Metabolic defects known to occur in these steps that trim, extend, and modify the N-glycans are listed in Table 2.2.

The synthesis of N-linked oligosaccharides involves many more steps than there are currently recognized defects, suggesting that there are many more CDGs to be defined. Of greater importance, why and how abnormal N-linked glycosylation leads to abnormal brain and eye development, growth, and nutrient handling; skeletal calcification and growth; endocrine hormone and receptor function; coagulation cascade function; and hematologic abnormalities opens the door to many possible areas of research.

N-Linked Oligosaccharide Function

Essentially every membrane bound and secreted protein, except albumin, is N-glycosylated, as are most proteins within vesicles. This list includes extracellular matrix proteins, cell

TABLE 2.2 **Clinical Findings Described in the Different Subtypes of N-linked Glycosylation Disorders or Disorders of Multiple Pathways Including the N-linked Pathway**

N-Linked Glycosylation Disorders[a] or Disorders of Multiple Pathways Including the N-Linked Pathway				Clinical Spectrum												
Disorder	Functional Defect	Gene	OMIM	ID/DD/Autism	Seizures/Epilepsy	Hypotonia	Eye Anomalies or RP	Skeletal Defects	Liver Dysfunction or Elevated Liver Function Tests	Connective Tissue or Ichthyosis	Hematological or Coagulopathy	Myopathy	Deafness	Cardiac Involvement	Recurrent Infections	Gastrointestinal/Failure to thrive
Type I defects																
PMM2-CDG	Phosphomannomutase Man-6-P→Man-1-P	*PMM2*	212065	√	√	√	√	√	√		√			√		√
MPI-CDG	Phosphomannose isomerase Fru-6-P<->Man-6-P	*MPI*	601785						√		√					√
ALG6-CDG[a]	α-1,3-glucosyltransferase	*ALG6*	603147	√	√	√	√		√		√					
ALG3-CDG[a]	α-1,3-mannosyltransferase	*ALG3*	601110	√	√	√	√				√		√			
DPM1-CDG	Dolichol-P-Man synthase	*DPM1*	603503	√	√	√	√		√		√	√				
MPDU1-CDG[a]	Dolichol-P sugar utilization protein	*MPDU1*	604041	√	√	√	√			√						
ALG12-CDG[a]	α-1,6-mannosyltransferase	*ALG12*	607143	√		√		√			√		√	√	√	√
ALG8-CDG[a]	α-1,3-glucosyltransferase	*ALG8*	608104	√		√			√		√				√	√
ALG2-CDG[a]	α-1,3-mannosyltransferase	*ALG2*	607906	√	√		√		√		√	√				
DPAGT1-CDG[a]	GlcNAc-1-P transferase	*DPAGT1*	608093	√	√	√	√						√			√
ALG1-CDG[a]	β-1,4-mannosyltransferase	*ALG1*	608540	√	√	√			√		√			√	√	√
ALG9-CDG[a]	α-1,2-mannosyltransferase	*ALG9*	608776	√	√	√			√		√	√				
DOLK-CDG	Dolichol kinase	*DOLK/DK1*	610768	√	√	√				√		√				
RFT1-CDG[a]	Man (5)GlcNAc Flippase	*RFT1*	612015	√	√	√			√		√		√			
DPM3-CDG	Dolichol-P-Man synthase	*DPM3*	612937								√	√		√		
DPM2-CDG	Dolichol-P-Man synthase	*DPM2*	615042	√	√	√	√	√	√		√	√				
TUSC3-CDG[a]	Subunit of the OST complex	*TUSC3*	611093	√												√
MAGT1-CDG[a]	Subunit of the OST complex	*MAGT1*	300716	√												√
DDOST-CDG[a]	Subunit of the OST complex	*DDOST*	614507	√		√	√	√	√		√			√		√
STT3A-CDG[a]	Subunit of the OST complex	*STT3A*	NA	√	√	√	√									√
STT3B-CDG[a]	Subunit of the OST complex	*STT3B*	NA	√	√	√	√		√		√					√
SSR4-CDG[a]	Subunit of the TRAP complex	*SSR4*	NA	√	√	√										
ALG11-CDG[a]	α-1,2-mannosyltransferase	*ALG11*	613661	√	√	√	√						√			√
ALG13-CDG[a]	Subunit of UDP-N-acetylglucosamine transferase complex	*ALG13*	300884	√	√	√	√	√	√		√					√

(continued)

TABLE 2.2 Continued

N-Linked Glycosylation Disorders[a] or Disorders of Multiple Pathways Including the N-Linked Pathway				Clinical Spectrum												
Disorder	Functional Defect	Gene	OMIM	ID/DD/Autism	Seizures/Epilepsy	Hypotonia	Eye Anomalies or RP	Skeletal Defects	Liver Dysfunction or Elevated Liver Function Tests	Connective Tissue or Ichthyosis	Hematological or Coagulopathy	Myopathy	Deafness	Cardiac Involvement	Recurrent Infections	Gastrointestinal/Failure to thrive
Type I defects																
ALG14-CDG[a]	Subunit of UDP-N-acetylglucosamine transferase complex	ALG14	NA									√				
SRD5A3-CDG	5-α steroid reductase (polyprenol reductase)	SRD5A3	612379	√			√		√	√	√			√		
DHDDS-CDG	Dehydrodolichyl Diphosphate synthase	DHDDS	613861				√									
GMPPA-CDG	Homologue of GDP-mannose pyrophosphorylase	GMPPA	NA	√												
Type II defects																
MGAT2-CDG[a]	N-acetylglucosaminyl transferase II	MGAT2	212066	√	√		√				√					√
B4GALT1-CDG	β-1,4-galactosyltransferase	B4GALT1	607091	√		√						√	√			
Epileptic encephalopathy 15 non-syndromic ID 12	β-Galactoside-α-2,3-sialyltransferase-III	ST3GAL3	611090 615006	√	√											
I-cell disease[a]	GlcNAc-1-P transferase	GNPTAB	252500	√			√	√		√				√		
GCS1-CDG[a]	α-1,2- Glucosidase I	GCS1	601336	√	√	√			√	√						√
Autosomal Dominant Polycystic liver disease[a]	Glucosidase II subunit β	PRKCSH	174050						√							
MAN1B1-CDG[a]	α-1,2-mannosidase	MAN1B1	614202	√	√											
NGLY1-CDG[a]	N-glycanase-1	NGLY1	615273	√	√	√			√							
SLC35A1-CDG	CMP-sialic acid transporter	SLC35A1	603585								√				√	
SLC35A2-CDG	UDP-galactose transporter	SLC35A2	300896	√	√	√	√	√			√				√	√
SLC35A3-CDG	UDP-GlcNAc transporter	SLC35A3	N/A	√	√			√								
SLC35C1-CDG	GDP-fucose transporter	FUCT1	266265	√		√					√				√	
Autosomal Dominant Polycystic liver disease	ER translocation	SEC63	174050						√							
Congenital dyserythropoietic anaemia II (CDA II)	ER-Golgi protein trafficking	SEC23B	224100								√					

(continued)

TABLE 2.2 Continued

Disorder	Functional Defect	Gene	OMIM	ID/DD/Autism	Seizures/Epilepsy	Hypotonia	Eye Anomalies or RP	Skeletal Defects	Liver Dysfunction or Elevated Liver Function Tests	Connective Tissue or Ichthyosis	Hematological or Coagulopathy	Myopathy	Deafness	Cardiac Involvement	Recurrent Infections	Gastrointestinal/Failure to thrive
Type II defects																
Cranio-lenticulo-sutural dysplasia (CLSD)	ER-Golgi protein trafficking	SEC23A	607812				√	√								
COG1-CDG	Conserved oligomeric Golgi Subunit 1	COG1	611209	√			√	√	√	√				√		√
COG4-CDG	Conserved oligomeric Golgi Subunit 4	COG4	613489	√	√	√			√	√	√				√	√
COG5-CDG	Conserved oligomeric Golgi Subunit 5	COG5	613612	√		√										
COG6-CDG	Conserved oligomeric Golgi Subunit 6	COG6	614576	√	√	√			√		√					√
COG7-CDG	Conserved oligomeric Golgi Subunit 7	COG7	608779	√	√	√			√	√					√	√
COG8-CDG	Conserved oligomeric Golgi Subunit 8	COG8	611182	√	√	√					√					√
Achondrogenesis Type 1A	Golgi structure	GMAP-210	200600					√								
ATP6V0A2-CDG	Golgi pH regulator	ATP6V0A2	219200	√	√	√			√		√					
TMEM165-CDG	Golgi pH regulator/calcium homeostasis	TMEM165	614727	√	√				√	√	√					√
PGM1-CDG Glycogen storage disease 14	Glucose 1P ←→ Glucose 6P	PGM1	614921 612934						√			√		√		
Glycogen Storage Disease Ib and Ic	Glucose-6-phosphate transporter	G6PT1	232240						√						√	
Severe congenital neutropenia 4/Dursun syndrome	Glucose-6-phosphatase catalytic, 3	G6PC3	612541	√					√					√	√	√
Congenital myasthenia syndrome	Glutamine-fructose-6-P transaminase	GFAT1	610542									√				

Note. [a]Disorders only disrupting the N-linked pathway of glycosylation.

surface sugar, ion transporters, and lysosomal enzymes. Each of these proteins can have multiple sugar chain structures at different sites on the protein. This generates enormous structural diversity. In some cases, a very specific set of structures is required for function. A good example is I-cell disease in which the presence of mannose-6-P on multiple enzymes is required for their targeting to the lysosome. Absence of mannose-6-P dispatches these critical enzymes to the blood and results in the accumulation of undigested material in the lysosomes and clinical pathology.[46] Absence of whole sugar chains on a protein can result in the rapid degradation of that protein. The conceptually difficult aspect of glycosylation is that the effects of omitting glycan chains or making the wrong glycan structure must be considered separately for each protein. Many are indifferent or tolerant of major change in the N-glycan structure. For others, such as the case of I-cell disease, the change is devastating to the protein's function or half-life. It is a daunting task to determine which specific underglycosylated protein causes various phenotypes. The impact on specific target proteins depends on the type of cell/tissue and their overall glycosylation demands.

There are some aspects of the function of N-linked glycosylation that can be generalized. One of the most important roles of N-linked oligosaccharides is to encourage proper protein folding during synthesis. They also play major roles in proofreading properly folded proteins. The $Glc_3Man_9GlcNAc_2$ glycan transferred from dolichol donor to protein is trimmed to $Glc_1Man_9GlcNAc_2$ in the ER. This glycan is recognized by chaperones, calnexin, and calreticulin, which usher it along the pathway to the Golgi. If N-glycans are missing, the proteins can be degraded before leaving the ER. N-glycans can also help proteins form multimeric complexes in the ER. The glycans can also determine the residence time of a protein on the cell surface, and in cases where signaling within and between cells require a threshold amount, poor glycosylation may make receptors unavailable. This is especially important during brain development or at times when growth factors are required. A defect in any of these functions leads to the embryologic and biologic consequences seen in individuals affected with CDG. Clearly, the phenotypes of affected individuals highlight the importance of glycosylation for pre- and postnatal life. Experts in many fields should see that this group of glycosylation disorders presents opportunities to better understand embryology, growth, neurodevelopmental biology, hematology, bone biology, and endocrinology.

The importance of N-linked glycans in the nervous system is underscored by the findings of abnormal neurologic development seen in almost all types of CDG. Current literature documents that carbohydrate-carrying proteins have important roles during neurodevelopment, regeneration, and synaptic plasticity. Both the wide structural diversity of glycan chains and their concentrated localization on the neuronal cell surface underscore their role in the interaction between cells and the matrix that surrounds it. It is known that while high mannose structures are considered an intermediate in the synthesis of fully processed N-linked glycans, the high mannose structures are actually carried to the cell surface in brain cells as recognition molecules such as L1, neural cell adhesion molecule, and adhesion molecule on glia.[47] The abnormal glycosylation on these proteins in the brains of children and adults with CDG may lead to abnormal brain development, for example the cerebellar hypoplasia in brains of children with PMM2-CDG.

The turnover of serum glycoproteins, including the coagulation cascade, Antithrombin-III, Protein C, and Protein S, is also dependent on correct N-linked glycosylation. The hepatic asialoglycoprotein receptor binds liver derived serum glycoproteins without the proper sialic acid terminus. In CDG, incorrectly synthesized N-linked glycoproteins are inappropriately endocytosed by the liver endothelia lowering levels of circulating serum glycoproteins. This impacts both the pro- and anticoagulant serum proteins leading to low serum levels, an unpredictable balance between these functionally opposed groups of proteins, and the clinical risk of either inappropriate bleeding or clotting.

Glycoproteins are involved in virtually every endocrine axis. Protein glycosylation can affect the stability, binding affinity, and ligand specificity of peptide hormones, hormone carrier proteins, and hormone receptors. Many individuals with CDG have failure to thrive, hypoglycemia, osteopenia, and delayed or incomplete pubescence, implicating the functional importance of glycosylation on these hormones peptides and their receptors. It is, however, a complex story. For example, the glycosylation status of the follicle-stimulating hormone receptor has been shown to affect its production and may affect its ligand binding affinity. In contrast, the unglycosylated LG receptor has normal ligand binding and signal transduction activity.

O-Linked Disorders

Although N-linked glycosylation disorders have been in the limelight for about 20 years, more recently defects in a different set of oligosaccharide synthetic pathways, the O-linked glycan pathways, have emerged as the underlying pathologic mechanism for other groups of disorders with a fascinating spectrum of clinical issues. In O-linked glycosylation, the sugar chains (ranging from single monosaccharides to large polymers) are bound to the hydroxyl group of either serine or threonine in the recipient protein. Defects have been identified in the biosyntheses of several different types of O-linked glycosylation, including O-xylose, O-GalNAc, O-GlcNAc, O-fucose, and O-mannose. The biological roles of the O-linked chains are very diverse and often organ specific. Some occur on a broad range of proteins (e.g., O-GalNAc), whereas others seem confined to a small specific set of proteins (e.g., O-mannosylation of mainly α-dystroglycan[48]). The different disorders caused by mutations in these pathways are discussed below.

Clinical Disorders Resulting from Defective O-Linked Oligosaccharide Synthesis

O-Mannose Pathway Defects and Other Myopathic Glycosylation Disorders

α-Dystroglycansopathies

The description of POMGNT1 glycosyltransferase deficiency, as the underlying cause in muscle-eye-brain (MEB) disease, was the first identified defect in the synthesis of O-mannose glycan chains. This group of clinical disorders is now recognized as the α-dystroglycanopathies,[49]

TABLE 2.3 Clinical Findings Described in the Different Subtypes of Dystroglycan-Glycosylation Disorders

Disorder	Enzymatic Defect	Gene	OMIM	Brain anomalies	Seizures / Epilepsy	Hypotonia	Eye Anomalies or Retinitis	ID/DD	Myopathy	Cardiomyopathy	Visceral involvement	Hematological or Coagulopathy
MDDGA1-C1	O-mannosyltransferase	*POMT1*	A = 236670 B = 613155 C = 609308	√	√	√	√	√	√	√		
MDDGA2-C2	O-mannosyltransferase	*POMT2*	A = 613150 B = 613156 C = 613158	√	√	√	√	√	√	√		
MDDGA3-C3	GlcNAc transferase	*POMGnT1*	A = 253280 B = 613151 C = 613157	√	√	√	√	√	√			
MDDGA4-C4	Putative glycosyltransferase (Fukutin)	*FKTN*	A = 253800 B = 613152 C = 611588	√	√	√	√	√	√			
MDDGA5-C5	Putative glycosyltransferase (Fukutin related protein)	*FKRP*	A = 613153 B = 606612 C = 607155	√		√	√	√	√	√		
MDDGA6-B6	Combined xylosyl- and glucuronyltransferases	*LARGE*	A = 613154 B = 608840	√		√		√	√			
MDDGA7	Isoprenoid synthesis	*ISPD*	A = 614643	√		√	√	√	√	√		
MDDGA8	GlcNAc transferase	*GTDC2*	A = 614830	√		√	√		√			
MDDGA10	Putative glycosyltransferase	*TMEM5*	A = 615041	√		√	√		√			√
MDDGA11	GalNAc transferase	*B3GALNT2*	A = 615181	√	√	√	√	√	√			
MDDGA12	GalNac-GlcNac-Man-(6-P)-*O*-protein mannosyl kinase	*SGK196*	A = 615249	√		√	√	√	√			
MDDGA13	β1,3-GlcNAc transferase 1	*B3GNT1*	A = 615287	√	√	√	√	√	√		√	
MDDGA14-C14	GDP-Man Pyrophosphorylase B	*GMPPB*	A = 615350 B = 615351 C = 615352	√	√	√	√	√	√	√		
DOLK-CDG	Dolichol kinase	*DOLK*	A = 610768		√	√			√		√	√
DPM1-CDG	Dol-P-Man synthase subunit 1	*DPM1*	A = 608799	√	√	√			√	√		√
DPM2-CDG	Dol-P-Man synthase subunit 2	*DPM2*	A = 615042	√	√	√			√	√		√
DPM3-CDG	Dol-P-Man synthase subunit 3	*DPM3*	A = 612937						√	√	√	√

Note. MDDGA = muscular dystrophy/dystroglycanopathy—severe form (Walker Warburg syndrome, muscle-eye-brain disease, and Fukuyama congenital muscular dystrophy like phenotypes); MDDGB = muscular dystrophy/dystroglycanopathy—intermediate form; MDDGC = muscular dystrophy/dystroglycanopathy—mild form (limb-girdle muscular dystrophy like phenotype).

as the underlying pathology revolves around defective glycosylation of α-dystroglycan. The group presently contains 13 genetically different disorders as shown in Table 2.3. The clinical spectrum is wide, ranging from very severe (including Walker Warburg syndrome [WWS], MEB, and Fukuyama congenital muscular dystrophy [FCMD]) to milder forms of limb-girdle muscular dystrophy.[50] All show muscular involvement (muscular dystrophy), whereas the more severe forms also affect the eyes and the brain. Brain findings include abnormalities ranging from white-matter changes on MRIs to cerebellar hypoplasia or congenital brain malformations. Congenital eye anomalies are also seen ranging from glaucoma and myopia or cataracts to microphthalmia. Although each of these disorders has its own clinical picture, there is significant overlap of clinical findings, reminiscent of the shared underlying pathology. In fact, genetic testing shows that the clinical distinctions result more from the impact of the mutation on the gene function than the gene identity. The deficiencies can be recognized when muscle biopsies or immunoblots are probed with a glycan-directed monoclonal antibody. Like transferrin for N-glycan disorders, this is a key diagnostic tool.

The classification of the α-dystroglycanopathies is either based on the pure clinical phenotype (WWS, MEB, FCMD, etc.) or a combination of severity and genetic cause (as suggested by OMIM[51]). In this classification, an α-dystroglycanopathy is referred to as a muscular dystrophy-dystroglycanopathy (MDDG) and separated into three severity groups: A= severe (e.g., WWS, MEB, and FCMD); B = intermediate (e.g., MDC1D); C = mild (e.g., limb-girdle muscular dystrophy 2I), followed by a number indicating the defective gene (1 = POMT1, 2 = POMT2, 3 = POMGNT1, etc). A classical case of WWS is thus referred to as MDDGA1 or 2 and MEB is MDDGA3.

WWS (mainly MDDGA1-2) is most often caused by mutations in the *POMT1* or *POMT2* genes and is the most severe type of α-dystroglycanopathy. These genes encode the two subunits of the protein-O-mannosyltransferase, the enzyme that initiates the O-mannose glycan formation.[52] However, mutations in at least nine other glycosylation-related genes (*POMGNT1, FKTN, FKRP, LARGE, ISPD, GTDC2, SGK196, TMEM5, B3GNT1*) have been shown to be causative in patients with this disease,[53-56] underscoring the genetic heterogeneity of these syndromes. The pathogenesis involves abnormal neuronal migration, affecting the brain and eye, and results in brain lesions such as severe hydrocephalus, agenesis of the *corpus callosum*, agyria or cobblestone lissencephaly, and cerebellar hypoplasia. WWS progresses rapidly, and patients usually die within a year. They have severe muscular dystrophy without motor development and ophthalmopathies (congenital cataracts, micropthalmia, and buphthalmos).[57,58]

MEB (mainly MDDGA3) usually results from mutations in the gene *POMGNT1* encoding O-mannosyl-α-1,2-N-acetylglucosaminyltransferase; the enzyme catalyzes the second step in the synthesis of the *O*-mannose glycans. However, distinct mutations in many of the other α-dystroglycanopathy-related genes also can cause this disease. MEB is similar to WWS but is somewhat milder in its course. Patients have generalized muscle weakness from birth, intellectual disability, and eye conditions such as pallor of the optic discs, congenital myopia, and glaucoma. Multiple CNS malformations are known, including fronto-parietal pachygyria, polymicrogyria, and cerebellar hypoplasia. The disease progress is slow, and most patients survive into adulthood.[57]

Recently, exome sequencing has revealed several more genes that affect dystroglycan mannosylation, and, so far, defects in 10 more genes are known to cause an α-dystroglycanopathy (*FKTN, FTRP, LARGE, SGK196, TMEM5, GTDC2, ISPD, B3GNT1, B3GALNT2, GMPPB*[54,55,59-65]), some of which still possess unknown biochemical functions (*FKTN, FTRP*, and *TMEM5*). Nevertheless, all 10 defects impair synthesis of the O-mannose linked glycan on α-dystroglycan. Also, muscular dystrophy has been a leading symptom in patients where the defective gene is involved in the biosynthesis of dolichol monophosphate mannose (*DPM1, DPM2, DPM3*),[66-68] a step that is also crucial for N-linked glycosylation and GPI-anchor synthesis. These are examples of genes that affect multiple glycosylation steps and thus may cause a mixed symptomatology, different from that seen in "strict" α-dystroglycanopathies.

Other Myopathic Glycosylation Disorders

Hereditary inclusion body myopathy, caused by defects in *GNE*, lead to a progressive muscle weakness with onset in early adulthood. Typically the quadriceps appear to be spared even in the later stages of the disease. *GNE* encodes the bifunctional enzyme that catalyzes the first two committed steps in the biosynthesis of sialic acid, and abnormal glycosylation of α-dystroglycan has been shown in affected individuals. Mutations in GFAT1 (encoding glutamine-fructose-6P transaminase 1) causes an autosomal recessive congenital myasthenic syndrome characterized by limb-girdle pattern weakness with tubular aggregates in muscle biopsies.[69] The enzyme is rate-limiting in the hexosamine biosynthesis. The patients respond well to acetylcholine esterase inhibitors. Finally, mutations in additional genes that typically cause severe CDG-I phenotypes (DPAGT1, ALG2, ALG13) have also been found to cause myasthenic syndromes. The reason for this dramatic phenotypic distinction is unknown.

O-Fucose and O-GlcNAc Pathway Defects

O-fucosylation is a rare type of O-linked modification that can occur on proteins with either EGF-like or trombospondin type 1 repeats (TSR).[70] The most well-studied proteins carrying this modification are of the Notch family.[71,72]

One patient with autosomal recessive spondylocostal dysostosis type 3 was shown to carry functional mutations in *LFNG*, the human homolog of lunatic fringe. This gene encodes an enzyme that adds GlcNAc to O-fucose residues on EGF modules on Notch, a critical signaling molecule in many phases of development.[73] Patients with Peters Plus syndrome have prenatal growth delay, intellectual disability, short stature, brachymorphism, short limbs, and sometimes cleft palate.[74] This condition is caused by defects in a α-1,3-Glucosyltransferase (*B3GALTL*) that adds glucose to O-fucose glycans located in a TSR. Protein-O-fucosyltransferases (encoded by *POFUT1* and *POFUT2*) are specific for the EGF-like and TSR pathways, respectively. A deficiency in *POFUT1* was recently shown to cause the autosomal dominant dermatological condition Dowling-Degos disease 2.[75] Other defects in the O-fucosylation pathway are likely to follow.

O-GlcNAcylation, the addition of a single N-acetyl glucosamine to a protein, is a peculiar type of glycosylation that was long thought to occur on intracellular proteins only.[76] It influences the stability of a number of proteins and regulates their role in various mechanisms, including protein trafficking, intracellular signaling in response to environmental stimuli, such as nutrition and stress, and epigenetic and transcriptional regulation. All intracellular O-GlcNAcylations are catalyzed by a single enzyme, OGT, whereas another enzyme, OGA, counteracts its action. Recently, an ER-located OGT (EOGT) that adds O-GlcNAc on extracellular bound proteins was discovered.[77] A main target of this enzyme is the EGF-like repeats in the Notch receptor.

Deficiency in EOGT was recently shown to cause Adams-Oliver syndrome in three unrelated families. The syndrome is primarily characterized by *aplasia cutis congenita* and terminal transverse limb defects, but other defects have been described.[78]

O-Xylose Pathway Defects (Glycosaminoglycan Synthesis Defects)

Table 2.4 shows defects in glycosaminoglycans (heparin, heparan sulfate, chondroitin sulfate, dermatan sulfate, and keratan sulfate) biosynthesis. The glycosaminoglycans are attached to a defined group of specific core proteins through an O-β-xylose linkage to form proteoglycans. All these (except some keratan sulfate species) share a common core of GlcA-β1,3-Gal-β1,3-Gal-β1,4- added to xylose. Heparan sulfate is composed of repeating disaccharides GlcNAc-α1,4-GlcA-β1,4-, chondroitin sulfate and dermatan sulfate are composed of GalNAc-β1,4-GlcA-β1,3- repeats, and keratan sulfate has a lactosamine core. A host of polymer-specific sulfotransferases and epimerases converting GlcA to iduronic acid modify the chains during synthesis. A large number of disorders have been identified in synthesis and delivery of the substrates, synthesis of the core unit, chain polymerization, and sulfation.[79] Each of the disorders has unique presentations. As with other glycosylation disorders, the mutations tend to be hypomorphic rather than null.

Linkage Region Defects

Several defects in the synthesis of the common linkage region have been found in patients. Deficiency in the first reaction, formation of the xylose-O-protein stub (by xylosyltransferase), due to mutations in *XYLT1*, was found in two related consanguineous patients with short stature, characteristic facial features, alterations of fat distribution, and intellectual disability.[80] Mutations in the next step, addition of a β1,4-Gal (*B4GALT7*) causes an Ehlers-Danlos syndrome variant with progeriod features.[81,82] Further, the addition of the second Gal (encoded by *B3GALT6*) was deficient in a group of patients from three independent families with a pleiotropic Ehlers-Danlos-like syndrome including "skin fragility, delayed wound healing, joint hyperlaxity and contractures, muscle hypotonia, intellectual disability, and a spondyloepimetaphyseal dysplasia with bone fragility and severe kyphoscoliosis."[83] The last step of the linkage region synthesis, addition of a β1,3-linked GlcA, which is catalyzed by a gluconyltransferase (encoded by *B3GAT3*), was deficient in patients with a Larsen-like syndrome.[8] These patients exhibited a phenotype including joint dislocations and congenital heart defects, (bicuspid aortic valve and aortic root dilatation).

TABLE 2.4 Clinical Findings Described in the Different Subtypes of Glycosaminoglycan Biosynthesis Disorders

Disorder	Enzymatic Defect	Gene	OMIM	ID/DD	Seizures / Epilepsy	Hypotonia	Eye Anomalies or Retinitis	Skeletal Defects	Connective Tissue or Ichthyosis	Hematological or Coagulopathy	Myopathy	Endocrine	Cardiac Involvement
Autosomal recessive short stature with moderate intellectual disability	Xylosyltransferase 1	XYLT1	N/A	√				√				√	
Progeroid EDS	Xylosylprotein β-1,4- galactosyltransferase	B4GALT7	130070 604327	√	√			√					√
Progeroid EDS/ Spondyloepimetaphyseal dysplasia with joint laxity	Galactosyltransferase 2	B3GALT6	615349 271640	√	√			√	√				√
Recessive joint dislocations and congenital heart defects	Glucuronyltransferase 1	B3GAT3	245600					√	√				√
Multiple hereditary exostoses	Heparan sulfate co-polymerase	EXT1, EXT2	133700 133701					√					
Idiopathic hypogonadotropic hypogonadism (Kallmann syndrome)	HS 6-O-sulfotransferase 1	HS6ST1	614880									√	
Spondyloepimetaphyseal dysplasia (Omani Type)	Chondroitin sulfate 6-sulfotransferase	CHST3	143095					√					√
Adducted thumb-clubfoot syndrome/ Musculocontractural EDS type I	N-acetylgalactosamine 4-O-sulfotransferase 1	CHST14	601776	√	√	√	√	√	√				√
Musculocontractural EDS type II	Dermatan sulfate epimerase-1	DSE	615539	√	√	√	√						√
Schneckenbecken dysplasia	UDP-GlcA / UDP-GalNAc Golgi Transporter	SLC35D1	610804					√					
Peeling skin syndrome	GalNAc-4-O-sulfatotransferase	CHST8	N/A						√				
Diastrophic dysplasia achondrogenesis	Anion (sulfate) transporter	DTDST	606718 600972					√					
Spondyloepimetaphyseal dysplasia	3′-phosphoadenosine-5′-phosphosulphate synthase	ATPSK2	603005					√					
Macular corneal dystrophy I	GlcNAc 6-O-sulfotransferase	CHST6	217800				√						

Note. EDS = Ehlers-Danlos syndrome.

Heparan Sulfate Defects

One of the few autosomal dominant disorders in a glycobiologic synthetic pathway, hereditary multiple exostoses is caused by mutations in *EXT1/EXT2*, the heparan sulfate co-polymerase. Patients have recurrent, painful osteochondromas typically at the end of long bones that must be surgically removed. Histology of the growth plate shows a characteristic disorganization in these patients. The osteochondroma develop due to loss of heterozygosity in the *EXT* genes and the outgrowths contain a substantial population of cells with only a single mutated gene.[85,86] The patients are at increased risk to develop osteosarcomas.[87] Further, mutations in HS6ST1, encoding a heparan sulfate 6-O-sulfotransferase, affect the formation of the olfactory nerve and the associated GnRH-releasing neurons, which leads to a variant of Kallmann syndrome.[88]

Chondroitin Sulfate/Dermatan Sulfate Defects

Spondylo-epimetaphyseal dysplasia results from mutations in chondroitin sulfate specific 6-O-sulfotransferase (encoded by *CHST3*) with clinical manifestations of short stature, progressive kyphoscoliosis, and arthritic changes with joint dislocations.[89] Mutations in *CHST8*, encoding a GalNAc 4-O-sulfotransferase that among others transfer sulfate groups to chondroitin sulfate (and also N-linked oligosaccharides), cause a variant of peeling skin syndrome.[90] Ehlers-Danlos syndrome (type VIB), also called adducted thumb-clubfoot syndrome, is caused by a defect in the GalNAc-4-sulfotransferase I coded for by the gene *CHST14*.[91] In addition, patients have facial clefting, coagulopathy with thin translucent skin along with intestinal, kidney, and heart defects. Further, a deficiency in the gene for dermatan sulfate epimerase, the protein responsible for the formation of iduronic acid from glucuronic acid in the dermatan sulfate chain, causes a musculocontractural Ehlers-Danlos-like phenotype.[92] In Schneckenbecken dysplasia, mutations in the UDP-GlcA/UDP-GalNAc Golgi transporter (*SLC35D1*) limits the amount of substrates available for chondroitin sulfate synthesis. These patients have multiple skeletal abnormalities, including bell-shaped thorax, metaphyseal flaring, and narrowing of the interpediculate distance along with severe delay of vertebral body ossification. Gene-deficient mouse models show the gene is critical for prenatal skeletal development.[93]

Miscellaneous

A series of allelic chondrodysplasias result from mutations in the diastrophic dysplasia sulfate transporter and from mutations of phosphoadenosine 5-prime-phosphosulfate synthase (*ATPSK2*), the synthase of the proximate activated sulfate donor.[94] Deficiency in *CHST6*, encoding a GlcNAc 6-O-sulfotransferase that adds a 6-O-sulfate to keratan sulfate, causes macular corneal dystrophy.[95]

Defects in GPI Anchor Synthesis and Glycosphingolipid Synthesis

GPI-Anchor Synthesis Deficiencies

GPI-anchors are a group of glycolipids that link many plasma membrane proteins to the cell surface in place of a transmembrane domain.[96] Mutations in eight genes in GPI-anchor synthesis have been shown to affect the multistep pathway in which GlcNAc, several mannose units, and phosphoethanolamine are added step-wise to phosphatidylinositol to build a precursor, which is transferred to proteins following their synthesis in the ER.[97–105]

PIGA encodes a GlcNAc transferase and is the first step in the GPI pathway. Somatic mutations in *PIGA* in hematopoietic precursors cause acquired paroxysmal nocturnal hemoglobinuria with partial or complete loss of GPI-linked membrane proteins. The cells carrying the mutation overtake the unaffected populations and cause intravascular hemolysis.[97] Interestingly, germline mutations in the same gene can give rise to several different presentations: the X-linked multiple congenital anomalies-hypotonia-seizures syndrome 2, a disorder with dysmorphic features, hypotonia, myoclonic seizures, and variable congenital anomalies[102]; a neurodegenerative epileptic encephalopathy with systemic iron overload[106]; and accelerated linear growth, elevated alkaline phosphatase, and progressive CNS abnormalities.[107] Other multiple congenital anomalies-hypotonia-seizures syndromes (1 and 3) are caused by mutations in *PIGN*[100] and *PIGT*,[104] respectively. *PIGN* encodes GPI ethanolamine phosphate transferase-1 whereas *PIGT* encodes GPI transamidase. These two disorders are, in contrast to multiple congenital anomalies-hypotonia-seizures syndrome 2, inherited in an autosomal recessive mode.

Mutations in *PIGM*, which codes for the first mannosyltransferase in GPI-anchor synthesis, led to venous thrombosis and seizures in affected individuals.[98] In lymphoblasts from a PIGM patient with the mutation confined to the promoter region of the gene, treatment with sodium butyrate corrected *PIGM* transcription and cell surface GPI expression. Further, two weeks of providing sodium phenylbutyrate, a histone deacetylase inhibitor, eliminated seizures, and improved motor skills in affected individuals.[108]

PIGV encodes the second mannosyltransferase in GPI anchors. Mutations in this gene cause hyperphosphatasia and intellectual impairment and is also known as Mabry syndrome. These patients show a large increase in plasma alkaline phosphatase, a GPI-anchored protein, along with unusual facial features, variable seizures, and muscular hypotonia.[99,109] As expected, patients' leukocytes had reduced surface expression of GPI-anchored proteins. Three other genes involved in the GPI anchor synthesis have recently been implicated in hyperphosphatasia: intellectual impairment (*PIGO*[103] and *PGAP2*[105]) and West's syndrome (*PIGW*[110]). *PIGO* encodes PGI ethanolamine phosphate transferase, and *PGAP2* and PIGW code for proteins involved in is involved in fatty-acid GPI-anchor remodeling.

CHIME syndrome (colobomas, heart defects, ichthyosiform dermatosis, mental retardation, and ear anomalies) is an ultra-rare condition caused by mutations in *PIGL*.[101] *PIGL* encodes for the GlcNAc-phosphoinositol-de-N-acetylase that precedes flipping the growing GPI-anchor precursor form the cytosolic to the luminal side of ER.

It is very likely that additional disorders of GPI anchor synthesis will be found, but clearly the phenotypic spectrum will be quite broad based on the examples seen to date. Levels of CD59 and CD55, known as the decay accelerating factor, are two members of the complement system that may be good markers to search for GPI-anchor deficiencies.

TABLE 2.5 Clinical Findings Described in the Different Subtypes of GPI-Anchor Biosynthesis Disorders or Other Miscellaneous Glycosylation Disorders

GPI-Anchor and Other Miscellaneous Glycosylation Disorders				Clinical Spectrum										
Disorder	Enzymatic Defect	Gene	OMIM	ID/DD	Seizures / Epilepsy	Hypotonia	Eye involvement	Skeletal Defects	Connective Tissue or skin	Hematological or Coagulopathy	Intestine or urinary tract malforma	Elevated alkaline phosphatase	Cardiac Involvement	Visceral involvement
NPH/X-linked multiple congenital anomalies-hypotonia-seizures syndrome 2	Subunit of GPI GlcNAc transferase	PIGA	300818 300868	√	√	√		√		√	√	√	√	√
X-linked multiple congenital anomalies-hypotonia-seizures syndrome 1	GPI ethanolamine phosphate transferase-1	PIGN	614080	√	√	√	√						√	√
X-linked multiple congenital anomalies-hypotonia-seizures syndrome 3	GPI transamidase	PIGT	615398	√	√	√	√						√	√
Inherited GPI deficiency	GPI mannosyltransferase 1	PIGM	610293	√						√				
Hyperphosphasia with mental retardation syndrome 1	GPI mannosyltransferase 2	PIGV	239300	√	√	√		√	√			√	√	
Hyperphosphasia with mental retardation syndrome 2	GPI ethanolamine-P transferase	PIGO	614730	√	√			√	√			√	√	√
Hyperphosphasia with mental retardation syndrome 3	GPI anchor modification	PGAP2	614207	√	√	√						√	√	√
CHIME syndrome	GPI GlcNAc-phosphoinositol-de-N-acetylase	PIGL	280000	√	√		√		√				√	
Hyperphosphasia with mental retardation and West's syndrome	GPI anchor modification	PIGW	N/A	√	√			√				√		
Amish infantile epilepsy syndrome	GM3 synthase (sialyltransferase-9)	SIAT9	609056	√	√		√	√						√
Spastic paraplegia 26	GM2/GD2 synthase	B4GALNT1	609195	√	√									
Hyperphosphatemic familial tumoral calcinosis	UDP-GalNAc transferase	GALNT3	211900						√	√	√			
Spondylocostal dysostosis AR 3	Fucose-specific β-1,3-GlcNAc transferase	LFNG	609813					√						
Peter's Plus syndrome	β-1,3-glucosyltransferase	B3GALTL	261540	√				√						
Dowling-Degos disease 2	Protein-O-fucosyltransferase 1	POFUT1	607491						√					

Note. GPI = glycosylphosphatidylinositol.

Glycosphingolipid Synthesis Defects

Only two defects are known in glycosphingolipid synthesis in contrast to their catabolic counterparts (glycosphingolipid hydrolases), whose deficiencies constitute a large part of the lysosomal disorders. Children with Amish infantile epilepsy have developmental delay, seizures, and blindness, which has been shown to be caused by nonsense mutations in *SIAT9*, a sialyltransferase that makes ganglioside GM3 (Siaα2,3Galβ1,4Glc-ceramide) from lactosylceramide (Galβ1,4Glc-ceramide). Patients accumulate nonsialylated plasma glycosphingolipids, which are GM3 precursors.[111] It was recently shown that mutations in the same gene can cause "salt and pepper syndrome" in which patients display dysmorphic facial features, severe intellectual disability, choreoathetosis, epilepsy, scoliosis, and altered dermal pigmentation.[112] Mutations in the GM2/GD2 synthase (encoded by *B4GALNT1*) cause an autosomal recessive form of spastic paraplegia with lower limb spasticity, hyperreflexia, muscle weakness, and mild to moderate intellectual disability.[113] The onset of the disease is in the first or second decade of life.

Defects in Mucin Type Glycosylation

Hyperphosphatemic familial tumoral calcinosis results in calcium deposits in the periarticular spaces, soft tissues, and sometimes bone as well as hyperphosphatemia (Table 2.5). *GALNT3* is mutated in hyperphosphatemic familial tumoral calcinosis and encodes a UDP-GalNAc transferase that adds GalNAc to initiate a mucin type O-glycosylation to a serine or threonine. Over 20 genes encode homologous enzymes, but *GALNT3* has specificity not typical of other family members. One of these is a growth factor, FGF23, and when it is not O-glycosylated, is nonfunctional.[114]

Defects in Multiple Glycosylation Pathways

Defects in substrate synthesis and delivery can affect several different pathways. Good examples are the transporters that carry activated nucleotide sugars into the Golgi. The pathways affected depend on the glycosylation burden of the cells. A chondrocyte needs to make large amounts of chondroitin sulfate. Defects that could impact several pathways will be more easily seen in those pathways with the highest demand. Of particular interest is a recent group of ER and Golgi trafficking proteins that insure proper distribution and recycling of the glycosylation machinery within the cell. Notable among this trafficking system are six of eight proteins that comprise the COG complex. It is thought to act as a tether for guiding one set of vesicles containing Golgi enzymes to the right place so it can then fuse with the receiving membrane. A series of other proteins called Golgins and SEC proteins also have roles in trafficking. Defects in these members of the COG complex have been seen in individuals that present with hypotonia and failure to thrive.[115]

Therapy and Model Systems

There are only four CDGs with known treatment options despite much work directed toward therapeutic options. These include MPI-CDG, SLC35C1-CDG, PGM1-CDG, and PIGM-CDG. Treatment of MPI-CDG with oral mannose has been ongoing for many years in some affected individuals.[38] The therapeutic rationale is that hexokinases phosphorylate mannose to mannose 6-phosphate bypass the defect and provide sufficient substrate to synthesize GDP-mannose. Some individuals with SLC35C1-CDG, a GDP-fucose transporter deficiency show some immune response when given oral fucose. Galactose was recently shown to improve the clinical course in PGM1-CDG. Butyrate, a deacetylase inhibitor, has been given to increase *PIGM* transcription and decrease seizure activity in a small number of patients.

A few of the usual model systems, such as mice, fish, flies, and worms, are becoming available to study these disorders.[116–120] Unfortunately, knocking out single genes in mice for essential glycosylation pathways are frequently an embryonic lethal. An alternative is to knock in corresponding patient mutations in mice. These studies are in progress for both PMM2-CDG and MPI-CDG.

Final Thoughts

When looking for new glycosylation disorders, what should you look for? This is probably the most challenging question. Scores of papers conclude that transferrin glycosylation testing should be done on any individual with an unexplained multisystemic disorder. How often will these results be abnormal? Current data show that transferrin testing is abnormal 1% to 3% of the time, which equals or exceeds the frequency of the most commonly tested metabolic disorders. This fact alone should convince clinicians to order transferrin glycosylation analysis early in their diagnostic testing, especially for infants and children.

However, abnormal transferrin analysis does not indicate the defective gene and must be combined with whole exome or full genome sequencing to improve the odds of identifying the defective gene. Whole genome sequencing is likely to revolutionize diagnosis of rare disorders. Ever-expanding databases, falling costs, and improved bioinformatics will contribute to refining the candidate genes. Insertions, deletions, and substitutions that generate premature stop signals and highly deleterious mutations will likely be helpful in narrowing the candidates. In many instances, they will remain candidates unless and until appropriate functional assays are developed that confirm the mutations' functional impact. It will be vital for the glycobiology community to provide appropriate assays for the potential glycosylation deficiencies. Clinicians will need to work closely with basic scientists since many of these genes are not likely to have convenient, simple enzymatic assays for their products.

Once the defective genes are identified, whether familiar or novel, what are the therapeutic options? In a few types, such as MPI-CDG, SLC35C1-CDG, and PGM1-CDG, dietary supplements of simple sugars proved effective. This simple approach is unlikely to be useful for other types, and there is no rationale for their use at this time. It is important to caution that mannose may actually have negative side effects if used indiscriminately.

Another option for therapy is to identify small molecules that stabilize a misfolded or unstable protein to acquire a more stable and active conformation. This approach is now being developed for the common mutation (ΔF508) of the cystic fibrosis transmembrane conductance regulator. Identifying suitable stabilizers requires a robust marker for high throughput assays, and it may only stabilize selected hypomorphic mutations. Each mutation may require a different stabilizing molecule. This is important if model organisms are used as therapeutic assays; simple knockdown of the normal gene product would not be useful for most hypomorphic mutations.

Better patient care demands more extensive interactions between scientists and clinicians. These relationships will be vital to link mechanisms and therapeutics. The increasingly web-wise and determined family advocacy groups are a click away from our laboratories, offices, and clinics. They expect a high level of collaboration and will watch to make sure that we do so.

Acknowledgments

We thank Bobby Ng for his help in compiling the tables and to the families of the patients with these disorders for their long-term collaboration with us, especially the CDG Family Network Foundation and more recently CDG United on Facebook. This work is supported by The Rocket Fund and R01DK55615 (HHF) and ALF (EAE).

References

1. Van Schaftingen E, Jaeken J. Phosphomannomutase deficiency is a cause of carbohydrate-deficient glycoprotein syndrome type I, *FEBS Lett*. 1995; 377: 318–320.
2. Freeze HH. Genetic defects in the human glycome. *Nat Rev Genet*. 2006; 7: 537–551.
3. Jaeken J, Hennet T, Matthijs G, Freeze HH. CDG nomenclature: time for a change! *Biochim Biophys Acta*. 2009; 1792: 825–826.
4. Grunewald S. The clinical spectrum of phosphomannomutase 2 deficiency (CDG-Ia). *Biochim Biophys Acta*. 2009; 1792: 827–834.
5. Truin G, Guillard M, Lefeber DJ, et al. Pericardial and abdominal fluid accumulation in congenital disorder of glycosylation type Ia. *Mol Genet Metab*. 2008; 94: 481–484.
6. van de Kamp JM, Lefeber DJ, Ruijter GJ, et al. Congenital disorder of glycosylation type Ia presenting with hydrops fetalis. *J Med Genet*. 2007; 44: 277–280.
7. Coman D, McGill J, MacDonald R, Morris D, Klingberg S, Jaeken J, Appleton D. Congenital disorder of glycosylation type 1a: three siblings with a mild neurological phenotype, *J Clin Neurosci*. 2007; 14: 668–672.
8. Miossec-Chauvet E, Mikaeloff Y, Heron D, et al. Neurological presentation in pediatric patients with congenital disorders of glycosylation type Ia, *Neuropediatrics*. 2003; 34: 1–6.
9. Pancho C, Garcia-Cazorla A, Varea V, et al. Congenital disorder of glycosylation type Ia revealed by hypertransaminasemia and failure to thrive in a young boy with normal neurodevelopment. *J Pediatr Gastroenterol Nutr*. 2005; 40: 230–232.
10. Damen G, de Klerk H, Huijmans J, den Hollander J, Sinaasappel M. Gastrointestinal and other clinical manifestations in 17 children with congenital disorders of glycosylation type Ia, Ib, and Ic. *J Pediatr Gastroenterol Nutr*. 2004; 38: 282–287.
11. Hertz-Pannier L, Dechaux M, Sinico M, et al. Congenital disorders of glycosylation type I: a rare but new cause of hyperechoic kidneys in infants and children due to early microcystic changes, *Pediatr Radiol*. 2006; 36: 108–114.
12. Footitt EJ, Karimova A, Burch M, et al. Cardiomyopathy in the congenital disorders of glycosylation (CDG): a case of late presentation and literature review. *J Inherit Metab Dis*. 2009; 32(Suppl. 1): S313–S319.
13. Jensen H, Kjaergaard S, Klie F, Moller HU. Ophthalmic manifestations of congenital disorder of glycosylation type 1a. *Ophthalmic Genet*. 2003; 24: 81–88.
14. Coman D, Bostock D, Hunter M, et al. Primary skeletal dysplasia as a major manifesting feature in an infant with congenital disorder of glycosylation type Ia. *Am J Med Genet A*. 2008; 146: 389–392.

15. Miller BS, Freeze, HH. New disorders in carbohydrate metabolism: congenital disorders of glycosylation and their impact on the endocrine system. *Rev Endocr Metab Disord*. 2003; 4: 103–113.
16. Bohles, H, Sewell AA, Gebhardt B, Reinecke-Luthge A, Kloppel G, Marquardt T. Hyperinsulinaemic hypoglycaemia—leading symptom in a patient with congenital disorder of glycosylation Ia (phosphomannomutase deficiency). *J Inherit Metab Dis*. 2001; 24: 858–862.
17. Krasnewich D, O'Brien K, Sparks S. Clinical features in adults with congenital disorders of glycosylation type Ia (CDG-Ia). *Am J Med Genet C, Semin Med Genet*. 2007; 145C: 302–306.
18. Stibler H, Blennow G, Kristiansson B, Lindehammer H, Hagberg B. Carbohydrate-deficient glycoprotein syndrome: clinical expression in adults with a new metabolic disease. *J Neurol Neurosurg Psychiatry*. 1994; 57: 552–556.
19. Jaeken J. Congenital disorders of glycosylation. *Ann NY Acad Sci*. 2010; 1214: 190–198.
20. Chantret I, Dupre T, Delenda C, et al. Congenital disorders of glycosylation type Ig is defined by a deficiency in dolichyl-P-mannose:Man7GlcNAc2-PP-dolichyl mannosyltransferase. *J Biol Chem*. 2002; 277: 25815–25822.
21. Schollen E, Frank CG, Keldermans L, et al. Clinical and molecular features of three patients with congenital disorders of glycosylation type Ih (CDG-Ih) (ALG8 deficiency), *J Med Genet*. 2004; 41: 550–556.
22. Eklund EA, Sun L, Westphal V, Northrop JL, Freeze HH, Scaglia F. Congenital disorder of glycosylation (CDG)-Ih patient with a severe hepato-intestinal phenotype and evolving central nervous system pathology. *J Pediatr*. 2005; 147: 847–850.
23. Morava E, Wevers RA, Cantagrel V, et al. A novel cerebello-ocular syndrome with abnormal glycosylation due to abnormalities in dolichol metabolism. *Brain*. 2010; 133: 3210–3220.
24. Jaeken J, Imbach T, Schenk B, Smeets E, Carchon H. A newly recognized glycosylation defect with psychomotor retardation, ichthyosis and dwarfism. *J. Inherit. Metab. Dis*. 2000; 23 (Suppl.1): 186.
25. Kranz C, Denecke J, Lehrman MA, et al. A mutation in the human MPDU1 gene causes congenital disorder of glycosylation type If (CDG-If). *J Clin Invest*. 2001; 108: 1613–1619.
26. Kranz C, Jungeblut C, Denecke J, et al. A defect in dolichol phosphate biosynthesis causes a new inherited disorder with death in early infancy. *Am J Hum Genet*. 2007; 80: 433–440.
27. Kranz C, Denecke J, Lehrman M, et al. A mutation in the human MPDU1 gene causes congenital disorder of glycosylation type If (CDG-If). *J Clin Invest*. 2001; 108:1613–1619.
28. Kranz C, Sun L, Eklund EA, Krasnewich D, Casey JR, Freeze HH. CDG-Id in two siblings with partially different phenotypes. *Am J Med* Genet A. 2007; 143A: 1414–1420.
29. Thiel C, Schwarz M, Peng J, et al. A new type of congenital disorders of glycosylation (CDG-Ii) provides new insights into the early steps of dolichol-linked oligosaccharide biosynthesis. *J Biol Chem*. 2003; 278: 22498–22505.
30. Cantagrel V, Lefeber DJ, Ng BG, et al. SRD5A3 is required for converting polyprenol to dolichol and is mutated in a congenital glycosylation disorder, Cell, 142 203–217.
31. Morava E, Wevers RA, Cantagrel V, et al. A novel cerebello-ocular syndrome with abnormal glycosylation due to abnormalities in dolichol metabolism. *Brain*. 2010; 133: 3210–3220.
32. Eklund EA, Newell JW, Sun L, et al. Molecular and clinical description of the first US patients with congenital disorder of glycosylation Ig. *Mol Genet Metab*. 2005; 84: 25–31.
33. Reynders E, Foulquier F, Leao Teles E, et al. Golgi function and dysfunction in the first COG4-deficient CDG type II patient. *Hum Mol Genet*. 2009; 18: 3244–3256.
34. Etzioni A, Sturla L, Antonellis A, et al. Leukocyte adhesion deficiency (LAD) type II/carbohydrate deficient glycoprotein (CDG) IIc founder effect and genotype/phenotype correlation. *Am J Med Genet*. 2002; 110: 131–135.
35. Lubke T, Marquardt T, Etzioni A, Hartmann E, von Figura K, Korner C. Complementation cloning identifies CDG-IIc, a new type of congenital disorders of glycosylation, as a GDP-fucose transporter deficiency. *Nat Genet*. 2001; 28: 73–76.
36. Martinez-Duncker I, Dupre T, Piller V, et al. Genetic complementation reveals a novel human congenital disorder of glycosylation of type II, due to inactivation of the Golgi CMP-sialic acid transporter. *Blood*. 2005; 105: 2671–2676.
37. Zuchner S, Dallman J, Wen R, et al. Whole-exome sequencing links a variant in DHDDS to retinitis pigmentosa. *Am J Hum Genet*. 2011; 88: 201–206.
38. de Lonlay P, Seta N. The clinical spectrum of phosphomannose isomerase deficiency, with an evaluation of mannose treatment for CDG-Ib. *Biochim Biophys Acta*. 2009; 1792: 841–843.

39. Thiel C, Messner-Schmitt D, Hoffmann GF, Korner C. Screening for congenital disorders of glycosylation in the first weeks of life. *J Inherit Metab Dis.* 2013; 36: 887–892.
40. Mandato C, Brive L, Miura Y, et al. Cryptogenic liver disease in four children: a novel congenital disorder of glycosylation. *Pediatr Res.* 2006; 59: 293–298.
41. Kranz C, Denecke J, Lehle L, et al. Congenital disorder of glycosylation type Ik (CDG-Ik): a defect of mannosyltransferase I. *Am J Hum Genet.* 2004; 74: 545–551.
42. Wopereis S, Grunewald S, Morava E, et al. Apolipoprotein C-III isofocusing in the diagnosis of genetic defects in O-glycan biosynthesis. *Clin Chem.* 2003; 49: 1839–1845.
43. Faid V, Chirat F, Seta N, Foulquier F, Morelle W. A rapid mass spectrometric strategy for the characterization of N- and O-glycan chains in the diagnosis of defects in glycan biosynthesis. *Proteomics.* 2007; 7: 1800–1813.
44. Sturiale L, Barone R, Garozzo D. The impact of mass spectrometry in the diagnosis of congenital disorders of glycosylation. *J Inherit Metab Dis.* 2011; 34: 891–899.
45. Guillard M, Morava E, van Delft FL, et al. Plasma N-glycan profiling by mass spectrometry for congenital disorders of glycosylation type II. *Clin Chem.* 2011; 57: 593–602.
46. Kollmann K, Pohl S, Marschner S, et al. Mannose phosphorylation in health and disease. *Eur J Cell Biol.* 2010; 89: 117–123.
47. Hanisch G, Breloy I. Protein-specific glycosylation: signal patches and cis-controlling peptidic elements. *Biol Chem.* 2009; 390: 619–626.
48. Wells, L. The O-mannosylation pathway: glycosyltransferases and proteins implicated in congenital muscular dystrophy. *J Biol Chem.* 2013; 288: 6930–6935.
49. Muntoni F, Voit T. The congenital muscular dystrophies in 2004: a century of exciting progress. *Neuromuscul Disord.* 2004; 14: 635–649.
50. Godfrey C, Foley AR, Clement E, Muntoni F. Dystroglycanopathies: coming into focus. *Curr Opin Genet Dev.* 2011; 21: 278–285.
51. Amberger J, Bocchini C, Hamosh A. A new face and new challenges for Online Mendelian Inheritance in Man (OMIM(R)). *Hum Mutat.* 2011; 32: 564–567.
52. Akasaka-Manya K, Manya H, Nakajima A, Kawakita M, Endo T. Physical and functional association of human protein O-mannosyltransferases 1 and 2. *J Biol Chem.* 2006; 281: 19339–19345.
53. van Reeuwijk J, Grewal PK, Salih MA, et al. Intragenic deletion in the LARGE gene causes Walker-Warburg syndrome. *Hum Genet.* 2007; 121: 685–690.
54. de Bernabe DB, van Bokhoven H, van Beusekom E, et al. A homozygous nonsense mutation in the fukutin gene causes a Walker-Warburg syndrome phenotype. *J Med Genet.* 2003; 40: 845–848.
55. Beltran-Valero de Bernabe D, Voit T, Longman C, et al. Mutations in the FKRP gene can cause muscle-eye-brain disease and Walker-Warburg syndrome. *J Med Genet.* 2004; 41: e61.
56. Yoshida-Moriguchi T, Willer T, Anderson ME, et al. SGK196 is a glycosylation-specific O-mannose kinase required for dystroglycan function. *Science.* 2013; 341: 896–899.
57. Clement E, Mercuri E, Godfrey C, et al. Brain involvement in muscular dystrophies with defective dystroglycan glycosylation. *Ann Neurol.* 2008; 64: 573–582.
58. Hewitt JE. Abnormal glycosylation of dystroglycan in human genetic disease. *Biochim Biophys Acta.* 2009; 1792: 853–861.
59. Jae LT, Raaben M, Riemersma M, et al. Deciphering the glycosylome of dystroglycanopathies using haploid screens for lassa virus entry. *Science.* 2013; 340: 479–483.
60. Stevens E, Carss KL, Cirak S, et al. Mutations in B3GALNT2 cause congenital muscular dystrophy and hypoglycosylation of alpha-dystroglycan. *Am J Hum Genet.* 2013; 92: 354–365.
61. Manzini MC, Tambunan DE, Hill RS, et al. Exome sequencing and functional validation in zebrafish identify GTDC2 mutations as a cause of Walker-Warburg syndrome. *Am J Hum Genet.* 2012; 91: 541–547.
62. Willer T, Lee H, Lommel M, et al. ISPD loss-of-function mutations disrupt dystroglycan O-mannosylation and cause Walker-Warburg syndrome. *Nat Genet.* 2012; 44: 575–580.
63. Roscioli T, Kamsteeg EJ, Buysse K, et al. Mutations in ISPD cause Walker-Warburg syndrome and defective glycosylation of alpha-dystroglycan *Nat Genet.* 2012; 44: 581–585.
64. Buysse K, Riemersma M, Powell G. et al. Missense mutations in beta-1,3-N-acetylglucosaminyltransferase 1 (B3GNT1) cause Walker-Warburg syndrome. *Hum Mol Genet* 2013; 22: 1746–1754.
65. Carss KJ, Stevens E, Foley AR, et al. Mutations in GDP-mannose pyrophosphorylase B cause congenital and limb-girdle muscular dystrophies associated with hypoglycosylation of alpha-dystroglycan. *Am J Hum Genet.* 2013; 93: 29–41.

66. Yang AC, Ng BG, Moore SA, et al. Congenital disorder of glycosylation due to DPM1 mutations presenting with dystroglycanopathy-type congenital muscular dystrophy. *Mol Genet Metab* 2013; 110: 345–351.
67. Barone R, Aiello C, Race V, et al. DPM2-CDG: a muscular dystrophy-dystroglycanopathy syndrome with severe epilepsy. *Ann Neurol*. 2012; 72: 550–558.
68. Lefeber DJ, Schonberger J, Morava E, et al. Deficiency of Dol-P-Man synthase subunit DPM3 bridges the congenital disorders of glycosylation with the dystroglycanopathies. *Am J Hum Genet*. 2009; 85: 76–86.
69. Senderek J, Muller JS, Dusl M, et al. Hexosamine biosynthetic pathway mutations cause neuromuscular transmission defect. *Am J Hum Genet*. 2011; 88: 162–172.
70. Chen CI, Keusch JJ, Klein D, Hess D, Hofsteenge J, Gut H. Structure of human POFUT2: insights into thrombospondin type 1 repeat fold and O-fucosylation. *EMBO J*. 2012; 31: 3183–3197.
71. Guruharsha KG, Kankel MW, Artavanis-Tsakonas S. The Notch signalling system: recent insights into the complexity of a conserved pathway. *Nat Rev Genet*. 2012; 13: 654–666.
72. Haines N, Irvine KD. Glycosylation regulates Notch signalling. *Nat Rev Mol Cell Biol*. 2003; 4:786–797.
73. Sparrow DB, Chapman G, Wouters MA, et al. Mutation of the LUNATIC FRINGE gene in humans causes spondylocostal dysostosis with a severe vertebral phenotype. *Am J Hum Genet*. 2006; 78: 28–37.
74. Hess D, Keusch JJ, Oberstein SA, Hennekam RC, Hofsteenge J. Peters Plus syndrome is a new congenital disorder of glycosylation and involves defective Omicron-glycosylation of thrombospondin type 1 repeats. *J Biol Chem*. 2008; 283: 7354–7360.
75. Li M, Cheng R, Liang J, et al. Mutations in POFUT1, encoding protein O-fucosyltransferase 1, cause generalized Dowling-Degos disease. *Am J Hum Genet*. 2013; 92: 895–903.
76. Hanover JA, Krause MW, Love DC. The hexosamine signaling pathway: O-GlcNAc cycling in feast or famine. *Biochim Biophys Acta*. 2010; 1800: 80–95.
77. Sakaidani Y, Ichiyanagi N, Saito C, et al. O-linked-N-acetylglucosamine modification of mammalian Notch receptors by an atypical O-GlcNAc transferase Eogt1. *Biochem Biophys Res Commun*. 2012; 419: 14–19.
78. Shaheen R, Aglan M, Keppler-Noreuil K, et al. Mutations in EOGT confirm the genetic heterogeneity of autosomal-recessive Adams-Oliver syndrome. *Am J Hum Genet*. 2013; 92: 598–604.
79. Mizumoto S, Ikegawa S, Sugahara K. Human genetic disorders caused by mutations in genes encoding biosynthetic enzymes for sulfated glycosaminoglycans. *J Biol Chem*. 2013; 288: 10953–10961.
80. Schreml J, Durmaz B, Cogulu O, et al. The missing "link": an autosomal recessive short stature syndrome caused by a hypofunctional XYLT1 mutation. *Hum Genet*. 2014; 133: 29–39.
81. Quentin E, Gladen A, Roden L, Kresse H. A genetic defect in the biosynthesis of dermatan sulfate proteoglycan: galactosyltransferase I deficiency in fibroblasts from a patient with a progeroid syndrome. *Proc Natl Acad Sci USA*. 1990; 87: 1342–1346.
82. Faiyaz-Ul-Haque M, Zaidi SH, Al-Ali M, et al. A novel missense mutation in the galactosyltransferase-I (B4GALT7) gene in a family exhibiting facioskeletal anomalies and Ehlers-Danlos syndrome resembling the progeroid type. *Am J Med* Genet A. 2004; 128A: 39–45.
83. Malfait F, Kariminejad A, Van Damme T, et al. Defective initiation of glycosaminoglycan synthesis due to B3GALT6 mutations causes a pleiotropic Ehlers-Danlos syndrome-like connective tissue disorder. *Am J Hum Genet*. 2013; 92: 935–945.
84. Baasanjav S, Al-Gazali L, Hashiguchi T, et al. Faulty initiation of proteoglycan synthesis causes cardiac and joint defects. *Am J Hum Genet*. 2011; 89: 15–27.
85. Matsumoto K, Irie F, Mackem S, Yamaguchi Y. A mouse model of chondrocyte-specific somatic mutation reveals a role for Ext1 loss of heterozygosity in multiple hereditary exostoses. *Proc Natl Acad Sci USA*. 2010; 107: 10932–10937.
86. Zak BM, Schuksz M, Koyama E, et al. Compound heterozygous loss of Ext1 and Ext2 is sufficient for formation of multiple exostoses in mouse ribs and long bones. *Bone*. 2011; 48: 979–987.
87. Heinritz W, Huffmeier U, Strenge S, et al. New mutations of EXT1 and EXT2 genes in German patients with multiple osteochondromas. *Ann Hum Genet*. 2009; 73: 283–291.
88. Tornberg J, Sykiotis GP, Keefe K, et al. Heparan sulfate 6-O-sulfotransferase 1, a gene involved in extracellular sugar modifications, is mutated in patients with idiopathic hypogonadotrophic hypogonadism. *Proc Natl Acad Sci USA*. 2011; 108: 11524–11529.
89. Tuysuz B, Mizumoto S, Sugahara K, Celebi A, Mundlos S, Turkmen S. Omani-type spondyloepiphyseal dysplasia with cardiac involvement caused by a missense mutation in CHST3. *Clin Genet*. 2009; 75: 375–383.

90. Cabral RM, Kurban M, Wajid M, Shimomura Y, Petukhova L, Christiano AM. Whole-exome sequencing in a single proband reveals a mutation in the CHST8 gene in autosomal recessive peeling skin syndrome. *Genomics*. 2012; 99: 202–208.
91. Shimizu K, Okamoto N, Miyake N, et al. Delineation of dermatan 4-O-sulfotransferase 1 deficient Ehlers-Danlos syndrome: observation of two additional patients and comprehensive review of 20 reported patients. *Am J Med* Genet A. 2011; 155A: 1949–1958.
92. Muller T, Mizumoto S, Suresh I, et al. Loss of dermatan sulfate epimerase (DSE) function results in musculocontractural Ehlers-Danlos syndrome. *Hum Mol Genet*. 2013; 22: 3761–3772.
93. Hiraoka S, Furuichi T, Nishimura G, et al.Nucleotide-sugar transporter SLC35D1 is critical to chondroitin sulfate synthesis in cartilage and skeletal development in mouse and human. *Nat Med*. 2007; 13: 1363–1367.
94. Dwyer E, Hyland J, Modaff P, Pauli RM. Genotype–phenotype correlation in DTDST dysplasias: atelosteogenesis type II and diastrophic dysplasia variant in one family. *Am J Med* Genet A. 2010; 152A: 3043–3050.
95. Akama To, Nishida K, Nakayama J, et al. Macular corneal dystrophy type I and type II are caused by distinct mutations in a new sulphotransferase gene. *Nat Genet*. 2000; 26: 237–241.
96. Paulick MG, Bertozzi CR. The glycosylphosphatidylinositol anchor: a complex membrane-anchoring structure for proteins. *Biochemistry*. 2008; 47: 6991–7000.
97. Takeda J, Miyata T, Kawagoe K, et al. Deficiency of the GPI anchor caused by a somatic mutation of the PIG-A gene in paroxysmal nocturnal hemoglobinuria *Cell*. 1993; 73:703–711.
98. Almeida AM, Murakami Y, Layton DM, et al. Hypomorphic promoter mutation in PIGM causes inherited glycosylphosphatidylinositol deficiency. *Nat Med*. 2006; 12: 846–851.
99. Krawitz PM, Schweiger MR, Rodelsperger C, et al. Identity-by-descent filtering of exome sequence data identifies PIGV mutations in hyperphosphatasia mental retardation syndrome. *Nat Genet*. 2010; 42: 827–829.
100. Maydan G, Noyman I, Har-Zahav A, et al. Multiple congenital anomalies-hypotonia-seizures syndrome is caused by a mutation in PIGN.*J Med Genet*. 2011; 48: 383–389.
101. Ng BG, Hackmann K, Jones MA, et al. Mutations in the glycosylphosphatidylinositol gene PIGL cause CHIME syndrome. *Am J Hum Genet*. 2012; 90: 685–688.
102. Johnston JJ, Gropman AL, Sapp JC, et al. The phenotype of a germline mutation in PIGA: the gene somatically mutated in paroxysmal nocturnal hemoglobinuria. *Am J Hum Genet*. 2012; 90: 295–300.
103. Krawitz PM, Murakami Y, Hecht J, et al. Mutations in PIGO, a member of the GPI-anchor-synthesis pathway, cause hyperphosphatasia with mental retardation. *Am J Hum Genet*. 2012; 91: 146–151.
104. Kvarnung M, Nilsson D, Lindstrand A, et al. A novel intellectual disability syndrome caused by GPI anchor deficiency due to homozygous mutations in PIGT. *J Med Genet*. 2013; 50: 521–528.
105. Krawitz PM, Murakami Y, Riess A, et al. PGAP2 mutations, affecting the GPI-anchor-synthesis pathway, cause hyperphosphatasia with mental retardation syndrome. *Am J Hum Genet*. 2013; 92: 584–589.
106. Swoboda KJ, Margraf RL, Carey JC, et al. A novel germline PIGA mutation in Ferro-Cerebro-Cutaneous syndrome: a neurodegenerative X-linked epileptic encephalopathy with systemic iron-overload. *Am J Med* Genet A. 2013; 164A: 17–28.
107. van der Crabben SN, Harakalova M, Brilstra EH, et al. Expanding the spectrum of phenotypes associated with germline PIGA mutations: a child with developmental delay, accelerated linear growth, facial dysmorphisms, elevated alkaline phosphatase, and progressive CNS abnormalities. *Am J Med* Genet A. 2013; 164: 29–35.
108. Almeida AM, Murakami Y, Baker A, et al. Targeted therapy for inherited GPI deficiency. *N Engl J Med*. 2007; 356: 1641–1647.
109. Horn D, Schottmann G, Meinecke P. Hyperphosphatasia with mental retardation, brachytelephalangy, and a distinct facial gestalt: delineation of a recognizable syndrome. *Eur J Med Genet*. 2010; 53: 85–88.
110. Chiyonobu T, Inoue N, Morimoto M, Kinoshita T, Murakami Y. Glycosylphosphatidylinositol (GPI) anchor deficiency caused by mutations in PIGW is associated with West syndrome and hyperphosphatasia with mental retardation syndrome. *J Med Genet*. 2013; 51: 203–207.
111. Simpson MA, Cross H, Proukakis C, et al. Infantile-onset symptomatic epilepsy syndrome caused by a homozygous loss-of-function mutation of GM3 synthase. *Nat Genet*. 2004; 36: 1225–1229.

112. Boccuto L, Aoki K, Flanagan-Steet H, et al. A mutation in a ganglioside biosynthetic enzyme, ST3GAL5, results in salt & pepper syndrome, a neurocutaneous disorder with altered glycolipid and glycoprotein glycosylation, *Hum Mol Genet.* 2013; 23: 418–433.
113. Boukhris A, Schule R, Loureiro JL, et al. Alteration of ganglioside biosynthesis responsible for complex hereditary spastic paraplegia. *Am J Hum Genet.* 2013; 93: 118–123.
114. Chefetz I, Sprecher E. Familial tumoral calcinosis and the role of O-glycosylation in the maintenance of phosphate homeostasis. *Biochim Biophys Acta.* 2009; 1792: 847–852.
115. Freeze HH, Ng BG. Golgi glycosylation and human inherited diseases. *Cold Spring Harb Perspect Biol.* 2011; 3: a005371.
116. Thiel C, Korner C. Mouse models for congenital disorders of glycosylation. *J Inherit Metab Dis.* 2011; 34: 879–889.
117. Sharma V, Ichikawa M, He P et al. Phosphomannose isomerase inhibitors improve n-glycosylation in selected phosphomannomutase-deficient fibroblasts. *J Biol Chem.* 2011; 286: 39431–39438.
118. Kubota Y, Nishiwaki K. C. elegans as a model system to study the function of the COG complex in animal development. *Biol Chem.* 2006; 387: 1031–1035.
119. Berninsone, PM. Carbohydrates and glycosylation. *WormBook.* 2006; 1–22.
120. Ishikawa HO, Higashi S, Ayukawa T, et al. Notch deficiency implicated in the pathogenesis of congenital disorder of glycosylation IIc. *Proc Natl Acad Sci USA.* 2005; 102: 18532–18537.

3

Gluconeogenesis

ERIN M. COFFEE AND DEAN R. TOLAN

The many inborn errors in metabolism that affect gluconeogenesis are reviewed in this chapter. This central metabolic pathway is responsible for glucose homeostasis and for providing intermediates for glycogen storage, ribose synthesis, phospholipid metabolism, and more. Many of these metabolic diseases have been well documented, and recent reviews of individual diseases arising from the genes encoding the enzymes in this pathway are available.[1-8] This chapter does not duplicate these efforts; instead, it attempts to describe the many gaps in our overall understanding of the pathway(s) involved in the whole organism and the roles played by the many isozymes that exist for these gluconeogenic enzymes. The chapter is divided into three parts. The first part describes the diseases arising from defects in the four enzymes that distinguish this pathway from the glycolytic pathway; pyruvate carboxylase (PC), phosphoenolpyruvate carboxykinase (PCK), fructose-1,6-bishosphatase (FBP), and glucose-6-phosphatase (G6PC). The second part describes defects in enzymes common to both gluconeogenesis and glycolysis but for which there are liver-specific forms that have evolved to perform gluconeogenesis in this tissue. The third part describes defects in enzymes that must operate in both gluconeogenesis and glycolysis for which liver-specific isozymes do not exist. Table 3.1 lists the enzymes involved in this pathway and the corresponding isozymes, alternative names, OMIM numbers, and gene IDs. In addition, inborn errors in metabolism that affect gluconeogenesis but in which the defects are not in gluconeogenic or glycolytic enzymes are discussed. The study of these inborn errors in metabolism and their animal models has enlightened our understanding of glucose homeostasis and the critical nature of this pathway.

Gluconeogenesis is a vital pathway in many mammalian cells where it culminates in providing a pool of glucose 6-phosphate (Glc 6-P) for glycogen synthesis and the oxidative arm of the pentose phosphate shunt. These pathways provide for energy storage and reduced NADPH for biosynthesis, respectively. Moreover, in certain tissues there is the capacity for production of free glucose, which is central for maintaining glucose

TABLE 3.1 **Human Enzymes Involved in Gluconeogenesis**

Enzyme[a]	Gene	Other Names	GENE Ref[b]	OMIM Disease Refs[c]
Pyruvate Carboxylase	PC		5091	266150
Phosphoenolpyruvate Carboxykinase	PCK1	PEPCK1, PEPCKC	5105	261680
	PCK2	PEPCK2, PEPCKM	5106	261650
Enolase	ENO1	Enolase α, Tau-crystallin	2023	172430
	ENO2	Enolase γ, Neuron specific enolase, NSE	2026	
	ENO3	Enolase β, Muscle specific enolase, MSE	2027	612932
Phosphoglycerate Mutase	PGAM1	PGAMA, PGAM brain, PGAMB	5223	
	PGAM2	PGAM muscle, PGAMM	5224	261670
Phosphoglycerate Kinase	PGK1	PGKA	5230	300653
Glyceraldehyde-3-phosphate dehydrogenase	GAPDH	GAPD, G3PD	2597	138400
Triosphosphate isomerase	TPI	TIM	7167	190450
Aldolase	ALDOA	Aldolase 1, ALDA	226	611881
	ALDOB	Aldolase 2, ALDB	229	229600
	ALDOC	Aldolase 3, ALDC	230	
Fructose-1,6-bisphosphatase	FBP1	FBPase1	2203	229700
	FBP2	FBPase2	8189	
Glucose-6-phosphate Isomerase	GPI	Phosphoglucose isomerase, PGI, glucosephosphate isomerase, Autocrine motility factor, AMF, Neuroleukin, NLK	2821	172400
Glucose-6-phosphatase System	G6PC	G6Pase α	2538	232200
	G6PC2	IGRP	57818	
	G6PC3	UGRP, G6Pase β	92579	611045
	G6PT1	Glucose-6-phosphate Transporter, Solute Carrier Member Family 4, SLC37A4, G6P Translocase	2542	232220, 232240

[a]Enzymes in bold are those specific to gluconeogenesis. [b]ID numbers are GeneIDs for those in the "gene" database at the National Center for Biotechnology Information. [c]Numbers only for those where a deficiency has been described. No number is given if the deficiency is unknown (see Table 3.2).

homeostasis in the organism. In addition, the pathway provides other intermediates. For example, fructose 6-phosphate (Fru 6-P) is important for the shunting between trioses and pentoses in the pentose phosphate shunt, dihydroxyacetone phosphate (DHAP) is important for glycerol phosphate production in lipid metabolism (membrane lipids and storage fats), and the phosphoglycerates are important for many specialized roles in biosynthesis (e.g., 3-phosphoglycerate in serine biosynthesis and 2,3-bisphosphoglycerate for hemoglobin regulation). Figure 3.1 depicts the pathway from pyruvate to Glc 6-P and its many fates, as well as the role gluconeogenesis has in providing necessary metabolic precursors for other pathways.

As reviewed here, perturbation of glucose homeostasis is not the major outcome arising from inborn errors in metabolism among the 11 enzymes directly involved in generation

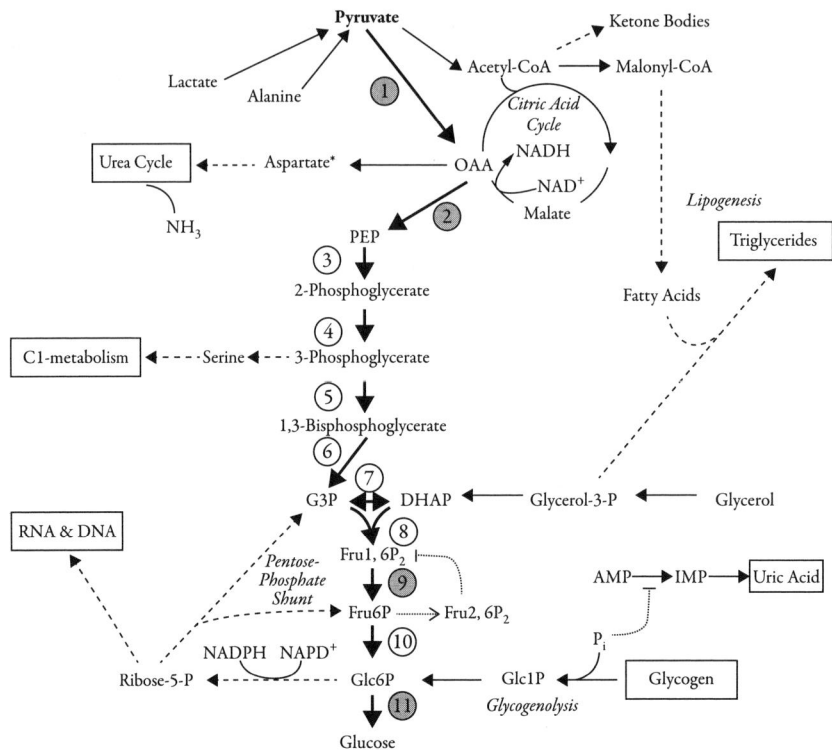

FIGURE 3.1 **Gluconeogenesis and the Inter-Dependent Pathways.** All arrows are indicated in the direction needed for glucose production. Thick arrows indicate a catalytic step in gluconeogenesis (Pyruvate to Glucose). Thin arrows indicate reactions intersecting with gluconeogenesis. Dashed arrows indicate reaction pathways with multiple steps. Dotted lines indicate synthesis and action of regulatory molecules. Boxes indicate end products. Numbered circles indicate reactions catalyzed by gluconeogenic enzymes. Gray circles indicate those reactions that are specific to gluconeogenesis. Numbers are 1= PC, 2 = PCK, 3 = ENO, 4 = PGAM, 5 = PGK, 6 = GAPDH, 7 = TPI, 8 = aldolase, 9 = FBP, 10 = GPI, and 11 = Glucose-6-phosphatase system. Asterisk (*) indicates that this cataplerotic reaction also occurs for other non-essential amino acids such as glutamate and eventually glutamine and asparagine.

of glucose from pyruvate. Due to the critical function that this central metabolic pathway has in the cell, most of the diseases arising from defects in gluconeogenic enzymes are relatively rare. Overall, the prevalence is less than 1:50,000 (Table 3.2) with G6Pase deficiency being the most common disease.[3]

Defects in Enzymes That Distinguish Gluconeogenesis From Glycolysis

The four enzymes needed to reverse the pathway between glucose and pyruvate are, in order, PC, PCK, FBP, and G6PC. The study of both inborn errors in metabolism and animal models that led to deficiencies in these enzymes has revealed the importance of the gluconeogenic pathway in lipid, nitrogen, redox, and purine metabolism as well as its clear role in glucose homeostasis (see Figure 3.1). In addition, careful analysis of the symptoms presenting from

TABLE 3.2 Prevalence of Inborn Errors in Metabolism Due to Defects in Genes for Gluconeogenesis

Disease[a]	Gene	Prevalence or Number of Cases
Pyruvate Carboxylase deficiency	PC	
Group A		25
Group B		<50
Group C		1
PCK1 deficiency	PCK1	1
PCK2 deficiency	PCK2	4
ENO1 deficiency	ENO1	<5
ENO2 deficiency	ENO2	unknown
Glycogen Storage Disease Type XIII[b]	ENO3	1
PGAM1 deficiency	PGAM1	unknown
Glycogen Storage Disease Type X[b]	PGAM2	<10
PGK1 deficiency	PGK1	<20
GAPDH deficiency	GAPDH	3
TPI deficiency	TPI	<30
Glycogen Storage Disease Type XII[b]	ALDOA	3
Hereditary Fructose Intolerance	ALDOB	1:20,000
ALDOC deficiency	ALDOC	unknown
FBP1 deficiency	FBP1	35
FBP2 deficiency	FBP2	unknown
GPI deficiency	GPI	<50
Glycogen Storage Disease Type Ia	G6PC1	1:100,000
G6PC2 deficiency	G6PC2	unknown
G6PC3 deficiency	G6PC3	<6
Glycogen Storage Disease Type Ib	G6PT1	1:400,000
Glycogen Storage Disease Type Ic		<6[c]
Glycogen Storage Disease Type Id		<2[c]

[a]Enzymes in bold are those specific to gluconeogenesis. [b]Also known as the various enzyme deficiencies (e.g., ALDOA deficiency). All lead to hereditary nonspherocytic hemolytic anemia. [c]Most of these patients were subsequently found to have mutations in the G6PT1 gene.[82]

metabolic diseases involving these enzymes updates the longstanding dogma concerning the regulation of gluconeogenic flux.

Pyruvate Carboxylase

Pyruvate carboxylase catalyzes the conversion of pyruvate to oxaloacetate (OAA) in the mitochondria. By the incorporation of carbon dioxide at the expense of adenosine triphosphate hydrolysis, this is considered the first step in gluconeogenesis, although this is not a committed step. PC is known as an anaplerotic enzyme as it provides intermediates for several pathways; the exit of acetyl-CoA from the mitochondria for fatty acid biosynthesis, the conversion to aspartate for amino-group removal via the urea cycle, and the replenishing of OAA for the citric acid cycle (see Scheme 1[9]). In addition, it has an important role in astrocytes for the biosynthesis of neurotransmitters.[10,11] A single PC gene (*pc*) in humans expresses a nuclear-encoded mitochondrial homotetrameric enzyme of 127 kDa subunits.[12,13] It is highly expressed in the liver and kidney as well as many other cells and tissues,[9,12] belying its strategic position at the intersection for several metabolic pathways. It is often said to be a key regulatory enzyme in gluconeogenesis,[14] lipogenesis, and neurotransmitter synthesis, although its only known allosteric effector is acetyl-CoA,[15] which indicates that its regulation for lipid metabolism is more important than its ability to regulate gluconeogenesis.

PC deficiency is a rare disorder that manifests as severe lactic acidemia.[16] There are three groups (A, B, and C) of the disorder distinguished by the severity and pervasiveness of the symptoms. Those with as little as 2% residual PC activity show lactic acidemia and a psychomotor retardation (Group A). These children do not survive childhood. Those with no PC cross-reacting material and/or no PC activity have more severe symptoms that additionally involve amino acid and redox metabolism (Group B). These patients die within the first three months. The third group is rarer and presents only as acute lactic acidosis with survival and normal development (Group C). For all groups, the lactic acidemia results from a clear inability to convert lactate beyond pyruvate in the liver. There have been reports of hypoglycemic episodes, although it is not a major problem.[17] Though purported to be a key regulatory enzyme for gluconeogenesis,[16] the effect of PC deficiency on glucose homeostasis is not severe. Moreover, when PC is absent there are effects on urea metabolism (see Figure 3.1). Patients have hyperammonemia and cannot convert excess ammonia to urea due to depletion of the OAA/aspartate pool. This indicates that PC has a crucial role in the liver and kidney in providing OAA for cycling aspartate out of the mitochondria. This symptom is not observed in Group A patients, who retain as little as 2% residual PC activity. In astrocytes, PC provides a pool of OAA that is used for neurotransmitter synthesis (Glu, Gln, and γ-aminobutyric acid).[10,11] Furthermore, the OAA is used for cycling acetyl-CoA out of the mitochondria for lipid biosynthesis, and depletion of this pool results in poor myelin formation. Patients from Group A suffer neurological sequela due to the importance of PC in astrocytes. This is a further indication of the role of the gluconeogenic pathway in providing precursors for biosynthesis that is beyond its role in glucose homeostasis.

Phosphoenolpyruvate Carboxykinase

PCK is a gluconeogenic-specific enzyme that catalyzes the conversion of OAA to phosphoenolpyruvate. Two isoforms exist; a cytosolic form (PCK 1) and a mitochondrial form (PCK 2), which share 70% identity at the amino acid level.[18] PCK1 and PCK2 differ in their levels of expression and regulation. Controversy exists over the distribution of these two isoforms in various cells with reports suggesting the PCK1 is anywhere from 50% to over 95% of PCK activity in the liver.[19,20] While PCK1 is regulated by hormones such as insulin, glucagon, cAMP, and glucocorticoids, these same hormones have no effect on PCK2 expression, as this mitochondrial form is constitutively expressed.[21] For the enzyme believed to be the "rate-limiting" enzyme for gluconeogenesis, it is interesting that neither isoform of PCK is allosterically regulated. In addition to being expressed in the liver and kidney, known sites of gluconeogenesis, PCK is present in many tissues that are not thought to produce glucose (i.e., white and brown adipose tissue, heart, lung, muscle, and brain).[22] Further characterization of its metabolic role in tissues that do not produce glucose has not been well defined.

PCK deficiency has been reported in less than half a dozen individuals, can occur in either isoform, and generally results in death in infancy.[23–27] PCK deficiencies have been reported to be one underlying cause of SIDS.[28,29] All patients have presented with severe hypoglycemia with some presenting with lactic acidemia,[25,27] unlike PC deficiency, in which the opposite is observed (see above). In addition, postmortem analysis of patient liver and kidney shows massive fatty acid deposition.[23–27] Diagnosis is performed by measuring PCK activity in liver biopsy samples or by analysis of cultured fibroblasts. It has been reported that cultured fibroblasts only express the mitochondrial form (PCK2),[23] and PCK1 deficiency could be missed when using cultured fibroblasts for the diagnosis.

Mouse models of PCK deficiency that lack PCK1 mimic the phenotypes reported in humans.[2,20,30] These *pck1*[-/-] mice are not embryonic lethal as PCK1 expression does not appear until birth.[31] However, these mice die within two to three days of birth, and while their severe hypoglycemia seems the obvious culprit,[20] the exact cause has not been determined. Administration of intraperitoneal glucose could not rescue these mice from death, which suggests that the morbidity is more likely due to a larger role of PCK in metabolism. To understand the implications in overall metabolism brought on by fasting, liver-specific *pck1*[-/-] mice (*pck*[lox/lox]+Alb*cre*) were created.[20] Like PCK deficiency in humans, liver-specific *pck1*[-/-] mice had a marked increase in hepatic lipid accumulation (fatty liver). The concentration of triglycerides in the liver and blood of *pck1*[-/-] mice was increased two-fold.[2] This fatty liver was somewhat surprising, and it has illuminated the many critical roles of PCK. PCK is not only involved in the removal of OAA from the citric acid cycle but in providing phosphoenolpyruvate for synthesis of serine (and other reactions dependent on one-carbon metabolism) and in the synthesis of glycerol 3-phosphate for triglyceride synthesis (see Figure 3.1).

Many aspects of these *pck1*[-/-] mice remain a mystery. Most surprisingly, the liver-specific *pck1*[-/-] mice are euglycemic after a 24-hr fast. This could be due to gluconeogenesis from glycerol, bypassing the first part of the pathway.[30,32] However, the role other tissues have in playing a major, or at least redundant, part (kidney, small intestine, maybe others) in glucose production remains a question.[33] This is consistent with reports in humans where removal of the liver causes only 50% reduction in glucose production.[34,35] Mice lacking PCK in the liver have only a slight decrease in glucose turnover rates.[30] In addition, the underlying cause of lipid accumulation (fatty liver) is unclear. When PCK is deficient, OAA builds up, and the OAA is converted to malate (malate is increased 10-fold in the livers of *pck1*[-/-] mice[30]) with subsequent increases in most of the citric acid cycle intermediates.[32] There is an important and subsequent decrease in the rate of the citric acid cycle due to allosteric inhibition caused by this buildup as well as the known increase in the NADH/NAD$^+$ ratio in the mitochondria.[32] The loss of citric acid cycling leads to pyruvate buildup, with subsequent lactic acidemia and increases in acetyl-CoA. The acetyl-CoA cannot be burned to carbon dioxide and ends up generating fatty acids and ketone bodies. This lipogenesis is exacerbated by the high levels of mitochondrial NADH, which inhibits β-oxidation, along with the inhibition of β-oxidation by malonyl-CoA from fatty acid biosynthesis. Whether it is inhibition of β-oxidation or activation of lipogenesis that predominates in the liver is unclear. It is thought that liver plays a role in glyceroneogenesis where glycerol 3-P is produced. If the liver is involved in gluconeogenesis from glycerol 3-phosphate, then its depletion explains the excess free fatty acids in the blood of both total *pck1*[-/-] mice and liver-specific *pck1*[-/-] mice.[20] However, free fatty acids are normally taken up by the liver and then condensed with glycerol-3-P to make triglycerides. If glycerol 3-phosphate is being used for gluconeogenesis, then this intermediate would not be readily available for triglyceride formation, which is clearly happening in both the blood[2,20] and the liver of total *pck*[-/-] mice[2] as well as liver-specific *pck1*[-/-] mice.[20] The source of the gluconeogenesis and the triglycerides in PCK deficiency remains a mystery. Nevertheless, the decreased citric acid cycle flux is likely playing a part in stimulating triacylglyceride formation.

Moreover, the decreased flux of the citric acid cycle causes increases in amino acids, such as Asp, Asn, Glu, Gln, Ala, and Gly, in the blood of *pck1*[-/-] mice.[2] This can be explained in two ways. The buildup of their α-ketoacid backbones in the form of citric acid cycle intermediates can lead to increase in amino acid biosynthesis and/or the inability of these amino acids to enter the citric acid cycle for degradation due to the lower rate of the cycle. Either explains the increase in these nonessential amino acids in the blood in *pck1*[-/-] mice.[30]

While PCK has long been thought to be the rate-limiting enzyme responsible for controlling glucose production through gluconeogenesis, work done with mouse models over the past decade has proven this false.[2,20,30] From these studies, it is clear that PCK plays an important role in regulating flux through many pathways. As seen with PC deficiency, studies on PCK deficiency have highlighted the importance of the gluconeogenic pathway as a central stream for providing intermediates for biosynthesis and not solely associated with glucose homeostasis.

Fructose-1,6-Bisphosphate 1-Phosphohydrolase

FBP catalyzes the hydrolysis of fructose 1,6-bisphosphate (Fru 1,6-P_2) to Fru 6-P and inorganic phosphate (P_i). This enzyme reverses the key step in glycolysis catalyzed by phosphofructokinase. In mammals, there appear to be two isozymes, sometimes termed for their tissue of highest expression, liver and muscle.[36] Although patients with defects in the muscle FBP2 gene (*fbp2*) are unknown, those with defects in the gene for the liver isozyme (*fbp1*) have fructose-1,6-bisphosphatase deficiency.[37] This disorder is of unknown prevalence with diagnosis made most often in the newborn period. The disorder is manifested by recurrent attacks of hypoglycemia and metabolic acidosis, usually associated with fasting or illness. It often first presents itself in the clinic by episodes of hyperventilation caused by acute acidosis due to the buildup of lactate and OAA. There are also reports of apnea, tachycardia, hypotonia, ketosis, and coma. The hypoglycemia and ketosis arise from similar metabolic disturbances as seen in G6PC deficiency (see below). Although the disorder may be lethal in the newborn period, proper treatment of avoiding fasting and sugars (sucrose and fructose) yields an excellent prognosis.[38,39] After survival of the newborn period, the acute hypoglycemia wanes, which has led to the speculation that there may be many adults living undiagnosed.[37] Due to the loss of gluconeogenesis as a source for blood glucose, the severity and even the onset of symptoms depends on the available glycogen stores. Therefore, the hypoglycemia is unresponsive to glucagon.[40] An interesting observation that demonstrates the crossroads of fructose and glucose metabolism is the effect that fructose ingestion has on those suffering from FBP deficiency.[37,41] Although not as drastic as in hereditary fructose intolerance (HFI), there is an excessive dependence on glycogenolysis for normal glucose production.[37] After ingestion of fructose or sorbitol, the build up of fructose 1-phosphate (Fru 1-P) has deleterious effects on the levels of phosphate, alanine, bicarbonate, and glucose, which lead to increases in the levels of lactate and urate (see glucose-6-phosphatase, below). Similar effects are seen after oral glycerol or dihydroxyacetone administration. These effects on glycogenolysis can be explained by the inhibition of liver phosphorylase-a by lack of P_i, which is pronounced in the presence of intermediates that build up in FBP deficiency after ingestion of these sugars; Fru 1-P, Fru 1,6-P_2, and glycerol 3-phosphate.[42–45]

There are no animal models for this disease. While the incidence of the disease is unknown, there have been several dozen patients diagnosed by demonstrating enzyme deficiency in liver biopsy specimens or by mutational analysis. Because the newborn is more dependent on gluconeogenesis,[46,47] diagnosis is normally made this time. Adults learn to avoid fasting, although sugars such as sorbitol and fructose can cause issues.

Glucose 6-Phosphate 6-Phosphohydrolase

G6PC catalyzes the hydrolysis of Glc 6-P to free glucose and P_i. This enzyme reverses the initial step in glycolysis catalyzed by hexokinase and is the key enzyme in the gluconeogenic pathway, as well as the glycogenolytic pathway, necessary for glucose homeostasis. In mammals, three isozymes of the hydrolase have been described, although this crucial and final step in gluconeogenesis involves more than just these isozymes, and it is sometimes termed the G6PC system.[48] Unlike the other enzymes in the pathway, G6PC is associated with the endoplasmic reticulum (ER) and is a trans-membrane protein with nine membrane-spanning helices.[49] The other parts of the system likely include transporters for Glc 6-P (G6PT), glucose, and P_i. Genes and cDNAs for three G6PC homologs have been characterized and one for G6PT. The identity of genes for the proposed glucose and P_i transporters remains elusive. One model that is currently favored for this final step in gluconeogenesis is depicted in Figure 3.2. This model is still controversial with several components of the system relatively undefined, as described below.

The three homologs for the G6PC are termed glucose-6-phosphatase, catalytic-1 (G6PC1), G6PC2, and G6PC3. The enzyme found in liver and kidney is expressed from the G6PC1 gene. The product of the G6PC2 gene is sometimes called the islet-specific G6PC-related protein(IGRP). This protein is found exclusively in the pancreatic islet cells, and clear demonstration of catalytic activity has been equivocal.[48,50,51] The third homolog, G6PC3, is sometimes termed the ubiquitously expressed G6PC (UGRP or G6Pase-β).[52] The later two proteins are 50% and 36% identical to the G6PC1, respectively, and all have the same gene structure and protein size (357, 355, and 346 amino acid residues, respectively).[52] The major functional enzyme in glucose homeostasis is the G6PC1 in the liver and kidney. The G6PC3 isozyme is apparently less active,[53–57] and the gene (*g6pc3*) is expressed in most tissues examined. The tissues with highest to lowest levels are skeletal muscle, heart, brain, placenta,

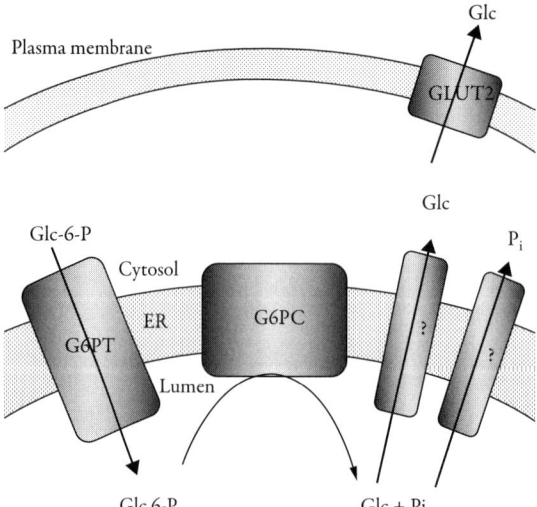

FIGURE 3.2 **Model of the Glucose-6-phosphatase System (Arion's model).** Both ER and plasma membranes are indicated (grey bars). Shadowed boxes indicate the membrane proteins. The characterized catalytic enzyme and transporter are indicated by gene name. Putative transporters are indicated by question marks. Arrows indicate the reactions of Glc 6-P, Glc, and P_i.

kidney, colon, thymus, spleen, pancreas, liver, lung, small intestine, and leukocytes.[58] Null mice (*g6pc3*[-/-]) are unaffected in glucose homeostasis but show[52] affects in G6Pase activity in the brain, growth in females, and neutropenia,[59] which was confirmed in humans.[60] Interestingly, G6PC3 does not possess the ER-retention motif present in both G6PC1 and G6PC2.[58]

The G6PT1 is arguably the most important component of the G6PC system. It is the rate-limiting step in the system.[61] This situation may have evolved because if Glc 6-P is needed for other pathways (pentose-phosphate shunt, glycogen synthesis, etc.; see Figure 3.1), it does not enter the ER and become committed for export as free glucose. The transporter was discovered in 1997[62] and is also known as the solute carrier family 37, member 4 (SLC37A4) or as the G6P translocase. The protein is a 46-kDa peptide with 10 transmembrane helices. The gene (*slc37a4*) is most highly expressed in the liver, kidney, and progenitor blood cells.[63,64] Tissue-specific expression of several splice variants, with an interesting exon 7-containing isoform (adding 22 amino acid residues to a cytoplasmic loop), is present in brain, heart, and skeletal muscle.[63] It's not clear what activity these variants possess.

The scheme depicted in Figure 3.2, first proposed in 1975 by Arion et al.,[65] shows the presence of proteins in the ER that are predicted to return free glucose and P_i to the cytosol. The identity of these two transporter proteins remains obscure.[33] The glucose transporter in the ER could be one of the plasma membrane GLUT transporters[3] that have been described in a family that now numbers about 13 to 14[66,67](Zhang & Tolan, unpublished data). There have yet to be any ER-retained GLUTs described, although this has been an active area of investigation.[68,69] It had been reported that GLUT7 was a hepatic microsomal glucose transport protein perhaps responsible for the facilitated release of glucose from the ER lumen,[69] but subsequent research has contradicted this as there has been no appreciable GLUT7 mRNA found in the liver.[68,70] An additional GLUT family member, GLUT10, has been proposed to export glucose due to its recent identification of localization to the ER in various cell lines[71]; however, its function has yet to be determined. Additionally, it remains possible that alternative plasma membrane transporters may function as glucose transporters in the ER membrane.[72] Finally, data using liver microsomes suggest the ability of glucose to freely permeate the ER membrane.[73–75] The mechanism for P_i release from the ER is equally elusive. The P_i transporter has been predicted to be the same as the Na/P_i cotransporter 4, which is expressed in the liver and kidney and localizes to the ER.[76] However, other transporters have been suggested,[48] including the mitochondrial P_i/PP_i transporter.[77] G6PT1 itself has been suggested as a glucose/P_i antiporter,[78] but recent studies have not confirmed this activity.[79] Last, perhaps the anion channels that allow P_i permeability through the sarcoplasmic reticulum membrane could serve a similar role in the liver ER membrane.[80] The lack of a complete molecular description, including the reconstitution of the system described in Figure 3.2, has led to other hypotheses regarding the export of free glucose from the cell. The use of exocytosis of glucose-containing vesicles[81] has been proposed based on the observation that mice missing the glucose transporter at the liver plasma membrane (*glut2*$^{-/-}$) have normal glucose homeostasis. However, other active glucose transporters, besides GLUT2, may be present in mouse liver.[48] Another model that attributes most of the activities to G6PC without a specific Glc-6-P transporter is called the conformational-flexibility/substrate-transport model.[82–85] This model is supported by kinetics,[82] specificity changes (ratio of activity toward mannose 6-phosphate versus Glc 6-P)[84], and inhibition of the G6PC affecting uptake of Glc 6-P.[86,87] This model purports that G6PC is in contact with a pore molecule that allows free diffusion of products and binding of substrate from outside the ER. The activity of the enzyme changes in response to different substrates through conformational changes.[88] Clearly, the discovery of the Glc-6-P-specific transporter contradicts this model. However, until all of the components of the G6PC system have been purified and studied in isolation and in combination, our understanding of this physiologically important step in gluconeogenesis will be lacking. It is interesting that so many of the studies on this system have been done in liver microsomes, which are at best only isolated fragments of the ER. The use of a more realistic system that uses intact ER, such as permeabilized hepatocytes[89,90] in combination with purified systems of recombinant proteins in artificial vesicles, should clarify many of the remaining questions.

Humans afflicted with mutations in genes involved in the G6PC system lead to one of the many glycogen storage diseases (GSD). Specifically, GSD Type I (GSDI), also known as von Gierke disease,[3] is the major inborn error in metabolism affecting gluconeogenesis.[3] Although first described in 1929, deficiencies in the G6PC system were not demonstrated until 1952.[91] This autosomal recessive disorder has been classified further as Type Ia, Ib, Ic, and Id.[3] This subdivision was needed after the discovery of individuals with ample G6PC activity. About 80% of the cases of G6PC deficiency are Type Ia, and most of the remaining cases are Type Ib. Those with Type Ia have mutations in the G6PC1 gene (*g6pc1*) with dozens of mutations having been identified.[92] Those individuals with Type Ib were thought to have defects in the transporter gene (*g6pt1*), which was clearly demonstrated in 1980.[93] The existence of distinct forms Ic and Id are in some doubt with only a few cases reported.[3,94] One reason for this doubt comes from studies of several patients with Ic who have subsequently been found with mutations in *g6pt1*.[95-97] Only one patient has been reported who is thought deficient in the ER glucose transporter, but this analysis was incomplete.[98]

There are slight differences in clinical presentation among the forms of GSD Type I. Like other GSDs that involve the liver, all GSD Type I patients present with hepatomegaly and hypoglycemia. The laboratory findings for all GSDI types include a dangerous lactic acidemia, hyperlipidemia, and hyperuricemia.[3] In addition to these symptoms, those with GSDIb suffer from recurrent infections due to neutropenia and neutrophil dysfunction.[99] These symptoms are explained by the difference in expression of *g6pt1*, found in progenitor blood cells, and *g6pc1*, which is not expressed there.[64] No symptomatic differences between Ib and Ic have been described. Neonates are in the most danger of severe pathology and death, having less tolerance to fasting and higher needs for gluconeogenesis.[46,47] Gluconeogenesis is needed for both blood glucose homeostasis and cell growth in providing precursors for biosynthesis. However, studies of GSDI patients show that the capability of producing blood glucose is not lost.[100-102] Rates of glucose production were half of normal, with near normal rates in adult patients. This ability may be the root of the lower prevalence of hypoglycemia in adults with GSDI. The mechanism for this glucose production is unknown, although the role of the ubiquitously expressed G6PC3 in this mechanism is supported by expression studies of *g6pc3* and *g6pt1*, where both are expressed in skeletal muscle, colon, and brain[55,57] (Coffee, Ma, & Tolan, unpublished data).

Mouse models for GSDIa have been developed.[87,103] These mice ($g6pc1^{-/-}$) recapitulate the GSDIa symptoms quite closely with hepatomegaly, hypoglycemia, hyperuricemia, and hyperlipidemia, including the lack of hypoglycemia in a liver-specific knockout.[103] Models for GSDIa have also been developed in dogs.[104] The mouse model for GSDIb ($g6pt1^{-/-}$) mimics the disruption in glucose homeostasis as well as the neutropenia that distinguishes it from GSD1a.[105] Attempts to mimic GSDIb in a cell line by reducing *g6pt1* expression using RNA interference, as well as the inhibition of G6PT1 by the anticancer drug curcumin, in U87 glioma cells have been reported.[61] Both treatments induced necrosis and late apoptosis. This curcumin-induced cell death could be rescued by overexpression of *g6pt1*. Again, this result could be an indication of the central role that the gluconeogenic pathway plays in the overall metabolism of the cell. An interesting murine model with homozygous deletion of the liver glucose transporter $glut2^{-/-}$ has been reported.[81] This model should show defects in both glucose uptake as well as gluconeogenesis; however, these mice had normal gluconeogenesis. Humans with GLUT2 deficiency (Fanconi-Bickel syndrome) have been reported to have liver glycogenesis defects and renal Fanconi syndrome.[106,107] Although there are no defects in sugar absorption by the intestine, the response of blood glucose to fasting has not been noted. Clearly there may be other sugar transporters involved in the intestine, and the liver may use other transporters or mechanisms for exporting glucose (see above).

The pathophysiology of the hypoglycemia seen in GSDI is more or less obvious, with the question of where residual glucose production occurs being more intriguing (see above). The lactic acidosis arises from the increase in glycolysis, which is brought on by the buildup of Glc 6-P and Fru 6-P. The increase in Fru 6-P triggers the increase in the synthesis of the positive allosteric effector, fructose 2,6-bisphosphate, which activates phosphofructokinase[3] (see Figure 3.1). Since glycogen stores are depleted, the only route for the Glc 6-P is to pyruvate, which continues on to large supplies of acetyl-CoA and lactate, plus increases in NADH. The role of the gluconeogenic pathway in providing intermediates for lipid metabolism in the form of glycerol 3-phosphate is highlighted by the hyperlipidemia seen in GSDIa patients.[3] With the aforementioned supplies of acetyl-CoA and NADH/NADPH from the TCA cycle and the pentose-phosphate shunt, there are all the necessary precursors for fatty acid biosynthesis. The excess glycerol 3-phosphate is easily converted to triglycerides. In addition, acetyl-CoA is easily shunted out of the mitochondria in the form of citrate by the abundance of OAA, which is formed after glucagon stimulation of PC.[9] The block in recycling of P_i due to its sequestration in Glc 6-P leads to the hyperuricemia. A decrease in intracellular P_i signals that nucleotides and nucleosides are overly abundant relative to the amount of available P_i. Liver AMP-deaminase is activated under these conditions, thus starting the degradation of purines, which ends with uric acid (see Figure 3.1). This phenomenon is similar in many other metabolic disorders in which organophosphate precursors build up, such as in HFI, galactosemia, and FBP deficiency.[37,108]

Summary

Textbooks describe the first committed step in the gluconeogenic pathway as that catalyzed by PCK, and therefore it should affect the production of glucose. Although the gene for PCK is highly regulated, as would be consistent with a "rate-limited step," the information to date does not support a large role for PCK in glucose homeostasis. Rather, the enzymes at the end of the pathway, FBP and G6PC in particular, have much larger roles in the production of glucose. This is not surprising when considering other biosynthetic pathways such as amino acid biosynthesis, wherein the control of these pathways is attributed at the export steps.[109] The dogma regarding control of gluconeogenesis by PCK highlights one of the tenants of metabolic control analysis and the concept of distributed control of metabolic flux.[110] Furthermore, it is clear that this pathway is additionally a wellspring for other pathways and cannot be considered in isolation. Certainly, a more integrated approach that should be derived from use of systems biology should benefit our understanding of metabolism and its inborn errors.

Enzymes Common to Both Gluconeogenesis and Glycolysis With Liver-Specific Isoforms

Of the 11 enzymes in the gluconeogenic pathway, only one plays a role in glycolysis, with isozymes that have evolved for a particular role in gluconeogenesis in the liver and kidney.

Fructose-1,6-Bisphosphate Aldolase (Aldolase)

Fructose-1,6-bisphosphate aldolase catalyzes the synthesis of fructose-1,6-bisphosphate (Fru 1,6-P_2) from DHAP and glyceraldehyde 3-phosphate (G3P) during gluconeogenesis. Aldolase also performs the reverse reaction during glycolysis and can breakdown Fru 1-P into DHAP and glyceraldehyde during fructose metabolism.[37] Aldolase exists as three isoforms located on separate genes.[111] The aldolase A gene (*aldoA*) is ubiquitously expressed and is the isoform found in the erythrocytes and muscle. It is the most well suited isoform for glycolysis as it has the highest k_{cat} for Fru-1,6-P_2 cleavage. The aldolase B gene (*aldoB*) is expressed in the liver and kidney where it plays a critical function in fructose metabolism as it has the highest k_{cat} for Fru-1-P cleavage. Due to its tissue-specific expression pattern in the liver, aldolase B is the isoform responsible for gluconeogenesis. This is supported by the lower K_m values that aldolase B has toward both DHAP and G3P compared to the other isozymes.[112] Patients with an aldolase-A deficiency suffer from symptoms affecting the red blood cells (hemolytic anemia) and muscle (rhabdomyolysis).[113] Patients with *aldoA* mutations have mild missense mutations,[114] and there are no reports of patients harboring two null alleles. Patients with aldolase-B deficiency are unable to metabolize ingested fructose and suffer from hereditary fructose intolerance (HFI).[115] HFI can result in liver and kidney failure and even death if not diagnosed.[37] HFI is not to be confused with fructose malabsorption, a common affliction that is reported to affect one in three people[116] and results from an inability to absorb fructose by the intestinal epithelium.

Patients with HFI often present with hypoglycemia, hypophosphatemia, hyperuricemia, and failure to thrive. However, these symptoms appear only following fructose ingestion.[37] In the liver, fructose metabolism starts with transport by GLUT2 followed by phosphorylation by ketohexokinase at carbon-1. Without aldolase B activity, the levels of Fru 1-P increase, thus sequestering P_i. This causes inhibition of phosphorylase-a by low P_i levels preventing glycogenolysis. Glucose formation is prevented further by the Fru 1-P inhibition of the glucose 1-phosphate to Glc 6-P conversion catalyzed by phosphoglucomutase. This results in the hypoglycemia seen following fructose ingestion. The hyperuricemia is caused indirectly by the hypophosphatemia, which activates AMP deaminse and begins the conversion of AMP to IMP and eventually to uric acid (see Figure 3.1).[117] This same pathophysiology is seen in FBP deficiency and GSDI (see above).

An interesting enigma is seen in HFI patients. Aldolase-B deficiency manifests symptoms only upon fructose ingestion, while gluconeogenesis appears to be unaffected, even in the fasted state.[40,118] Specifically, HFI patients are able to maintain blood glucose levels after an overnight fast and can readily form glucose from DHAP and glycerol. Both suggest that a loss of aldolase B does not inhibit gluconeogenesis.[118,119] This enigma could be explained by the activation of the gene(s) for aldolase A or C in the liver[120] and/or that gluconeogenesis is not limited to the liver and kidney and is occurring in tissues that express aldolase A or C.[121,122] An animal model for aldolase-B deficiency that could answer these remaining questions about gluconeogenesis, is being developed (Coffee & Tolan, unpublished data).

Enzymes Common to Both Pathways With One Isoform

The remaining six enzymes of gluconeogenesis must also be active for glycolysis, and there is no liver-specific form or one that has evolved for gluconeogenic function required in pertinent tissues. The entire pathway is shown in Figure 3.3 and distinguishes each enzyme in the pathway in the way that separates those involved specifically in gluconeogenesis and those involved in glycolysis as described here.

Enolase

Enolase catalyzes the interconversion of phosphoenolpyruvate to 2-phosphoglycerate. Enolase exists as three homodimeric isoforms that differ in their tissue expression patterns and biochemical properties.[123] Enolase 1 (ENO1), or alpha, is expressed in nearly all tissues including during embryonic development. In addition, this embryonic isoform was identified as being tau-crystallin.[124] Enolase 2 (ENO2), or gamma, is a neuron-specific isoform. Enolase 3 (ENO3), or beta, is a muscle-specific isoform found in high amounts in adult skeletal muscle. Partial deficiencies of ENO1 have been reported with variable clinical symptoms.[125,126] Hereditary red cell enolase deficiency is associated with a spherocytic phenotype and hemolytic anemia. Deficiencies in ENO3 are now classified as GSD Type XIII with one patient reported to have adult onset exercise-induced

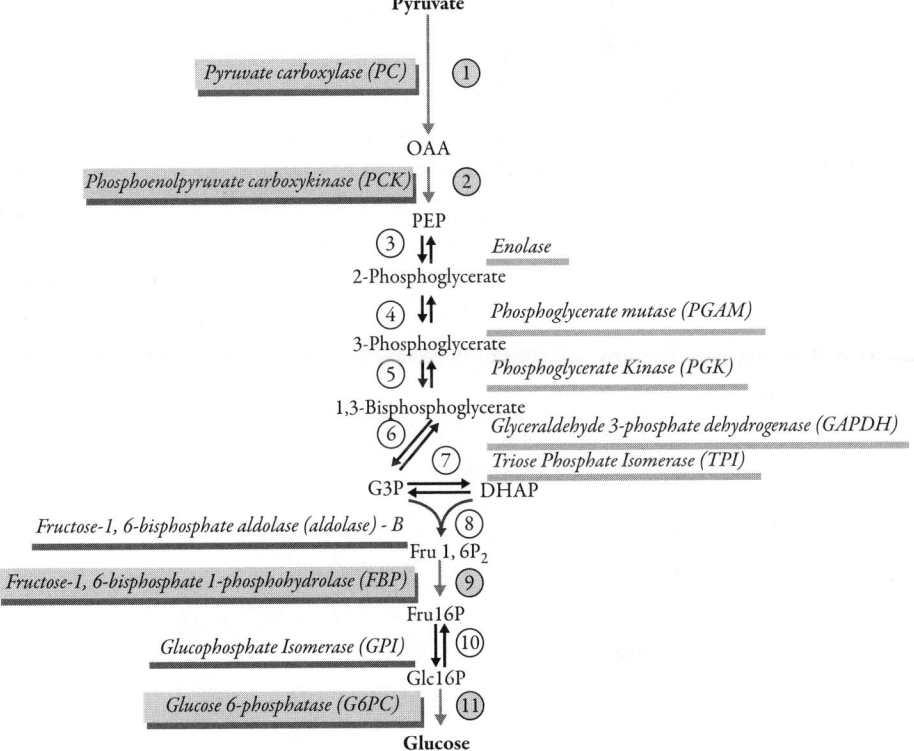

FIGURE 3.3 **Summary of Gluconeogenic Pathway.** The pathway is indicated with arrows corresponding to the classification of enzymes (numbered as in Fig. 3.1) as described in the text. The enzymes distinct for gluconeogenesis are indicated with gray arrows and gray-boxed names. Indicated in dark gray arrows and underlined name is the enzyme common to both gluconeogenesis and glycolysis, but with liver-specific isoforms adapted for gluconeogenesis. Indicated with black double arrows are the enzymes that are common to both gluconeogenesis and glycolysis without an isoform adapted for the liver.

myalgias, muscle weakness, and fatigability.[127] No enolase deficiencies report problems with gluconeogenesis.

Phosphoglycerate Mutase

Phosphoglycerate mutase (PGAM) catalyzes the interconversion of 2-phosphoglycerate and 3-phosphoglycerate. PGAM exists as two isozymes: PGAM1 (PGAM-A, PGAMB [brain]) and PGAM2 (PGAMM [muscle]).[128] The two isozymes can homo- and hetero-dimerize in different tissues. PGAM1 homo-dimer is present in the brain, liver, erythrocytes, and leukocytes.[128] The PGAM2 homo-dimer is found in high amounts in muscle. In cardiac tissue, all three dimeric forms, the two homo-dimers and the hybrid PGAM1/PGAM2 hetero-dimer, are present, although the PGAM2 homo-dimer predominates. Deficiencies of PGAM2 have been reported to cause GSD Type X.[129,130] Patients present with exercise intolerance with exercise-induced muscle pain and cramps, pigmenturia following exercise, and, in some cases, increased serum creatine kinase levels.[129-132] There are no reports of deficiencies in glucose production or other difficulties in gluconeogenesis with PGAM2 deficiency. There are no reports of deficiencies in PGAM1 indicating perhaps its essential role in the cell.

Phosphoglycerate Kinase

Phosphoglycerate kinase (PGK) catalyzes the conversion of 3-phosphoglycerate to 1,3-phosphoglycerate and the gene (*pgk1*) is located on the X chromosome.[133] In addition to its expression in most tissues, tumor cells also secrete PGK1. It is believed to have a role in angiogenesis whereby acting as a disulfide reductase.[134] PGK1 deficiency is an X-linked recessive disorder that results in highly variable clinical phenotypes. Patients can suffer from chronic nonspherocytic hemolytic anemia, muscle involvement in the form of rhabdomyolysis, and neurological impairment. Patients may present with any one or all three of these symptoms.[135] Attempts to explain the variability of symptoms based on genotype-phenotype studies is still ongoing.[4] Unlike the other gluconeogenic enzyme deficiencies, PGK deficiency is X-linked, with male patients being affected more severely and usually culminate in death in infancy. There are no reports of deficiencies in glucose production or other difficulties in gluconeogenesis with PGK1 deficiency.

Glyceraldehyde 3-Phosphate Dehydrogenase

Glyceraldehyde-3-phosphate dehydrogenase (GAPDH) catalyzes the reversible conversion of 1,3-bisphosphoglycerate to G3P. This reaction also yields NAD^+ and P_i. GAPDH exists as an ubiquitous enzyme synthesized from a single gene.[136] GAPDH is considered the preeminent "housekeeping" gene whose expression is crucial not only in glycolysis but has been identified as having many essential, albeit unrelated (moonlighting), roles in phosphotransferase activity, membrane dynamics, microtubule complexes, RNA transport, DNA replication, and DNA repair.[137] There are only two reports of a GAPDH deficiency[138,139] in which the loss of activity was mild and caused hereditary nonspherocytic hemolytic anemia. Complete absence of GAPDH would be expected to be developmentally lethal.

Recently, GAPDH-mutant mouse lines were created and characterized.[140] Not surprisingly, nearly all lines homozygous for mutations that lead to complete loss of GAPDH activity resulted in GAPDH knockouts, which proved embryonically lethal with mortality occurring shortly after implantation. Given the critical and diverse roles of GAPDH, it follows that organisms cannot survive without this enzyme. However, heterozygotes were viable and quantification of GAPDH levels was measured. These mice showed no significant phenotype associated with as little as 10% GAPDH activity and had no symptoms of hemolytic anemia. The effects of this GAPDH deficiency on blood glucose levels after fasting were not investigated. Therefore, it is difficult to know what effect reduced GAPDH expression/activity might have on gluconeogenesis. One could imagine maintenance of glucose homeostasis is prohibited, but this is likely secondary to the global and devastating effects on energy metabolism and the critical role GAPDH plays at the intersection of lipid and carbohydrate metabolism (see Figure 3.1).

Triose Phosphate Isomerase

Triose phosphate isomerase (TPI) is a ubiquitous enzyme that catalyzes the interconversion of G3P and DHAP. TPI deficiency is a rare autosomal recessive disorder[1]. Patients exhibit hemolytic anemia, increased susceptibility to infection, progressive neuromuscular impairment, and marked neurological degeneration. Most patients have low levels of residual TPI activity, while no reports have identified patients as being null; therefore, those with TPI deficiency have rather mild effects on the enzyme.[141] Based on the heterozygote frequency of 1 in 25 to 500, one would expect a higher number of TPI deficient cases than has been observed.[142,143] This could likely be due to embryonic lethality or lack of diagnosis due to the mild affects of mutant alleles on patients. Consistent with the former possibility, a deficiency of TPI is embryonically lethal in *tpi*[-/-] mice, while heterozygotes with 50% reduced activity showed no difference in physiological functions.[144] The hemolytic anemia is explained by the loss of the glycolytic enzyme, as seen for many other glycolytic enzyme defects.

Because TPI only equilibrates one-half of the glycolytic intermediates, whether or not TPI deficiency is a metabolic or conformational disease remains unclear. Studies performed on *Drosophila* models have concluded there was no bioenergetic deficit as adenosine triphosphate levels remain normal.[145] However, minimal work has been done on brain tissues of humans with TPI deficiency to determine the basis of the neurological component of disease symptoms. It is known that DHAP can decompose to methylglyoxal, which can form advanced glycation end products, and in particular is toxic to neurons.[146] Alternative theories for the neurological symptoms have been postulated. Some suggest that mutant TPI proteins are forming aggregates in the brain[147] leading to similar phenotypes seen in diseases such as Alzheimer's and Parkinson's. TPI is known to bind to microtubules,[148] which is a large component of neuronal axons, and mutations resulting in perturbation of this binding could cause structural defects.

The TPI deficiency is one of the most severe of any glycolytic enzyme deficiencies with the underlying causes being controversial. Nevertheless, there are no reports of symptoms related to gluconeogenesis.[1]

Glucophosphate Isomerase

Glucophosphate isomerase (GPI), also known as phosphoglucose isomerase, exists as an ubiquitous enzyme that catalyzes the interconversion of Fru 6-P and Glc 6-P. GPI deficiency has been reported in approximately 50 individuals with patients having hemolytic anemia with variable levels of severity and a few patients reported with neurological dysfunction,[149] unlike the more common neurological defects in TPI deficiency. Patients generally harbor missense mutations in the GPI gene (*gpi*) and have varying amounts of residual enzyme activity. Mice with a deficiency of GPI activity were found in mutagenic experiments, and they were shown to serve as an animal model for GPI deficiency.[150] Mice with 10% to 20% residual activity were characterized, and they mimicked the hemolytic syndrome seen in humans with GPI deficiency. Decreased viability for some homozygous mice indicated that complete loss of GPI activity is lethal. No reports of patients harboring two null alleles have ever been identified,[151] suggesting that loss of GPI, like aldolase A, GAPDH, and TPI, would be incompatible with development. Neither patients nor these animals were studied under conditions that would test the effect of GPI deficiency on gluconeogenesis and/or glucose homeostasis.

Summary

The American College of Medical Genetics and the March of Dimes Foundation recommends that newborns have blood taken within a few days of birth and standard analysis be performed for 29 disorders.[152] Currently, none of the disorders/deficiencies reported in this chapter on gluconeogenesis are included. When suspected, the diagnosis of these enzyme deficiencies is performed by mutational analysis, including whole exome sequencing and next-generation sequencing, or measuring enzyme activity in a liver biopsy samples, or, in some cases, measuring activity in fibroblasts cultured from patients.

Gluconeogenesis, while a major pathway for maintaining glucose homeostasis, is also an integral means for providing multiple intermediates required for overall biosynthesis. Loss of function of the gluconeogenic pathway-specific enzymes, PC, PCK, FBP, and G6PC, cause rare diseases that, as expected, manifest in the liver and cause multiple disruptions in nitrogen, redox, and lipid metabolism, in addition to hypoglycemia. Defects in the enzymes common to glycolysis generally show pathologies in cells where generation of adenosine triphosphate is crucial (erythrocytes, in the form of hemolytic anemia and muscle in the form of rhabdomyolysis) and in the brain, where it is likely many of these enzymes are exerting various moonlighting functions. In nearly all cases, questions regarding gluconeogenesis remain. Are the liver and kidney the only sites of glucose production from pyruvate? Evidence taken from liver-specific *pck*$^{-/-}$ mice, patients diagnosed with FBP deficiency, and HFI suggests not. To what degree gluconeogenesis interfaces with other pathways is still unfolding. It is clear that metabolic pathways are intricately linked whereby a change in one pathway can redirect flux resulting in dramatic and sometimes surprising outcomes.

Deficiencies in Other Pathways That Affect Gluconeogenesis

Multiple enzymes and transporters are necessary for proper fatty acid oxidation. Mutations in any of these proteins can cause serious defects. While these enzymes are not involved in gluconeogenesis specifically, the disease symptoms can manifest as hypoglycemia, which at first glance could be seen as deficiencies of gluconeogenesis. Carnitine palmitoyl transferase (CPT type IA) is located on the inner mitochondrial membrane and is essential for the transport of long-chain fatty acids from the cytoplasm into the mitochondrial matrix. The acyl-CoA dehydrogenases (VLCAD, LCAD, MCAD, and SCAD) are responsible for starting the sequential degradation of fatty acids to acetyl-CoA to be used in the liver for ketone-body synthesis or in the muscle as part of the citric acid cycle. A deficiency of hepatic CPT type IA,[153] VLCAD, LCAD, MCAD, and SCAD[154] can cause severe hypoglycemia indirectly due to the physiological demand for glucose by tissues that normally utilize ketone bodies (heart, brain, and muscle). With the loss of acetyl-CoA, the ability of the liver to synthesize ketone bodies is impaired. Tissues that prefer ketone bodies for energy production resort to using glucose, and the extra demand leads to hypoglycemia.

References

1. Orosz F, Olah J, Ovadi J. Triosephosphate isomerase deficiency: facts and doubts. *IUBMB Life*. 2006; 58; 703–715.
2. Hakimi P, Johnson MT, Yang J, et al. Phosphoenolpyruvate carboxykinase and the critical role of cataplerosis in the control of hepatic metabolism. *Nutr Metab*. 2005; 2: 33.
3. Chen Y-T. Glycogen storage diseases. In: Scriver CR, Beaudet AL, Sly WS, Valle D, eds. *The Metabolic and Molecular Basis of Inherited Disease*. New York: McGraw-Hill; 2001:1521–1551.
4. Spiegel R, Gomez EA, Akman HO, et al. Myopathic form of phosphoglycerate kinase (PGK) deficiency: a new case and pathogenic considerations. *Neuromuscul Disord*. 2009; 19: 207–211.
5. Beutler E. PGK deficiency. *Br J Haematol*. 2007; 136: 3–11.
6. Naini A, Toscano A, Musumeci O, et al. Muscle phosphoglycerate mutase deficiency revisited. *Arch Neurol*. 2009; 66: 394–398.
7. Climent F, Roset F, Repiso A, Perez de la Ossa P. Red cell glycolytic enzyme disorders caused by mutations: an update. *Cardiovasc Hematol Disord Drug Targets*. 2009; 9: 95–106.
8. Monnot S, Serre V, Chadefaux-Vekemans B, et al. Structural insights on pathogenic effects of novel mutations causing pyruvate carboxylase deficiency. *Hum Mutat*. 2009; 30: 734–740.
9. Jitrapakdee S, Booker GW, Cassady AI, Wallace JC. Cloning, sequencing and expression of rat liver pyruvate carboxylase. *Biochem J*. 1996; 316 (Pt 2): 631–637.
10. Benjamin AM, Quastel JH. Fate of L-glutamate in the brain. *J Neurochem*. 1974; 23: 457–464.
11. Cooper AJ, Plum F. Biochemistry and physiology of brain ammonia. *Physiol Rev*. 1987; 67: 440–519.
12. Wexler ID, Du Y, Lisgaris MV, et al. Primary amino acid sequence and structure of human pyruvate carboxylase. *Biochim Biophys Acta*. 1994; 1227: 46–52.
13. Barden RE, Scrutton MC. Pyruvate carboxylase from chicken liver: effects of univalent and divalent cations on catalytic activity. *J Biol Chem*. 1974; 249: 4829–4838.
14. Barrit GJ. Resolution of gluconeogenic flux by pyruvate carboxylase. In: Keech, DB, Wallace JC, eds. *Pyruvate Carboxylase*. Boca Raton, FL: CRC Press; 1985: 141–155.
15. von Glutz G, Walter P. Regulation of pyruvate carboxylation by acetyl-CoA in rat liver mitochondria. *FEBS Lett*. 1976; 72: 299–303.
16. Robinson BH. Lactic acidemia: disorders of pyruvate carboxylase and pyruvate dehydrogenase. Scriver CR, Beaudet AL, Sly WS, Valle D, eds. *The Metabolic and Molecular Basis of Inherited Disease*. New York: McGraw-Hill; 2001: 2275–2295.
17. Robinson BH, Oei J, Saudubray JM, et al. The French and North American phenotypes of pyruvate carboxylase deficiency, correlation with biotin containing protein by 3H-biotin incorporation, 35S-streptavidin labeling, and Northern blotting with a cloned cDNA probe. *Am J Hum Genet*. 1987; 40: 50–59.
18. Modaressi S, Christ B, Bratke J, et al. Molecular cloning, sequencing and expression of the cDNA of the mitochondrial form of phosphoenolpyruvate carboxykinase from human liver. *Biochem J*. 1996; 315 (Pt 3): 807–814.

19. Modaressi S, Brechtel K, Christ B, Jungermann K. Human mitochondrial phosphoenolpyruvate carboxykinase 2 gene: structure, chromosomal localization and tissue-specific expression. *Biochem J*. 1998; 333 (Pt 2): 359–366.
20. She P, Shiota M, Shelton KD, et al. Phosphoenolpyruvate carboxykinase is necessary for the integration of hepatic energy metabolism. *Mol Cell Biol*. 2000; 20: 6508–6517.
21. Hanson RW, Reshef L. Regulation of phosphoenolpyruvate carboxykinase (GTP) gene expression. *Annu Rev Biochem*. 1997; 66: 581–611.
22. Hanson RW, Patel YM. Phosphoenolpyruvate carboxykinase (GTP): the gene and the enzyme. *Adv Enzymol Relat Areas Mol Biol*. 1994; 69: 203–281.
23. Clayton PT, Hyland K, Brand M, Leonard JV. Mitochondrial phosphoenolpyruvate carboxykinase deficiency. *Eur J Ped*. 1986; 145: 46–50.
24. Vidnes J, Sovik O. Gluconeogenesis in infancy and childhood. III: deficiency of the extramitochondrial form of hepatic phosphoenolpyruvate carboxykinase in a case of persistent neonatal hypoglycaemia. *Acta Pediatr Scand*. 1976; 65: 307–312.
25. Robinson BH, Taylor J, Sherwood, WG. The genetic heterogeneity of lactic acidosis: occurrence of recognizable inborn errors of metabolism in pediatric population with lactic acidosis. *Pediat Res*. 1980; 14: 956–962.
26. Hommes FA, Bendien K, Elema JD, Bremer HJ, Lombeck I. Two cases of phosphoenolpyruvate carboxykinase deficiency. *Acta Pediatr Scand*. 1976; 65: 233–240.
27. Atkin BM, Buist NR, Utter MF, Leiter AB, Banker BQ. Pyruvate carboxylase deficiency and lactic acidosis in a retarded child without Leigh's disease. *Pediat Res*. 1979; 13: 109–116.
28. Sturner WQ, Susa JB. Sudden infant death and liver phosphoenolpyruvate carboxykinase analysis. *Forensic Sci Int*. 1980; 16: 19–28.
29. Prandota J. Possible pathomechanisms of sudden infant death syndrome: key role of chronic hypoxia, infection/inflammation states, cytokine irregularities, and metabolic trauma in genetically predisposed infants. *Am J Ther*. 2004; 11: 517–546.
30. She P, Burgess SC, Shiota M, et al. Mechanisms by which liver-specific PEPCK knockout mice preserve euglycemia during starvation. *Diabetes*. 2004; 52: 1649–1654.
31. Ballard FJ, Hanson RW. Phosphoenolpyruvate carboxykinase and pyruvate carboxylase in developing rat liver. *Biochem J*. 1967; 104: 866–871.
32. Burgess SC, Hausler N, Merritt M, et al. Impaired tricarboxylic acid cycle activity in mouse livers lacking cytosolic phosphoenolpyruvate carboxykinase. *J Biol Chem*. 2004; 279: 48941–48949.
33. Marcolongo P, Fulceri R, Gamberucci A, et al. Multiple roles of glucose-6-phosphatases in pathophysiology: state of the art and future trends. *Biochim Biophys Acta*. 2012; 1830: 2608–2618.
34. Joseph SE, Heaton N, Potter D, et al. Renal glucose production compensates for the liver during the anhepatic phase of liver transplantation. *Diabetes*. 2000; 49: 450–456.
35. Lauritsen TL, Grunnet N, Rasmussen A, Secher NH, Quistorff B. The effect of hepatectomy on glucose homeostasis in pig and in man. *J Hepatol*. 2002; 36: 99–104.
36. Tillmann H, Eschrich K. Isolation and characterization of an allelic cDNA for human muscle fructose-1,6-bisphosphatase. *Gene*. 1998; 212: 295–304.
37. Steinmann B, Gitzelmann R, Van den Berghe G. Disorders of fructose metabolism. In: Scriver CR, Beaudet AL, Sly WS, Valle D, eds. *The Metabolic and Molecular Basis of Inherited Disease*. New York: McGraw-Hill; 2001:1489–1520.
38. Kikawa Y, Inuzuka M, Jin BY, et al. Identification of genetic mutations in Japanese patients with fructose-1,6-bisphosphatase deficiency. *Am J Hum Genet*. 1997; 61: 852–861.
39. Matsuura T, Chinen Y, Arashiro R, et al. Two newly identified genomic mutations in a Japanese female patient with fructose-1,6-bisphosphatase (FBPase) deficiency. *Mol Genet Metab*. 2002; 76: 207–210.
40. Baerlocher K, Gitzelmann R, Nussli R, Dumermuth G. Infantile lactic acidosis due to hereditary fructose1,6-diphosphatase deficiency. *Helv Paediat Acta*. 1971; 26: 489–506.
41. Nagai T, Yokoyama T, Hasegawa T, Tsuchiya Y, Matsuo N. Fructose and glucagon loading in siblings with fructose-1,6-diphosphatase deficiency in fed state. *J Inherit Metab Dis*. 1992; 15: 720–722.
42. Van den Berghe G., Hue L., Hers HG. Effect of the administration of fructose on the glycogenolytic action of glycogen. Biochem J. 1973; 134: 637.
43. Maddaiah VT, Madsen NB. Kinetics of purified liver phosphorylase. *J Biol Chem*. 1996; 241: 3873–3881.

44. Kaufmann U, Froesch ER. Inhibition of phosphorylase-a by fructose-1-phosphate, alpha-glycerophosphate and fructose-1,6-diphosphate: explanation for fructose-induced hypoglycaemia in hereditary fructose intolerance and fructose-1,6-diphosphatase deficiency. *Eur J Clin Invest*. 1973; 3: 407–413.
45. Thurston JH, Jones EM, Hauhart RE. Decrease and inhibition of liver glycogen phosphorylase after fructose: an experimental model for the study of hereditary fructose intolerance. *Diabetes*. 1974; 23: 597–604.
46. Pagliara AS, Karl IE, Haymond M, Kipnis DM. Hypoglycemia in infancy and childhood. II. *J Ped*. 1973; 82: 558–577.
47. Pagliara AS, Karl IE, Haymond M, Kipnis DM. Hypoglycemia in infancy and childhood. I. *J Ped*. 1973; 82: 365–379.
48. van Schaftingen E, Gerin I. The glucose-6-phosphatase system. *Biochem J*. 2002; 362: 513–532.
49. Pan CJ, Lei KJ, Annabi B, Hemrika W, Chou JY. Transmembrane topology of glucose-6-phosphatase. *J Biol Chem*. 1998; 273: 6144–6148.
50. Petrolonis AJ, Yang Q, Tummino PJ, et al. Enzymatic characterization of the pancreatic islet-specific glucose-6-phosphatase-related protein (IGRP). *J Biol Chem*. 2004; 279: 13976–13983.
51. Martin CC, Bischof LJ, Bergman B, et al. Cloning and characterization of the human and rat islet-specific glucose-6-phosphatase catalytic subunit-related protein (IGRP) genes. *J Biol Chem*. 2001; 276: 25197–25207.
52. Wang Y, Oeser JK, Yang C, et al. Deletion of the gene encoding the ubiquitously expressed glucose-6-phosphatase catalytic subunit-related protein (UGRP)/glucose-6-phosphatase catalytic subunit-beta results in lowered plasma cholesterol and elevated glucagon. *J Biol Chem*. 2006; 281: 39982–39989.
53. Guionie O, Clottes E, Stafford K, Burchell A. Identification and characterisation of a new human glucose-6-phosphatase isoform. *FEBS Lett*. 2003; 551: 159–164.
54. Ghosh A, Shieh JJ, Pan CJ, Chou JY. Histidine 167 is the phosphate acceptor in glucose-6-phosphatase-beta forming a phosphohistidine enzyme intermediate during catalysis. *J Biol Chem*. 2004; 279: 12479–12483.
55. Shieh JJ, Pan CJ, Mansfield BC, Chou JY. A potential new role for muscle in blood glucose homeostasis. *J Biol Chem*. 2004; 279: 26215–26219.
56. Shieh JJ, Pan CJ, Mansfield BC, Chou JY. A glucose-6-phosphate hydrolase, widely expressed outside the liver, can explain age-dependent resolution of hypoglycemia in glycogen storage disease type Ia. *J Biol Chem*. 2003; 278: 47098–47103.
57. Ghosh A, Cheung YY, Mansfield BC, Chou JY. Brain contains a functional glucose-6-phosphatase complex capable of endogenous glucose production. *J Biol Chem*. 2005; 280: 11114–11119.
58. Martin CC, Oeser JK, Svitek CA, et al. Identification and characterization of a human cDNA and gene encoding a ubiquitously expressed glucose-6-phosphatase catalytic subunit-related protein. *J Mol Endocrinol*. 2002; 29: 205–222.
59. Cheung YY, Kim SY, Yiu WH, et al. Impaired neutrophil activity and increased susceptibility to bacterial infection in mice lacking glucose-6-phosphatase-beta. *J Clin Invest*. 2007; 117: 784–793.
60. Boztug K, Appaswamy G, Ashikov A, et al. A syndrome with congenital neutropenia and mutations in G6PC3. *N Engl J Med*. 2009; 360: 32–43.
61. Belkaid A, Copland IB, Massillon D, Annabi B. Silencing of the human microsomal glucose-6-phosphate translocase induces glioma cell death: potential new anticancer target for curcumin. *FEBS Lett*. 2006; 580: 3746–3752.
62. Gerin I, Veiga-da-Cunha M, Achouri Y, Collet JF, Van Schaftingen E. Sequence of a putative glucose 6-phosphate translocase, mutated in glycogen storage disease type Ib. *FEBS Lett*. 1997; 419: 235–238.
63. Ihara K, Nomura A, Hikino S, Takada H, Hara T. Quantitative analysis of glucose-6-phosphate translocase gene expression in various human tissues and haematopoietic progenitor cells. *J Inherit Metab Dis*. 2000; 23: 583–592.
64. Gerin I, Veiga-da-Cunha M, Noel G, Van Schaftingen E. Structure of the gene mutated in glycogen storage disease type Ib. *Gene*. 1999; 227: 189–195.
65. Arion WJ, Wallin BK, Lange AJ, Ballas LM. On the involvement of a glucose 6-phosphate transport system in the function of microsomal glucose 6-phosphatase. *Mol Cell Biochem*. 1975; 6: 75–83.
66. Stuart CA, Yin D, Howell ME, et al. Hexose transporter mRNAs for GLUT4, GLUT5, and GLUT12 predominate in human muscle. *Am J Physiol Endocrinol Metab*. 2006; 291: E1067–1073.
67. Thorens B, Mueckler M. Glucose transporters in the 21st Century. *Am J Physiol Endocrinol Metab*. 2010; 298: E141–145.

68. Burchell A. A re-evaluation of GLUT 7. *Biochem J.* 1998; 331 (Pt 3): 973.
69. Waddell ID, Zomerschoe AG, Voice MW, Burchell A. Cloning and expression of a hepatic microsomal glucose transport protein: comparison with liver plasma-membrane glucose-transport protein GLUT 2. *Biochem J.* 1992; 286 (Pt 1): 173–177.
70. Karim S, Adams D, Lalor P. Hepatic expression and cellular distribution of the glucose transporter family. *World J Gastroenterol.* 2012; 18: 6771–6781.
71. Segade F. Glucose transporter 10 and arterial tortuosity syndrome: the vitamin C connection. *FEBS Lett.* 2010; 584: 2990–2994.
72. Takanaga H, Frommer WB. Facilitative plasma membrane transporters function during ER transit. *Faseb J.* 2010; 24: 2849–2858.
73. Meissner G, Allen R. Evidence for two types of rat liver microsomes with differing permeability to glucose and other small molecules. *J Biol Chem.* 1981; 256: 6413–6422.
74. Marcolongo P, Fulceri R, Giunti R, Burchell A, Benedetti A. Permeability of liver microsomal membranes to glucose. *Biochem Biophys Res Commun.* 1996; 219: 916–922.
75. Banhegyi G, Marcolongo P, Burchell A, Benedetti A. Heterogeneity of glucose transport in rat liver microsomal vesicles. *Arch Biochem Biophys.* 1998; 359: 133–138.
76. Melis D, Havelaar AC, Verbeek E, et al. NPT4, a new microsomal phosphate transporter: mutation analysis in glycogen storage disease type Ic. *J Inherit Metab Dis.* 2004; 27: 725–733.
77. Waddell ID, Lindsay JG, Burchell A. The identification of T2; the phosphate/pyrophosphate transport protein of the hepatic microsomal glucose-6-phosphatase system. *FEBS Lett.* 1988; 229: 179–182.
78. Chen SY, Pan CJ, Nandigama K, et al. The glucose-6-phosphate transporter is a phosphate-linked antiporter deficient in glycogen storage disease type Ib and Ic. *Faseb J.* 2008; 22: 2206–2213.
79. Marcolongo P, Fulceri R, Giunti R, et al. The glucose-6-phosphate transport is not mediated by a glucose-6-phosphate/phosphate exchange in liver microsomes. *FEBS Lett.* 2012; 586: 3354–3359.
80. Laver DR, Lenz GK, Dulhunty AF. Phosphate ion channels in sarcoplasmic reticulum of rabbit skeletal muscle. *J Physiol.* 2001; 535: 715–728.
81. Guillam MT, Burcelin R, Thorens B. Normal hepatic glucose production in the absence of GLUT2 reveals an alternative pathway for glucose release from hepatocytes. *Proc Natl Acad Sci USA.* 1998; 95: 12317–12321.
82. Berteloot A, Vidal H, van de Werve G. Rapid kinetics of liver microsomal glucose-6-phosphatase: evidence for tight-coupling between glucose-6-phosphate transport and phosphohydrolase activity. *J Biol Chem.* 1991; 266: 5497–5507.
83. Vidal H, Berteloot A, Larue MJ, St-Denis JF, van de Werve G. Interaction of mannose-6-phosphate with the hysteretic transition in glucose-6-phosphate hydrolysis in intact liver microsomes. *FEBS Lett.* 1992; 302: 197–200.
84. St-Denis JF, Berteloot A, Vidal H, Annabi B, van de Werve G. Glucose transport and glucose 6-phosphate hydrolysis in intact rat liver microsomes. *J Biol Chem.* 1995; 270: 21092–21097.
85. Xie W, van de Werve G, Berteloot A. An integrated view of the kinetics of glucose and phosphate transport, and of glucose 6-phosphate transport and hydrolysis in intact rat liver microsomes. *J Membr Biol.* 2001; 179: 113–126.
86. St-Denis JF, Comte B, Nguyen DK, et al. A conformational model for the human liver microsomal glucose-6-phosphatase system: evidence from rapid kinetics and defects in glycogen storage disease type 1. *J Clin Endocrinol Metabol.* 1994; 79: 955–959.
87. Lei KJ, Chen H, Pan CJ, et al. Glucose-6-phosphatase dependent substrate transport in the glycogen storage disease type-1a mouse. *Nat Genet.* 1996; 13: 203–209.
88. Foster JD, Nordlie RC. The biochemistry and molecular biology of the glucose-6-phosphatase system. *Exp Biol Med* (Maywood). 2002; 227: 601–608.
89. Jorgenson RA, Nordlie RC. Multifunctional glucose-6-phosphatase studied in permeable isolated hepatocytes. *J Biol Chem.* 1980; 255: 5907–5915.
90. Nordlie RC, Jorgenson RA. Latency and inhibitability by metabolites of glucose-6-phosphatase of permeable hepatocytes from fasted and fed rats. *J Biol Chem.* 1981; 256: 4768–4771.
91. Cori GT, Cori CF. Glucose-6-phosphatase of the liver in glycogen storage disease. *J Biol Chem.* 1952; 199: 661–667.
92. Chou JY, Mansfield BC. Mutations in the glucose-6-phosphatase-alpha (G6PC) gene that cause type Ia glycogen storage disease. *Hum Mutat.* 2008; 29: 921–930.

93. Lange AJ, Arion WJ, Beaudet AL. Type Ib glycogen storage disease is caused by a defect in the glucose-6-phosphate translocase of the microsomal glucose-6-phosphatase system. *J Biol Chem*. 1980; 255: 8381–8384.
94. Nordlie RC, Sukalski KA, Munoz JM, Baldwin JJ. Type Ic, a novel glycogenosis: underlying mechanism. *J Biol Chem*. 1983; 258: 9739–9744.
95. Burchell A, Gibb L. Diagnosis of type 1B and 1C glycogen storage disease. *J Inherit Metab Dis*. 1991; 14: 305–307.
96. Lin B, Hiraiwa H, Pan CJ, Nordlie RC, Chou JY. Type-1c glycogen storage disease is not caused by mutations in the glucose-6-phosphate transporter gene. *Hum Genet*. 1999; 105: 515–517.
97. Lei KJ, Shelly LL, Lin B, et al. Mutations in the glucose-6-phosphatase gene are associated with glycogen storage disease types 1a and 1aSP but not 1b and 1c. *J Clin Invest*. 1995; 95: 234–240.
98. Veiga-da-Cunha M, Gerin I, Chen YT, et al. The putative glucose 6-phosphate translocase gene is mutated in essentially all cases of glycogen storage disease type I non-a. *Eur J Hum Genet*. 1999; 7: 717–723.
99. Gitzelmann R, Bosshard NU. Defective neutrophil and monocyte functions in glycogen storage disease type Ib: a literature review. *Eur J Ped*. 1993; 152 (Suppl. 1): S33–S38.
100. Collins JE, Bartlett K, Leonard JV, Aynsley-Green A. Glucose production rates in type 1 glycogen storage disease. *J Inherit Metab Dis*. 1990; 13: 195–206.
101. Tsalikian E, Simmons P, Gerich JE, Howard C, Haymond MW. Glucose production and utilization in children with glycogen storage disease type I. *Am J Physiol*. 1984; 247: E513–E519.
102. Kalhan SC, Gilfillan C, Tserng KY, Savin SM. Glucose production in type I glycogen storage disease. *J Ped*. 1982; 101: 159–160.
103. Mutel E, Abdul-Wahed A, Ramamonjisoa N, et al. Targeted deletion of liver glucose-6 phosphatase mimics glycogen storage disease type 1a including development of multiple adenomas. *J Hepatol*. 2011; 54: 529–537.
104. Kishnani PS, Faulkner E, VanCamp S, et al. Canine model and genomic structural organization of glycogen storage disease type Ia (GSD Ia). *Vet Pathol*. 2001; 38: 83–91.
105. Chen LY, Shieh JJ, Lin B, et al. Impaired glucose homeostasis, neutrophil trafficking and function in mice lacking the glucose-6-phosphate transporter. *Hum Mol Genet*. 2003; 12: 2547–2558.
106. Santer R, Schneppenheim R, Dombrowski A, et al. Mutations in GLUT2, the gene for the liver-type glucose transporter, in patients with Fanconi-Bickel syndrome. *Nat Genet*. 1997; 17: 324–326.
107. Garty R, Cooper M, Tabachnik E. The Fanconi syndrome associated with hepatic glycogenosis and abnormal metabolism of galactose. *J Ped*. 1974; 85: 821–823.
108. Kogut MD, Roe TF, Ng W, Nonnel GN. Fructose-induced hyperuricemia: observations in normal children and in patients with hereditary fructose intolerance and galactosemia. *Pediat Res*. 1975; 9: 774–778.
109. Hermann T, Kramer R. Mechanism and regulation of isoleucine excretion in Corynebacterium glutamicum. *Appl Environ Microbiol*. 1996; 62: 3238–3244.
110. Fell DA. Metabolic control analysis: a survey of its theoretical and experimental development. *Biochem J*. 1992; 286: 313–330.
111. Tolan DR, Niclas J, Bruce BD, Lebo RV. Evolutionary implications of the human aldolase-A, -B, -C, and -pseudogene chromosome locations. *Am J Hum Genet*. 1987; 41: 907–924.
112. Penhoet EE, Rutter WJ. Catalytic and immunochemical properties of homomeric and heteromeric combinations of aldolase subunits. *J Biol Chem*. 1971; 246, 318–323.
113. Beutler E, Scott S, Bishop A, et al. Red cell aldolase deficiency and hemolytic anemia: a new syndrome. *Trans Assoc Am Phys*. 1973; 86: 154–166.
114. Yao DC, Tolan DR, Murray M, et al. Hemolytic anemia and severe rhabdomyolysis due to compound heterozygous mutations of the gene for erythrocyte/muscle isozyme of aldolase: ALDOA$^{(Arg303X/Cys338Tyr)}$. *Blood* 2003; 203: 2401–2403.
115. Hers HG, Joassin G. Anomalie de l'aldolase hepatique dans l'intolerance au fructose. *Enzymol Biol Clin*. 1961; 1: 4–14.
116. Beyer PL, Caviar EM, McCallum RW. Fructose intake at current levels in the United States may cause gastrointestinal distress in normal adults. *J Am Diet Assoc*. 2005; 105: 1559–1566.
117. Tolan DR. Molecular basis of hereditary fructose intolerance: mutations and polymorphisms in the human aldolase B gene. *Hum Mutat*. 19995; 6: 210–218.
118. Gentil C, Colin J, Valette AM, Alagille D, LeLong M. Étude du métabolisme glucidique au cours de l'intolérance héréditaire au fructose: essai d'interprétation de l'hypoglucosémie. *Rev Fr Etud Clin Biol*. 1964; 9: 596–607.

119. Steinmann B, Baerlocher K, Gitzelmann R. Hereditäre Störungen des Fruktosestoffwechsels: belastungsproben mit Fruktose, Sorbitol, und Dihydroxyaceton. *Nutritional Metabolism.* 1975; 18 (Suppl. 1): 115.
120. Schapira F, Hatzfeld A, Gregori C. Studies on liver aldolases in hereditary fructose intolerance. *Enzyme.* 1974; 18: 73–83.
121. Funari VA, Crandall JE, Tolan DR. Fructose metabolism in the cerebellum. *Cerebellum.* 2007; 6: 130–140.
122. Funari VA, Herrera VLM, Freeman D, Tolan DR. Genes required for fructose metabolism are expressed in purkinje cells in the cerebellum. *Molec Brain Res.* 2005; 142: 115–122.
123. Pancholi V. Multifunctional alpha-enolase: its role in diseases. *Cell Mol Life Sci.* 2001; 58: 902–920.
124. Wistow GJ, Lietman T, Williams LA, et al. Tau-crystallin/alpha-enolase: one gene encodes both an enzyme and a lens structural protein. *J Cell Biol.* 1988; 107: 2729–2736.
125. Lachant NA, Tanaka KR. Enolase kinetic properties in partial erythrocyte enolase deficiency. *Clinical Research.* 1987; 35: 426a.
126. Lachant NA, Jennings MA, Tanaka KR. Partial erythrocyte enolase deficiency: a hereditary disorder with variable clinical expression. *Blood.* 1986; 68: 55a.
127. Comi GP, Fortunato F, Lucchiari S, et al. Beta-enolase deficiency, a new metabolic myopathy of distal glycolysis. *Ann Neurol.* 2001; 50: 202–207.
128. de Atauri P, Repiso A, Oliva B, et al. Characterization of the first described mutation of human red blood cell phosphoglycerate mutase. *Biochim Biophys Acta.* 2005; 1740: 403–410.
129. Tsujino S, Shanske S, Sakoda S, Fenichel G, DiMauro S. The molecular genetic basis of muscle phosphoglycerate mutase (PGAM) deficiency. *Am J Hum Genet.* 1993; 52: 472–477.
130. Hadjigeorgiou GM, Kawashima N, Bruno C, et al. Manifesting heterozygotes in a Japanese family with a novel mutation in the muscle-specific phosphoglycerate mutase (PGAM-M) gene. *Neuromuscul Disord.* 1999; 9: 399–402.
131. Bresolin N, Ro YI, Reyes M, Miranda AF, DiMauro S. Muscle phosphoglycerate mutase (PGAM) deficiency: a second case. *Neurol.* 1983; 33: 1049–1053.
132. DiMauro S, Miranda AF, Khan S, Gitlin K, Friedman R. Human muscle phosphoglycerate mutase deficiency: newly discovered metabolic myopathy. *Science.* 1981; 212: 1277–1279.
133. Grzeschik KH, Allderdice PW, Grzeschik A, et al. Cytological mapping of human X-linked genes by use of somatic cell hybrids involving an X-autosome translocation (mouse-hamster-human X-linked markers). *Proc Natl Acad Sci USA.* 1972; 69: 69–73.
134. Lay AJ, Jiang XM, Kisker O, et al. Phosphoglycerate kinase acts in tumour angiogenesis as a disulphide reductase. *Nature.* 2000; 408: 869–873.
135. Shirakawa K, Takahashi Y, Miyajima H. Intronic mutation in the PGK1 gene may cause recurrent myoglobinuria by aberrant splicing. *Neurol.* 2006; 66: 925–927.
136. Edwards YH, Clark P, Harris, H. Isozymes of glyceraldehyde-3-phosphate dehydrogenase in man and other mammals. *Ann Hum Genet.* 1976; 40: 67–77.
137. Sirover MA. New insights into an old protein: the functional diversity of mammalian glyceraldehyde-3-phosphate dehydrogenase. *Biochim Biophys Acta.* 1999; 1432: 159–184.
138. Harkness DR. A new erythrocytic enzyme defect with haemolytic anemai: glyceraldehyde-3-phosphate dehdrogenase deficiency. *J Lab Clin Med.* 1966; 68: 879–880.
139. Oski FA, Whaun J. Hemolytic anemia and red cell glyceraldehyde-3-phosphate dehydrogenase (G-3-PD) deficiency. *Clin Res.* 1969; 17: 601.
140. Pretsch W, Favor J. Genetic, biochemical, and molecular characterization of nine glyceraldehyde-3-phosphate dehydrogenase mutants with reduced enzyme activity in Mus musculus. *Mammal Genom.* 2007; 18: 686–692.
141. Schneider AS. Triosephosphate isomerase deficiency: historical perspectives and molecular aspects. *Baillieres Best Pract Res Clin Haematol.* 2000; 13: 119–140.
142. Eber SW, Dunnwald M, Heinemann G, et al. Prevalence of partial deficiency of red cell triosephosphate isomerase in Germany—A study of 3000 people. *Hum Genet.* 1984; 67: 336–339.
143. Mohrenweiser HW, Fielek S. Elevated frequency of carriers for triosephosphate isomerase deficiency in newborn infants. *Pediat Res.* 1982; 16: 960–963.
144. Merkle S, Pretsch W. Characterization of triosephosphate isomerase mutants with reduced enzyme activity in Mus musculus. *Genet.* 1989; 123: 837–844.

145. Celotto AM, Frank AC, Seigle JL, Palladino MJ. Drosophila model of human inherited triosephosphate isomerase deficiency glycolytic enzymopathy. *Genet.* 2006; 174: 1237–1246.
146. Kikuchi S, Shinpo K, Takeuchi M, et al. Glycation—a sweet tempter for neuronal death. *Brain Res Brain Res Rev.* 2003; 41: 306–323.
147. Ovadi J, Orosz F, Hollan S. Functional aspects of cellular microcompartmentation in the development of neurodegeneration: mutation induced aberrant protein-protein associations. *Mol Cell Biochem.* 2004; 256-257: 83–93.
148. Knull HR, Walsh JL. Association of glycolytic enzymes with the cytoskeleton. *Current Topics in Cell Regulation.* 1992; 33: 15–30.
149. Kugler W, Breme K, Laspe P, et al. Molecular basis of neurological dysfunction coupled with haemolytic anaemia in human glucose-6-phosphate isomerase (GPI) deficiency. *Hum Genet.* 1998; 103: 450–454.
150. Merkle S, Pretsch W. Glucose-6-phosphate isomerase deficiency associated with nonspherocytic hemolytic anemia in the mouse: an animal model for the human disease. *Blood.* 1993; 81: 206–213.
151. Kugler W, Lakomek M. Glucose-6-phosphate isomerase deficiency. *Baillieres Best Pract Res Clin Haematol.* 2000; 13: 89–101.
152. Watson MS, Lloyd-Puryear MA, Mann MY, Rinaldo P, Howell RR. Newborn screening: toward a uniform screening panel and system. *Genet Med.* 2006; 8 (Suppl. 1): 1S–252S.
153. Bonnefont JP, Demaugre F, Prip-Buus C, et al. Carnitine palmitoyltransferase deficiencies. *Mol Genet Metab.* 1999; 68: 424–440.
154. Gregersen N, Bross P, Andresen BS. Genetic defects in fatty acid beta-oxidation and acyl-CoA dehydrogenases: molecular pathogenesis and genotype-phenotype relationships. *Eur J Biochem.* 2004; 271: 470–482.

4

Branched Chain Amino Acid Disorders

Irini Manoli and Charles P. Venditti

Basic Biochemical Pathways, Clinical Presentation, Diagnosis and Treatment

Overview of Branched Chain Amino Acids—Biochemistry, Metabolism, Regulation

The branched chain amino acids (BCAAs), leucine, isoleucine, and valine, are three of the nine essential amino acids and comprise almost 20% to 25% of dietary protein intake.[1,2] They can be glucogenic (valine), ketogenic (leucine and isoleucine), or both (isoleucine), since their end products succinyl-CoA and/or acetyl-CoA can (i) enter the Krebs cycle for energy generation and gluconeogenesis through conversion of succinyl-CoA to pyruvate, and/or (ii) act as precursors for lipogenesis or ketone body production through acetyl-CoA and acetoacetate. These amino acids are also critical participants in interorgan metabolic cycles. For example, in the muscle they can serve as nitrogen donors for the synthesis of glutamine and alanine, which are subsequently transferred to the liver for ureagenesis or gluconeogenesis, respectively.[3]

BCAA catabolism has distinct characteristics compared to the metabolism of other essential or nonessential amino acids. Leucine, isoleucine, and valine share the first two steps in their degradation: (1) the readily reversible transamination by BCAA aminotransferases (BCAT), a pyridoxal-phosphate dependent enzyme with cytosolic (BCATc) and mitochondrial (BCATm) isoforms and (2) the irreversible oxidative decarboxylation and coupled thioesterification of the respective ketoacids by the single mitochondrial branched chain keto-acid dehydrogenase (BCKD) complex to form coenzyme A derivatives, which commits them to oxidative metabolism. A detailed biochemical pathway overviewing oxidative BCAA metabolism is provided in Figure 4.1.[4] Circulating BCAA largely escape first-pass hepatic metabolism, due to the low level expression of the mitochondrial

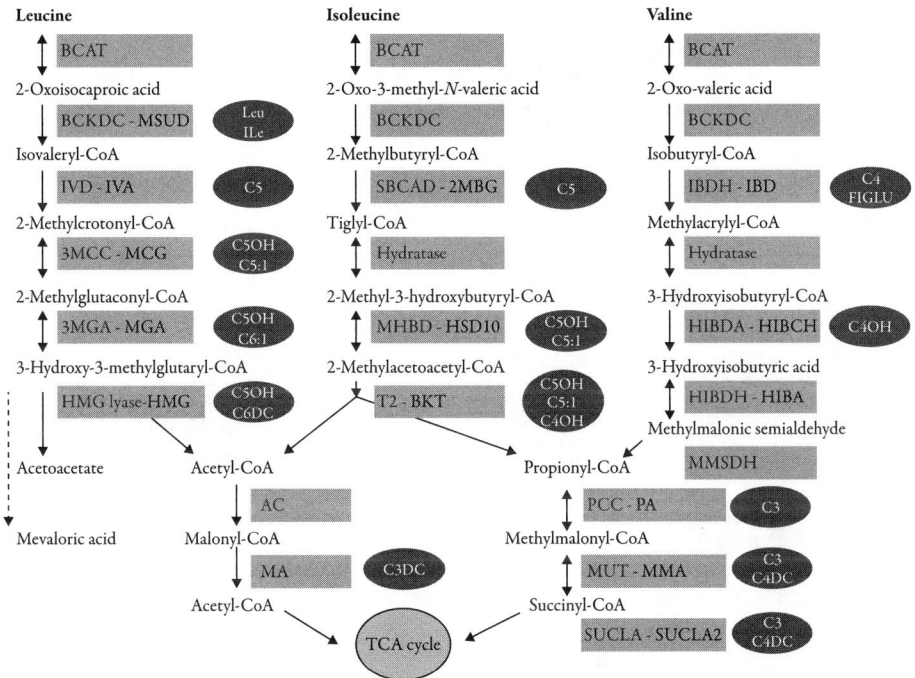

FIGURE 4.1 **Biochemical Pathways of Branched Chain Amino Acid Metabolism.** The enzymatic steps for the metabolism of leucine, isoleucine and valine are provided. Shaded boxes include the acronyms of the enzymes and the associated inborn errors, while ovals depict the metabolites (acylcarnitines or amino acid elevations) used for their detection at newborn screening. *Abbreviations:* BCAT = branched chain amino acid aminotransferase; BCKDC: branched chain α-keto-acid dehydrogenase complex; MSUD = maple syrup urine disease; IVD: isovaleryl CoA dehydrogenase; IVA = isovaleric acidemia; 3-MCC = 3-methylcrotonyl-CoA carboxylase; MCG: 3-methylcrotonylglycinuria; 3-MGA = 3-methylglutaconic aciduria type I; HMGL = 3-hydroxy-3-methylglutaryl-CoA lyase deficiency; SBCAD = methylbutyryl CoA dehydrogenase; 2MBG: 2-Methylbutyrylglycinuria; MHBD–HSD1 = 2-methyl-3-hydroxyisobutyric aciduria; BKT = mitochondrial acetoacetyl-CoA thiolase deficiency; IBDH = isobutyryl-CoA dehydrogenase/deficiency; HIBDA: 3-hydroxy-isobutyryl-CoA deacylase (hydrolase) HIBCH = 3-hydroxyisobutyryl- CoA deacylase deficiency; HIBDH: 3-hydroxyisobutyrate dehydrogenase: HIBA = 3-hydroxyisobutyric aciduria; MMSDH = methylmalonic semialdehyde dehydrogenase deficiency; PCC: propionyl-CoA carboxylase; PA = propionic acidemia; MUT: methylmalonyl-CoA mutase; MMA = methylmalonic acidemia; SUCLA: succinyl-CoA ligase; SUCLA2: *SUCLA2*-related mitochondrial DNA (mtDNA) depletion syndrome; TCA cycle: tricarboxylic acid cycle (Krebs).

BCAT2 or BCATm in the liver; hence, they are primarily metabolized in the skeletal muscle and adipose tissue. Because BCAA are large neutral amino acids (phenylalanine, tryptophan, leucine, methionine, isoleucine, tyrosine, histidine, valine, and threonine), they are transported into the brain and other organs primarily by the L1-neutral amino acid transporter. Therefore, the relative concentrations of and competition for the same transporter affect brain amino acid uptake and the downstream synthesis of various neurotransmitters,[5] an effect with significant pathophysiological and therapeutic implications for the diseases in the BCAA metabolic pathway. BCAAs, especially leucine, have been proven to participate in numerous signaling pathways (Figure 4.2). Leucine is a potent stimulator of the mammalian target of rapamycin complex 1 and downstream targets, including the ribosomal S6 kinase 1 (S6K1) and eukaryotic initiation factor 4E binding

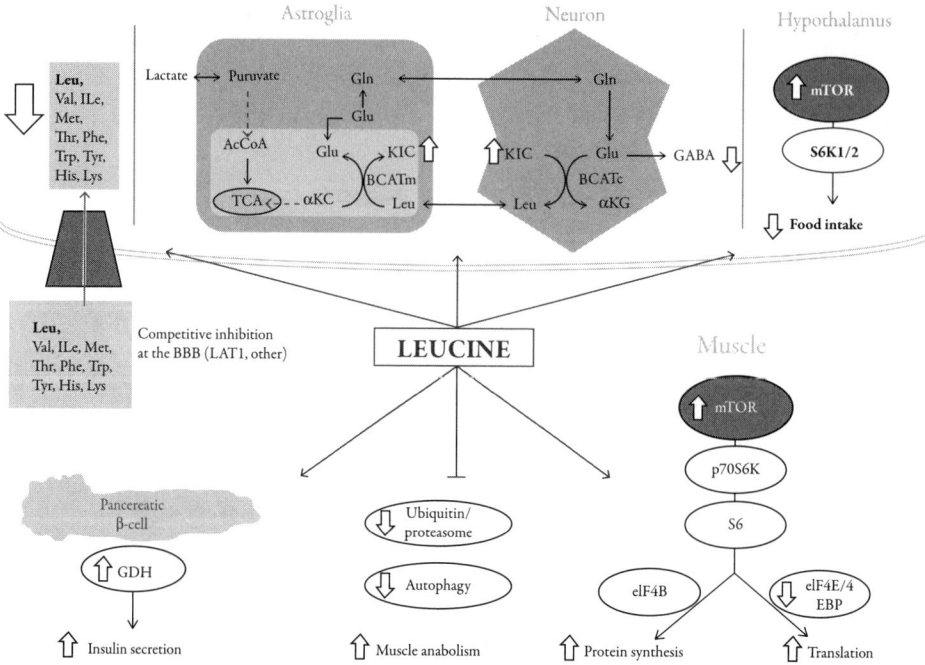

FIGURE 4.2 **Leucine Effects on Different Organ Systems.** In the central nervous system, leucine a) competes for the transport of other large neutral amino acids (tyrosine, phenylalanine, tryptophan, isoleucine, valine, histidine, methionine, glutamine, and threonine) across the blood–brain barrier, because of the low Km of leucine for their shared transporter (L1-neutral amino acid transporter, LAT1); b) disturbs the glutamate/GABA/glutamine cycle between the astrocytes and neurons, depleting the neuronal synapses of glutaminergic neurotransmitters, while increasing the production of ketoisocaproic and leucine and causing secondary mitochondrial dysfunction; c) increases hypothalamic mTOR signaling and decreases food intake. In skeletal muscle, leucine acts through the mammalian target of rapamycin complex 1 pathway to enhance protein synthesis. In addition, it interacts with the ubiquitin-proteasome and the autophagy-lysosome system to promote anabolism. In the pancreas, leucine stimulates insulin secretion from the β-cell and activates glutamate dehydrogenase.

protein 1. The former, in turn, stimulates eukaryotic elongation factor 2 and enhances translation elongation and protein synthesis.[6–8] In addition, leucine may act as an inhibitor of muscle protein breakdown via interactions with the ubiquitin-proteasome and the autophagy-lysosome system.[9] Furthermore, leucine stimulates insulin secretion from the pancreatic β-cell serving as metabolic fuel as well as an allosteric activator of glutamate dehydrogenase.[10–14] Leucine also plays a role in central nervous system food intake regulatory circuits and feeding behavior.[15,16]

The third step in the BCAA metabolic pathway is dehydrogenation of the activated ketoacid by either isovaleryl-CoA dehydrogenase (leucine metabolism) or the α-methyl-branched chain dehydrogenase (isoleucine and valine metabolism). After these first three steps, the metabolism of each of the BCAAs diverges (Figure 4.1) and eventually yields acetyl-CoA and/or propionyl-CoA. Terminal valine metabolism is unique because a free acid, 3-hydroxyisobutyric acid, forms after the hydrolysis of the corresponding thioester. 3-hydroxyisobutyric acid is then dehydrogenated and reacylated to complete metabolism. Rare patients with 3-hydroxyisobutyryl-CoA deacylase (hydrolase)[17,18] or methylmalonic semialdehyde dehydrogenase[19,20] deficiency shed light to the pathophysiology of these complex reactions at the terminal steps of valine metabolism.

The oxidation of BCAAs and BCKAs is tightly regulated primarily at the BCKD step (i) by products of the reaction or substrate analogs, (ii) by phosphorylation, and (c) at the level of transcription; altogether these factors determine the synthesis and activity state of the BCKD complex.[1,4,21] The complex shares many structural and biochemical features with the pyruvate and α-ketoglutarate dehydrogenases.

(a) The BCKD multienzyme complex in the inner mitochondrial membrane is subject to feedback inhibition by branched chain acyl-CoAs, as well as by an increase in the ratio of NADH:NAD+. For example, the addition of oleate and the subsequent increased NADH:NAD+ ratio results in suppression of the oxidative phosphorylation of ketoisocaproate (KIC).

(b) BCKD enzyme activity is tightly regulated through reversible phosphorylation of the E1α at the residue Ser 293. This is achieved by the opposing effects of a kinase, BDK, that inactivates the enzyme and by a mitochondrial type 2C phosphatase (PP2Cm) that activates it. Different tissues have variable percentages of active enzyme, with the heart being the highest and the kidney the lowest percentage of active BCKD in humans.[22] Diet composition and hormonal effects are known modulators of BCKD activity; a high-protein diet, adrenaline, and glucagon stimulate (dephosphorylating) the enzyme complex. Phenylbutyrate has also been found to prevent the inactivation (phosphorylation) of the E1α subunit of the complex, thus enhancing its activity and lowering BCAA levels in maple syrup urine disease (MSUD) patients.[23] The *PP2Cm* knockout mouse model exhibits an intermediate MSUD phenotype, providing yet another potential genetic cause for intermittent or intermediate MSUD in humans.[24]

(c) At the gene expression level, the three different subunits seem to be differentially regulated by a variety of factors, such as glucose, dexamethasone, cAMP, and insulin, among others.[25,26]

MSUD is the only BCAA disorder that can be detected by plasma amino acid analysis, as it is caused by a defect in the second step of BCAA metabolism, resulting in massive plasma elevations of primarily leucine but also isoleucine and valine, as well as their BCKAs, alpha-ketoisocaproate (α-KIC), α-keto-β-methylvaleric, and α-ketoisovaleric acid, deriving from leucine, isoleucine, and valine, respectively. Impaired metabolism of isoleucine leads to the endogenous formation of L-alloisoleucine, which is pathognomonic for MSUD.

For the rest of the disorders described here, the defect lies distal to the nonreversible BCKD reaction, and therefore amino acids and 2-oxo-acids do not accumulate. In contrast, most subsequent reactions in all three pathways of BCAA metabolism lead to accumulation of several intermediates above the block in the respective pathway, resulting in identifiable patterns for each enzyme defect. These inborn errors are detected by tandem mass spectrometry analysis of plasma carnitine esters that are in equilibrium with the respective CoA esters, which is the method used for extended newborn screening, or by gas chromatography-mass-spectrometry analysis of organic acids in the urine and are therefore referred to as organic acidurias.

These include the deficiencies of each of the four enzymes in the catabolism of leucine: isovaleric acidemia, isolated 3-methylcrotonyl-CoA carboxylase deficiency, 3-methylglutaconic aciduria, and 3-hydroxy-2-methylglutaryl-CoA lyase deficiency; three disorders in the metabolism of isoleucine: mitochondrial acetoacetyl-CoA thiolase deficiency, short/branched chain acyl-CoA dehydrogenase deficiency, and 2-methyl-3-hydroxybutyryl-CoA dehydrogenase deficiency; and four disorders of the catabolism of valine: isobutyryl-CoA dehydrogenase deficiency, 3-hydroxyisobutyryl-CoA hydrolase deficiency, 2-hydroxyisobutyric aciduria, and methylmalonic semialdehyde dehydrogenase deficiency. Propionic and methylmalonic acidemia result from a defect in propionyl-CoA oxidation, which represents the final step of the metabolism of valine and isoleucine, as well as other propiogenic substrates, such as methionine, threonine, odd-chain fatty acids, and cholesterol.

For the purpose of this chapter we divide the BCAA metabolic lesions into early (MSUD) versus late (organic acidurias) defects and disorders with conjugation/detoxification (isovaleric acidemia [IVA]) versus not (propionic acidemia [PA], methylmalonic acidemia [MMA]). More common inborn errors, such as MSUD, IVA, 3-methylcrotonyl-CoA carboxylase deficiency (3-MCC), 3-methylglutaconic aciduria (3-MGA), PA, and MMA, will be described in more detail, while descriptions of differential diagnosis, clinical presentation, and treatment for all other disorders are provided in Tables 4.1, 4.2, and 4.3.

Diagnosis by Newborn Screening Versus Symptomatic Presentation

The development of acylcarnitine detection by tandem mass spectrometry (MS/MS) and its widespread implementation for newborn screening has marked a new era in our understanding of many inherited inborn errors of metabolism, as early detection and treatment is changing the natural history of these disorders. On the other hand, many previously unrecognized and possibly benign disease variants now come to medical attention, and it is imperative to achieve a better understanding of their long-term significance in order to develop appropriate follow-up and/or treatment guidelines.

A detailed description of the metabolites and the suggested follow-up algorithms are provided in Table 4.1, while for the most updated information readers are referred to the American College of Medical Genetics' screening ACT sheets and confirmatory algorithms (http://www.acmg.net).

The biggest positive impact by newborn screening has been noted in MSUD, where early detection of classic MSUD infants, comprising about 80% of the MSUD cases, has led to improved management and markedly improved neurological outcome.[27–29] Patients detected by newborn screening are confirmed earlier, have significantly lower concentrations of leucine in their plasma AA analysis on presentation, and require less extracorporeal detoxification methods for initial treatment.[29,30] Concerns, though, have been raised about missing the milder variants of the disease due to insufficient accumulation of toxic

TABLE 4.1 **Symptomatic Diagnosis of BCAA Disorders and Long-Term Outcome**

Disorder	Presenting Symptoms	Clinical Spectrum	Outcome
MSUD	*Classic*: maple syrup odor in cerumen, poor feeding, lethargy/irritability, progressive encephalopathy, opisthotonus, coma *Intermediate*: metabolic intoxication and encephalopathy with stress, anorexia, growth failure, intellectual disability *Intermittent*: normal early development, episodic decompensations with stress *Thiamine responsive*: similar to intermediate, improved biochemical profile with thiamine *Type III, E3 deficient*: Leigh-type encephalopathy, lactic acidosis, often lethal	Cognitive impairment Transient encephalopathy, hyperactivity, focal dystonia, choreoathetosis, ataxia Iatrogenic amino acid or other nutritional deficiencies, osteoporosis, Candida infections, pancreatitis	Intellectual disability depending on time of diagnosis and long-term control ADHD, anxiety, depression
IVA	*Acute*: Metabolic ketoacidosis, hyperammonemia, neutropenia, thrombocytopenia, pancytopenia, poor feeding, vomiting, encephalopathy, "sweaty feet" odor *Chronic intermittent*: Exacerbations during periods of stress or high protein intake with vomiting, dehydration, metabolic ketoacidosis resembling diabetic ketoacidosis *Asymptomatic*: common recurring missense mutation identified at newborn screening, 932C>T (A282V), with partial reduction in IVD activity	Failure to thrive, pancreatitis, pancytopenia with acidotic episodes, myeloproliferative syndrome, Fanconi syndrome, cardiac arrhythmias, intellectual disability	Intellectual disability if diagnosis/treatment is delayed
3-MCC	Acute hypoglycemia, episodic metabolic acidosis, seizures, hypotonia, coma, developmental delay)—rare cases Completely asymptomatic adults (i.e., affected mothers detected through newborn screening)		Intellectual disability in severely affected patients
3-MGA	Intellectual disability, seizures, hepatomegaly, hypotonia	Optic atrophy, dysarthria, ataxia, dementia	Adult-onset progressive leukoencephalopathy
3-Methylglutaconic aciduria type II (Barth syndrome)	X-linked dilated cardiomyopathy, cyclic neutropenia, skeletal myopathy, and mitochondrial respiratory chain dysfunction	Growth retardation	
3-Methylglutaconic aciduria type III (Costeff optic atrophy)	Infantile optic atrophy, extrapyramidal signs, spasticity, ataxia, dysarthria		Intellectual disability
3-Methylglutaconic aciduria type IV: "unclassified"	Encephalomyopathic, hepatocerebral, cardiomyopathic, myopathic forms with mitochondrial respiratory chain dysfunction, MEGDEL association	Cataracts, cardiomyopathy, deafness, lactic acidosis, facial dysmorphism	Intellectual disability

(continued)

TABLE 4.1 Continued

Disorder	Presenting Symptoms	Clinical Spectrum	Outcome
HMGL	Nonketotic hypoglycemia, metabolic acidosis, sensitivity to dietary leucine	Hepatomegaly, early death	
MHBD–HSD1	Chronic or progressive encephalopathy, few cases with acute metabolic decompensation, milder phenotype in female patients	Seizures, optic atrophy, retinopathy, deafness, ataxia, di- or tetraplegia, cardiomyopathy, facial dysmorphism	Static or progressive encephalopathy
SBCAD	Common in the Hmong; detected by newborn screening; affecteds are asymptomatic		Patients manifest with biochemical perturbations only
BKT	Acute intermittent ketoacidosis, vomiting, coma		Intellectual disability (small percentage of patients); mostly excellent outcome with dietary restriction
IBDH	Anemia	Dilated cardiomyopathy	
HIBCH	Congenital malformations, failure to thrive, developmental delay	Failure to thrive	Intellectual disability
HIBA	Brain dysgenesis, multiple congenital malformations, acute ketoacidosis	Failure to thrive	Intellectual disability
MMSDH	Mild clinical symptoms	Asymptomatic	
Malonic aciduria	Developmental delay, hypotonia, hypoglycemia	Seizures, hypertrophic cardiomyopathy	Intellectual disability
PA	Recurrent ketoacidosis, hyperglycinemia, hyperammonemia, coma, neutropenia, thrombocytopenia, hypotonia	Cardiomyopathy, seizures, osteoporosis, pancreatitis	Intellectual disability, spastic quadriparesis, choreoathetosis, dystonia
MMA	Recurrent ketoacidosis, anorexia, failure to thrive, hepatomegaly, hyperglycinemia, hyperammonemia, coma, pancytopenia, hypotonia	Chronic renal failure, renal tubular acidosis, recurrent pancreatitis, osteoporosis, metabolic stroke of the globus pallidus, optic nerve atrophy Bulls' eye maculopathy and blindness (in cblC disease)	Intellectual disability, spastic quadriparesis, choreoathetosis, dystonia

Note. BCAA = branched chain amino acids; MSUD = maple syrup urine disease; IVA = isovaleric acidemia; 3-MCC = 3-methylcrotonyl-CoA carboxylase deficiency; 3-MGA = 3-methylglutaconic aciduria type I; HMGL = 3-hydroxy-3- methylglutaryl-CoA lyase deficiency; MHBD–HSD1 = 2-methyl-3-hydroxyisobutyric aciduria; SBCAD = methylbutyryl CoA dehydrogenase deficiency; BKT = mitochondrial acetoacetyl-CoA thiolase deficiency; IBDH = isobutyryl-CoA dehydrogenase deficiency; HIBCH = 3-hydroxyisobutyryl- CoA deacylase deficiency; HIBA = 3-hydroxyisobutyric aciduria; MMSDH = methylmalonic semialdehyde dehydrogenase deficiency; PA = propionic acidemia; MMA = methylmalonic acidemia.

TABLE 4.2 Differential Diagnosis and Follow-Up of BCAA Disorders Detected by Newborn Screening

Metabolite	Differential Diagnosis	Follow-Up Testing
Leu	MSUD	• Plasma amino acids (leucine, isoleucine, valine, and alloisoleucine), urine ketones and ketoacids (methoximated urine organic acids, dinitrophenylhydrazine test) • Sequencing of the *BCKDHA, BCKDHB, DBT, DLD** genes
	Hydroxyprolinemia (benign)	• Urine organic acids (hydroxyproline)
C5	IVA	• Urine organic acids (IVG), acylglycine and acylcarnitine analysis (isovalerylglycine) • c.932C>T (p.A282V) mutation assay • Sequencing of *IVD* gene
	SBCAD	• Urine organic acids (2MBG), acylglycine and acylcarnitine analysis (2-methylbutyrylglycine, 2-ethylhydracrylic acid) • BCAA metabolism in fibroblasts/lymphocytes • Sequencing of *ACADSB* gene
	Pivalic containing antibiotics	• Urine organic acids (PIV)
C5OH	3-MCC	• Urine organic acids (3-MCC) • Biotinidase assay • Plasma carnitine analysis • Testing of mother (urine organic acids, plasma acylcarnitines) • Enzyme assay in lymphocytes or fibrablasts • Sequencing of *MCC1* or *MCC2* genes
	3-MGA	• Urine organic acids (MGA) • Sequencing of *AUH* gene
	3-Methylglutaconic aciduria type II (Barth syndrome)	• Urine organic acids (MGA) • Sequencing of *TAZ* gene (*X-linked*)
	3-Methylglutaconic aciduria type III (Costeff optic atrophy)	• Urine organic acids (MGA) • Sequencing of *OPA3* gene
	3-Methylglutaconic aciduria type IV	• Sequencing of *POLG1, SUCLA2, DNAJC19, TMEM70*, mtDNA deletion testing
	HMGL	• Urine organic acids (HMG-CoA) • Sequencing of *HMGCL*
	MHBD	• Urine organic acids (2M3HBA, TG, EHA, no 2MAA) • Sequencing of *HSD17B10* gene *(X-linked)*
	T2	• Urine organic acids (ketones, 2MAA, 2M3HBA, TG) • Sequencing of *ACAT1* gene
	Multiple carboxylase deficiency	• Urine organic acids, • Biotinidase and holocarboxylase synthetase activity assays
C4OH	SCHAD deficiency	• Urine organic acids (OH-DCA) • Plasma insulin • Sequencing of *HAD1* gene
	T2	• Urine organic acids (Ketones, 2MAA, 2M3HBA, TG) • Sequencing of *ACAT1* gene
	HIBCH	• Urine organic acids • Sequencing of *HIBCH* gene
C4	SCAD or IBDH	• Urine organic acids (EMA in SCAD) • Urine acylcarnitine and acylglycine analysis • Sequencing of *ACADS, ACAD8, ETHE1*
C4DC	Mitochondrial DNA depletion syndrome-5 and 9	• Urine organic acids (MMA), lactic acidosis • Sequencing of *SUCLA2, SUCLG1* genes
	PA	• Urine organic acids (3-OH-propionic, methylcitrate) • Propionyl-CoA enzyme assay • Sequencing of *PCCA, PCCB*

(continued)

TABLE 4.2 Continued

Metabolite	Differential Diagnosis	Follow-Up Testing
C3	MMA	• Urine organic acids (MMA, 3-OH-propionic, methylcitrate) • Serum B12 level, hydroxocobalamin responsiveness • Plasma homocysteine and MMA concentrations • Mut enzyme assay • Complementation studies • Sequencing of *MUT, MMAA, MMAB, MMACH, MMACHC*, etc.
C3DC	Malonic aciduria	• Urine organic acids (MMA < malonic) • MCD enzyme assay • Sequencing *MLYCD*

Note. BCAA = branched chain amino acids; MSUD = maple syrup urine disease; IVA = isovaleric acidemia; SBCAD = short branched-chain acyl CoA dehydrogenase deficiency; 3-MCC = 3-methylcrotonyl-CoA carboxylase deficiency; 3-MGA = 3-methylglutaconic aciduria type I; HMGL = 3-hydroxy-3-methylglutaryl-CoA lyase deficiency; MHBD = 2-methyl-3-hydroxybutyryl-CoA deficiency; T2 = mitochondrial acetoacetyl-CoA thiolase deficiency; HIBCH = 3-hydroxyisobutyryl- CoA deacylase deficiency; SCAD = short-chain acyl-CoA dehydrogenase deficiency; IBDH = isobutyryl-CoA dehydrogenase deficiency; PA = propionic acidemia; MMA = methylmalonic acidemia; MCD = malonyl-CoA decarboxylase.

metabolites in the immediate neonatal period.[31–33] An increased ratio of Leu/Phe or Leu/Ala and second-tier testing for allo-isoleucine have been proposed to increase sensitivity, but some of the intermediate and intermittent variants of MSUD are expected to escape detection and serve to emphasize the limitations of expanded newborn screening in the diagnosis of all affecteds.

Patients with IVA or beta-ketothiolase deficiency can be detected by newborn screening prior to the onset of symptoms. For both disorders, early initiation of appropriate preventative therapy is expected to significantly reduce morbidity and mortality.

A somewhat more complicated picture is emerging for the disorders in the propionate pathway, where newborn screening may help identify and change the course in the milder patients with methylmalonic (*mut*⁻, cobalamin A and B of isolated MMA or other types of combined MMA and homocystinuria of the cobalamin metabolism pathways) and propionic acidemia but will have little effect on the most severe and devastating end of the spectrum. Early-onset MMA and PA patients may present before screening is initiated in the immediate neonatal period with massive metabolite elevations and hyperammonemia resulting in demise or significant brain damage.[34,35] Despite that fact, though, screening even in those cases of early neonatal lethality will help achieve the diagnosis of an inborn error of metabolism that otherwise might not have been suspected. There also remains a small group of patients with milder variants missed by newborn screening (false negatives), and efforts to develop methods that will improve sensitivity and specificity and integrate secondary markers into screening are underway.[34,36,37]

The application of expanded newborn screening has also resulted in the identification of a number of milder variants of patients with classic organic acidurias, including:

• Patients with IVA (detected by elevated isovaleryl or 3-methylbutyrylcarnitine, C5), who carry a common mutation in the *IVDH* gene 932C>T; A282V in heterozygous or homozygous form that results in partially reduced isovalery-CoA dehydrogenase activity and

TABLE 4.3 **Treatment of BCAA Metabolism Disorders: Conventional Practice and Research Options**

Disorder	Treatment	Research Options
General measures	Fasting avoidance, continuous feeds via G-tube High-caloric diet based on carbohydrate and fat, restriction of branched chain amino acids Micronutrient enrichment L-Carnitine or glycine for conjugation Hemodialysis for removal of toxic metabolites (hyperammonemia) Multidisciplinary care	Organ or cell transplantation Gene therapy Mitochondria-targeted therapies Anaplerotic agents
MSUD	Leucine restriction, high-caloric BCAA-free formulas Valine and isoleucine, glutamine/alanine supplementation (as needed) Thiamine (according to genotype) Multivitamin, minerals Liver transplantation (classic patients)	LNAT analogs (norleucine) for antagonism of brain uptake of leucine Phenylbutyrate to increase enzyme activity in iMSUD Enzyme replacement (TAT-mediated E3 delivery to mitochondria)
IVA	Leucine restriction Glycine supplementation L-Carnitine Multivitamin, minerals	
3-MCC	Fasting avoidance L-Carnitine (Biotin, glycine or leucine restriction—no evidence-based recommendations)	
3-MGA	Leucine restriction L-Carnitine	
HMGL	Leucine and fat restriction L-Carnitine	
MHBD	Isoleucine restriction Antioxidant therapy	
SBCAD	No treatment needed	
BKT	Protein restriction	
IBDH	L-Carnitine	
HIBCH	Protein restriction L-Carnitine	N-acetylcysteine Antioxidants
HIBA	Protein restriction L-Carnitine	
MMSDH	Protein restriction L-Carnitine	
Malonic aciduria	High-carbohydrate, low-fat diet L-Carnitine	
PA	Protein restriction Valine, isoleucine, methionine, threonine free formula L-Carnitine (biotin) Bicarbonate replacement Metronidazole or neomycin for reduction of propiogenic gut flora Liver transplantation	Gene therapy Carglumic acid Mitochondria-targeted treatments Growth hormone

(continued)

TABLE 4.3 Continued

Disorder	Treatment	Research Options
MMA	Protein restriction Valine, isoleucine, methionine, threonine free formula L-Carnitine Bicarbonate replacement Metronidazole or neomycin for reduction of propiogenic gut flora OHCbl (cblA, mut- responsive patients) OHCbl and betaine (in cblC disease) Liver and/or kidney transplant (selected patients)	Gene therapy Antioxidants Mitochondria-targeted treatments Growth hormone Read-through agents (stop mutations)

Note. BCAA = branched chain amino acids; MSUD = maple syrup urine disease; IVA = isovaleric acidemia; 3-MCC = 3-methylcrotonyl-CoA carboxylase deficiency; 3-MGA = 3-methylglutaconic aciduria type I; HMGL = 3-hydroxy-3- methylglutaryl-CoA lyase deficiency; MHBD = 2-methyl-3-hydroxybutyryl-CoA deficiency; SBCAD = methylbutyryl CoA dehydrogenase deficiency; BKT = mitochondrial acetoacetyl-CoA thiolase deficiency; IBDH = isobutyryl-CoA dehydrogenase deficiency; HIBCH = 3-hydroxyisobutyryl-CoA deacylase deficiency; HIBA = 3-hydroxyisobutyric aciduria; MMSDH = methylmalonic semialdehyde dehydrogenase deficiency; PA = propionic acidemia; MMA = methylmalonic acidemia.

mildly increased isovaleryl-CoA derivatives. These individuals have remained completely asymptomatic up to at least 10 years of age[38,39] and comprise up to 47% of the mutant alleles in a reported series of 19 cases detected by newborn screening.[39] The need for follow-up or treatment of these patients is debatable.

- Patients with 3MCC deficiency, detected by elevated C5OH, which is stated to be the most common inborn error of metabolism identified by newborn screening with an incidence of 1:36,000 live births.[40] Most infants detected remain asymptomatic and develop normally, while many affected, apparently healthy, mothers were diagnosed based on the findings of a positive newborn screen in the babies. Despite previous reports describing patients, who present in neonatal crisis, it has been suggested that MCCD is a condition with low clinical expressivity and penetrance that should be excluded from newborn screening to avoid unnecessary psychological and financial burden to families and metabolic care centers.[41] It seems, though, that some affected individuals remain at risk for metabolic crises during severe stress, with the range of presentation varying widely even within the same families.[40, 42–44] Consensus clinical practice protocols have been developed and are awaiting validation from larger clinical trials.[40]

- Patients with short branched-chain acyl-CoA dehydrogenase deficiency (detected by elevated isovaleryl or 3-methylbutyrylcarnitine, C5) can present with a wide phenotypic spectrum, ranging from severe neonatal acidosis[45,46] to transient hypotonia or even completely asymptomatic individuals, especially in the subgroup of patients of Hmong descent.[47,48] This disorder is now considered a biochemical genetic finding only because patients detected through newborn screening are asymptomatic and do not need dietary or cofactor therapy.

- Patients with either short-chain acyl-CoA dehydrogenase deficiency (SCAD) or isobutyryl-CoA dehydrogenase deficiency detected by elevated butyrylcarnitine, C4. Similar to 3-MCC, SCAD is a very frequently detected biochemical disease, with a prevalence of about 1:50,000 live-births and with symptoms that are nonspecific, often transient, and relatively mild, with questionable relation to the biochemical abnormality, while C4 elevations can also be found in completely asymptomatic individuals. Furthermore, two SCAD gene (*ACADS*) variants (511C>T and 625G>A) occur in homozygous or compound heterozygous states in up to 7% of the general population and their clinical importance is uncertain. This represents yet another disease entity about which there is debate in the newborn screening platforms.[49,50] Last, isobutyryl-CoA dehydrogenase deficiency deficiency is a disorder in the valine metabolic pathway caused by a defect in the acyl-CoA dehydrogenase 8, or *IBD* gene.[51-53] A small number of mostly asymptomatic individuals have been reported, with few exceptions, including a patient with anemia, cardiomyopathy, and secondary carnitine deficiency.[54] Algorithms for the follow-up of elevated C4 to include ethylmalonic encephalopathy in the differential diagnosis that can also present with elevated C4 and C5 acylcarnitines have been developed.[55]

Differential Diagnoses and Approaches for Secondary Work-Up

Newborn screening provides a unique opportunity to identify patients with defects in these pathways early in the disease process, leading to accurate diagnosis, initiation of disease-specific diet, and other treatment and better outcomes.

Algorithms outlining the differential diagnosis to consider following detection of abnormal metabolites at newborn screening are increasingly developed to guide physicians in the field and beyond. An outline of the abnormal metabolites detected at newborn screening and the indicated work-up to confirm the diagnosis is provided in Table 4.2. Readers are referred to the American College of Medical Genetics website for the most updated guidelines for follow-up of a positive newborn screening result (https://www.acmg.net/ACMG/Resources/ACT_Sheets_and_Confirmatory_Algorithms/)

A detailed description of the differential diagnosis for each of the disorders is outside the scope of this chapter.

Outcomes and Treatments

In general, early detection and vigilant metabolic control maximizes the chances to avoid significant insults to the developing brain and achieve an optimal outcome for each patient. Caloric support with high-fat and carbohydrate-based diets and special medical foods devoid of offensive amino acids, in order to avoid the generation of toxic by-products in the metabolic pathways, remain the mainstay of dietary management. Overnight feeds by a gastrostomy or jejunostomy tube have been increasingly implemented in the management of patients with organic acidemias and have allowed successful fasting avoidance and easy access for fluid replacement. While the search for small molecules that could minimize disease complications and improve quality of life is ongoing, more drastic treatment options, such as gene and cell therapy and organ transplantation, are being pursued. Similar to the previous section, outcomes and current guidelines for therapy for each of the disorders in the BCAA metabolism are summarized in Tables 4.1 and 4.3. Current therapeutic guidelines and research options are discussed in detail later.

Current Paradigm on Pathogenesis and Interaction With Other Metabolic Pathways

Understanding of the pathophysiology behind the clinical presentation of the various disorders in these pathways has improved significantly with recent studies on an increasing number of disease-specific animal models. For clarity of discussion, we divide the disorders into those in which toxicity from accumulating toxic metabolites proximal to the enzymatic defect plays the key role in the pathogenesis and those in which downstream secondary targets are disrupted, resulting in perturbed cellular physiology, including mitochondrial dysfunction.[56] One of the most well-studied disorders is MSUD, which is the prototype for the first of these disease mechanisms, while distal enzymopathies, including methylmalonic and propionic acidemias, are better represented in the second group, even though massive elevations of abnormal metabolites are present.

Maple Syrup Urine Disease

The acute elevations of leucine and α-KIC during intercurrent illness or other physiologic stress in individuals with MSUD can cause severe acute metabolic encephalopathy and life-threatening cerebral edema, while chronic imbalance in the plasma levels of BCAAs or protein overrestriction can lead to abnormal brain amino acid uptake with subsequent decreased myelin and neurotransmitter synthesis, causing further brain damage manifesting as chronic encephalopathy.[57]

One hypothesis about the metabolism of leucine in the central nervous system is that leucine is transaminated in the astrocytes with α-ketoglutarate to α-KIC and glutamate via the mitochondrial BCAA transaminase reaction (Figure 4.2). Glutamate is subsequently converted to glutamine. The glutamine and α-KIC are released from the astrocytes and taken up in the neurons, where glutamine is converted to glutamate via phosphate-dependent glutaminase and α-KIC is converted back to leucine and pyruvate by reversal of a cytosolic, in this case, BCAA transamination reaction, which is released and transported back to astrocytes, completing the so-called "leucine-glutamate cycle."[58-61] Glutamine produced in glia is thus an essential precursor for the production of glutamate and g-amino-butyric acid (GABA) in the glutamate/GABAergic neurons.

In MSUD accumulation of branched-chain ketoacids (α-KIC) within astrocytes and neurons may drive the reverse transamination toward α-ketoglutarate, resulting in increased α-KG/glutamate ratios. This mechanism may underlie the deficiencies in cerebral glutamate, GABA, glutamine, and aspartate that have been described in MSUD mouse models, as well as postmortem brain of an infant with MSUD.[62,63] This can also inhibit the malate/aspartate shuttle and result in an increased NADH/NAD+ ratio and impaired conversion of lactate to pyruvate,[64] while high α-KIC can inhibit pyruvate dehydrogenase and α-ketoglutarate dehydrogenase, resulting in Krebs cycle dysfunction.[65,66] Defective oxidative phosphorylation is consistent with the high cerebral lactate levels observed in mice and humans during a metabolic crisis.[62,67]

High plasma levels of leucine result in competitive inhibition of the transport of other large neutral amino acids (tyrosine, phenylalanine, tryptophan, isoleucine, valine, histidine, methionine, glutamine, and threonine) across the blood–brain barrier through their shared transporter (L1-neutral amino acid transporter).[62,68,69] Reduced levels of these essential amino acids inhibit protein and neurotransmitter synthesis, such as dopamine, serotonin, histamine, and S-AdoMet, by limiting available precursors. Furthermore, deficiency of branched-chain ketoacid dehydrogenase impairs the production of ketone bodies from leucine that are essential for myelin synthesis. Combined with impaired protein synthesis, this leads to severe dysmyelination.[70,71]

The illustration of the above mechanisms for the pathogenesis of acute and chronic brain injury in MSUD and, more important, the implementation of that knowledge for the development of improved special metabolic formulas, has yielded evidence-based guidelines for the management of this challenging condition.[27,72,73]

Organic Acidurias

In contrast to the "intoxication" from excess leucine that plays a primary role in the pathogenesis of MSUD, the pathophysiology of each of the subsequent blocks in the BCAA metabolic pathways is less well characterized. Following the same paradigm, initial studies have focused on establishing the effects of the accumulation of toxic metabolites proximal to the block in many of the remaining disorders.

In methylmalonic acidemia, deficient activity of methylmalonyl-CoA mutase results in significant accumulation of methylmalonic acid, as well as of propionyl-CoA derived metabolites, such as 3-OH-propionate, 2-methylcitrate (product of the reaction of propionyl-CoA with oxaloacetate), and propionylglycine. Original studies focused on methylmalonic acid as the primary toxin, while subsequent studies suggested a key role for 3-OH-propionate and 2-methylcitrate for the various secondary biochemical alterations seen in MMA, including lactic acidosis, hyperglycinemia, hyperammonemia, and hypoglycemia. It has been proposed that methylmalonyl-CoA, a known inhibitor of pyruvate carboxylase, blocks the formation of oxaloacetate and phosphoenolpyruvate, an important substrate for gluconeogenesis in the liver, thereby increasing lipid catabolism and resulting in hypoglycemia and ketoacidosis.[74] MMA has structural similarities to malonate, a known inhibitor of complex II of the respiratory chain (succinate dehydrogenase) and was shown to induce neuronal damage in vitro, as well as striatal lesions and seizures after intrastriatal administration in rats[75–79]; MMA was also shown to impair the transmitochondrial malate shuttle, another key step in gluconeogenesis, while the formation of methylcitrate disrupts the Krebs cycle, further contributing to the bioenergetic problems that manifest in MMA patients.[80–82] Propionyl-CoA accretion leads to a competitive inhibition of N-acetylglutamate synthase through the excess production of N-propionylglutamate, which in turn leads to the failure of CPS-1 to synthesize carbamoylphosphate, the first step in the urea cycle. Furthermore, Krebs cycle dysfunction caused by (i) the decreased production of succinate due to the block and (ii) the depletion of oxaloacetate via the formation of 2-methylcitrate may result in insufficient α-ketoglutarate (glutamate precursor) production and underlie the paradoxical hyperammonemia in the presence of low glutamate/glutamine that is observed in propionic and methylmalonic acidemia patients during metabolic crises.[83–85] Toxic metabolites also cause decreased H-protein activity resulting in inhibition of the glycine cleavage system and hyperglycinemia.[86,87]

Based on the "toxic metabolite" hypothesis, treatment with protein restriction to reduce the load of the offensive metabolites, as well as supplementation with glycine and/or carnitine to promote the synthesis and excretion of less toxic conjugates, have been the mainstay of treatment for organic acidemias. Disorders for which such conjugation occurs more efficiently, like isovaleric acidemia, are therefore more biochemically responsive compared to defects like propionic or methylmalonic acidemia.

It seems, though, that deficiencies of intermediates downstream the metabolic block, as well as other secondary effects on associated pathways, like the Krebs cycle and oxidative phosphorylation, may have a more significant role in the pathogenesis of these group of disorders (Figure 4.3). Moreover, although they are often grouped together and managed in a similar fashion, it is obvious that they are very different diseases with unique characteristics distinguishing even defects in nearby metabolic steps, such as propionic and methylmalonic acidemia. Despite the similarities in their clinical phenotypes, propionic and methylmalonic acidemia patients have notable differences, with propionic acidemia commonly associated with dilated cardiomyopathy and methylmalonic acidemia with early-onset chronic kidney failure characterized by tubulointerstitial nephritis, both not as common occurrences in the other disorder. The difference in the renal phenotype has led to theories about more nephrotoxic effects of MMA compared to the other metabolic intermediates shared by the two diseases, or effects involving antagonism and inhibition of glutathione uptake by MMA via the dicaboxyclic acid transporter in the proximal tubules leading to glutathione depletion in the mitochondria and increased oxidative stress.[88–90]

Intracellular CoA ester accumulation is considered a key pathogenetic mechanism for many of the organic acidemias and other disorders leading to coenzyme A sequestration,

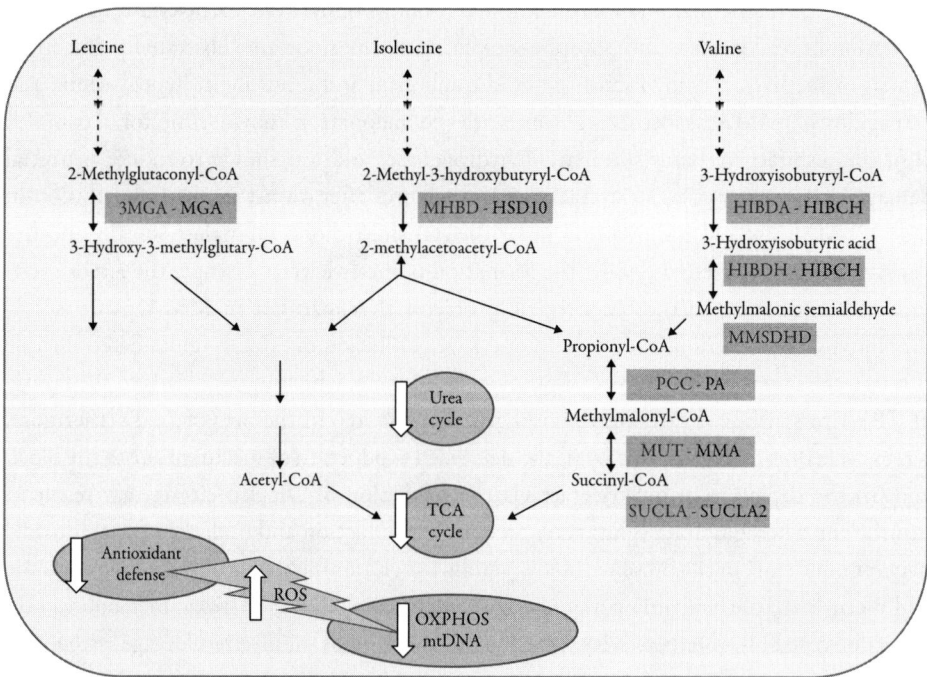

FIGURE 4.3 **Secondary Mitochondrial Dysfunction is Associated with Enzymatic Defects in the Terminal Steps of Branched Chain Amino Acid Metabolism.** Dysfunction of the urea or Krebs cycle and the oxidative phosphorylation or mtDNA maintenance, as well as increased reactive oxygen species (ROS) formation with depletion of antioxidant pools (glutathione), have been observed in disorders caused by defects in distant steps of BCAA metabolic pathways.

toxicity or redistribution (also known as CASTOR).[91] The high concentration of the acyl-CoA substrate of the respective enzyme and/or the subsequent depletion of acetyl- or CoA-SH species may lead to detrimental effects that are primarily localized inside the mitochondria and are characterized by cell autonomy and organ specificity.[91]

Studies in the $Mut^{-/-}$ knock-out and transgenic mice have established that cell-specific mitochondrial ultrastructural changes in the liver, the proximal tubules, and the pancreas are present. Moreover, structural pathology was associated with decreased complex IV (cytochrome c oxidase) enzymatic activity in the liver or the proximal tubules, and increased serum and/or urine markers of oxidative stress, both in mice and patients with MMA.[56,90,92] Subsequent studies confirmed increased oxidative stress (decreased glutathione levels in tissue and plasma levels), decreased OXPHOS enzymatic activities, and mtDNA levels in patients with propionic or mut^0 methylmalonic acidemia[93–97] and suggested a benefit of antioxidants or other mitochondria-targeted therapies in these patients.

A similar picture, where secondary mitochondrial dysfunction is considered a key player in the pathophysiology of the disorder, is observed in the late defects of each of the three biochemical pathways of BCAA metabolism, including 3-MGA, 2-methyl-3-hydroxybutyryl-CoA dehydrogenase, 3-hydroxyisobutyryl-CoA hydrolase, and 3-Hydroxyisobutyric aciduria (HIBA), suggesting a need to study these disorders outside the classic biochemical pathway of BCAA metabolism and rather focus on the intramitochondrial effects caused by the metabolic block. This would also move the treatment target away from dietary modifications and cofactors and into mitochondrial-targeted therapeutic approaches.

3-Methylglutaconic aciduria caused by a deficiency in 3-methylglutaconyl-CoA hydratase, the enzyme converting 3-methylglutaconyl–CoA to 3 hydroxy-3-methylglutaryl-CoA in the last step of leucine metabolism, is the cause for 3-MGA type I. Four more types of 3-MGA have been described and are characterized by various degrees of mitochondrial dysfunction and are very remotely, if at all, linked to leucine metabolism.[98,99] How mitochondrial dysfunction leads to increased 3-MGA is also unclear. Type I 3-MGA presents with nonspecific symptoms, such as seizures and mental retardation in childhood, while recently an adult-onset slowly progressive leukoencephalopathy was added to the clinical manifestations of this poorly defined entity.[100] 3-MGA type II or Barth syndrome is an X-linked recessive form of the disease, caused by mutations in the TAZ gene, encoding the protein taffazin. The pathognomonic finding in the disease is the abnormal cardiolipin profile in the patient's cells. Clinical symptoms include cardiomyopathy, cyclic neutropenia, skeletal myopathy associated with mitochondrial OXPHOS dysfunction, increased 3-MGA excretion, and low plasma cholesterol levels.[101] In these patients, 3-MGA excretion is not related to protein loading, and it is thought to derive through a mevalonate shunt.[102]

3-MGA type III or Costeff syndrome is characterized by infantile bilateral optic nerve atrophy, dysarthria, ataxia, and extrapyramidal signs and is caused by mutations in *OPA3*, which encodes for a protein localized in the outer membrane of the mitochondrion with critical role in mitochondrial fission and apoptosis.[103] 3-MGA type V is caused by mutations in a mitochondrial inner membrane translocase, *DNAJC19*, and presents as dilated cardiomyopathy with ataxia and in the Canadian Dariusleut Hutterite population, with testicular dysgenesis and growth failure. The remaining undefined cases with 3-MGA secretion are classified as type IV and encompass a variety of disorders affecting mitochondrial function that have as a secondary marker increased 3-MGA. Mutations in *POLG1, SUCLA2, DNAJC19, TMEM70,* and mtDNA have all been described to cause elevated 3-MGA in the urine organic acid analysis.

2-Methyl-3-hydroxybutyryl-CoA dehydrogenase deficiency is a newly identified enzyme defect in the pathway of isoleucine metabolism, caused by an interesting enzyme with different substrates besides short-branched chain acyl-CoAs. These include 17β/3α-hydroxysteroids, compounds that play a role in sex hormone and neurosteroid metabolism, and is therefore also referred to as 17β-hydroxysteroid dehydrogenase (17β-HSD10). It also shows affinity for amyloid-β-peptide and has the additional designation of endoplasmic reticulum-associated amyloid-β-binding protein.[104] The disease presentation is that of a mitochondrial disorder with progressive neurodegeneration in the more severely affected males. More studies are needed to investigate the role of isoleucine restriction or antioxidant therapies in the management of these patients.[105–107]

3-Hydroxyisobutyryl-CoA hydrolase deficiency is a very rare disease described in three families in the literature. The first patient presented with congenital malformations, including vertebral abnormalities, tetralogy of Fallot, and agenesis of the cingulate gyrus and corpus callosum, poor feeding, gross motor delay, and neurological regression in infancy.[108] The subsequent cases displayed progressive infantile neurodegeneration as well as episodes of ketoacidosis and Leigh-like changes in the basal ganglia associated with a combined deficiency of multiple mitochondrial respiratory chain enzymes and pyruvate dehydrogenase in one set of siblings.[18,109] This defect involves an exceptional step in valine metabolism where free acids are generated in contrast to all other intermediates that are CoA thioesters. Patients had increased secretion of *S*-2-carboxypropyl-cysteamine and *S*-2-carboxypropyl-cysteine and persistently elevated C4-OH acylcarnitine that led to the identification of mutations in the *HIBCH* gene.[109] Methacrylyl-CoA formed because of the block is a highly reactive compound that reacts with thiol groups, such as glutathione, cysteine, or cysteamine, causing significant oxidative stress.

The last enzymatic steps in the valine degradation pathway convert 3-hydroxyisobutyrate to (S)-methylmalonic semialdehyde by 3-hydroxyisobutyrate dehydrogenase and (S)-methylmalonic semialdehyde to propionyl-CoA by the methylmalonate semialdehyde dehydrogenase enzyme (MMSDH). Thymine metabolism on the other hand generates (R)-aminoisobutyric acid, which is then deaminated to (R)-methylmalonic semialdehyde. Both S- and R-methylmalonic semialdehyde are then handled by MMSDH, which catalyzes their oxidative decarboxylation to propionyl-CoA, suggesting that a single enzyme is involved in the catabolism of valine, thymine, and uracil. Pathogenic mutations in the gene encoding MMSDH (*ALDH6A1*) have been identified in patients that displayed 3-hydroxyisobutyric aciduria,[110] while others also manifested transient methylmalonic acidemia/uria.[20]

Over the years, 3-hydroxyisobutyric aciduria and methylmalonic semialdehyde deficiency have been recognized as heterogenous conditions, both clinically and biochemically. The small number of patients with 3-hydroxyisobutyric aciduria described presented with dysmorphic features, including a triangular face, low-set ears, long philtrum and microcephaly, and widely different phenotypes ranging from mild vomiting attacks with normal cognitive development to profound intellectual impairment and early death.[111–113] Enzymatic or molecular testing of the predicted human cDNA for 3-hydroxyisobutyrate dehydrogenase were negative in some of these patients.[114] Whether previously described but untested patients will harbor mutations in *ALDH6A1* or other gene(s) remains unknown.

Methylmalonyl semialdehyde deficiency can present at newborn screening as hypermethioninemia and is associated with developmental delay, hypotonia, and dysmorphic features.[115,116] The urine metabolic pattern is variable, including beta-alanine, 3-hydroxypropionic acid, both isomers of 3-amino- and 3-hydroxyisobutyric acid, and mild methylmalonic aciduria. Mutations in *ALDH6A1* have been identified only in a subset of patients with these biochemical findings.[19]

Approaches to Therapy
Dietary Management

Therapy of all the disorders in these biochemical pathways is based on dietary restriction of protein and particularly the offensive amino acids, leucine for MSUD and IVA or valine and isoleucine for PA and MMA, among the other less frequent disorders in the respective pathways, with regular clinical assessments of growth and monitoring of specific biochemical biomarkers. Primary goals of dietary management include (a) the promotion of growth and anabolism, avoiding fasting or energy imbalance that may result in metabolic decompensation; this is achieved by providing a high caloric intake, continuous feeds through gastrostomy tube, and hospitalization for parenteral nutrition during intercurrent illness; (b) the reduction of toxic intermediates through the provision of medical foods deficient in the offensive amino acids or antibiotics to reduce precursor generation from propiogenic gut flora; (c) the enhancement of excretion of toxic metabolites through the provision of substrates for conjugation, such as carnitine for the acyl-CoA species or glycine in the case of IVA to form isovalerylglycine; (d) the administration of cofactors where indicated, such as thiamine in thiamine-responsive MSUD or hydroxocobalamin in MMA; and (e) vigilant monitoring for nutritional deficiencies, such as micronutrients, vitamins, and essential amino and fatty acids.

There are no evidence-based guidelines for each of the above therapeutic measures employed. This is reflected in the wide range of practices recorded in multicenter studies and the controversies surrounding even the few available therapeutic measures, such as carnitine supplementation. Furthermore, there are only few carefully conducted studies that document the actual dietary requirements and outcomes for these patients.[117–121]

The experience gained in MSUD in recent years from clinical and animal studies has led to the design of improved formulas, which are enriched in amino acids that compete with leucine for brain uptake (such as Tyr, Trp, Phe, Met, Thr, His) and in essential fatty acids and micronutrients observed to be deficient with current management (omega-3 polyunsaturated fatty acids, zinc, and selenium). Use of this modified formula resulted in improved metabolic control and biochemical parameters, fewer hospitalizations, and normal growth and development of the patients.[122] Based on the same pathophysiological paradigm, a synthetic analog of leucine, norleucine, was shown to effectively compete for brain uptake of leucine, improving survival and biochemical aberrations and delaying the encephalopathy symptoms of different mouse models for classic and intermediate MSUD,[62] making this an interesting candidate treatment approach for the patients.

Carnitine supplementation has been widely accepted as a means to restore the depleted intramitochondrial free CoA pool and help excrete toxic acyl-CoA compounds in the urine as carnitine esters, for example propionyl-CoA in the form of the less toxic propionylcarnitine, and thereby also prevent secondary carnitine deficiency.[123–125] The efficacy of this approach given the renal handling of supplemental carnitine has been debated.[126] However, a combination of L-carnitine with glycine conjugation in severe forms of isovaleric acidemia was found to provide an efficient means to eliminate isovaleryl-CoA.[127,128] More recently, treatment with phenylbutyrate was shown to increase the dephosphorylated active form of the E1a subunit by preventing its phosphorylation by the BCKD kinase. This results in reduced BCAA and BCKA levels in cases with iMSUD.[23]

Mitochondria-Targeted Therapies

Given the secondary mitochondrial dysfunction affecting various aspects of mitochondrial metabolism that has been documented in an increasing number of disorders in the BCAA metabolic pathway, agents targeting the mitochondria could hold significant therapeutic benefit for these patients.

The use of antioxidants has been evaluated mainly in experimental animal models of organic acidemias, including MSUD,[129] isovaleric acidemia,[130] 3-hydroxyisobutyric acidemia,[131] 3-MGA,[132] and methylmalonic acidemia,[90,133] among others. Glutathione deficiency was documented during a metabolic crisis in a patient with isolated MMA, who responded to ascorbate therapy,[134] while a regimen including coenzyme Q_{10} and vitamin E has been shown to prevent progression of acute optic nerve involvement in a different MMA patient.[135] Despite these encouraging case reports, systematic randomized multicenter studies addressing the role of antioxidants in the acute or chronic management of MMA or other disorders in these pathways are currently lacking. This is a well-recognized shortcoming in treatment studies for mitochondrial disorders of all principles, where only very few well-conducted randomized controlled studies were able to convincingly show benefit of such therapeutic interventions.[136–139]

It is evident from the current acute management guidelines that we are using a rather oversimplified approach in the acute management of most of the disorders discussed herein, where patients are uniformly treated with caloric support and protein restriction until their own defense mechanisms achieve a new equilibrium. The expectation from ongoing research studies on animal models is that through gaining a better understanding of the pathophysiology underlying the mitochondrial involvement of each of these disorders, we will be able to design better disease-specific therapies.

A representative example of such a mitochondria-targeted specific therapeutic approach is the recent transcriptional activator of transcription peptide-mediated enzyme replacement therapy in a mouse model of the lipoamide dehydrogenase or E3 deficiency. The peptide is able to aid delivery into the mitochondria as well as achieve delivery through the blood-brain-barrier into the brain tissue.[140] This approach may be applicable to other disorders in these pathways.

Organ Transplantation

Liver transplantation has been used to cure different inborn errors of metabolism, including urea cycle defects, tyrosinemia, familial hypercholesterolemia, primary hyperoxaluria, Wilson disease, Criggler-Najar syndrome, and others. Among the BCAA metabolism disorders, classic MSUD is probably the only condition where liver transplantation has been shown to have a significant therapeutic, though not completely curative, effect.

Maple Syrup Urine Disease

Liver transplantation has been reported to greatly improve the metabolic instability and allow protein intake liberalization in MSUD patients.[141,142] It is suggested that the donor liver introduces sufficient BCKD activity in the body that is also subject to physiologic regulation, resulting in the maintenance of near-normal plasma BCAA and α–KIC levels through various dietary and physiological challenges. Patients can liberalize their protein intake and are less vulnerable during intercurrent illnesses, although significant leucinosis can occur during periods of stress. Although there is no further deterioration, existing neurocognitive dysfunction or behavioral problems cannot be reversed.

There have been a number of cases where classical MSUD patient livers were successfully transplanted into a recipient ("domino" transplantation) with no adverse consequences for peripheral amino acid homeostasis on unrestricted protein intake.[141,143] Such a utilization of explanted organs from patients with MSUD or other organic acidurias may alleviate some of the ethical controversies surrounding allograft distribution.

Propionic Acidemia

There have been several reported cases of successful liver transplantation in PA.[144–146] Furthermore, it has been shown to restore cardiac function in cases with propionic acidemia complicated by dilated cardiomyopathy.[147] There have been fewer cases of early elective transplants in this disorder to prospectively address its effects on neurological outcome for these patients.

Methylmalonic Acidemia

Although renal transplant has an absolute indication for patients with MMA in end-stage renal failure, the benefits of elective liver, kidney, or combined liver and kidney transplantation are less conclusive.[148–152] While organ transplant stabilizes the patients and decreases the frequency of admissions associated with metabolic decompensations, it does not completely prevent devastating neurological complications, such as the metabolic stroke.[153] Levels of plasma MMA post-transplantation remain significantly elevated, most likely due to extrahepatorenal MMA production from tissues such as the muscle and brain.[92] Continued dietary restriction is therefore strongly recommended post-transplant.

Gene and Cell Therapies

Results from gene therapy studies in mouse models of both methylmalonic and propionic acidemias have been very encouraging, making this a realistic therapeutic intervention that may be rapidly translated into clinical studies. A single intrahepatic or systemic injection of an adeno-associated virus designed to express the *Mut* gene has resulted in complete rescue from early neonatal lethality and long-term phenotypic correction in knock-out mouse models of methylmalonic acidemia.[154] Moreover, selective expression in the liver[155] or administration of a different serotype (rAAV9)[156] were both similarly effective, providing evidence for the effects of hepatocyte-specific correction or the ability to transduce the kidney and preserve kidney morphology and glomerular filtration rate, which have obvious therapeutic implications for this disorder.

The potential for expanding these observations to other disorders in these metabolic pathways was evidenced by the efficacy of a similar approach in propionic acidemia.[157] Gene therapy approaches may offer an alternative treatment approach for these devastating and often lethal multisystemic disorders that are in great need of new therapeutic options.

The promising results of liver-directed gene expression, whether by a rAAV gene delivery under the control of a liver-specific promoter or an orthotopic liver transplantation, makes alternative options of hepatocyte correction, such as hepatocyte or stem-cell delivery, another appealing treatment consideration for patients with many of the disorders in the BCAA metabolism pathways.[158–161]

References

1. Harper AE, Miller RH. Block KP. Branched-chain amino acid metabolism. *Annu Rev Nutr*. 1984; 4: 409–454.
2. Layman DK. The role of leucine in weight loss diets and glucose homeostasis. *J Nutr*. 2003; 133: 261S–267S.
3. Brosnan JT, Brosnan ME. Branched-chain amino acids: enzyme and substrate regulation. *J Nutr*. 2006; 136: 207S–211S.
4. Chuang DT, Wynn RM, Shih VE. *Maple Syrup Urine Disease (Branched-Chain Ketoaciduria*. New York: McGraw Hill; 2008.
5. Hargreaves KM, Pardridge WM. Neutral amino acid transport at the human blood-brain barrier. *J Biol Chem*. 1988; 263: 19392–19397.
6. Kimball SR, Shantz LM, Horetsky RL, Jefferson LS. Leucine regulates translation of specific mRNAs in L6 myoblasts through mTOR-mediated changes in availability of eIF4E and phosphorylation of ribosomal protein S6. *J Biol Chem*. 1999; 274: 11647–11652.
7. Beugnet A, Tee AR, Taylor PM, Proud CG. Regulation of targets of mTOR (mammalian target of rapamycin) signalling by intracellular amino acid availability. *Biochem J*. 2003; 372: 555–566.
8. Gingras AC, Raught B, Sonenberg N. Regulation of translation initiation by FRAP/mTOR. *Genes Dev*. 2001; 15: 807–826.
9. Frost RA, Lang CH. mTor signaling in skeletal muscle during sepsis and inflammation: where does it all go wrong? *Physiology (Bethesda)*. 2011; 26: 83–96.
10. Malaisse WJ, Huttn JC, Carpinelli AR, Herchuelz A, Sener A. The stimulus-secretion coupling of amino acid-induced insulin release: metabolism and cationic effects of leucine. *Diabetes*. 1980; 29: 431–437.
11. Sener A, Malaisse WJ. L-leucine and a nonmetabolized analogue activate pancreatic islet glutamate dehydrogenase. *Nature*. 1980; 288: 187–189.
12. Henquin JC, Dufrane D, Nenquin M. Nutrient control of insulin secretion in isolated normal human islets. *Diabetes*. 2006; 55: 3470–3477.
13. Gao Z, et al. Distinguishing features of leucine and alpha-ketoisocaproate sensing in pancreatic beta-cells. *Endocrinology*. 2003; 144: 1949–1957
14. Patti ME, Brambilla E, Luzi L, Landaker EJ, Kahn CR. Bidirectional modulation of insulin action by amino acids. *J Clin Invest*. 1998; 101: 1519–1529.

15. Ropelle ER, et al. A central role for neuronal AMP-activated protein kinase (AMPK) and mammalian target of rapamycin (mTOR) in high-protein diet-induced weight loss. *Diabetes.* 2008; 57: 594–605.
16. Cota D, et al. Hypothalamic mTOR signaling regulates food intake. *Science.* 2006; 312: 927–930.
17. Loupatty FJ, et al. Mutations in the gene encoding 3-hydroxyisobutyryl-CoA hydrolase results in progressive infantile neurodegeneration. *Am J Hum Genet.* 2007; 80: 195–199.
18. Ferdinandusse S, et al. HIBCH mutations can cause Leigh-like disease with combined deficiency of multiple mitochondrial respiratory chain enzymes and pyruvate dehydrogenase. *Orphanet J Rare Dis.* 2013; 8: 188.
19. Chambliss KL, Gray RG, Rylance G, Pollitt RJ, Gibson KM. Molecular characterization of methylmalonate semialdehyde dehydrogenase deficiency. *J Inherit Metab Dis.* 2000; 23: 497–504.
20. Marcadier JL, et al. Mutations in ALDH6A1 encoding methylmalonate semialdehyde dehydrogenase are associated with dysmyelination and transient methylmalonic aciduria. *Orphanet J Rare Dis.* 2013; 8: 98.
21. Shimomura Y, Obayashi M, Murakami T, Harris RA. Regulation of branched-chain amino acid catabolism: nutritional and hormonal regulation of activity and expression of the branched-chain alpha-keto acid dehydrogenase kinase. *Curr Opin Clin Nutr Metab Care.* 2001; 4: 419–423.
22. Suryawan A, et al. A molecular model of human branched-chain amino acid metabolism. *Am J Clin Nutr.* 1998; 68: 72–81.
23. Brunetti-Pierri N, et al. Phenylbutyrate therapy for maple syrup urine disease. *Hum Mol Genet.* 2011; 20: 631–640.
24. Lu G, et al. Protein phosphatase 2Cm is a critical regulator of branched-chain amino acid catabolism in mice and cultured cells. *J Clin Invest,* 2009; 119: 1678–1687.
25. Chinsky JM, Bohlen LM, Costeas PA. Noncoordinated responses of branched-chain alpha-ketoacid dehydrogenase subunit genes to dietary protein. *FASEB J.* 1994; 8: 114–120.
26. Chicco AG, Adibi SA, Liu WQ, Morris SM Jr, Paul HS. Regulation of gene expression of branched-chain keto acid dehydrogenase complex in primary cultured hepatocytes by dexamethasone and a cAMP analog. *J Biol Chem.* 1994; 269: 19427–19434.
27. Morton DH, Strauss KA, Robinson DL, Puffenberger EG, Kelley RI. Diagnosis and treatment of maple syrup disease: a study of 36 patients. *Pediatrics.* 2002; 109: 999–1008.
28. Kaplan P, et al. Intellectual outcome in children with maple syrup urine disease. *J Pediatr.* 1991; 119: 46–50.
29. Simon E, et al. Maple syrup urine disease: favourable effect of early diagnosis by newborn screening on the neonatal course of the disease. *J Inherit Metab Dis.* 2006; 29:L 532–537.
30. Heldt K, Schwahn B, Marquardt I, Grotzke M, Wendel U. Diagnosis of MSUD by newborn screening allows early intervention without extraneous detoxification. *Mol Genet Metab.* 2005; 84: 313–316.
31. Puckett RL, et al. Maple syrup urine disease: further evidence that newborn screening may fail to identify variant forms. *Mol Genet Metab.* 2010; 100: 136–142.
32. Oglesbee D, et al. Second-tier test for quantification of alloisoleucine and branched-chain amino acids in dried blood spots to improve newborn screening for maple syrup urine disease (MSUD). *Clin Chem.* 2008; 54: 542–549.
33. Fingerhut R, Simon E, Maier EM, Hennermann JB, Wendel U. Maple syrup urine disease: newborn screening fails to discriminate between classic and variant forms. *Clin Chem.* 2008; 54: 1739–1741.
34. Leonard JV, Vijayaraghavan S, Walter JH. The impact of screening for propionic and methylmalonic acidaemia. *Eur J Pediatr.* 2003; 162 (Suppl. 1):, S21–S24.
35. Dionisi-Vici C, Deodato F, Roschinger W, Rhead W, Wilcken B. "Classical" organic acidurias, propionic aciduria, methylmalonic aciduria and isovaleric aciduria: long-term outcome and effects of expanded newborn screening using tandem mass spectrometry. *J Inherit Metab Dis.* 2006; 29: 383–389.
36. Lindner M, et al. Newborn screening for methylmalonic acidurias—optimization by statistical parameter combination. *J Inherit Metab Dis.* 2008; 31: 379–385.
37. Turgeon CT, et al. Determination of total homocysteine, methylmalonic acid, and 2-methylcitric acid in dried blood spots by tandem mass spectrometry. *Clin Chem.* 2010; 56: 1686–1695.
38. Vockley J, Ensenauer R. Isovaleric acidemia: new aspects of genetic and phenotypic heterogeneity. *Am J Med Genet C, Semin Med Genet* 2006; 142C: 95–103.
39. Ensenauer R, et al. A common mutation is associated with a mild, potentially asymptomatic phenotype in patients with isovaleric acidemia diagnosed by newborn screening. *Am J Hum Genet.* 2004; 75: 1136–1142.

40. Arnold GL, et al. A Delphi-based consensus clinical practice protocol for the diagnosis and management of 3-methylcrotonyl CoA carboxylase deficiency. *Mol Genet Metab.* 2008; 93: 363–370.
41. Stadler SC, et al. Newborn screening for 3-methylcrotonyl-CoA carboxylase deficiency: population heterogeneity of MCCA and MCCB mutations and impact on risk assessment. *Hum Mutat.* 2006; 27: 748–759.
42. Roschinger W, et al. 3-Hydroxyisovalerylcarnitine in patients with deficiency of 3-methylcrotonyl CoA carboxylase. *Clin Chim Acta.* 1995; 240: 35–51.
43. Ficicioglu C, Payan I. 3-Methylcrotonyl-CoA carboxylase deficiency: metabolic decompensation in a noncompliant child detected through newborn screening. *Pediatrics.* 2006; 118: 2555–2556.
44. Oude Luttikhuis HG, et al. Severe hypoglycaemia in isolated 3-methylcrotonyl-CoA carboxylase deficiency; a rare, severe clinical presentation. *J Inherit Metab Dis.* 2005; 28: 1136–1138.
45. Gibson KM, et al. 2-Methylbutyryl-coenzyme A dehydrogenase deficiency: a new inborn error of L-isoleucine metabolism. *Pediatr Res.* 2000; 47: 830–833.
46. Andresen BS, et al. Isolated 2-methylbutyrylglycinuria caused by short/branched-chain acyl-CoA dehydrogenase deficiency: identification of a new enzyme defect, resolution of its molecular basis, and evidence for distinct acyl-CoA dehydrogenases in isoleucine and valine metabolism. *Am J Hum Genet.* 2000; 67: 1095–1103.
47. Matern D, et al. Prospective diagnosis of 2-methylbutyryl-CoA dehydrogenase deficiency in the Hmong population by newborn screening using tandem mass spectrometry. *Pediatrics.* 2003; 112: 74–78.
48. Alfardan J, et al. Characterization of new ACADSB gene sequence mutations and clinical implications in patients with 2-methylbutyrylglycinuria identified by newborn screening. *Mol Genet Metab.* 2010; 100: 333–338.
49. van Maldegem BT, et al. Clinical, biochemical, and genetic heterogeneity in short-chain acyl-coenzyme A dehydrogenase deficiency. *JAMA.* 2006; 296: 943–952.
50. van Maldegem BT, Wanders RJ, Wijburg FA. Clinical aspects of short-chain acyl-CoA dehydrogenase deficiency. *J Inherit Metab Dis.* 2010; 33: 507–511.
51. Nguyen TV, et al. Identification of isobutyryl-CoA dehydrogenase and its deficiency in humans. *Mol Genet Metab.* 2002; 77: 68–79.
52. Sass JO, Sander S, Zschocke J. Isobutyryl-CoA dehydrogenase deficiency: isobutyrylglycinuria and ACAD8 gene mutations in two infants. *J Inherit Metab Dis.* 2004; 27: 741–745.
53. Koeberl DD, et al. Rare disorders of metabolism with elevated butyryl and isobutyryl carnitine detected by tandem mass spectrometry newborn screening. *Pediatr Res.* 2003; 54: 219–223.
54. Roe CR, et al. Isolated isobutyryl-CoA dehydrogenase deficiency: an unrecognized defect in human valine metabolism. *Mol Genet Metab.* 1998; 65: 264–271.
55. Oglesbee D, et al. Development of a newborn screening follow-up algorithm for the diagnosis of isobutyryl-CoA dehydrogenase deficiency. *Genet Med.* 2007; 9: 108–116.
56. Chandler RJ, et al. Mitochondrial dysfunction in mut methylmalonic acidemia. *FASEB J.* 2009; 23: 1252–1261.
57. Strauss KA, Puffenberger EG, Morton DH. Maple syrup urine disease. In: Pagon RA, Bird TC, Dolan CR, Stephens K, eds. *GeneReviews.* Seattle: University of Washington; Published January 30, 2006. Updated December 15, 2009
58. Yudkoff M, et al. Astrocyte leucine metabolism: significance of branched-chain amino acid transamination. *J Neurochem.* 1996; 66: 378–385.
59. Yudkoff M, et al. Brain amino acid requirements and toxicity: the example of leucine. *J Nutr.* 2005; 135: 1531S-1538S.
60. Yudkoff M. Brain metabolism of branched-chain amino acids. *Glia.* 1997; 21: 92–98.
61. Hutson SM, Lieth E, LaNoue KF. Function of leucine in excitatory neurotransmitter metabolism in the central nervous system. *J Nutr.* 2001; 131: 846S-850S.
62. Zinnanti WJ, et al. Dual mechanism of brain injury and novel treatment strategy in maple syrup urine disease. *Brain.* 2009; 132: 903–918.
63. Prensky AL, Moser HW. Brain lipids, proteolipids, and free amino acids in maple syrup urine disease. *J Neurochem.* 1966; 13: 863–874.
64. McKenna MC, et al. Alpha-ketoisocaproate alters the production of both lactate and aspartate from [U-13C]glutamate in astrocytes: a 13C NMR study. *J Neurochem.* 1998; 70: 1001–1008.

65. Shestopalov AI, Kristal BS. Branched chain keto-acids exert biphasic effects on alpha-ketoglutarate-stimulated respiration in intact rat liver mitochondria. *Neurochem Res.* 2007; 32: 947–951.
66. Amaral AU, et al. Alpha-ketoisocaproic acid and leucine provoke mitochondrial bioenergetic dysfunction in rat brain. *Brain Res.* 2010; 1324: 75–84.
67. Jan W, et al. MR diffusion imaging and MR spectroscopy of maple syrup urine disease during acute metabolic decompensation. *Neuroradiology* 2003; 45: 393–399.
68. Smith QR, Takasato Y, Sweeney DJ, Rapoport SI. Regional cerebrovascular transport of leucine as measured by the in situ brain perfusion technique. *J Cereb Blood Flow Metab.* 1985; 5: 300–311.
69. Smith QR, Takasato Y. Kinetics of amino acid transport at the blood–brain barrier studied using an in situ brain perfusion technique. *Ann N Y Acad Sci.* 1986; 481: 186–201.
70. Schonberger S, Schweiger B, Schwahn B, Schwarz M, Wendel U. Dysmyelination in the brain of adolescents and young adults with maple syrup urine disease. *Mol Genet Metab.* 2004; 82: 69–75.
71. Treacy E, et al. Maple syrup urine disease: interrelations between branched-chain amino-, oxo- and hydroxyacids; implications for treatment; associations with CNS dysmyelination. *J Inherit Metab Dis.* 1992; 15: 121–135.
72. Strauss KA, et al. Classical maple syrup urine disease and brain development: principles of management and formula design. *Mol Genet Metab.* 2010; 99: 333–345.
73. Strauss KA, Morton DH. Branched-chain ketoacyl dehydrogenase deficiency: maple syrup disease. *Curr Treat Options Neurol.* 2003; 5: 329–341.
74. Utter MF, Keech DB, Scrutton MC. A possible role for acetyl CoA in the control of gluconeogenesis. *Adv Enzyme Regul.* 1964; 2: 49–68.
75. McLaughlin BA, Nelson D, Silver IA, Erecinska M, Chesselet MF. Methylmalonate toxicity in primary neuronal cultures. *Neuroscience.* 1998; 86: 279–290.
76. Kolker S, Ahlemeyer B, Krieglstein J, Hoffmann GF. Methylmalonic acid induces excitotoxic neuronal damage in vitro. *J Inherit Metab Dis.* 2000; 23: 355–358.
77. de Mello CF, et al. Intrastriatal methylmalonic acid administration induces rotational behavior and convulsions through glutamatergic mechanisms. *Brain Res.* 1996; 721: 120–125.
78. Malfatti CR, et al. Intrastriatal methylmalonic acid administration induces convulsions and TBARS production, and alters Na+,K+-ATPase activity in the rat striatum and cerebral cortex. *Epilepsia.* 2003; 44: 761–767.
79. Malfatti CR, et al. Convulsions induced by methylmalonic acid are associated with glutamic acid decarboxylase inhibition in rats: a role for GABA in the seizures presented by methylmalonic acidemic patients? *Neuroscience.* 2007; 146: 1879–1887.
80. Cheema-Dhadli S, Leznoff CC, Halperin ML. Effect of 2-methylcitrate on citrate metabolism: implications for the management of patients with propionic acidemia and methylmalonic aciduria. *Pediatr Res.* 1975; 9: 905–908.
81. Halperin ML, Schiller CM, Fritz IB. The inhibition by methylmalonic acid of malate transport by the dicarboxylate carrier in rat liver mitochondria: A possible explantation for hypoglycemia in methylmalonic aciduria. *J Clin Invest.* 1971; 50: 2276–2282.
82. Okun JG, et al. Neurodegeneration in methylmalonic aciduria involves inhibition of complex II and the tricarboxylic acid cycle, and synergistically acting excitotoxicity. *J Biol Chem.* 2002; 277: 14674–14680.
83. Oberholzer VG, Levin B, Burgess EA, Young WF. Methylmalonic aciduria: An inborn error of metabolism leading to chronic metabolic acidosis. *Arch Dis Child.* 1967; 42: 492–504.
84. Coude FX, Sweetman L, Nyhan WL. Inhibition by propionyl-coenzyme A of N-acetylglutamate synthetase in rat liver mitochondria: A possible explanation for hyperammonemia in propionic and methylmalonic acidemia. *J Clin Invest.* 1979; 64: 1544–1551.
85. Filipowicz HR, Ernst SL, Ashurst CL, Pasquali M, Longo N. Metabolic changes associated with hyperammonemia in patients with propionic acidemia. *Mol Genet Metab.* 2006; 88: 123–130.
86. Hayasaka K, et al. Glycine cleavage system in ketotic hyperglycinemia: a reduction of H-protein activity. *Pediatr Res.* 1982; 16: 5–7.
87. Hayasaka K, Tada K. Effects of the metabolites of the branched-chain amino acids and cysteamine on the glycine cleavage system. *Biochem Int.* 1983; 6: 225–230.
88. Kolker S, Okun JG. Methylmalonic acid—an endogenous toxin? *Cell Mol Life Sci.* 2005; 62: 621–624.

89. Morath MA, et al. Neurodegeneration and chronic renal failure in methylmalonic aciduria—a pathophysiological approach. *J Inherit Metab Dis.* 2008; 31: 35–43.
90. Manoli I, et al. Targeting proximal tubule mitochondrial dysfunction attenuates the renal disease of methylmalonic acidemia. *Proc Natl Acad Sci USA.* 2013; 110: 13552–13557.
91. Mitchell GA, et al. Hereditary and acquired diseases of acyl-coenzyme A metabolism. *Mol Genet Metab.* 2008; 94: 4–15.
92. Chandler RJ, et al. Metabolic phenotype of methylmalonic acidemia in mice and humans: the role of skeletal muscle. *BMC Med Genet.* 2007; 8: 64.
93. Schwab MA, et al. Secondary mitochondrial dysfunction in propionic aciduria: a pathogenic role for endogenous mitochondrial toxins. *Biochem J.* 2006; 398: 107–112.
94. Atkuri KR, et al. Inherited disorders affecting mitochondrial function are associated with glutathione deficiency and hypocitrullinemia. *Proc Natl Acad Sci USA.* 2009; 106: 3941–3945.
95. de Keyzer Y, et al. Multiple OXPHOS deficiency in the liver, kidney, heart, and skeletal muscle of patients with methylmalonic aciduria and propionic aciduria. *Pediatr Res.* 2009; 66: 91–95.
96. Valayannopoulos V, et al. Multiple OXPHOS deficiency in the liver of a patient with CblA methylmalonic aciduria sensitive to vitamin B(12). *J Inherit Metab Dis.* 2009; 32: 159–162.
97. Mc Guire PJ, Parikh A, Diaz GA. Profiling of oxidative stress in patients with inborn errors of metabolism. *Mol Genet Metab.* 2009; 98: 173–180.
98. Gunay-Aygun M. 3-Methylglutaconic aciduria: a common biochemical marker in various syndromes with diverse clinical features. *Mol Genet Metab.* 2005; 84: 1–3.
99. Wortmann SB, Kluijtmans LA, Engelke UF, Wevers RA, Morava E. The 3-methylglutaconic acidurias: what's new? *J Inherit Metab Dis.* 2010; 35: 13–22.
100. Wortmann SB, et al. 3-Methylglutaconic aciduria type I redefined: a syndrome with late-onset leukoencephalopathy. *Neurology.* 2010; 75: 1079–1083.
101. Kelley RI, et al. X-linked dilated cardiomyopathy with neutropenia, growth retardation, and 3-methylglutaconic aciduria. *J Pediatr.* 1991; 119: 738–747.
102. Di Rosa G, et al. Hypertrophic cardiomyopathy, cataract, developmental delay, lactic acidosis: a novel subtype of 3-methylglutaconic aciduria. *J Inherit Metab Dis.* 2006; 29: 546–550.
103. Ryu SW, Jeong HJ, Choi M, Karbowski M, Choi C. Optic atrophy 3 as a protein of the mitochondrial outer membrane induces mitochondrial fragmentation. *Cell Mol Life Sci.* 2010; 67: 2839–2850.
104. Lustbader JW, et al. ABAD directly links Abeta to mitochondrial toxicity in Alzheimer's disease. *Science.* 2004; 304: 448–452.
105. Zschocke J, et al. Progressive infantile neurodegeneration caused by 2-methyl-3-hydroxybutyryl-CoA dehydrogenase deficiency: a novel inborn error of branched-chain fatty acid and isoleucine metabolism. *Pediatr Res.* 2000; 48: 852–855.
106. Perez-Cerda C, et al. 2-Methyl-3-hydroxybutyryl-CoA dehydrogenase (MHBD) deficiency: an X-linked inborn error of isoleucine metabolism that may mimic a mitochondrial disease. *Pediatr Res.* 2005; 58: 488–491.
107. Korman SH. Inborn errors of isoleucine degradation: a review. *Mol Genet Metab.* 2006; 89: 289–299.
108. Brown GK, et al. Beta-hydroxyisobutyryl coenzyme A deacylase deficiency: a defect in valine metabolism associated with physical malformations. *Pediatrics.* 1982; 70: 532–538.
109. Loupatty FJ, et al. Mutations in the gene encoding 3-hydroxyisobutyryl-CoA hydrolase results in progressive infantile neurodegeneration. *Am J Hum Genet.* 2007; 80: 195–199.
110. Sass JO, et al. 3-Hydroxyisobutyrate aciduria and mutations in the ALDH6A1 gene coding for methylmalonate semialdehyde dehydrogenase. *J Inherit Metab Dis.* 2012; 35: 437–442.
111. Ko FJ, Nyhan WL, Wolff J, Barshop B, Sweetman L. 3-Hydroxyisobutyric aciduria: an inborn error of valine metabolism. *Pediatr Res.* 1991; 30: 322–326.
112. Chitayat D, et al. Brain dysgenesis and congenital intracerebral calcification associated with 3-hydroxyisobutyric aciduria. *J Pediatr.* 1992; 121: 86–89.
113. Boulat O, Benador N, Girardin E, Bachmann C. 3-hydroxyisobutyric aciduria with a mild clinical course. *J Inherit Metab Dis.* 1995; 18: 204–206.
114. Loupatty FJ, et al. Clinical, biochemical, and molecular findings in three patients with 3-hydroxyisobutyric aciduria. *Mol Genet Metab.* 2006; 87: 243–248.
115. Pollitt RJ, Green A, Smith R. Excessive excretion of beta-alanine and of 3-hydroxypropionic, R- and S-3-aminoisobutyric, R- and S-3-hydroxyisobutyric and S-2-(hydroxymethyl)butyric acids probably due to a defect in the metabolism of the corresponding malonic semialdehydes. *J Inherit Metab Dis.* 1985; 8: 75–79.

116. Gibson KM, Lee CF, Bennett MJ, Holmes B, Nyhan WL. Combined malonic, methylmalonic and ethylmalonic acid semialdehyde dehydrogenase deficiencies: an inborn error of beta-alanine, L-valine and L-alloisoleucine metabolism? *J Inherit Metab Dis*. 1993; 16: 563–567.
117. Yannicelli S, et al. Improved growth and nutrition status in children with methylmalonic or propionic acidemia fed an elemental medical food. *Mol Genet Metab*. 2003; 80: 181–188.
118. Hauser NS, Manoli I, Graf JC, Sloan J, Venditti CP. Variable dietary management of methylmalonic acidemia: metabolic and energetic correlations. *Am J Clin Nutr*. 2011; 93: 47–56.
119. Touati G, et al. Methylmalonic and propionic acidurias: management without or with a few supplements of specific amino acid mixture. *J Inherit Metab Dis*. 2006; 29: 288–298.
120. de Baulny HO, et al. Methylmalonic and propionic acidaemias: management and outcome. *J Inherit Metab Dis*. 2005; 28: 415–423.
121. Zwickler T, et al. Diagnostic work-up and management of patients with isolated methylmalonic acidurias in European metabolic centres. *J Inherit Metab Dis*. 2008; 31: 361–367.
122. Strauss KA, et al. Classical maple syrup urine disease and brain development: principles of management and formula design. *Mol Genet Metab*. 2010; 99: 333–345.
123. Roe CR, Millington DS, Maltby DA, Bohan TP, Hoppel CL. L-carnitine enhances excretion of propionyl coenzyme A as propionylcarnitine in propionic acidemia. *J Clin Invest*. 1984; 73: 1785–1788.
124. Chalmers RA, Roe CR, Stacey TE, Hoppel CL. Urinary excretion of l-carnitine and acylcarnitines by patients with disorders of organic acid metabolism: evidence for secondary insufficiency of l-carnitine. *Pediatr Res*. 1984; 18: 1325–1328.
125. Sauer SW, Okun JG, Hoffmann GF, Koelker S, Morath MA. Impact of short- and medium-chain organic acids, acylcarnitines, and acyl-CoAs on mitochondrial energy metabolism. *Biochim Biophys Acta*. 2008; 1777: 1276–1282.
126. Stanley CA, et al. Renal handling of carnitine in secondary carnitine deficiency disorders. *Pediatr Res*. 1993; 34: 89–97.
127. Chalmers RA, et al. L-carnitine and glycine therapy in isovaleric acidaemia. *J Inherit Metab Dis*. 1985; 8 (Suppl. 2): 141–142.
128. de Sousa C, et al. The response to L-carnitine and glycine therapy in isovaleric acidaemia. *Eur J Pediatr*. 1986; 144: 451–456.
129. Mescka C, et al. In vivo neuroprotective effect of L-carnitine against oxidative stress in maple syrup urine disease. *Metab Brain Dis*. 2011; 26: 21–28.
130. Ribeiro CA, et al. Creatine administration prevents Na+,K+-ATPase inhibition induced by intracerebroventricular administration of isovaleric acid in cerebral cortex of young rats. *Brain Res*. 2009; 1262: 81–88.
131. Viegas CM, et al. Evidence that 3-hydroxyisobutyric acid inhibits key enzymes of energy metabolism in cerebral cortex of young rats. *Int J Dev Neurosci*. 2008; 26: 293–299.
132. Ribeiro CA, Hickmann FH, Wajner M. Neurochemical evidence that 3-methylglutaric acid inhibits synaptic Na+,K+-ATPase activity probably through oxidative damage in brain cortex of young rats. *Int J Dev Neurosci*. 2011; 29: 1–7.
133. Fernandes CG, et al. Experimental evidence that methylmalonic acid provokes oxidative damage and compromises antioxidant defenses in nerve terminal and striatum of young rats. *Cell Mol Neurobiol*. 2011; 31: 775–785.
134. Treacy E, et al. Glutathione deficiency as a complication of methylmalonic acidemia: response to high doses of ascorbate. *J Pediatr*. 1996; 129: 445–448.
135. Pinar-Sueiro S, Martinez-Fernandez R, Lage-Medina S, Aldamiz-Echevarria L, Vecino E. Optic neuropathy in methylmalonic acidemia: the role of neuroprotection. *J Inherit Metab Dis*. 2010; 33 (Suppl. 3): S199–S203.
136. Kerr DS. Treatment of mitochondrial electron transport chain disorders: a review of clinical trials over the past decade. *Mol Genet Metab*. 2010; 99: 246–255.
137. Klopstock T, et al. A randomized placebo-controlled trial of idebenone in Leber's hereditary optic neuropathy. *Brain*. 2011; 134 (Pt 9): 2677–2686.
138. Glover EI, et al. A randomized trial of coenzyme Q10 in mitochondrial disorders. *Muscle Nerve*. 2010; 42: 739–748.
139. Tarnopolsky MA, Roy BD, MacDonald JR. A randomized, controlled trial of creatine monohydrate in patients with mitochondrial cytopathies. *Muscle Nerve*. 1997; 20: 1502–1509.

140. Rapoport M, Salman L, Sabag O, Patel MS, Lorberboum-Galski H. Successful TAT-mediated enzyme replacement therapy in a mouse model of mitochondrial E3 deficiency. *J Mol Med* (Berl). 2011; 89: 161–170.
141. Mazariegos GV, et al. Liver transplantation for classical maple syrup urine disease: long-term follow-up in 37 patients and comparative United Network for Organ Sharing experience. *J Pediatr.* 2011; 160: 116–121.
142. Strauss KA, et al. Elective liver transplantation for the treatment of classical maple syrup urine disease. *Am J Transplant.* 2006; 6: 557–564.
143. Barshop BA, Khanna A. Domino hepatic transplantation in maple syrup urine disease. *N Engl J Med.* 2005; 353: 2410–2411.
144. Vara R, et al. Liver transplantation for propionic acidemia in children. *Liver Transpl.* 2011; 17: 661–667.
145. Saudubray JM, et al. Liver transplantation in propionic acidaemia. *Eur J Pediatr.* 1999; 158 (Suppl. 2): S65–S69.
146. Barshes NR, et al. Evaluation and management of patients with propionic acidemia undergoing liver transplantation: a comprehensive review. *Pediatr Transplant.* 2006; 10: 773–781.
147. Romano S, et al. Cardiomyopathies in propionic aciduria are reversible after liver transplantation. *J Pediatr.* 2010; 156: 128–134.
148. Leonard JV, Walter JH, McKiernan PJ. The management of organic acidaemias: the role of transplantation. *J Inherit Metab Dis.* 2001; 24: 309–311.
149. Nyhan WL, Gargus JJ, Boyle K, Selby R, Koch R. Progressive neurologic disability in methylmalonic acidemia despite transplantation of the liver. *Eur J Pediatr.* 2002; 161: 377–379.
150. Kasahara M., et al. Current role of liver transplantation for methylmalonic acidemia: a review of the literature. *Pediatr Transplant.* 2006; 10: 943–947.
151. Kaplan P, Ficicioglu C, Mazur AT, Palmieri MJ, Berry GT. Liver transplantation is not curative for methylmalonic acidopathy caused by methylmalonyl-CoA mutase deficiency. *Mol Genet Metab.* 2006; 88: 322–326.
152. Mc Guire PJ, et al. Combined liver-kidney transplant for the management of methylmalonic aciduria: a case report and review of the literature. *Mol Genet Metab.* 2008; 93: 22–29.
153. Chakrapani A, Sivakumar P, McKiernan PJ, Leonard JV. Metabolic stroke in methylmalonic acidemia five years after liver transplantation. *J Pediatr.* 2002; 140: 261–263.
154. Chandler RJ, Venditti CP. Long-term rescue of a lethal murine model of methylmalonic acidemia using adeno-associated viral gene therapy. *Mol Ther.* 2010; 18: 11–16.
155. Carrillo-Carrasco N, Chandler RJ, Chandrasekaran S, Venditti CP. Liver-directed recombinant adeno-associated viral gene delivery rescues a lethal mouse model of methylmalonic acidemia and provides long-term phenotypic correction. *Hum Gene Ther.* 2010; 21: 1147–1154.
156. Senac JS, Chandler RJ, Sysol JR, Li L, Venditti CP. Gene therapy in a murine model of methylmalonic acidemia using rAAV9-mediated gene delivery. *Gene Ther.* 2011; 19(4): 385–389.
157. Chandler RJ, et al. Adeno-associated virus serotype 8 gene transfer rescues a neonatal lethal murine model of propionic acidemia. *Hum Gene Ther.* 2011; 22: 477–481.
158. Meyburg J, et al. One liver for four children: first clinical series of liver cell transplantation for severe neonatal urea cycle defects. *Transplantation.* 2009; 87: 636–641.
159. Horslen SP, et al. Isolated hepatocyte transplantation in an infant with a severe urea cycle disorder. *Pediatrics.* 2003; 111: 1262–1267.
160. Meyburg J, Hoffmann GF. Liver, liver cell and stem cell transplantation for the treatment of urea cycle defects. *Mol Genet Metab.* 2010; 100 (Suppl. 1): S77–S83.
161. Skvorak KJ, et al. Hepatocyte transplantation improves phenotype and extends survival in a murine model of intermediate maple syrup urine disease. *Mol Ther.* 2009; 17: 1266–1273.

5

Glycolysis

AREEG EL-GHARBAWY AND DWIGHT KOEBERL

Basic Biochemical Pathway, Clinical Presentation, Diagnosis, and Treatment

Glycolysis accomplishes the phosphorylation of two molecules of adenosine triphosphate (ATP) from adenosine diphosphate (ADP) for every molecule of glucose traversing the Embden-Myerhof pathway (Figure 5.1). Glycolysis in erythrocytes is regulated by three rate-limiting enzymes—hexosekinase (HK), phosphofructokinase (PFK), and pyruvate kinase (PK)—and by the availability of nicotinamide adenine dinucleotide and ATP. Some glycolytic enzymes are allosterically stimulated (eg, fructose-1,6-bisphosphate for PK) or inhibited (e.g., glucose-6-phosphate [G6P] for HK) by intermediate products of the pathway.[1] Unlike other major pathways for the production of cellular energy in the form of ATP, glycolysis does not involve mitochondrial oxidative phosphorylation and is termed anerobic. The rate of ATP production from anaerobic glycolysis far exceeds that of oxidative phosphorylation, when glycolysis is activated to meet acute energy needs. Thus any impairment of glycolysis has a marked effect on those tissues with uniquely high and variable energy requirements such as skeletal muscle.[2]

Inherited disorders of glycolysis impair the inducible, rapid-onset production of cellular energy and affect multiple organ systems. Specific defects of glycolysis cause some or all of the following involvements, including hemolysis resulting in nonspherocytic anemia, recurrent myoglobinuria, or neurocognitive impairment (Table 5.1). These clinical manifestations are clinically obvious, and a great number of patients have been described especially for hemolysis phenotype, which can be readily diagnosed by enzyme testing performed on a blood sample. The myoglobinuria phenotype is less readily ascertained, at least in part due to the invasiveness of muscle sampling and to delays in the recognition of the clinical presentation with rhabdomyolysis.

However, with the advent of next generation sequencing technology, this group of disorders has become more readily diagnosable using the massively parallel sequencing approach to analyze multiple genes associated with energy metabolism disorders causing rhabdomyolysis at the same time.

At least 13 unique enzyme deficiencies of glycolysis have been described (Table 5.1). The related tissue involvement stems from the failure to quickly generate ATP by anaerobic metabolism of glucose. Erythrocytes are especially reliant on glycolysis due to the loss of nuclei and mitochondria while maturing from reticulocyte precursors, whereas reticulocytes retain functional oxidative phosphorylation as an alternative route for ATP production and are relatively spared from hemolysis.[3] Furthermore, myofibers in skeletal muscle are uniquely dependent on glycolysis for the rapid-onset generation of ATP during vigorous exercise, termed anaerobic exercise, and rhabdomyolysis results from membrane instability associated with ATP depletion.

The pattern of involvement for specific defects in glycolysis cannot be readily predicted based on the position in glycolysis where a defect occurs, because the most proximal deficiencies cause either isolated hemolysis (HK) or myopathy (phosphoglucomutase 1/PGM1), and the most distal deficiency, PK, causes isolated hemolysis.[3] Rather, the pattern of tissue expression for each enzyme in question determines the related pathophysiology (Table 5.1). For example, deficiency of one of three isozymes for PFK, PFK-M (muscle), causes myoglobinuria and compensated hemolysis. PFK-M is the sole isozyme for PFK expressed in

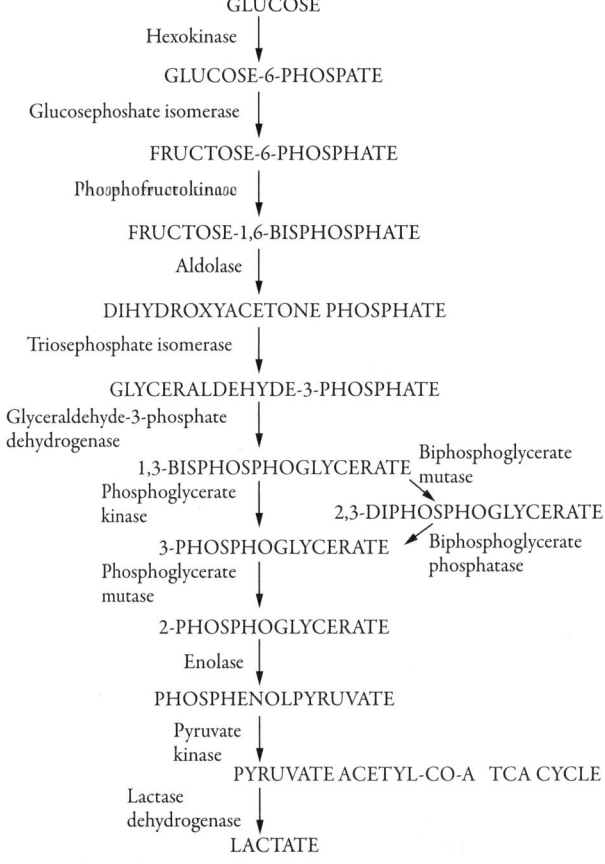

FIGURE 5.1 **Enzymes of Glycolysis.** Intermediates of glycolysis are shown in uppercase, and enzyme steps as arrows with the enzyme name adjacent.

TABLE 5.1 **Enzyme Deficiencies of Glycolysis**

Enzyme (GSD Type/GSD#)	OMIM	Gene	Locus	Inheritance[1]	Common Mutation	Ethnic Predisposition	Clinical Presentation[2]
Phosphoglucomutase 1 (GSD XIV)	*171900	PGM1	1p31	AR	Unknown	Unknown	M
Hexokinase	*142600	HK1	10q22	AR	None	None	H
Glucose-6-phosphate isomerase	*172400	GPI	19q13.1	AR	None	None	H, N, M
PFK (muscle) (GSD VII)	*610681	PFK-M	12q13.3	AR	Δ5/g>a (61%); del2003C (33%)	Ashkenazi Jewish	H, M
Phosphoglycerate mutase (GSD X)	*612931	PGAM2	7p13-p12.3	AR	W78X	African American	M
Aldolase (GSD XII)	*103850	ALDOA	16q11.2	AR	None	None	H, m
Triosephosphate isomerase	*190450	TPI1	12p13	AR	Glu104Asp (77%)	None	H, N
Phosphoglycerate kinase	*311800	PGK1	Xq13	XL	None	None	H, N, m
Diphosphoglycerate mutase	*613896	BPGM	7q22-34	AR	Arg89Cys; del205C	African-American	H, E, m
Enolase (GSD XIII)	*131370	ENO3	17pter-p12	AR	None	None	M
Pyruvate kinase	*609712	PKLR	1q21	AR	Arg510Gln (30%)	None	H
Lactate dehydrogenase (GSD XI)	*150000	LDHA	11p15.4	AR			M
Phosphoglucomutase (GSD XIV)	*171900	PGM1	1p31	AR	None	None	M

Note. GSD = glycogen storage disease; PFK = phosphofructokinase; AR = autosomal recessive; XL = X-linked; H = hemolytic anemia, common; N = neurologic, common; M = myopathic, common; m = myopathic, infrequent; E = erythrocytosis, common.

muscle, and it is co-expressed with PFK-L (liver) in erythrocytes. Pyruvate kinase, liver and RBC (PKLR), defects reduce PK activity in the liver and in erythrocytes but not in muscle, explaining isolated hemolysis in this disorder. One of the most severe disorders, phosphoglycerate kinase (PGK) deficiency, results from defects in a gene (PGK-1) that is expressed in all tissues other than spermatozoa, and this disorder causes hemolysis, myoglobinuria, and progressive central nervous system dysfunction.[3]

Hemolysis Phenotype: Pyruvate Kinase deficiency

Mature red blood cells (RBCs) are dependent on glycolysis for energy. PK is one of the rate-limiting enzymes critical for control of the metabolic flux in the second part of glycolysis. Thus mature RBCs with deficient PK activity undergo energy crises due to ATP depletion, ultimately affecting their life term viability.[4] PK deficiency (OMIM *609712) is the most frequent enzyme abnormality of the glycolytic pathway and the most common cause of hereditary nonspherocytic hemolytic anemia, together with G6P dehydrogenase deficiency.[3] The PKLR gene (over 9.5 Kb) is located on chromosome 1q21,[5] where it directs tissue specific transcription for both the liver and RBC (RPK) PK isoenzymes by alternate promoters.[6] The prevalence of PK deficiency is 1:20,000 in the general white population,[7] low erythrocyte activity was found in 1:697 of newborn infants in the United States[8] and in 37:3069 of Japanese.[9] The PK defect leads to accumulation of glycolytic intermediates proximal to the metabolic block, particularly 2,3 diphosphoglycerate (2,3-DPG), which may increase up to threefold and further impair the glycolytic flux through the inhibition of hexokinase. The clinical hallmark of PK deficiency is chronic hemolysis.[3,7,10] The anemia of infancy gradually improves with age, whereas the anemia of adulthood is stable with the exception of exacerbations during acute infections or pregnancy. The anemia in PK deficient patients is thought to be relatively well tolerated because of the increased red cell 2,3-DPG content, which is responsible for a rightward shift in the oxygen dissociation curve of hemoglobin. Complications of PK deficiency include gall stones even after splenectomy, aplastic crises following parvovirus B19 infection, kernicterus, chronic leg ulcers, acute pancreatitis secondary to biliary tract disease, splenic abscess, and extramedullary hematopoietic tissue.[3] Iron overload is a known complication, the pathogenesis of which is multifactorial in PK deficiency and related to hemolysis and the need for frequent transfusions.[3] It has also been postulated that iron overload is exacerbated by mutations involving either one or both alleles of the hemochromatosis gene. Hematological features of PK deficiency are not distinctive and can occur in other forms of nonspherocytic hemolytic anemia. Reticulcytosis is a typical feature of hemolytic anemias; however, in contrast to other disorders, in PK deficiency reticulocytes are not proportional to the severity of hemolysis. Instead, young erythrocytes deficient in PK are selectively sequestered by the spleen. Splenectomy results in a rise of reticulocytes, even when the anemia improves, and this may be a clue for the diagnosis of PK deficiency.[11] A definitive diagnosis of PK deficiency is made by measurement of enzyme activity. Particular caution must be taken to ensure removal of white blood cells; also, the presence of reticulocytosis with "age dependent enzymes," including PK, may mask the deficiency in the rest of RBC population and may result in false assessment of the actual level of enzyme activity.[12] Genotype–phenotype correlations have been described: clinical studies indicated that severe disease (hemoglobin <8 g/dl and or >50 transfusions) was more commonly associated with missense mutations as 994A and 1529A in the homozygous state, or with disruptive mutations in the first part of the protein, such as a stop codon, for example Glu241stop, frameshift and splicing mutations, or missense mutations involving the terminal part of the protein.[10] A mild phenotype with hemoglobin concentration ≥10 g/dl is more commonly seen in patients with the Arg486Trp mutation. Clinical outcome prediction based on molecular findings remains limited due to complex interactions between physiological and environmental factors, which include, in addition to the genetic background, concomitant functional polymorphisms of other enzymes; posttranslational or epigenetic modifications; and variability due to the occurrence of intercurrent infections, ineffective erythropoiesis, and differences in splenic function.[13]

Treatment of PK deficiency consists of folate supplementation, blood transfusions, and splenectomy.[3] RBC transfusions are required in severely anemic cases. As the delivery of oxygen to tissues is highly efficient because of the high 2,3-DPG content and associated low hemoglobin oxygen affinity, the decision to transfuse a PK-deficient patient would be based on the clinical condition and the presence of comorbidities. Splenectomy results in an increase of 1 to 3 g/dl of hemoglobin but does not arrest hemolysis; however, it reduces or even eliminates in some cases the need for transfusions in transfusion-dependent patients. Iron chelation may be required as iron overload is relatively common in PK deficiency. Erythropoietin has been reported as an effective treatment in one patient.[14] Bone marrow transplantation has been successfully performed in one severely affected child.[15]

HK deficiency (OMIM *142600) and aldolase A deficiency (OMIM *103850) are also characterized by nonspherocytic hemolytic anemia. HK is a regulatory enzyme of the Embden-Meyerhof pathway, which catalyzes the phosphorylation of glucose to G6P by ATP.[3] HK is an age-dependent enzyme, because HK activity is much higher in reticulocytes than in mature cells and complicates the diagnosis of HK deficiency.

Aldolase A is found in red cells and muscle and is responsible for the conversion of fructose-1,6-bisphosphate into glyceraldehyde-3-phosphate and dihydroxyacetone phosphate (Figure 5.1) A predominantly myopathic form has been reported in a child with suspected hemolytic anemia.[16]

Myopathy Phenotype: Phosphofructokinase Deficiency

PFK deficiency (OMIM *610681) is the best characterized of the glycolysis defects with multisystem involvement. PFK is a rate limiting, acting at the third step of glycolysis, catalyzing the phosphorylation of fructose-6-phosphate to fructose-1,6-bisphosphate (Figure 5.1). A defect in PFK blocks muscle glycolysis and glycogenolysis, thus limiting ATP regeneration from glycoysis and impairing oxidative phosphorylation and energy production.[17] PFK is comprised of three subunits expressed in a tissue-specific manner: muscle (M), liver (L), and platelet (P). Deficiency of the M subunit results in myopathy, while partial loss of PFK activity in RBCs leads to compensated hemolysis, since the muscle type contributes to 50% of the total erythrocyte enzyme activity while the liver type contributes the other half.[17] Glycolysis is markedly abnormal in PFK deficiency, which explains the effect on erythrocytes and skeletal muscle. Downstream products of PFK were reduced in erythrocytes at rest in patients with Tarui disease, whereas exercise significantly increased the levels of intermediates of glycolysis in these patients in comparison with normals.[18] Four clinical forms of PFK deficiency have been characterized.[19] The classical form (glycogen storage disease [GSD] type VIIa) includes exercise intolerance, muscle cramps, muscle pain, and myoglobinuria after exercise. Patients with the late-onset form (GSD VIIb) usually develop fatigability or weakness during adult life, although the patient's ability to endure exercise is usually low beginning in childhood. Slow progressive weakness becomes prominent in the fifth decade, and this weakness leads to severe disability in daily life activity. The infantile form (GSD VIIc) presents soon after birth when infants are floppy and hypotonic. This is associated with either early demise or longer survival with developmental delay. The fourth features hereditary nonspherocytic hemolytic anemia with no muscle symptoms.[19]

An "out-of-wind" phenomenon has been observed in patients with Tauri disease, which correlates with increased glucose production and presumably decreased availability of free fatty acids and ketones for ATP production.[20] This feature distinguishes GSD VII from McArdle (GSD V) disease where the metabolic block is restricted to glycogenolysis, so patients develop a "second-wind phenomenon" (i.e., patients feel better when continuing exercise because elevated glucose utilization is supplied by increased blood flow during exercise). Other distinguishing features from GSD V include the presence of mild reticulocytosis and increased serum bilirubin.

Laboratory findings include marked elevation of the levels of serum enzymes released from skeletal muscle such as creatine kinase, lactate dehydrogenase, and aspartate transaminase. Mild reticulocytosis and increased serum bilirubin are typically present, along with elevated uric acid especially after exercise. Biochemical analysis of glycolytic intermediates in muscle biopsies demonstrate variable elevations of glycogen, glucose-1-phosphate, G6P, and fructose-6-phosphate, as well as decrease of fructose-1,6-bisphosphate and triose phosphates. Values for 2, 3-DPG, an important regulator of erythrocyte function, are markedly decreased, and therefore the affinity of hemoglobin for oxygen is increased.[18]

Enzymatic activity of PFK in muscle is usually completely lost with no clear evidence of a relationship between the residual PFK enzyme activity in skeletal muscle and phenotypic expression of the disease. The structure of glycogen accumulated in muscle is usually normal; however, in some cases of PFK deficiency, an abnormal polysaccharide (polyglucosan) is found in muscle fibers in addition to excess glycogen. The abnormal polysaccharide stains with periodic acid Schiff and is more often found in GSD VIIb.[19] Muscle histopathology may reveal vacuolar formation in the subsarcolemmal space.[21] Vacuolar myopathy has been reported in other GSDs, such as acid maltase deficiency, debrancher enzyme deficiency, and myophosphorylase deficiency. In PFK deficiency, the vacuoles could be red-rimmed, subsarcolemmal, and elongated and have acid phosphatase positive deposits that increase with age, suggesting increased lysosomal activity as the disease progresses.[22] Two mutations comprise the great majority of Tarui disease alleles among Ashkenazi Jewish patients: an exon five splicing defect and a single base deletion leading to a frameshift mutation in exon 22.[23] Currently there is no specific form of treatment, and treatment is symptomatic, including the avoidance of strenuous exercise and aggressive treatment of myoglobinuria.[24] A novel approach to therapy was demonstrated when a patient with infantile PFK deficiency and arthrogryposis showed improvement on a ketogenic diet, suggesting that dietary therapy, including a high fat content, may be beneficial in patients with PFK deficiency and muscular involvement.[24]

Phosphoglycerate mutase (PGAM) deficiency (OMIM *612931/GSD X) is considered to be a relatively benign muscle glycogenosis.[26] PGAM is an enzyme of terminal glycolysis that catalyzes the reversible shift of the phosphate group between C-2 and C-3 of glycerate (Figure 5.1). The prevalence of the disease appears to be more common in African Americans; however, other cases have been reported involving patients from Italy, from Japan, and of Pakestani descent. One nonsense mutation (W78X) in exon1 of the PGAM2 gene encoding the muscle subunit has been commonly found in African-American patients, suggesting a founder effect in this population.[26] Patients are asymptomatic until they perform brief strenuous exercise that triggers myalgia, muscle cramps, and often muscle necrosis and myoglobinuria. The benign clinical phenotype has been attributed to the remaining PGAM activity, which was thought to be sufficient to allow near normal oxidative capacity, and production of lactate during exercise—enough to prevent the occurrence of a "second wind" with continued exercise.[27] Creatine kinase may be elevated, and forearm ischemic exercise testing shows mildly increased venous lactate levels 1.3 to 1.5 times (reference range three- to five-fold increase).[28] Muscle biopsy shows normal to mild glycogen accumulation, with prominent tubular aggregates.

Muscle-specific enolase deficiency, or β-enolase deficiency (GSD XIII; OMIM *131370) blocks the conversion of 2-phospho-D-glycerate to 2-phospho-enolpyruvate, one of the terminal steps of glycolysis (Figure 5.1). *ENO3,* the gene encoding β-enolase, maps to chromosome 17pter-p11, contains 12 exons, and is translated in a protein of 433 residues.[29] Patients with β-enolase deficiency present by exercise-induced myalgia and increased CK levels after intense exercise. Symptoms may be episodic for years, with no lactate rise induced by ischemic exercise. The muscle biopsy does not show gross glycogen accumulation, although an increased amount of sarcoplasmic glycogen β particles may be detected by electron microscopy.[29] This last feature is also seen in aldolase A, PGAM, and lactate dehydrogenase (LDH)-M deficiencies and may be explained by expression of nonmuscle isozymes.[30] A distinguishing feature from other glycolytic defects, such as PFK and PGK deficiencies is the lack of nonmuscular tissues involvement, in accordance with the muscle-specific expression of the *ENO3* gene.[29]

LDH deficiency (GSD XI/OMIM *150000) is associated with metabolic myopathy. LDH is a tetrameric enzyme that consists of A and B subunits and plays a role in the final steps of glycolysis (Figure 5.1). LDH catalyzes the conversion of pyruvate to lactate with nicotinamide adenine dinucleotide (NAD) as cofactor. This enzyme reaction oxidizes nicotinamide adenine dinucleotide phosphate hydrogen (NADPH) and replenishes NAD, which is essential for the glycolytic conversion of glucose to pyruvate. LDHA is found predominantly in muscle (LDH-M).[31] Clinical features are related to diminished energy supply and impaired ability to sustain exercise due to muscle pain and stiffness. Patients present with intolerance to intense exercise, cramps, and recurrent myoglobinuria; the degree of severity of the symptoms varies from one case to the other. In LDH deficiency's myglobinuria episodes, the expectedly high levels of CK contrast with low levels of serum LDH.

PGM1 deficiency (GSD XIV/OMIM *171900) has been recently described in a patient with exercise-induced intolerance and episodes of rhabdomyolysis.[32] The patient had normal elevation of lactate and hyperammonemia on a forearm-exercise test. In vitro study of anaerobic glycogenolysis and glycolysis in muscle showed a metabolic block after formation of glucose-1-phosphate and before formation of G6P, indicating PGM1 deficiency. A muscle biopsy revealed abnormal subsarcolemmal and sarcoplasmic accumulations of normally structured, free glycogen. Biochemical investigation of muscle revealed marked reduction of PGM1 activity, whereas myophosphorylase and PFK activities were normal. Analysis of the PGM1 gene revealed de novo compound heterozygous mutations.[32]

The Combined Phenotype: Hemolysis and/or Neurological Manifestations (With or Without Myopathy)

The classical combined phenotype among glycolytic disorders is PGK deficiency (OMIM *311800), a multisystem disorder involving the RBC, the central nervous system and muscle. PGK deficiency is the only X-linked disorder of glycolysis.[33] PGK acts in the terminal glycolytic pathway yielding 3-phosphoglycerate and ATP (Figure 5.1). Manifesting females present with anemia, while hemizygous males have additional features suggestive of central nervous system and/or muscle disease. Central nervous system manifestations may be behavioral abnormalities, emotional lability, variable mental retardation, epilepsy, movement disorders, or hemiplegia and aphasia. A 4 base deletion in exon 6 of the PGK gene caused isolated exertional myopathy and myoglobinuria in an adult male.[34] As in other glycolytic disorders, the specific diagnosis is made by measuring PGK activity in muscle and erythrocytes. CK elevation occurs during the forearm ischemic exercise test; this reveals normal blood pyruvate and lactate in patients with the muscle phenotype. Although there is no specific treatment, a ketogenic was postulated to theoretically beneficial, since it would bypass the enzymopathy in glycolysis.[35]

Triose phosphate isomerase (TPI) deficiency (OMIM *190450) is a multisystem disorder characterized by being the most severe disorder of glycolysis. The majority of affected children die before the age of five years.[3] Genetic studies of multiple unrelated families have shown that a single mutation, G to C transversion at codon 104, accounts for 80% of mutant alleles, reflecting a founder effect.[36] TPI catalyzes the interconversion of dihydroxyacetone phosphate and glyceraldehyde-3-phosphate in the Embden-Meyerhof pathway (Figure 5.1). TPI deficiency may manifest as hemolytic anemia, progressive neurologic dysfunction, susceptibility to bacterial infection, and cardiomyopathy. The first symptom in newborns is nonspherocytic hemolytic anemia and neurologic symptoms, including dystonic movements, tremors, and pyramidal tract signs; spinal motor neuron involvement manifest between six and 24 months.[37] Currently there is no known effective treatment for TPI deficiency; splenectomy has not been helpful.[3] Successful metabolic correction of the defect in TPI-deficient cells after using culturing in the presence of exogenous enzymes suggested the feasibility of enzyme replacement therapy.[38]

Pathogenesis and Interaction With Other Metabolic Pathways

Hemolytic Phenotype: Congenital Nonspherocytic Hemolytic Anemia

Chronic hemolytic anemia is the only or predominant clinical manifestation in PK, hexokinase, and G6P isomerase deficiencies. Erythrocytes are essential for cellular vitality and oxygen transport. Devoid of nuclei, mitochondria, or ribosomes, erythrocytes lack protein, lipid synthesis, or oxidative phosphorylation. Consequently, erythrocytes are dependent on glycolysis for generation and storage of high energy phosphates in the form of ATP, as their unique metabolic source of energy. ATP is needed for maintaining membrane integrity, ionic composition, cell surface and volume, biconcave shape, and deformability.[3] Red cell enzymopathies due to defective anerobic glycolysis have features that distinguish them from hereditary spherocytosis: (a) Most are autosomal recessive (as opposed to dominant); (b) the red cells tend to lose potassium rather than gain sodium in vitro; (c) affected cells may show crenation but do not swell or become spherocytic in vivo; and (d) the membrane defect is sufficiently obvious so that the liver, rather than the spleen, is the primary site of destruction, and consequently hemolysis persists after splenectomy.[39]

Erythrocytes possess a unique glycolytic bypass for the production 2,3-DPG, called the Rapoport-Luebering shunt. This shunt bypasses the PGK step, which normally generates one molecule of ATP by catalyzing the reversible conversion of 1,3-bisphosphoglycerate to 3-phospho-glycerate (Figure 5.1), thus preventing the formation of the second ATP molecule.[39] The shunt is necessary for maintaining a high concentration of 2,3-DPG, an essential modulator of oxygen transport by hemoglobin and an energy buffer. Red cell enzymopathies affect the content of 2,3-DPG because of the pivotal position the shunt has in the glycolytic pathway.[39] Low levels of 2,3-DPG are found in enzymopathies affecting the early part of the pathway as in HK, PFK, and GPI deficiencies.[40] Generally speaking, high levels of 2,3-DPG occur in most anemias with or without reticulocytosis. Enzyme deficiencies proximal to the 2,3-DPG step (i.e., PGK and PK deficiency) show increased 2,3-DPG levels as a result of the respective metabolic blocks and of a retrograde accumulation of products of glycolysis. The increased 2,3-DPG levels result in a decreased oxygen affinity of hemoglobin so that oxygen is more readily transferred to tissue. Thus the anemia is ameliorated and exertional tolerance is improved. This beneficial effect is absent in the distal glycolytic enzyme defects HK, GPI, PFK, aldolase, and TPI deficiency, which all cause a decrease in 2,3-DPG levels.[1] Depletion of ATP is thought to be the primary cause of hemolysis in red cell enzymopathies of the anerobic glycolytic pathway, whereas changes of levels of glycolytic intermediates and 2,3-DPG, which can be very important, do not contribute to the hemolysis per se.[41] A physiologic response to compensate for anemia caused by hemolysis is increased erythrocyte production through reticulocytosis (reticulocytes normally comprise 0.5% to 2.5% of total erythrocytes). Reticulocytes still contain cytoplasmic organelles, including ribosomes and mitochondria, and are capable of synthesizing protein and producing ATP by oxidative phosphorylation. On the other hand, reticulocytes may be more severely compromised than mature erythrocytes in the spleen, particularly in patients with glycolytic enzymopathies.[3,11]

Myopathy Phenotype: Exercise Intolerance, Muscle Cramps, Myoglobinuria

The myopathy phenotype is associated with symptomatic presentation related to intense exertion causing myoglobinuria.[42] As in the hemolytic phenotype, impaired glycolysis prevents the adequate synthesis of ATP to maintain membrane stability. PFK deficiency prevents the generation of ATP from either glucose or glycogen, as does the downstream blocks in PGK deficiency. PFK deficiency impairs glycolysis more severely than GSD type V from myophosphorylase deficiency, which prevents ATP generation from glycogen but not glucose. The latter disorder is associated with a second-wind phenomenon due to enhanced hepatic glucose production during exercise, and no such adaptation is present in PFK deficiency.[43] The partial defect of PFK in erythrocytes of the patients is due to the lack of PFK-M isozyme, whereas PFK-L is still present and explains the compensated hemolytic anemia observed in PFK deficiency.[19] Therefore, PFK-M deficiency causes recurrent myoglobinuria due to lack of an alternative isoform in skeletal muscle that would provide an alternative source of PFK activity.

Hyperproduction of uric acid as a consequence of metabolic crises in the exercising muscle is referred to as "myogenic hyperuricemia." Hyperuricemia is a significant secondary abnormality in PFK deficient patients. An increase in the release of inosine and hypoxanthine from exercising muscle occurs due to accumulation of adenosine monophosphate (AMP) secondary to impaired glycolysis, increased degradation of ATP to ADP, and decreased synthesis of ATP from ADP. Inosine and hypoxanthine released from skeletal muscle are then used as substrates for uric acid production in the liver. Hyperproduction of uric acid as a consequence of metabolic crises in the exercising muscle is referred to as "myogenic hyperuricemia."[44]

Unanswered Questions, Future Directions, Impact on Common or Complex Traits

Potential for Population Screening to Achieve Early Detection of Glycolytic Disorders

Attempts to perform newborn screening for disorders of glycolysis would be complicated by the challenges of enzyme testing from a bloodspot on filter paper. In general, a blood sample must be deproteinized immediately to reliably assay glycolytic enzymes.[3] Alternatively, mutation screening could detect homozygous and heterozygous status for common mutations underlying inherited disorders of glycolysis (Table 5.1), followed by enzyme testing from a fresh blood sample to differentiate carrier from affected status. However, genetic testing as a method for newborn screening is complicated by the detection of unaffected carriers (false positives) and by missing rare mutations (false negatives) and has not been applied in absence of a complementary biochemical test.

Pyruvate Kinase Deficiency and Hemochromatosis

Secondary iron overload has been described in PK deficient patients with no or limited history of blood transfusions; this occurence is unusual in untransfused patients with other types of congenital hemolytic anemia. Traditional risk factors for hemosiderosis include recurrent blood transfusions, chronic hemolysis with increased cell turnover, splenectomy, and ineffective hematopoiesis.[45] Iron accumulation in PK deficiency has been postulated to be related to the fairly high incidence of hemochromatosis mutations C282Y and H63D.[46] Since hereditary hemochromatosis is a frequent disease in Caucasian populations, some patients with PK deficiency may also be homozygotes for the hemochromatosis gene.

Moreover, as the carrier rate of hereditary hemochromatosis can be as high as 1:10, it is even more likely that a patient with PK deficiency may also be a carrier of a hereditary hemochromatosis (HFE) gene mutation. In such cases, iron overload would be the consequence of an increased iron absorption due to both the presence of the hemochromatosis gene and the chronic hemolytic anemia.[45–47] In these patients, hemochromatosis was diagnosed after the third decade. A male with PK deficiency due to mutation of the H63D gene was treated successfully by phlebotomy, suggesting that phlebotomy did not worsen the anemia in PK deficient patients adequately transfused for hemolysis.[48] More patients with PK deficiency need to be studied for the presence of iron overload, and family studies must be conducted to look for the presence of hereditary hemochromatosis in order to test this hypothesis. Theoretically, the carrier state of hemochromatosis may increase the risk of hemochromatosis in a patient with PK deficiency by synergistic heterozygosity.

Altered Glycolysis in Skeletal Muscle Underlying Insulin Resistance

An initial report of type 2 diabetes mellitus (Type 2 DM) in affected relatives with PFK deficiency has stimulated investigation of the role for PFK-M in the pathogenesis of Type 2 DM.[49,50] Ristow et al. evaluated the hypothesis that homozygous mutations in PFK may lead to insulin resistance and diabetes. This case study revealed abnormal glucose tolerance in a father and son with PFK deficiency. Vertical transmission of PFK deficiency in this family was related to the mother carrying a common allele for PFK deficiency and represents pseudo-dominant inheritance of PFK deficiency. Furthermore, the mother had Type 2 DM and her other son was a carrier and demonstrated moderate resistance upon insulin tolerance testing.[49]

The basis for insulin resistance in PFK deficiency was hypothesized to be related to the regulatory role PFK plays in glycolysis. In PFK deficiency anaerobic glycolysis would be impaired and glucose tolerance would be affected. Biochemical studies of subjects with Type 2 DM have failed to reveal a causative role for PFK deficiency. Indeed, enzyme analyses of Type 2 DM muscle biopsies revealed normal or increased activity of PFK and other glycolytic enzymes.[51,52] Genetic studies of sibling pairs with Type 2 DM failed to reveal evidence for linkage to PFM or 18 other candidate genes.[53] Intriguingly, upregulation of PFK and other glycolytic enzymes following androgens in diabetic rats reduced hyperglycemia, indicating that compensatory increases in glycolysis might be adaptive or even therapeutic in diabetes mellitus.[54,55] Whether decreased expression of PFK and glycolysis underlies the pathogenesis of of Type 2 DM remains controversial, because gene expression analysis has revealed decreased PFK-L, hexokinase 2, and LDH-B RNA in the muscle of subjects with Type 2 DM,[56] in contrast with the evidence from biochemical investigations cited above.

Glycolysis and Apoptosis: Potential Role in Carcinogenesis

Glycolysis is critical to cellular energy production and therefore well situated to modulate the factors involved in cell survival. Increasingly glycolytic enzymes have been implicated as key players in carcinogenesis[57] and appear at least superficially to act both in

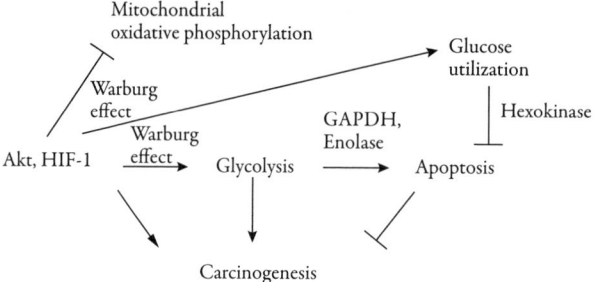

FIGURE 5.2 **Interrelationships of Cellular Metabolism and Cell Survival.** Akt and HIF-1 increase the activity of glycolysis and inhibit mitochondrial oxidative phosphorylation. Effects of the proteins depicted are shown, either stimulatory (arrows) or inhibitory (blunt arrows).

facilitative and repressive roles (Figure 5.2). The former role has been implied by the long-recognized upregulation of glycolysis in tumors, known as the Warburg effect, and more recently implicated by the induction of glycolysis by Akt and hypoxia inducible transcription factor 1 during carcinogenesis. The latter role has been recognized due to the multifaceted functions of glycolytic enzymes that include the induction of cell death through activation of apoptosis.

The implication of glycolytic enzymes in other functions, termed "moon-lighting," emphasizes the complexity of pathogenesis in common, multifactorial conditions such as cancer.[58] For instance, glyceraldehyde-3-phosphate dehydrogenase has at least 11 recognized functions, including the induction of apoptosis.[58] Elevated glyceraldehyde-3-phosphate dehydrogenase expression has been associated with increased apoptosis in the liver of GSD type Ia, where the block of G6P conversion to glucose drives high rates of glycolysis.[59] Although hepatocellular carcinoma occurs frequently in GSD type Ia,[60] increased apoptosis would seem to oppose carcinogenesis. However, increased glycolysis is recognized in many tumors and promotes glucose utilization in response to the hypoxic environment of tumor formation in response to hypoxia inducible transcription factor 1 expression.[57,61] Furthermore, increased mitochondrial hexokinase expression during enhanced glycolysis is associated with the suppression of apoptosis, consistent with carcinogenesis.[57] Overall, metabolism is controlled in cancer cells by Akt (Figure 5.2), which stimulates glycolysis stimulates and inhibits mitochondrial oxidative phosphorylation along with apoptosis.[62] The concept that cellular metabolism controls the fate of cancer cells has been extended to suggest that the activation of mitochondrial oxidative phosphorylation could be stimulated by dichloroacetate to enhance the effect of chemotherapy on tumors.[61] Yi et al. revealed a new mechanism for the regulation of metabolic pathways in cancer by inducing O-Gal NAc glycosylation at serine 529 of the PFK1 gene in response to hypoxia.[63] This approach led to inhibition of PFK1 regulation of glycolysis and diverted glucose through the pentose phosphate pathway thus favoring tumor growth and survival. The group also showed that blocking glycosylation at the same site reduced cancer cell proliferation in vitro and attenuated tumor formation, suggesting a possible target for therapeutic intervention. The observation that activation of PFK-1 occurs in tumor cells to increase glycolytic flux further supports the hypothesis that metabolism and cancer are linked and provides a rationale for inhibiting glycolysis during chemotherapy.[63]

Summary

Inherited disorders of glycogen are increasingly understood at the molecular and cellular levels, and new insights into common disorders such as diabetes and cancer have stemmed from a basic understanding of glycolysis. Ultimately new therapies for disorders of glycolysis will be available in the form of gene and cell therapy. Furthermore, manipulations of glycolysis could impact therapy for diabetes and cancer.

Acknowledgments

Dwight Koeberl was supported by NIH Grant R01 HL081122-01A1 from the National Heart, Lung, and Blood Institute.

References

1. van Wijk R, van Solinge WW. The energy-less red blood cell is lost: erythrocyte enzyme abnormalities of glycolysis. *Blood.* 2005; 106(13): 4034–4042.
2. DiMauro S, Bresolin N, Hays AP. Disorders of glycogen metabolism of muscle. *CRC Crit Rev Clin Neurobiol.* 1984; 1(2): 83–116.
3. Hirono A, Kanno H, Miwa S, Beutler E. Pyruvate kinase deficiency and other enzymopathies of the erythrocyte. In: Scriver CR, et al., eds. *The Metabolic and Molecular Bases of Inherited Disease,* 8th ed. New York: McGraw-Hill; 2001:4637–4664.
4. Zanella A, Fermo E, Bianchi P, Valentini G. Red cell pyruvate kinase deficiency: molecular and clinical aspects. *Br J Haematol.* 2005; 130(1): 11–25.
5. Satoh H, Tani K, Yoshida MC, Sasaki M, Miwa S, Fujii H. The human liver-type pyruvate kinase (PKL) gene is on chromosome 1 at band q21. *Cytogenet Cell Genet.* 1988; 47: 132–133.
6. Kanno H, Fujii H, Miwa S. Structural analysis of human pyruvate kinase L-gene and identification of the promoter activity in erythroid cells. *Biochem Biophys Res Commun.* 1992; 188(2): 516–523.
7. Beutler E, Gelbart T. Estimating the prevalence of pyruvate kinase deficiency from the gene frequency in the general white population. *Blood.* 2000; 95(11): 3585–3588.
8. Mohrenweiser HW. Frequency of enzyme deficiency variants in erythrocytes of newborn infants. *Proc Natl Acad Sci USA.* 1981; 78(8): 5046–5050.
9. Satoh C, Neel JV, Yamashita A, Goriki K, Fujita M, Hamilton HB. The frequency among Japanese of heterozygotes for deficiency variants of 11 enzymes. *Am. J. Hum. Genet.* 1983; 35: 656–674.
10. Zanella A, Bianchi P. Red cell pyruvate kinase deficiency: from genetics to clinical manifestations. *Baillieres Best Pract Res Clin Haematol.* 2000; 13(1): 57–81.
11. Mentzer WC, Baehner RL, Schmidt-Schonbeth H, Robinson SH, Nathan DG. Selective reticulocyte destruction in erythrocyte pyruvate kinase deficiency. *J Clin Invest* 1971; 50(3): 688–699.
12. Arya R, Layton DM, Bellingham AJ. Hereditary red cell enzymopathies. *Blood Rev.* 1995; 9(3):165–175.
13. Zanella A, Bianchi P, Fermo E. Pyruvate kinase deficiency. *Haematologica.* 2007; 92(6): 721–723.
14. Vukelja SJ. Erythropoietin in the treatment of iron overload in a patient with hemolytic anemia and pyruvate kinase deficiency. *Acta Haematol.* 1994; 91(4): 199–200.
15. Tanphaichitr VS, Suvatte V, Issaragrisil S, et al. Successful bone marrow transplantation in a child with red blood cell pyruvate kinase deficiency. *Bone Marrow Transpl.* 2000; 26(6): 689–690.
16. Kreuder J, Borkhardt A, Repp R, et al Brief report: inherited metabolic myopathy and hemolysis due to a mutation in aldolase A. *N Engl J Med.* 1996; 334(17): 1100–1104.
17. Tarui S. Glycolytic defects in muscle: aspects of collaboration between basic science and clinical medicine. *Muscle Nerve.* 1995; 3:S2–S9.
18. Shimizu T, Kono N, Kiyokawa H., et al. Erythrocyte glycolysis and its marked alterations by muscular exercise in type VII glycogenosis. *Blood.* 1988; 71(4): 1130–1134.
19. Nakajima H, Raben N, Hamaguchi T, Yamasaki T. Phosphofructokinase deficiency; past, present and future. *Curr Mol Med.* 2002; 2(2): 197–212.

20. Vissing J, Galbo H, Haller RG. Paradoxically enhanced glucose production during exercise in humans with blocked glycolysis caused by muscle phosphofructokinase deficiency. *Neurology.* 1996; 47(3): 766–771.
21. Agamanolis D, Askari AD, DiMauro S, et al. Muscle phosphofructokinase deficiency: two cases with unusual polysaccharide accumulation and immunologically active enzyme protein. *Muscle Nerve.* 1980; 3(6): 456–467.
22. Sivakumar K, Vasconcelos O, Goldfarb L, Dalakas MC Late-onset muscle weakness in partial phosphofructokinase deficiency: a unique myopathy with vacuoles, abnormal mitochondria, and absence of the common exon 5/intron 5 junction point mutation. *Neurology* 1996; 46(5): 1337–1342.
23. Sherman JB, Raben N, Nicastri C, et al. Common mutations in the phosphofructokinase-M gene in Ashkenazi Jewish patients with glycogenesis VII—and their population frequency. *Am J Hum Genet.* 1994; 55(2): 305–313.
24. Heyne N, Guthoff M, Weisel KC. Rhabdomyolysis and acute kidney injury. *N Engl J Med.* 2009; 61(14): 1412–1413.
25. Swoboda KJ, Specht L, Jones HR, Shapiro F, DiMauro S, Korson M.,Infantile phosphofructokinase deficiency with arthrogryposis: clinical benefit of a ketogenic diet. *J Pediatr.* 1997; 131(6): 932–934.
26. Naini A, Toscano A, Musumesi O, Vissing J, Akman HO, Di Mauro S., Muscle phosphoglycerate mutase deficiency revisited. *Arch Neurol.* 2009; 66(3): 394–398.
27. Vissing J, Quistorff B, Haller RG. Effect of fuels on exercise capacity in muscle phosphoglycerate mutase deficiency. *Arch Neurol.* 2005; 62(9): 1440–1443.
28. Henry JG, Stevens SM. Neuronal ceroid lipofuscinosis in the amaurotic retardate: electron microscopic confirmation. *Aust J Ophthalmol.* 1982; 10(3): 161–166.
29. Comi, GP, Fortunato F, Lucchiari S, et al. Beta-enolase deficiency, a new metabolic myopathy of distal glycolysis. *Ann Neurol.* 2001; 50(2): 202–207.
30. Tsujino S, Nonaka I, DiMauro S. Glycogen storage myopathies. *Neurol Clin.* 2000; 18(1): 125–150.
31. Takahashi Y,Miyajima H,Kaneko E. Genetic analysis of a family of lactate dehydrogenase A subunit deficiency, *Internal Med.* 1995; 34: 326–329.
32. Stojkovic T, et al. Muscle glycogenosis due to phosphoglucomutase 1 deficiency. *N Engl J Med.* 2009; 361(4): 425–427.
33. Tsujino S, Shanske S, DiMauro S. Molecular genetic heterogeneity of phosphoglycerate kinase (PGK) deficiency. *Muscle Nerve.* 1995; 3: S45–S49.
34. Hamano T, Mutoh H, Sugie H, Koga H, Kuriyama M. Phosphoglycerate kinase deficiency: an adult myopathic form with a novel mutation. *Neurology.* 2000; 54(5): 1188–1190.
35. De Vivo DC, Leary L, Wang D. Glucose transporter 1 deficiency syndrome and other glycolytic defects. *J Child Neurol.* 2002; 17 (Suppl 3): 3S15–3S23.
36. Arya R,Lalloz MRA, Nicolaides KH, Bellingham AJ,Layton DM. Evidence for founder effect of the Glu104Asp substitution and identification of new mutations in triosephosphate isomerase deficiency. *Hum Mutat.* 1997; 10(4): 290–294.
37. Poll-The BT, Aicardi J, Girot R, Rosa R. Neurological findings in triosephosphate isomerase deficiency. *Ann Neurol.* 1985; 17: 439–443.
38. Ationu A, Humphries A, Lalloz MR, et al. Reversal of metabolic block in glycolysis by enzyme replacement in triosephosphate isomerase-deficient cells. *Blood.* 1999; 94(9): 3193–3198.
39. Keitt AS. Pyruvate kinase deficiency and related disorders of red cell glycolysis. *Am J Med.* 1966; 41(5): 762–785.
40. Beutler E, Dyment PG, Matsumoto F. Hereditary nonspherocytic hemolytic anemia and hexokinase deficiency. *Blood.* 1978; 51(5): 935–940.
41. Valentine WN, Paglia DE. The primary cause of hemolysis in enzymopathies of anaerobic glycolysis: a viewpoint. *Blood Cells.* 1980; 6(4): 819–829.
42. Cornelio F, Di Donato S. Myopathies due to enzyme deficiencies. *J Neurol.* 1985; 232(6): 329–340.
43. Haller RG, Vissing J. No spontaneous second wind in muscle phosphofructokinase deficiency. *Neurology.* 2004; 62(1): 82–86.
44. Mineo I, Kono N, Hara N, et al. Myogenic hyperuricemia: A common pathophysiologic feature of glycogenosis types III, V, and VII. *N Engl J Med.* 1987; 317(2): 75–80.
45. De Braekeleer M, St Pierre C, Vigneault A, Simard H, De Medicis, E. Hemochromatosis and pyruvate kinase deficiency: report of a case and review of the literature. *Ann Hematol.* 1991; 62(5): 188–189.

46. Zanella A, Berzuini A, Colombo MB, et al. Iron status and HFE genotype in erythrocyte pyruvate kinase deficiency: study of Italian cases. *Blood Cells Mol Dis.* 2001; 27(3): 653–661.
47. Merryweather-Clarke AT, Pointon JJ, Shearman JD, Robson KJ. Global prevalence of putative haemochromatosis mutations. *J Med Genet.* 1997; 4(4): 275–278.
48. Arnold H, Blume KG. A rare combination of two inherited disorders in one patient: pyruvate kinase deficiency and hemochromatosis. *Ann Hematol.* 2009; 88(8): 815–816.
49. Ristow M, Vorgerd M, Möhlig M, Schatz H, Pfeiffer A. Deficiency of phosphofructo-1-kinase/muscle subtype in humans impairs insulin secretion and causes insulin resistance. *J Clin Invest.* 1997; 100(11): 2833–2841.
50. Ristow M, Vorgerd M, Möhlig M, Schatz H, Pfeiffer A. Insulin resistance and impaired insulin secretion due to phosphofructo-1-kinase-deficiency in humans. *J Mol Med.* 1999; 77(1): 96–103.
51. Simoneau JA, Kelley DE. Altered glycolytic and oxidative capacities of skeletal muscle contribute to insulin resistance in NIDDM. *J Appl Physiol.* 1997; 83(1): 166–171.
52. Vestergaard H, Lund S, Larsen FS, Bjerrum OJ, Pedersen O. Glycogen synthase and phosphofructokinase protein and mRNA levels in skeletal muscle from insulin-resistant patients with non-insulin-dependent diabetes mellitus. *J Clin Invest.* 1993; 91(6): 2342–2350.
53. Vionnet N, Hani EH, Lesage S, et al. Genetics of NIDDM in France: studies with 19 candidate genes in affected sib pairs. *Diabetes.* 1997; 46(6): 1062–1068.
54. Sato K, Iemitsu M, Aizawa K, Ajisaka R. Testosterone and DHEA activate the glucose metabolism-related signaling pathway in skeletal muscle. *Am J Physiol Endocrinol Metab.* 2008; 294(5): E961–E968.
55. Sato K, Iemitsu M, Aizawa K, Ajisaka R. DHEA improves impaired activation of Akt and PKC zeta/lambda-GLUT4 pathway in skeletal muscle and improves hyperglycaemia in streptozotocin-induced diabetes rats. *Acta Physiol (Oxf).* 2009; 197(3): 217–225.
56. Palsgaard J, Brøns C, Friedrichsen M, et al. Gene expression in skeletal muscle biopsies from people with type 2 diabetes and relatives: differential regulation of insulin signaling pathways. *PLoS One.* 2009; 4(8): e6575.
57. Kim JW, Dang CV. Multifaceted roles of glycolytic enzymes. *Trends Biochem Sci.* 2005; 30(3): 142–150.
58. Sriram G, Martinez JA, McCabe ER, Liao JC, Dipple KM. Single-gene disorders: what role could moonlighting enzymes play? *Am J Hum Genet* 2005; 76(6): 911–924.
59. Sun B, Li S, Yang L, et al. Activation of glycolysis and apoptosis in glycogen storage disease type Ia. *Mol. Genet Metab.* 2009; 97(4): 267–271.
60. Franco LM, Krishnamurthy V, Bali D, et al. Hepatocellular carcinoma in glycogen storage disease type Ia: a case series. *J Inherit Metab Dis.* 2005; 28(2): 153–162.
61. Michelakis ED, Webster L, Mackey JR. Dichloroacetate (DCA) as a potential metabolic-targeting therapy for cancer. *Br J Cancer* 2008; 99(7): 989–994.
62. Yeung SJ, Pan J, Lee MH. Roles of p53, MYC and HIF-1 in regulating glycolysis—the seventh hallmark of cancer. *Cell Mol Life Sci.* 2008; 65(24): 3981–3999.
63. Yi WC, et al. Phosphofructokinase 1 glycosylation regulates cell growth and metabolism. *Science.* 2012; 337(6097): 975–980.

6

Urea Cycle

Ureagenesis and Non-Ureagenic Functions

OLEG A. SHCHELOCHKOV, SANDESH C.S. NAGAMANI,
PHILIPPE M. CAMPEAU, AYELET EREZ, AND BRENDAN LEE

Introduction

Urea cycle disorders (UCDs) are inborn errors of metabolism characterized by the inability to efficiently dispose of waste nitrogen. Traditionally, UCDs were viewed as pediatric-onset diseases with unfavorable outcomes that ranged from chronic encephalopathy to death induced by hyperammonemia. The clinical presentation of patients with a block in ureagenesis was dominated by hyperammonemia that caused significant morbidity and mortality. The resulting devastating neurological outcomes often obscured the recognition of a broader clinical spectrum, including the long-term complications of UCDs. The introduction of arginine supplementation[1] and nitrogen-scavenging medications[2] along with universal newborn screening programs have dramatically improved the outcome of patients with severe forms of UCDs. This improved survival has led to the recognition of many late-onset manifestations that appear to be independent of hyperammonemia, such as liver dysfunction and essential hypertension in patients with argininosuccinate lyase deficiency and spastic paraplegia in those with arginase 1 deficiency.

These late-onset manifestations that occur in the context of specific biochemical defects have set the stage to appreciate the complexity of phenotypes in UCDs and provided an impetus to explore disease mechanisms beyond hyperammonemia. Recent studies have shown that some urea cycle enzymes serve additional functions in addition to their primary role in hepatic ureagenesis. The successful management of UCDs should hence not only consist of modalities that promote ureagenesis in the liver or facilitate nitrogen disposal by nitrogen-scavenging agents but also address compromised non-ureagenic functions of the urea cycle enzymes.

Since the first description of the urea cycle by Krebs and Henseleit in 1932, there has been a significant improvement in our understanding of its function, regulation, and complex interconnection with other metabolic pathways. In the first part of this chapter, we present an overview of ureagenesis as the primary function of the urea cycle in the liver and discuss the biochemical consequences of hyperammonemia. In the latter part, we enumerate the role of urea cycle enzymes in regulation of arginine metabolism, interconnection with the tricarboxylic acid (TCA) cycle, and the effects of altered metabolites' concentrations on the clinical manifestations of UCDs. The final section of this chapter focuses on the implications of the ureagenic and non-ureagenic functions in treatment of UCDs.

Ureagenesis: The Primary Function of the Urea Cycle

The urea cycle is the primary pathway to dispose of nitrogenous waste in mammals. It involves five catalytic enzymes, a cofactor-synthesizing enzyme, and at least two transport proteins that are involved in the facilitation of nitrogen transfer between subcellular compartments. The catalytic steps include (1) synthesis of carbamoyl phosphate from ammonia and bicarbonate by carbamoyl-phosphate synthase 1 (CPS1); (2) formation of citrulline from carbamoyl phosphate and ornithine by ornithine transcarbamylase (OTC); (3) synthesis of argininosuccinate from citrulline and aspartate by argininosuccinate synthase 1 (ASS1); (4) cleavage of argininosuccinate into arginine and fumarate by argininosuccinate lyase (ASL) and (5) hydrolysis of arginine into urea and ornithine by arginase 1 (ARG1) (Figure 6.1). Ornithine generated from the hydrolysis of arginine can re-enter the cycle by combining with carbamoyl phosphate to form citrulline. N-acetylglutamate synthase (NAGS) produces N-acetylglutamate, a cofactor of CPS1, the rate-limiting enzyme of the urea cycle. Ureagenesis spans two subcellular compartments, the mitochondria and the cytosol. Reactions catalyzed by CPS1 and OTC occur in the mitochondrial matrix, whereas the rest of the urea cycle enzymes reside in the cytosol, possibly adjacent to the outer mitochondrial membrane. The transport of ornithine into the mitochondria and citrulline into the cytosol across the semipermeable mitochondrial membrane is facilitated by ornithine transporters type 1, 2, 3 (ORNT1, ORNT2, and ORNT3; also known as SLC25A15, SLC25A2, and SLC25A29, respectively) through the ornithine/citrulline-proton antiport mechanism.[3-5]

The two nitrogen atoms of urea are incorporated at different steps in the cycle. Ammonia, the source of the first nitrogen atom in urea, originates mostly from hydrolysis of the amide group of glutamine that is catalyzed by glutaminase. The second nitrogen atom is derived from aspartate and often originates from the amino group of alanine or glutamate through reactions of transamination. Only hepatocytes express all of the components of the urea cycle at levels sufficient to meet the ureagenic requirements of mammals. Most other tissues express specific components of the urea cycle in order to serve functions unrelated to ureagenesis, as discussed later in this chapter.

To appreciate the physiological consequences of impaired ureagenesis, one needs to examine the role of urea cycle in the context of interorgan exchange of nitrogen. Under homeostatic conditions, protein turnover and excess protein from the diet result in nitrogenous waste. The nitrogen derived from amino acid catabolism is transported from peripheral organs to the liver in the form of amide group of glutamine and amino group of alanine (Figure 6.1). Impairments in nitrogen flux are hence often accompanied by elevations of the plasma pool of these amino acids in addition to hyperammonemia.[6] This has two important implications. First, elevated glutamine and alanine can be used as biomarkers of the long-term control of hyperammonemia. Second, conjugation and excretion of glutamine, the most abundant amino acid in human plasma, can be used to divert nitrogen away from the urea cycle. Stress, infections, fasting, and injury lead to increased protein catabolism and nitrogen turnover. In the presence of decreased flux through the urea cycle, these stressors cause elevations of glutamine, alanine, and ammonia.

The nitrogen flux through the urea cycle depends not only on the activity of the urea cycle enzymes but also on the interconnectedness of the urea cycle with other metabolic pathways, transporter proteins, and intermediate metabolites that facilitate nitrogen transport across subcellular compartments. Many conditions that alter the concentrations or the transport of intermediate metabolites of the urea cycle can present with impaired ureagenesis and hyperammonemia. Ornithine aminotransferase deficiency, hyperornithinemia-hyperammonemia-homocitrullinuria syndrome, Δ^1-pyrroline-5-carboxylate synthase deficiency, lysinuric protein intolerance, citrin deficiency, pyruvate carboxylase deficiency, organic acidemias, and fatty acid oxidation disorders are examples of such conditions.[7] Acquired causes of hyperammonemia include liver failure, drug intoxications, infections, and systemic illness. In ornithine aminotransferase deficiency, there is a deficiency in ornithine synthesis in the newborn period resulting in defective urea cycle function. Hyperornithinemia-hyperammonemia-homocitrullinuria syndrome is caused by mutations in *SLC25A15* encoding a mitochondrial ornithine transporter which leads to defective mitochondrial import of ornithine resulting in decreased substrate availability for OTC and ornithine aminotransferase. Carbamoyl phosphate can be diverted to alternate pathways resulting in generation of homocitrulline and orotic acid. Δ^1-pyrroline-5-carboxylate synthase deficiency results in decreased synthesis of proline, ornithine, and arginine from glutamate. The deficiencies of two important urea cycle intermediates, ornithine and arginine, leads to hyperammonemia. Lysinuric protein intolerance is caused by deficiency of SLC7A7, a component of the dibasic cationic amino acid transporter, which alters dibasic amino acid transport leading to decreased intestinal absorption and increased urinary loss of arginine, ornithine, and lysine. Depletion of intracellular arginine and ornithine results in decreased ureagenesis. Citrin is a mitochondrial aspartate-glutamate carrier, and its deficiency causes citrullinemia type II. Defective aspartate export from the mitochondria to the cytosol results in lower argininosuccinate synthesis from aspartate and citrulline leading to the accumulation of citrulline. Pyruvate carboxylase is a mitochondrial enzyme that converts pyruvate and carbon dioxide to oxaloacetate. Hence, deficiency of pyruvate carboxylase can lead to decreased generation of aspartate from oxaloacetate thus decreasing substrate availability to ASS1 thereby leading to elevation of citrulline levels. In patients with organic acidemias such as propionic acidemia, hyperammonemia can occur during episodes of clinical decompensation. Several mechanisms, including carnitine deficiency, inhibition of urea cycle enzymes by organic acids and α-ketoglutarate deficiency, have been suggested as the mechanisms underlying hyperammonemia.[8] In fatty acid oxidation defects, hyperammonemia is thought to result from a lack of energy in hepatocytes and a subsequent decrease in function of the urea cycle, which requires adenosine triphosphate for reactions catalyzed by CPS1 and ASS1.

Regulation of the Urea Cycle

The regulation of urea cycle enzymes is complex and involves allosteric regulation, transcriptional regulation, posttranslational modifications, substrate availability, and cellular compartmentalization. Insights into the mechanisms of regulation of the urea cycle enzymes has led to optimization of treatment in CPS1 deficiency and could potentially lead to improved treatment strategies in other UCDs.

The urea cycle in general is upregulated by deacetylation of CPS1 by SIRT5, and this is critical in situations of stress such as fasting, caloric restriction, and a high-protein diet.[9] N-acetylglutamate and carbamylglutamate are activators of CPS1 and have been shown to be effective as treatment in patients with hyperammonemia in the 1950s[10] and patients with NAGS deficiency in the 1990s.[11] Recently, its potential usefulness in treating hyperammonemia secondary to CPS1 deficiency and organic acidemias was described.[12]

Glucagon and dexamethasone regulate urea cycle enzymes by transcriptional activation of *ASS1* and *ASL*, stabilization of mRNA for *CPS1* and *ARG1*, and protein stabilization of OTC.[13] The specific additional regulation of ARG1 expression by cytokines and the nuclear receptor family of ligand-activated transcription factors is described in detail in a recent review.[14]

In addition to transcriptional regulation, urea cycle intermediates are subject to a compartmental regulation. The regulation of arginine utilization by compartmentalization starts at the organ level where each tissue can express a different set of urea cycle components necessary to triage arginine to ureagenesis, protein synthesis or synthesis of downstream small molecules. Arginine compartmentalization also occurs at the intracellular level. The phenomenon of cellular arginine regulation is best exemplified by the "arginine paradox," referring to the dependence of nitric oxide (NO) production on extracellular arginine despite of its apparently saturating intracellular levels.[17] While plasma and intracellular concentrations of arginine (140–200 μM)[18] far exceed the K_m of nitric oxide synthase (NOS) (2–20 μM),[19] many studies have shown that exogenously administered, extracellular sources of arginine are able to increase NO production, suggesting that arginine might be rate limiting in the specific subcellular compartment of NO production.[20]

Additionally, arginine itself regulates NO synthesis by (a) inhibiting the expression of inducible NOS (iNOS) at the translational level, through N^G-hydroxy-L-arginine, an intermediate in NO synthesis,[15] or (b) inhibiting arginase thereby upregulating NO synthesis.[16] Hence, it is possible that under different regulatory stimuli, components of the urea cycle dynamically respond to the constantly changing cellular needs to channel an intermediate metabolite from one enzyme's active site to another, thus forming a compartmental niche for the generation of specific metabolites.[21,22]

Acute Hyperammonemia as a Common Feature in Urea Cycle Disorders

Impaired ureagenesis leads to accumulation of free ammonia—hyperammonemia—the common clinical feature shared by all UCDs. Acute hyperammonemia results in increased synthesis of glutamine, dysregulation in the release of neurotransmitters and neuromodulators, mitochondrial dysfunction, and oxidative stress.

Infants with severe deficiencies of any of the urea cycle enzymes present in the neonatal period with the classic triad of hyperammonemia, encephalopathy, and respiratory alkalosis. Newborns typically appear normal in the first 24 hours but develop refusal to feed, vomiting, and increased lethargy over the next few days. The severity of hyperammonemia appears to depend at least in part on the proximity of the ureagenesis defect relative to the entry of nitrogen into the cycle. Defects in the enzymes NAGS, CPS1, and OTC—often referred to as "proximal UCDs"—result in a higher magnitude and longer duration of hyperammonemia.[23] The deficiencies of ASS1, ASL, and ARG1—referred to as "distal UCDs"—typically result in milder and often easier to control hyperammonemic episodes, because urea cycle intermediates like citrulline, argininosuccinic acid, and arginine can serve as nitrogen sinks (Figure 6.1). Tachypnea and respiratory alkalosis that are hypothesized to result from stimulation of the brain stem by ammonia are common early findings unless multiorgan failure ensues, leading to depressed respiration and metabolic acidosis. Failure to recognize and treat hyperammonemia leads to worsening lethargy, seizures, coma, and death. Patients with

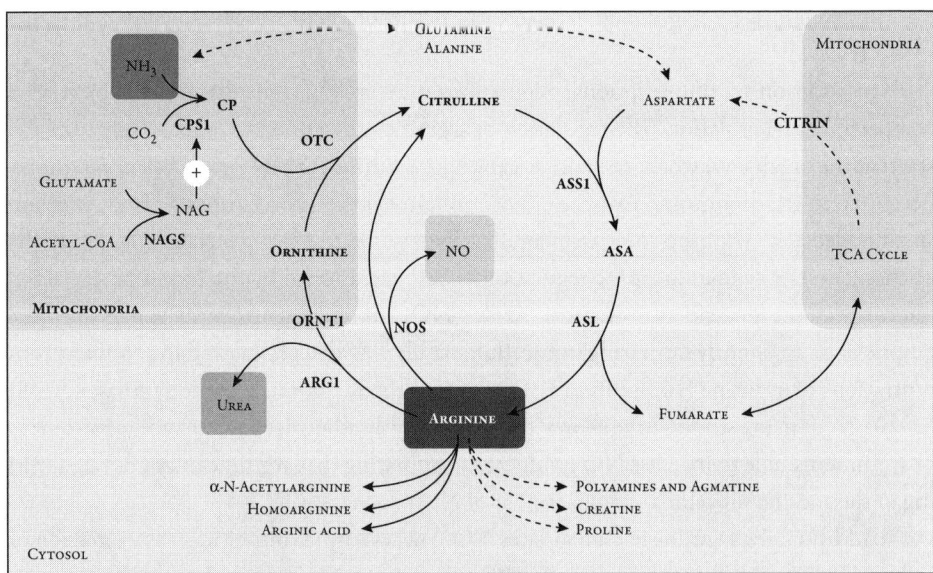

FIGURE 6.1 Urea Cycle and Its Nitrogen Exchange with Other Pathways. *Abbreviations:* ASA = argininosuccinic acid; ASL = argininosuccinate lyase; ASS1 = argininosuccinate synthase 1; ARG1 = arginase 1; CP = carbamoyl phosphate; CPS1 = carbamoyl-phosphate synthase 1; NAG = N-acetylglutamate; NAGS = N-acetylglutamate synthase; NO = nitric oxide; NOS = nitric oxide synthase; OTC = ornithine transcarbamylase; ORNT1 = ornithine transporter 1; TCA cycle = tricarboxylic acid cycle.

UCDs and residual enzymatic activity can present any time after the neonatal period. In contrast to those with neonatal-onset disease, patients with the late-onset forms present with episodic hyperammonemia that is more insidious and can manifest as irritability, disorientation, agitation, inattention, and psychosis.

The consequences of elevated ammonia are driven by the magnitude, duration, and frequency of hyperammonemic episodes.[24] Acute hyperammonemic injury is characterized by increased intracranial pressure due to cytotoxic and vasogenic cerebral edema. Astrocyte swelling is a characteristic cellular finding on autopsy. Prolonged exposure to ammonia can lead to transformation of astrocytes to Alzheimer type II glia, which are enlarged astrocytes with clear cytoplasm, large vesicular nuclei, and cytoplasmic accumulation of glycogen. Similar changes have been reproduced in astrocytes after exposure to high ammonia load *in vitro*.[25,26] The reasons for astrocyte swelling are complex and are likely related to their role as cells supporting neuronal metabolism and the integrity of blood–brain barrier. Since the mammalian brain does not express CPS1 and OTC to support ureagenesis, the incorporation of ammonia into glutamate to form glutamine via glutamine synthase is the primary method to temporarily sequester excess nitrogen.[27] Intracellular accumulation of glutamine, an osmotically active amino acid, is thought to contribute to astrocyte swelling. The efflux of glutamine into the intercellular space and subsequently into plasma results in the consistent observation of hyperglutaminemia in most patients with elevated ammonia.[28] Hyperammonemia has also been linked to decreased expression of astrocyte glutamate transporters and increased extracellular glutamate, a ligand for the N-methyl-D-aspartate receptor, that can trigger neuronal cell death.[29,30]

In addition to the deleterious effects of hyperammonemia on astrocytes and neurons, elevated ammonia alters the blood–brain barrier by affecting the transport of amino acids across the cell membranes. Experimental data suggest that increased efflux of glutamine is accompanied by intracellular accumulation of tyrosine, phenylalanine, tryptophan, methionine, and histidine.[31,32] As these amino acids are precursors of neurotransmitters (e.g. serotonin and dopamine) and neuromodulators (e.g., octapamine and phenylethylamine), it is hypothesized that altered neurotransmission contributes to the encephalopathy in hyperammonemia.[33,34]

Hyperammonemia is also accompanied by mitochondrial dysfunction and increased oxidative stress. Ammonia can suppress the activity of alpha-ketoglutarate dehydrogenase and inhibit the TCA cycle, thus leading to energy deficit.[35] Excess glutamine synthesized in the astrocyte cytoplasm can be transported into the mitochondria wherein it can undergo hydrolysis by glutaminase, thus releasing ammonia. Ammonia can in turn increase the permeability of the mitochondrial membranes to small molecules. These changes lead to the loss of electrochemical gradient, uncoupling of oxidative phosphorylation, depletion of adenosine triphosphate, production of reactive oxygen species, and nitrosative stress.[36]

In summary, hyperammonemic encephalopathy is a complex biochemical phenomenon driven by the direct effects of ammonia on the mitochondrial energy status, incorporation of ammonia into glutamine with far-reaching effects on the amino acid metabolism, neurotransmission, and altered intracellular osmotic balance.

Non-Ureagenic Functions of the Urea Cycle: The Arginine Connection

The urea cycle is intricately connected to other metabolic pathways. The metabolic fates of its intermediates can be traced to and from the TCA cycle, citrulline-NO cycle, creatine, polyamines, proline, alanine, and glutamine (Figure 6.1). The key branching points in the pathway are ornithine and arginine—two important metabolites that are critical for many other metabolic pathways. Arginine is involved in multiple metabolic processes and serves as the precursor for the synthesis of many biologically important compounds including NO, ornithine, polyamines, proline, glutamate, creatine, and agmatine. The sources of free arginine for mammals include diet, endogenous synthesis, and protein turnover. ASL, a urea cycle enzyme, is the only mammalian enzyme capable of synthesizing endogenous arginine. In contrast, four groups of enzymes use arginine as a substrate: arginase (types 1 and 2), arginine decarboxylase, NOS isoforms (NOS1, NOS2, NOS3), and arginine-glycine aminotransferase (Figure 6.1). Quantitatively, ARG1 and ARG2 are responsible for metabolizing most of arginine by conversion to urea and ornithine.[37] It is likely that complex mechanisms regulate the utilization of arginine by this competing pool of enzymes.

Liver is the major site of arginine metabolism, where it serves as an intermediary metabolite in the urea cycle that is rapidly converted to urea and ornithine. As ornithine reenters the urea cycle, there is in principle, no net synthesis of arginine and the liver does not contribute to the circulating pool of arginine. Approximately 60% of the net arginine synthesis in adult mammals occurs in the kidney, where citrulline is extracted from the blood and converted to arginine by ASS1 and ASL localized within the proximal tubules.[38] The majority of citrulline used in this process is produced by the intestine from the nonessential amino acid glutamine. However, most other tissues and cell types also express both ASL and ASS1, as these enzymes are necessary for generating arginine from citrulline.[39] Under conditions of metabolic stress or rapid protein accretion, the endogenous synthesis of arginine by ASS1 and ASL may not be sufficient to meet the metabolic requirements of the body, making arginine a semiessential amino acid.[40] A possible intriguing consequence is that the lack of urea cycle enzymes ASS1 or ASL can lead to arginine deficiency and alter the metabolism of its downstream metabolites in and outside the liver.

Undoubtedly, the most studied metabolite of arginine is NO. NO has important roles in many diverse processes, including vasodilatation, immune response, neurotransmission, and cell–cell interactions.[41,42] NO has been implicated in cardiovascular diseases,[41] disorders of central nervous system,[43] maternal–fetal tolerance, regulation of vascular changes in pregnancy, renal disease,[44] cancer,[45] infections,[46] and wound healing.[47] NO is generated by oxidation of arginine to citrulline by the three isoforms of NOS. Whereas two isoforms, eNOS (endothelial or NOS3) and nNOS (neuronal NOS or NOS1), are Ca^{2+}-dependent, localized to the cell membrane, and are constitutively expressed, the inducible isoform (iNOS or NOS2) expressed in macrophages and other cell types is Ca^{2+}-independent and is located in the cytosol. Although the affinity of NOS enzymes to arginine is a thousand-fold higher than arginase, the V_{max} of arginase is a thousand-fold higher than that of NOS enzymes. Hence, arginase can effectively compete with the NOS enzymes for substrate and thus limit NO production.[48]

Polyamines, synthesized from arginine via ornithine, share important roles in cell motility, proliferation, growth, and survival in addition to membrane trafficking and protein expression.[49] Ornithine is also a substrate for proline synthesis. Proline is a critical component of many proteins such as collagen and is able to modulate cell cycle, autophagy, and apoptosis.[50]

Arginine is also the precursor of creatine and agmatine. Creatine functions as an energy shuttle from mitochondrial sites of energy production to cytoplasmic sites of utilization. Hence, it is mainly found in cells with fluctuating energy demands, such as skeletal muscle, heart, and brain.[51] Finally, the lesser understood branch in arginine metabolism is that involving agmatine generated by decarboxylation, an intermediary in the polyamine synthesis. Though the exact function of agmatine is not known, it has been hypothesized to have effects on cell proliferation,[52] neurotransmission,[53] NO synthesis,[54] and possibly polyamine synthesis.[55]

ASL and ARG1 are the major enzymes involved in the generation and utilization of arginine, respectively. Deficiencies of these two enzymes lead to abnormal arginine metabolism and may provide the first non-ureagenic pathogenic mechanism for the complex phenotypes in UCDs.

In addition, the urea cycle is linked to the TCA cycle through oxaloacetate which after transamination and formation of aspartate enters the urea cycle to generate argininosuccinate that is converted by ASL to fumarate linking back to the TCA cycle. Recent evidence shows that alteration of flux through the TCA cycle due to fumarate hydratase deficiency leads to reversed ASL activity causing accumulation of argininosuccinate.[56] This alteration of metabolite fluxes through numerous interconnected cycles could add another layer of complexity to the mechanisms of UCDs and potentially explain some features that are independent of ureagenesis. The consequences of impaired non-ureagenic functions on metabolism and their contribution to the pathogenesis of complex phenotypes in UCD is discussed in the next section.

Urea Cycle Disorders as Complex Disorders

Although elevated ammonia is a common finding in all UCDs, the deficiency of each of the specific urea cycle enzymes demonstrate unique and recurrent features, which appear to be independent of hyperammonemia. These disease-specific associations arise from the unique biochemical profile of each disorder. Accumulation of metabolites upstream of the enzymatic block, a deficiency of metabolites downstream of the blockage, and interrupted flux of intermediary metabolites through the urea cycle or other metabolic pathways engender the disease-specific patterns of clinical and biochemical features in each UCD (Table 6.1). Our ability to make connections between these unique biochemical profiles and disease-specific phenotypic findings is important for at least two reasons. First, optimization of treatment of UCDs will require looking beyond the hyperammonemia and harnessing new strategies to correct biochemical imbalances in an organ-specific manner. Second, many of the complications of UCDs provide an opportunity to understand the biochemical underpinnings of more common human disorders.

TABLE 6.1 **Biochemical Abnormalities and Unique Clinical Features of Urea Cycle Disorders**

Disease	Biochemical Abnormalities and Unique Clinical Features
NAGS deficiency	Frequent and severe hyperammonemia Absence of urinary orotate The enzyme deficiency can be treated with carglumic acid supplementation
CPS1 deficiency	Frequent and severe hyperammonemia Absence of urinary orotate Evidence of NO dysregulation[a] CPS1 polymorphisms have been associated with pulmonary hypertension[a]
OTC deficiency	Frequent and severe hyperammonemia in males Elevated urinary orotate, low citrulline Liver dysfunction Possible risk factor in primary liver cancer[a]
ASS1 deficiency	Infrequent hyperammonemia Elevated urinary orotate, elevated citrulline, decreased arginine (in untreated patients)
ASL deficiency	Infrequent episodes of hyperammonemia Decreased arginine (in untreated patients) Dysregulation of NO biology[a] Liver dysfunction Trichorrhexis nodosa[a] Systemic hypertension[a] Intellectual disability independent of hyperammonemia[a]
ARG1 deficiency	Elevation of arginine Liver fibrosis Spastic paraplegia[a]

Note. NAGS = N-acetylglutamate synthase; CPS1 = carbamoyl-phosphate synthase 1; NO = nitric oxide; OTC = ornithine transcarbamylase; ASS1 = argininosuccinate synthase 1; ASL = argininosuccinate lyase; ARG1 = arginase 1.
[a]Likely due to compromised non-ureagenic functions.

Carbamoyl-Phosphate Synthase 1 and Pulmonary Hypertension

Increased pulmonary vascular pressure is a normal physiological phenomenon in the fetus. The amount of blood flow through the fetal pulmonary vasculature accounts for less than 10% of the right ventricular output. However, at birth, there is a dramatic cardiopulmonary transition characterized by a fall in pulmonary resistance and increase in the pulmonary blood flow. Failure of this normal circulatory transition at birth results in persistent pulmonary hypertension of the newborn. NO is one of the mediators that plays a role in the circulatory transition and regulation of pulmonary vascular resistance.[57–60] Thus, the ability to generate sufficient NO may be a determining factor in the circulatory transition. In fact, inhaled NO has been used as treatment for newborns with pulmonary hypertension. In a single center study, newborns with persistent pulmonary hypertension had lower levels plasma concentrations of arginine and NO metabolites[61] compared to those with respiratory distress but no pulmonary hypertension. Given the potential links between the urea cycle intermediates and NO production, it is plausible that variations in CPS1, the rate-limiting enzyme in ureagenesis, may determine the availability of intermediates and hence the output of NO. One particular single nucleotide polymorphism in CPS1 (p.T1405N) affects a critical N-acetylglutamate–binding domain and results in a 30% decrease in the efficiency of the enzyme. While there is no significant association between this single nucleotide polymorphism and persistent pulmonary hypertension, there is a statistically significant decrease in the rate of homozygosity for the Asn1405 allele that is associated with higher CPS1 activity. In a related study, the presence of even one Thr1405 allele independently conferred a significantly elevated risk of postoperative pulmonary hypertension in children with congenital heart disease as compared to those homozygous for Asn1405.[62]

Argininosuccinate Lyase and Nitric Oxide Deficiency

Patients with ASL deficiency demonstrate increased incidence of intellectual disability, hepatitis, cirrhosis, systemic hypertension, and trichorrhexis nodosa (coarse and brittle hair).[63,64] These manifestations can be seen even in the absence of significant hyperammonemia.[39,65–67] More specifically, patients with ASL deficiency have a significantly increased frequency of neurological abnormalities such as intellectual disability, seizures, attention deficit hyperactivity disorder, and learning disorders as compared to patients with other UCDs.[23,67] Hepatic involvement in ASL deficiency ranges from hepatomegaly and elevations of liver enzymes to severe liver fibrosis.[68–70] In addition, it has been observed that hypertension is more commonly observed in patients with ASL deficiency as compared to other UCDs.[71,72]

These data imply that the complex phenotype observed in ASL deficiency involves mechanisms beyond the blockage in ureagenesis. Studies in a novel mouse model and human subjects with ASL deficiency have shown that in addition to its function in ureagenesis, ASL is also critical not only for synthesis of endogenous arginine but also has a structural requirement for the formation of the NO synthesis complex. Hence, patients with ASL deficiency harboring mutations in its structural domains are unable to utilize exogenous arginine by NOS for NO production.[73] In addition, the lack of arginine substrate leads to uncoupling of NOS, which generates reactive oxygen species and oxidative stress that may contribute further to the vascular injury. Recently, we described that the deficiency of NOS-dependent NO generation is responsible in part for the hypertension in ASL deficiency. Importantly, treatment with NOS-independent NO donors normalized the blood pressure[73,74] and improved cognitive function in a single ASL-deficient patient. The finding that ASL is an important regulator for NO production opens avenues to explore modulation of ASL activity as a therapeutic intervention in many common disorders that result from dysregulation of NO.

Arginase 1 Deficiency and Spastic Paraplegia

ARG1 deficiency differs from the other UCDs in that hyperammonemic episodes are rare. Though rare patients with hyperammonemia in the neonatal period have been reported, neonatal presentation is uncommon, and generally the condition is minimally symptomatic in infancy.[75] Failure to thrive and delay in attainment of motor skills may be noted during early childhood. If untreated, a progressive course with loss of developmental milestones, progressive spasticity with upper motor neuron type of weakness, and exaggerated muscle reflexes may develop. In the majority of patients, these neurological findings may be limited to the lower limbs alone. Additionally, liver dysfunction and cirrhosis have also been reported. Hyperargininemia due to ARG1 deficiency presents a unique biochemical scenario, wherein excess arginine is diverted to the synthesis of guanidino compounds such as homoarginine, arginic acid, and alpha-N-acetylarginine. These toxic compounds can interfere with neurotransmission and Na^+/K^+-ATPase activity, thereby contributing to neurological injury.

In summary, the complex phenotypes in UCDs result from a combination of defective ureagenesis, altered arginine metabolism, abnormal flux of metabolites shared among different pathways, oxidative stress, generation of toxic intermediates, and perturbed neurotransmission. Thus, treatment of individuals with UCDs must not only focus on restoring disposal of waste nitrogen and repletion of the deficient enzyme's product but also address the non-ureagenic abnormalities.

Current and Future Treatment Strategies

Therapy for UCDs, both in the acute and chronic settings, has generally been focussed on two goals: (a) diversion of nitrogen waste away from urea cycle and (b) stimulation of impaired nitrogen flux through urea cycle. Diversion of nitrogen can be achieved by restriction of protein intake to decrease the nitrogen load, by promotion of anabolism to capture and retain nitrogen in the form of protein, and by stimulation of nitrogen disposal via alternate pathways.[76]

Introduction of specialized formulas composed of essential amino acids[77] or protein-free nutritional supplements have proven to be important elements in the long-term management of protein intake to promote anabolism without overloading the urea cycle with excess nitrogen.[78] Brusilow et al. first demonstrated the utility of alternative pathway to remove nitrogenous waste.[2] Nitrogen scavenging agents introduced by Brusilow, Batshaw, and collaborators over 30 years ago have remarkably decreased the mortality of patients with UCDs.[79,80] Phenylacetate is a common phenylalanine metabolite found at micromolar concentration in humans. It conjugates with glutamine forming phenylacetylglutamine that is excreted in the urine. Benzoate, a compound that conjugates with glycine to form hippuric acid, is another nitrogen scavenging agent. Both of these agents have been used successfully in the treatment of acute hyperammonemia and in long-term ammonia control. More recently, glyceryl tri-phenylbutyrate, a colorless, odorless formulation containing three molecules of phenylbutyric acid linked to glycerol was approved for treatment of UCDs. Treatment with glycerol phenylbutyrate is better tolerated and in an uncontrolled open-label extension study was associated with improved executive function.[81]

Supplementation with urea cycle intermediates citrulline or arginine promotes nitrogen excretion either as urea in cases of deficient proximal enzymes (NAGS, CPS1, and OTC) or as citrulline and argininosuccinate in ASS1 and ASL deficiencies, respectively. The discovery that supplementation with arginine leads to increased nitrogen disposal was made serendipitously by Brusilow.[1] Further studies showed that arginine was indeed an integral part of nitrogen disposal in patients with the neonatal forms of hyperammonemia. Since then, arginine supplementation (or citrulline in case of OTC deficiency) are considered standard of care in the management of UCDs.

As argininosuccinate contains the same two nitrogen atoms that become part of urea and has a very high renal clearance, it was hypothesized that this compound may serve as an alternative pathway for disposal of nitrogen in ASL deficiency. When large doses of arginine, typically in the range of 500 to 600 mg/kg/day are used, argininosuccinate accounts for up to 42% of urinary nitrogen. However, such high levels of argininosuccinate could cause liver toxicity, and hence a lower arginine dosage together with phenylbutyrate may be preferable in management of ASL deficiency.[82] In ASS1 deficiency, citrulline can be used as a waste nitrogen product. However, this seems less efficient than argininosuccinate because (a) citrulline has only one amide nitrogen and (b) even at very high levels of citrulline, the renal clearance is less than 20% of the glomerular filtration. In spite of these limitations, addition of arginine leads to increased citrulline production that can account for 30% of nitrogen in the urine.

Liver Transplantation

Liver transplantation in UCDs prevents recurrent episodes of metabolic decompensation. Preexisting neurological status that results from previous severe hyperammonemic episodes is a major factor in the final outcome.[83] In the 1980s and 1990s, liver transplantation was generally avoided in children younger than one year of age to prevent the potentially greater risks of death and morbidity resulting from surgical complications. Advances in surgical techniques and effective immunosuppressive agents now allow for transplantation at an earlier age with the mortality rates being no different from those of older children.[84] Five-year survival rate of 86% in children weighing less than 5 kg,[85] and one-year survival rate of 88% in infants less than 90 days of age, have been reported.[86]

In spite of these improvements, the five-year survival rate for transplantation from a deceased donor in all metabolic diseases combined is 80% ($N = 947$), and 84% for all liver diseases transplanted in children less than one year of age ($N = 686$).[87] Liver transplantation in UCDs has been performed in at least 59 patients, with an overall survival of 93% (mean follow-up of three years). Transplantation allows for a life free of hyperammonemic episodes, special diets, or alternative pathway medication, despite citrulline levels often remaining low in CPS1 and OTC deficiencies and high in ASS1 deficiency.[88] The long-term clinical significance of these alterations of the citrulline levels is not well understood. Further neurological deterioration is prevented by liver transplantation,[89] and the abnormalities observed on magnetic resonance spectroscopy are typically alleviated.[90] Residual neurological impairments were noted in five of 51 patients transplanted for various UCDs,[91] and these impairments can usually be attributed to pretransplantation neurological insults or transplantation complications.[89,92-94] In contrast, in a recent study of cognition among 92 nontransplanted children with UCDs by Krivitzky et al.,[95] the full-scale IQ in 13 patients with neonatal onset UCDs averaged 65 (average IQ ranged between 85 and 114).

Females with partial OTC deficiency have a better neurological outcome than other individuals with UCDs. Notably, in the study by Krivitzky et al., 13% of 26 females with OTC deficiency had intellectual disabilities, compared to a 33% rate of intellectual disability among males.[95] Studies focusing on partial OTC deficiency demonstrated that 82% of carriers can remain asymptomatic[99] and that, among symptomatic women, four out of 13 have IQs lower than 70[100] and 10 out of 23 have IQs lower than 80.[101] The 14 females with partial OTC deficiency reported to have been transplanted have all faired very well neurologically after liver transplantation.[66,91,94,96-98] When contrasting these data with the lower IQs in non-transplanted individuals stated above, it can be argued that liver transplantation may be considered in partial OTC deficiency if medical management fails to address hyperammonemic episodes.

Collectively, these data demonstrate that a combination of early liver transplantation, aggressive metabolic management, and early childhood intervention improve the neurologic outcome of children with UCDs.[102] However, an important question especially of the distal UCDs is whether the requirement of these enzymes in tissues outside of the liver may contribute to long-term morbidity that cannot be corrected by liver transplantation, including cognitive function.

Gene Transfer and Cell-Based Therapies

UCDs were one of the earliest conditions investigated for treatment with gene therapy. Early preclinical success using adenoviral vectors prompted phase I trials in humans. However, intrahepatic administration of 3×10^{11} vp/kg of a second-generation adenovirus vector in an OTC deficient patient resulted in an acute respiratory distress syndrome and death. This has limited the study of adenoviral vectors for targeting the liver. We and others have sought to decrease the toxicity of adenoviral gene therapy by using helper-dependent adenoviruses, by addressing the immune response with PEGylation of the adenoviruses, as well as with other approaches.[103–105] Using a liver-targeted *Asl* gene therapy in mice, we showed that restored ureagenesis corrects the metabolic defect thus normalizing growth and survival, but it is not sufficient to correct long-term complications such as hypertension, reflecting the tissue-specific requirement for ASL in extrahepatic tissues.[74] The use of adeno-associated virus and nonviral strategies are also being actively studied.[106] Notably, an adeno-associated virus vector was successfully used to treat the OTC deficiency model *spf*[a,b] mouse[107] and also in a model of more severe OTC deficiency generated by using an shRNA to *Otc* in the *spf*[ash] mouse.[108] The most recent success of gene therapy in a preclinical model is that of arginase deficiency using an adeno-associated virus vector.[109]

Liver cell transplantation is also being investigated as a bridge to liver transplantation in severely affected children. While the early results could be interpreted as encouraging,[110,111] quantitative assessments of efficacy are still pending. The risk-benefit question of proposing an invasive procedure and immunosuppression in clinically fragile children remains open especially with increasing pharmacotherapeutic options.

Another modality that has the potential to restore ureagenesis without the limitations that accompany cell- and gene-based therapies is enzyme replacement therapy (ERT). Whereas challenges facing ERT including delivery and targeting of the deficient protein to appropriate subcellular compartments of specific cells are well known, such therapy has been effective in the treatment of other genetic disorders. At least in the example of ARG1 deficiency, a peglyated form of human recombinant arginase could potentially be helpful for preventing the long-term complications of hyperarginiemia.[112,113]

Summary

The mechanisms underlying UCDs are complex. Hyperammonemia is the core feature common to all UCDs. The magnitude of hyperammonemic episodes to a large extent depends on the proximity of the affected enzyme in the urea cycle—more proximal defects engender a greater risk of hyperammonemic episodes. Hyperammonemia alone cannot explain all clinical findings in UCDs. Increasing evidence demonstrates the unique role of urea cycle in handling non-ureagenic functions tied to arginine metabolism. Defects in the urea cycle enzymes can affect downstream metabolites of arginine thus negatively affecting diverse cellular functions. The non-ureagenic functions of urea cycle enzymes appear to affect not only the liver but also other organs, as evidenced by a diverse gamut of extrahepatic symptoms, including intellectual disability and systemic hypertension. Liver transplantation, hepatocyte transplantation, and liver-directed gene therapy when safe for human use, could become effective approaches for correcting the hepatic ureagenesis defect common to all UCDs; however, these treatment modalities will not be able to address the problem of enzyme deficiency in other organs. Therefore, any comprehensive treatment strategy in the future will require restoration of ureagenesis in the liver and normalization of nitrogen flux and arginine metabolism in extra-hepatic organs. Undoubtedly, more studies aimed at deciphering the role and regulation of urea cycle enzymes outside of the liver will lead to further optimization of treatment as well as to a deeper understanding of the mechanisms underlying more common human disorders.

References

1. Walser M, Batshaw M, Sherwood G, Robinson B, Brusilow S. Nitrogen metabolism in neonatal citrullinaemia. *Clin Sci Mol Med.* 1977; 53: 173–181.
2. Brusilow SW, Valle DL, Batshaw M. New pathways of nitrogen excretion in inborn errors of urea synthesis. *Lancet.* 1979; 2: 452–454.
3. Camacho JA, Obie C, Biery B, et al. Hyperornithinaemia-hyperammonaemia-homocitrullinuria syndrome is caused by mutations in a gene encoding a mitochondrial ornithine transporter. *Nat Genet.* 1999; 22: 151–158.
4. Camacho JA, Rioseco-Camacho N. The human and mouse SLC25A29 mitochondrial transporters rescue the deficient ornithine metabolism in fibroblasts of patients with the hyperornithinemia-hyperammonemia-homocitrullinuria (HHH) syndrome. *Pediatr Res.* 2009; 66: 35–41.
5. Camacho JA, Rioseco-Camacho N, Andrade D, Porter J, Kong J. Cloning and characterization of human ORNT2: a second mitochondrial ornithine transporter that can rescue a defective ORNT1 in patients with the hyperornithinemia-hyperammonemia-homocitrullinuria syndrome, a urea cycle disorder. *Mol Genet Metab.* 2003; 79: 257–271.
6. Tuchman M, Lee B, Lichter-Konecki U, et al. Cross-sectional multicenter study of patients with urea cycle disorders in the United States. *Mol Genet Metab.* 2008; 94: 397–402.
7. Fernandes J, Saudubray JM, Van den Berghe G, Walter JH. *Inborn Metabolic Diseases: Diagnosis and Treatment.* New York: Springer; 2006.
8. Filipowicz HR, Ernst SL, Ashurst CL, Pasquali M, Longo N. Metabolic changes associated with hyperammonemia in patients with propionic acidemia. *Mol Genet Metab.* 2006; 88: 123–130.
9. Nakagawa T, Lomb DJ, Haigis MC, Guarente L. SIRT5 Deacetylates carbamoyl phosphate synthetase 1 and regulates the urea cycle. *Cell.* 2009; 137: 560–570.
10. Brown R, Manning R, Delp M, Grisolia S. Treatment of hepatocerebral intoxication. *Lancet* 1958; 271: 591–592.
11. Schubiger G, Bachmann C, Barben P, Colombo JP, Tönz O, Schüpbach D. N-acetylglutamate synthetase deficiency: diagnosis, management and follow-up of a rare disorder of ammonia detoxication. *Eur J Pediatr.* 1991; 150: 353–356.
12. Ah Mew N, McCarter R, Daikhin Y, Nissim I, Yudkoff M, Tuchman M. N-carbamylglutamate augments ureagenesis and reduces ammonia and glutamine in propionic acidemia. *Pediatrics* 2010; 126: e208–214.

13. Ulbright C, Snodgrass PJ. Coordinate induction of the urea cycle enzymes by glucagon and dexamethasone is accomplished by three different mechanisms. *Arch Biochem Biophys*. 1993; 301: 237–243.
14. Pourcet B, Pineda-Torra I. Transcriptional regulation of macrophage arginase 1 expression and its role in atherosclerosis. *Trends Cardiovasc Med*. 2013; 23(5): 143–152.
15. Lee J, Ryu H, Ferrante RJ, Morris SM, Ratan RR. Translational control of inducible nitric oxide synthase expression by arginine can explain the arginine paradox. *Proc Natl Acad Sci USA*. 2003; 100: 4843–4848.
16. Tenu JP, Lepoivre M, Moali C, Brollo M, Mansuy D, Boucher JL. Effects of the new arginase inhibitor N(omega)-hydroxy-nor-L-arginine on NO synthase activity in murine macrophages. *Nitric Oxide–Biol Ch*. 1999; 3: 427–438.
17. Kurz S, Harrison DG. Insulin and the arginine paradox. *J Clin Invest*. 1997; 99: 369–370.
18. Castillo L, Chapman TE, Sanchez M, et al. Plasma arginine and citrulline kinetics in adults given adequate and arginine-free diets. *Proc Natl Acad Sci USA*. 1993; 90: 7749–7753.
19. Wu G, Morris SM Jr. Arginine metabolism: nitric oxide and beyond. *Biochem J*. 1998; 336 (Pt 1): 1–17.
20. Vukosavljevic N, Jaron D, Barbee KA, Buerk DG. Quantifying the L-arginine paradox in vivo. *Microvasc Res*. 2006; 71: 48–54.
21. Cheung CW, Cohen NS, Raijman L. Channeling of urea cycle intermediates in situ in permeabilized hepatocytes. *J Biol Chem*. 1989; 264: 4038–4044.
22. Maher AD, Kuchel PW, Ortega F, de Atauri P, Centelles J, Cascante M. Mathematical modelling of the urea cycle: A numerical investigation into substrate channelling. *Eur J Biochem*. 2003; 270: 3953–3961.
23. Ah Mew N, Krivitzky L, McCarter R, Batshaw M, Tuchman M. Clinical outcomes of neonatal onset proximal versus distal urea cycle disorders do not differ. *J Pediatr*. 2013; 162: 324–329.
24. Enns GM. Neurologic damage and neurocognitive dysfunction in urea cycle disorders. *Semin Pediatr Neurol*. 2008; 15: 132–139.
25. Norenberg MD. A light and electron microscopic study of experimental portal-systemic (ammonia) encephalopathy: Progression and reversal of the disorder. *Lab Invest*. 1977; 36: 618–627.
26. Mossakowski MJ, Renkawek K, Krasnicka Z, Smialek M, Pronaszko A. Morphology and histochemistry of Wilsonian and hepatogenic gliopathy in tissue culture. *Acta Neuropathol*. 1970; 16: 1–16.
27. Cooper AJ, Plum F. Biochemistry and physiology of brain ammonia. *Physiol Rev*. 1987; 67: 440–519.
28. Tuchman M, Yudkoff M. Blood levels of ammonia and nitrogen scavenging amino acids in patients with inherited hyperammonemia. *Mol Genet Metab*. 1999; 66: 10–15.
29. Rodrigo R, Cauli O, Boix J, ElMlili N, Agusti A, Felipo V. Role of NMDA receptors in acute liver failure and ammonia toxicity: therapeutical implications. *Neurochem Int*. 2009; 55: 113–118.
30. de Knegt RJ, Schalm SW, van der Rijt CC, Fekkes D, Dalm E, Hekking-Weyma I. Extracellular brain glutamate during acute liver failure and during acute hyperammonemia simulating acute liver failure: an experimental study based on in vivo brain dialysis. *J Hepatol*. 1994; 20: 19–26.
31. Cangiano C, Cardelli-Cangiano P, James JH, et al. Brain microvessels take up large neutral amino acids in exchange for glutamine: Cooperative role of Na+-dependent and Na+-independent systems. *J Biol Chem*. 1983; 258: 8949–8954.
32. Inoue I, Gushiken T, Kobayashi K, Saheki T. Accumulation of large neutral amino acids in the brain of sparse-fur mice at hyperammonemic state. *Biochem Med Metab Biol*. 1987; 38: 378–386.
33. James JH, Ziparo V, Jeppsson B, Fischer JE. Hyperammonaemia, plasma aminoacid imbalance, and blood–brain aminoacid transport: a unified theory of portal-systemic encephalopathy. *Lancet*. 1979; 2: 772–775.
34. Skowronska M, Albrecht J. Alterations of blood–brain barrier function in hyperammonemia: an overview. *Neurotox Res*. 2012; 21: 236–244.
35. Felipo V, Butterworth RF. Mitochondrial dysfunction in acute hyperammonemia. *Neurochem Int*. 2002; 40: 487–491.
36. Rama Rao KV, Norenberg MD. Glutamine in the pathogenesis of hepatic encephalopathy: the Trojan horse hypothesis revisited. *Neurochem Res*. 2013; 39(3): 593–598.
37. Li X, Bazer FW, Gao H, et al. Amino acids and gaseous signaling. *Amino Acids* 2009; 37: 65–78.
38. Windmueller HG, Spaeth AE. Source and fate of circulating citrulline. *Am J Physiol*. 1981; 241: E473–E480.
39. Mori M, Gotoh T. Arginine metabolic enzymes, nitric oxide and infection. *J Nutr*. 2004; 134: 2820S–2825S; discussion 2853S.
40. Morris SM Jr. Recent advances in arginine metabolism: roles and regulation of the arginases. *Brit J Pharmacol*. 2009; 157: 922–930.

41. Naseem KM. The role of nitric oxide in cardiovascular diseases. *Mol Aspects Med*. 2005; 26: 33–65.
42. Malyshev IY, Shnyra A. Controlled modulation of inflammatory, stress and apoptotic responses in macrophages. *Curr Drug Targets Immune Endocr Metabol Disord*. 2003; 3: 1–22.
43. Bernstein H-G, Bogerts B, Keilhoff G. The many faces of nitric oxide in schizophrenia: A review. *Schizophr Res* 2005; 78: 69–86.
44. Tojo A, Onozato ML, Fujita T. Role of macula densa neuronal nitric oxide synthase in renal diseases. *Med Mol Morphol*. 2006; 39: 2–7.
45. Ekmekcioglu S, Tang C-H, Grimm, EA. NO news is not necessarily good news in cancer. *Curr Cancer Drug Targets*. 2005; 5: 103–115.
46. Proud D. Nitric oxide and the common cold. *Curr Opin Allergy Clin Immunol*. 2005; 5: 37–42.
47. Hackam DJ, Ford HR. Cellular, biochemical, and clinical aspects of wound healing. *Surg Infect* (Larchmt) 2002; 3 (Suppl 1): S23–S35.
48. Morris SM Jr. Arginine metabolism: boundaries of our knowledge. *J Nutr* 2007; 137: 1602S–1609S.
49. Coburn RF. Polyamine effects on cell function: Possible central role of plasma membrane PI(4,5)P2. *J Cell Physiol*. 2009; 221: 544–551.
50. Phang JM, Liu W, Zabirnyk O. Proline metabolism and microenvironmental stress. *Annu Rev Nutr*. 2010; 30: 441–463.
51. Brosnan JT, Brosnan ME. Creatine: endogenous metabolite, dietary, and therapeutic supplement. *Annu Rev Nutr*. 2007; 27: 241–261.
52. Satriano J, Matsufuji S, Murakami Y, et al. Agmatine suppresses proliferation by frameshift induction of antizyme and attenuation of cellular polyamine levels. *J Biol Chem*. 1998; 273: 15313–15316.
53. Reis DJ, Regunathan S. Is agmatine a novel neurotransmitter in brain? *Trends Pharmacol Sci*. 2000; 21: 187–193.
54. Galea E, Regunathan S, Eliopoulos V, Feinstein DL, Reis DJ. Inhibition of mammalian nitric oxide synthases by agmatine, an endogenous polyamine formed by decarboxylation of arginine. *Biochem J*. 1996; 316 (Pt 1): 247–249.
55. Morris SM Jr. Arginine: beyond protein. *Am J Clin Nutr*. 2006; 83: 508S–512S.
56. Adam J, Yang M, Bauerschmidt C, et al. A role for cytosolic fumarate hydratase in urea cycle metabolism and renal neoplasia. *Cell Rep*. 2013; 3(5): 1440–1448.
57. Abman SH, Chatfield BA, Hall SL, McMurtry IF. Role of endothelium-derived relaxing factor during transition of pulmonary circulation at birth. *Am J Physiol*. 1990; 259: H1921–1927.
58. Fineman JR, Wong J, Morin FC III, Wild LM, Soifer SJ. Chronic nitric oxide inhibition in utero produces persistent pulmonary hypertension in newborn lambs. *J Clin Invest*. 1994; 93: 2675–2683.
59. Lipsitz EC, Weinstein S, Smerling AJ, Stolar CJ. Endogenous nitric oxide and pulmonary vascular tone in the neonate. *J Pediatr Surg* 1996; 31: 137–140.
60. Nelin LD, Moshin J, Thomas CJ, Sasidharan P, Dawson CA. The effect of inhaled nitric oxide on the pulmonary circulation of the neonatal pig. *Pediatr Res*. 1994; 35: 20–24.
61. Pearson DL, Dawling S, Walsh WF, et al. Neonatal pulmonary hypertension—urea-cycle intermediates, nitric oxide production, and carbamoyl-phosphate synthetase function. *N Engl J Med*. 2001; 344: 1832–1838.
62. Canter JA, Summar ML, Smith HB, et al. Genetic variation in the mitochondrial enzyme carbamyl-phosphate synthetase I predisposes children to increased pulmonary artery pressure following surgical repair of congenital heart defects: a validated genetic association study. *Mitochondrion*. 2007;7(3):204–10.
63. Erez A, Nagamani SC, Lee B. Argininosuccinate lyase deficiency-argininosuccinic aciduria and beyond. *Am J Med Genet C, Semin Med Genet* 2011; 157: 45–53.
64. Nagamani SC, Erez A, Lee B. Argininosuccinate lyase deficiency. *Genet Med*. 2012; 14: 501–507.
65. Ficicioglu C, Mandell R, Shih VE. Argininosuccinate lyase deficiency: long-term outcome of 13 patients detected by newborn screening. *Mol Genet Metab*. 2009; 157: 45–53.
66. Saudubray JM, Touati G, Delonlay P, et al. Liver transplantation in urea cycle disorders. *Eur J Pediatr*. 1999; 158 (Suppl. 2): 55–59.
67. Tuchman M, Lee B, Lichter-Konecki U, et al. Cross-sectional multicenter study of patients with urea cycle disorders in the United States. *Mol Genet Metab*. 2008; 94: 397–402.
68. Billmeier GJ Jr, Molinary SV, Wilroy RS Jr, Duenas DA, Brannon ME. Argininosuccinic aciduria: investigation of an affected family. *J Pediatr*. 1974; 84: 85–89.
69. Zimmermann A, Bachmann C, Baumgartner R. Severe liver fibrosis in argininosuccinic aciduria. *Arch Pathol Lab Med*. 1986; 110: 136–140.

70. Mori T, Nagai K, Mori M, et al. Progressive liver fibrosis in late-onset argininosuccinate lyase deficiency. *Pediatr Dev Pathol.* 2002; 5: 597–601.
71. Brunetti-Pierri N, Erez A, Shchelochkov O, Craigen W, Lee B. Systemic hypertension in two patients with ASL deficiency: a result of nitric oxide deficiency? *Mol Genet Metab.* 2009; 98: 195–197.
72. Nagamani SCS, Erez A, Lee B. Argininosuccinate lyase deficiency. In: Pagon RA, Bird TD, Dolan CR, Stephens K, Adam MP, eds. *GeneReviews*. Seattle; University of Washington; 1993.
73. Erez A, Nagamani SC, Shchelochkov OA, et al. Requirement of argininosuccinate lyase for systemic nitric oxide production. *Nat Med.* 2011; 17: 1619–1626.
74. Nagamani SC, Campeau, PM, Shchelochkov OA, et al. Nitric-oxide supplementation for treatment of long-term complications in argininosuccinic aciduria. *Am J Hum Genet.* 2012; 90: 836–846.
75. Jain-Ghai S, Nagamani SC, Blaser S, Siriwardena K, Feigenbaum A. Arginase I deficiency: severe infantile presentation with hyperammonemia: more common than reported? *Mol Genet Metab.* 2011; 104: 107–111.
76. Enns GM, Berry SA, Berry GT, Rhead WJ, Brusilow SW, Hamosh A. Survival after treatment with phenylacetate and benzoate for urea-cycle disorders. *N Engl J Med.* 2007; 356: 2282–2292.
77. Snyderman SE, Sansaricq C, Phansalkar SV, Schacht RC, Norton PM. The therapy of hyperammonemia due to ornithine transcarbamylase deficency in a male neonate. *Pediatrics.* 1975; 56: 65–73.
78. Singh RH. Nutritional management of patients with urea cycle disorders. *J Inherit Metab Dis.* 2007; 30: 880–887.
79. Batshaw ML, Brusilow S, Waber L, et al. Treatment of inborn errors of urea synthesis: activation of alternative pathways of waste nitrogen synthesis and excretion. *N Engl J Med.* 1982; 306: 1387–1392.
80. Brusilow S, Tinker J, Batshaw ML. Amino acid acylation: a mechanism of nitrogen excretion in inborn errors of urea synthesis. *Science.* 1980; 207: 659–661.
81. Diaz GA, Krivitzky LS, Mokhtarani M, et al. Ammonia control and neurocognitive outcome among urea cycle disorder patients treated with glycerol phenylbutyrate. *Hepatology.* 2012; 57: 2171–2179.
82. Nagamani SC, Shchelochkov OA, Mullins MA, et al. A randomized controlled trial to evaluate the effects of high-dose versus low-dose of arginine therapy on hepatic function tests in argininosuccinic aciduria. *Mol Genet Metab.* 2012; 107: 315–321.
83. Meyburg J, Hoffmann GF. Liver transplantation for inborn errors of metabolism. *Transplantation* 2005; 80: 135–137.
84. Lee B, Goss J. Long-term correction of urea cycle disorders. *J Pediatr.* 2001;.138: 62–71.
85. Mekeel KL, Langham MR, Gonzalez-Peralta RP, Hemming AW. Liver transplantation in very small infants. *Pediatr Transplant.* 2007; 11: 66–72.
86. Sundaram SS, Alonso EM, Anand R. Outcomes after liver transplantation in young infants. *J Pediatr Gastroenterol Nutr.* 2008; 47: 486–492.
87. Organ Procurement and Transplantation Network and the Scientific Registry of Transplant Recipients. 2008 Annual Report of the U.S. Organ Procurement and Transplantation Network and the Scientific Registry of Transplant Recipients: Transplant Data 1998–2007. Rockville, MD: U.S. Department of Health and Human Services, Health Resources and Services Administration, Healthcare Systems Bureau, Division of Transplantation; 2008.
88. Leonard JV, McKiernan PJ. The role of liver transplantation in urea cycle disorders. *Mol Genet Metab.* 2004; 81 (Suppl. 1): S74–S78.
89. Busuttil AA, Goss JA, Seu P, et al. The role of orthotopic liver transplantation in the treatment of ornithine transcarbamylase deficiency. *Liver Transpl Surg.* 1998; 4: 350–354.
90. Takanashi J, Kurihara A, Tomita M, et al. Distinctly abnormal brain metabolism in late-onset ornithine transcarbamylase deficiency. *Neurology.* 2002; 59: 210–214.
91. Morioka D, Kasahara M, Takada Y, et al. Current role of liver transplantation for the treatment of urea cycle disorders: a review of the worldwide English literature and 13 cases at Kyoto University. *Liver Transpl.* 2005; 11: 1332–1342.
92. Broelsch CE, Emond JC, Whitington PF, Thistlethwaite JR, Baker AL, Lichtor JL. Application of reduced-size liver transplants as split grafts, auxiliary orthotopic grafts, and living related segmental transplants. *Ann Surg.* 1990; 212: 368–375.
93. Todo S, Starzl TE, Tzakis A, et al. Orthotopic liver transplantation for urea cycle enzyme deficiency. *Hepatology.* 1992; 15: 419–422.
94. Whitington PF, Alonso EM, Boyle JT, et al. Liver transplantation for the treatment of urea cycle disorders. *J Inherit Metab Dis.* 1998; 21 (Suppl. 1): 112–118.

95. Krivitzky L, Babikian T, Lee H-S, Thomas NH, Burk-Paull KL, Batshaw ML. Intellectual, adaptive, and behavioral functioning in children with urea cycle disorders. *Pediatr Res.* 2009; 66: 96–9101.
96. Largilliere C, Houssin D, Gottrand F, et al. Liver transplantation for ornithine transcarbamylase deficiency in a girl. *J Pediatr.* 1989; 115: 415–417.
97. Hasegawa T, Tzakis AG, Todo S, et al. Orthotopic liver transplantation for ornithine transcarbamylase deficiency with hyperammonemic encephalopathy. *J Pediatr Surg.* 1995; 30: 863–865.
98. Keskinen P, Siitonen A, Salo M. Hereditary urea cycle diseases in Finland. *Acta Paediatr.* 2008; 97: 1412–1419.
99. Batshaw ML, Msall M, Beaudet AL, Trojak J. Risk of serious illness in heterozygotes for ornithine transcarbamylase deficiency. *J Pediatr.* 1986; 108: 236–241.
100. Rowe PC, Newman SL, Brusilow SW. Natural history of symptomatic partial ornithine transcarbamylase deficiency. *N Engl J Med.* 1986; 314: 541–547.
101. Maestri NE, Brusilow SW, Clissold DB, Bassett SS. Long-term treatment of girls with ornithine transcarbamylase deficiency. *N Engl J Med.* 1996; 335: 855–859.
102. Campeau PM, Pivalizza PJ, Miller G, et al. Early orthotopic liver transplantation in urea cycle defects: follow up of a developmental outcome study. *Mol Genet Metab.* 2010; 100 (Suppl. 1): S84–S87.
103. Hu C, Cela RG, Suzuki M, Lee B, Lipshutz GS. Neonatal helper-dependent adenoviral vector gene therapy mediates correction of hemophilia A and tolerance to human factor VIII. *Proc Natl Acad Sci USA.* 2011; 108: 2082–2087.
104. Suzuki M, Cela R, Bertin TK, et al. NOD2 signaling contributes to the innate immune response against helper-dependent adenovirus vectors independently of MyD88 in vivo. *Hum Gene Ther.* 2011; 22: 1071–1082.
105. Suzuki M, Cerullo V, Bertin TK, et al. MyD88-dependent silencing of transgene expression during the innate and adaptive immune response to helper-dependent adenovirus. *Hum Gene Ther.* 2010; 21: 325–336.
106. Alexander IE, Kok C, Dane AP, Cunningham SC. Gene therapy for metabolic disorders: an overview with a focus on urea cycle disorders. *J Inherit Metab Dis.* 2012; 35: 641–645.
107. Cunningham SC, Dane AP, Spinoulas A, Logan GJ, Alexander IE. Gene delivery to the juvenile mouse liver using AAV2/8 vectors. *Mol Ther.* 2008; 16: 1081–1088.
108. Cunningham SC, Kok CY, Dane AP, et al. Induction and prevention of severe hyperammonemia in the spfash mouse model of ornithine transcarbamylase deficiency using shRNA and rAAV-mediated gene delivery. *Mol Ther.* 2011; 19: 854–859.
109. Lee EK, Hu C, Bhargava R, et al. AAV-based gene therapy prevents neuropathology and results in normal cognitive development in the hyperargininemic mouse. *Gene Ther.* 2013; 20(8): 785–796.
110. Meyburg J, Das AM, Hoerster F, et al. One liver for four children: first clinical series of liver cell transplantation for severe neonatal urea cycle defects. *Transplantation* 2009; 87: 636–641.
111. Meyburg J, Schmidt J, Hoffmann GF. Liver cell transplantation in children. *Clin Transplant.* 2009; 23 (Suppl. 21): 75–82.
112. Stone E, Chantranupong L, Gonzalez C, O'Neal L, Rani M, VanDenBerg C, Georgiou G. Strategies for optimizing the serum persistence of engineered human arginase I for cancer therapy. *J Cont Rel: Off J Control Rel Soc.* 2012;158:171–179.
113. Mauldin JP, Zeinali I, Kleypas K, et al. Recombinant human arginase toxicity in mice is reduced by citrulline supplementation. *Transl Oncol.* 2012;5:26–31.

7

Fatty Acid Metabolism and Defects

Marwan S. Shinawi and Lutfi A. Abu-Elheiga

Overview of Fatty Acid β-Oxidation

Fatty acid β-oxidation is a multistep process by which fatty acids (FAs) undergo catabolism to produce energy (Figure 7.1). Adipose tissue is the body's major fuel storage reserve, in which FAs are stored in the form of triacylglycerol. FAs utilized for β-oxidation originate from either plasma FAs bound to albumin or released from chylomicrons or very-low-density lipoproteins. Membrane uptake of long-chain FAs is the first step in cellular FA utilization and a point of regulation. FAs enter the cell via "flip-flop" diffusion[1] or by integral or membrane-associated transporters, including tissue specific fatty acid transport proteins (FATP), fatty acid translocase (FAT/CD36), and plasma-membrane-associated FA binding protein (FABPpm).[2] Once inside the cell, FAs are esterified by the fatty acyl-CoA synthetase to fatty acylCoA by adding a coenzyme A (CoA) group. The fatty acylCoA in the cytosol can then be converted and stored as triacylglycerol, or the acyl group transferred to carnitine via carnitine palmitoyltransferase I (CPT I). The acylcarnitine allows the FA to be shuttled across the inner mitochondrial membrane via carnitine-acylcarnitine translocase (CACT), which exchanges long-chain acylcarnitines for carnitine. The acylcarnitines are then converted back to long-chain acyl-CoA via carnitine palmitoyltransferase II (CPT II). In the mitochondrial matrix, the long-chain acyl-CoA enters the FA β-oxidation spiral reactions, producing acetyl-CoA, reduced flavin adenine dinucleotide (FADH2), reduced nicotinamide adenine dinucleotide (NADH), and shortening the acyl-CoA by two carbons in each cycle. Four mitochondrial enzymes are involved in this cycle: acyl-CoA dehydrogenase, 2-enoyl-CoA hydratase, L-3-hydroxyacyl-CoA dehydrogenase, and 3-ketoacyl-CoA thiolase. Acetyl-CoA can be fully oxidized to CO_2 and H_2O in the mitochondrial tricarboxylic (citric) acid (TCA) cycle or utilized for ketone body production. The NADH and FADH2 produced by both FA β-oxidation and the TCA cycle are used to generate adenosine triphosphate (ATP) by the mitochondrial electron transport chain.

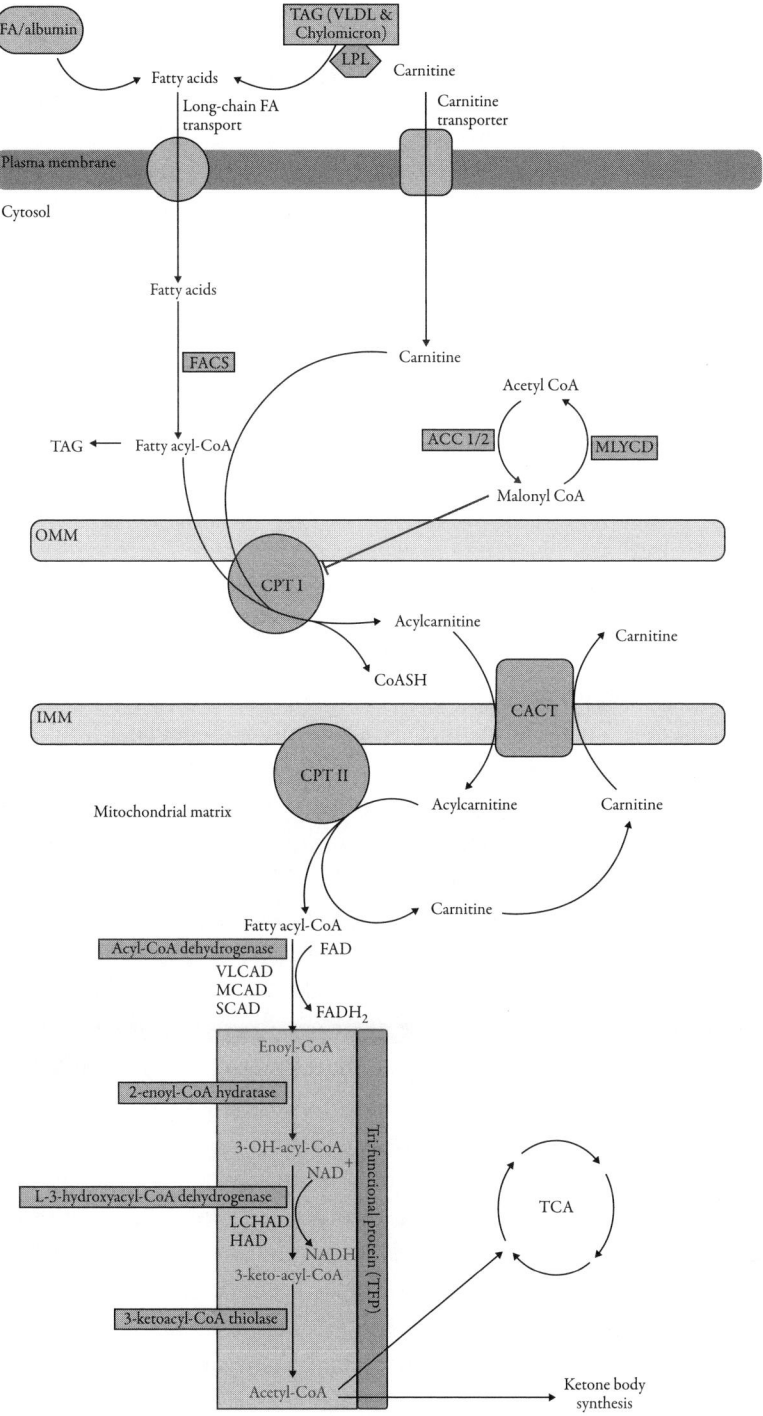

FIGURE 7.1 Overview of mitochondrial fatty acid β oxidation pathway. ACC, acetyl-CoA carboxylase; CACT, carnitine acylcarnitine translocase, CPT I, carnitine palmitoyltransferase I; CPT II, carnitine palmitoyltransferase II; CoA, Coenzyme A; FA, fatty acid; FACS, fatty acyl-CoA synthetase; FADH2 reduced flavin adenine dinucleotide; HAD, short- to medium-chain hydroxyacyl-CoA dehydrogenase; LCHAD, long-chain hydroxy-acyl-CoA dehydrogenase; LPL, lipoprotein lipase; MCAD, medium-chain acyl-CoA dehydrogenase; MLYCD, malonyl-CoA decarboxylase; NADH, reduced nicotinamide adenine dinucleotide; SCAD, short-chain acyl- CoA dehydrogenase; TAG, triacylglycerol; TCA, tricarboxylic acid cycle; VLCAD, very-long-chain acyl-CoA dehydrogenase; VLDL, very-low-density lipoprotein.

Fatty Acid Supply and Transport

Lipolysis is activated by β-adrenergic catecholamines and suppressed by insulin. During fasting, when plasma insulin is low, or at time of stress with high β-adrenergic stimulation, circulating free fatty acids are predominantly derived from adipocyte lipolysis. Postprandially, circulating plasma insulin levels are high, lipolysis is suppressed, and free fatty acids are predominantly derived from the action of lipoprotein lipase on very-low-density lipoproteins or chylomicrons.[3] The rate of FA release from adipose tissues is controlled by hormone-sensitive lipase (HSL), which is activated during fasting and suppressed by insulin and glucose.[4] HSL activity is regulated by cyclic adenosine monophosphate (AMP)- mediated serine phosphorylation.[5] HSL mediates lipolysis in response to β-adrenergic stimulation and is essential to normal structure of adipose tissue. However, the normal rate of lipolysis in unstimulated adipocytes from homozygous *hsl-/-* mice suggested that HSL-independent lipolytic pathway(s) exist in fat.[6] In fact, adipose triglyceride lipase (ATGL) was found to specifically hydrolyze long-chain FA triglycerides and is predominantly expressed in adipose tissue and, to a lesser extent, in heart, skeletal muscle, and testis.[7] Genetic inactivation of *Atgl* in mice increases adipose mass, glucose use and tolerance, and insulin sensitivity and leads to triacylglycerol deposition in multiple tissues, and defective cold adaptation.[8] Recently, it has been shown that the inhibition of lipolysis through genetic ablation of adipose *Atgl* or *Hsl* ameliorates certain features of cancer-associated cachexia.[9] In human, mutations in the *PNPLA2* gene, encoding the ATGL, cause the autosomal recessive neutral lipid storage disease with myopathy (MIM 610717).[10] The condition is characterized by systemic accumulation of triglycerides in cytoplasmic droplets, but individuals with this condition did not show obesity. Interestingly, mutations in the *ABHD5* gene that encodes a coactivator of ATGL cause Chanarin-Dorfman syndrome (MIM 275630), which also is characterized by neutral lipid storage disease in addition to ichthyosis, mild myopathy, and hepatomegaly.[11]

Intra-adipocytic lipid droplets, where triglycerides are stored within a unilocular droplet occupying up to 90% of the cell volume, are coated with several proteins. Perilipins (PLIN1-PLIN5) are the most abundant protein coating these droplets and serve important functions, including droplet formation and maturation, optimal triglyceride storage, and release of FFAs from the droplet.[12,13] It was found that phosphorylation of serine residues within perilipin A is required for HSL binding and maximal lipolysis.[14] Recent studies also showed that perilipin 5 regulates oxidative lipid droplet hydrolysis and controls local FA flux probably to protect mitochondria against excessive exposures to FAs during physiological stress.[15] Mutations in the *PLIN1* gene cause the autosomal dominant partial lipodystrophy type 4 (MIM 613877), characterized by lipodystrophy, severe dyslipidemia, and insulin-resistant diabetes.[16] Subcutaneous fat from patients with *PLIN1* mutations is characterized by smaller than normal adipocytes, macrophage infiltration, and their preadipocytes fail to increase triglyceride accumulation, highlighting the significant role of perilipins in the formation of lipid droplets in adipose tissue.[16] Interestingly, additional proteins involved in adipocyte lipid droplet formation and organization, including seipin, caveolin 1, and cavin, have been implicated in the etiology of other lipodystrophic syndromes.[17]

Once released, FAs are transported in blood in the form of unesterified FFAs with the majority attached to albumin. FAs enter cells through concentration-based flipping and via protein-mediated transport.[1,2,18,19] Fatty acyl-CoA synthetases are essential for the activation of FAs by catalyzing the formation of acyl-CoA from FAs, ATP, and CoA.[20] This activation process allows FAs participation in both anabolic and catabolic pathways. Twenty-six acyl-CoA synthetases genes/proteins have been identified so far[21,22]; 11 can activate the major long-chain FAs of 16 to 22 carbons, and these include members of the long-chain acyl-CoA synthetases and very long chain acyl-CoA synthetases.[23] These proteins are emerging also as likely players in FA transport and intracellular retention and trafficking mediated through vectorial acylation, which results in the formation of acyl-CoA concomitant with transport.[23,24] This process causes "trapping" of FA as an acyl-CoA within the cell and enables its use in downstream reactions.[23] All members of the very long chain acyl-CoA synthetases were also characterized as FATPs. Six distinct transmembrane FATPs in human were so far identified and they are designated FATP1 (SLC27A1), -2 (SLC27A2), -3 (SLC27A3), -4 (SLC27A4), -5 (SLC27A5), and -6 (SLC27A6).[25] FATPs are multifunctional proteins that mediate the uptake of FAs as well as catalyze the formation of CoA derivatives.[22,26] They facilitate high affinity and specific transport of FAs by cells such as cardiac muscle, hepatocytes, and adipocytes. There is increasing evidence that different FATP and long-chain acyl-CoA synthetases isoforms function individually and coordinately to channel distinct classes of acyl-CoAs into different metabolic pools and fates.[23,27,28] Mutations in the *FATP4* gene were found in patients with the ichthyosis prematurity syndrome (MIM 608649), an autosomal-recessive condition characterized by polyhydramnios, prematurity, respiratory complications, and a lifelong nonscaly ichthyosis with atopic manifestations.[29] The findings in this syndrome emphasize the critical role of FA metabolism for normal epidermal barrier function. FATP4 and ichthyin are expressed and closely interact in the upper stratum granulosum of epidermis to facilitate lipid deposition in the cornified layer.[30] It was hypothesized that FATP4 acts as an Mg^{2+}-dependent acyl-CoA synthetase, requiring ichthyin for Mg^{2+} recruitment.[30] Currently, there are no additional clinical phenotypes associated so far with the other FATPs.

The Carnitine Cycle

Carnitine (β-hydroxy-γ-trimethylammonium butyrate), a name derived from the Latin caro (flesh), is widely distributed and is particularly abundant in cardiac and skeletal muscle. Although muscle tissue harbors the highest concentrations; it cannot synthesize carnitine and therefore must acquire carnitine from blood.[31] Major dietary sources of carnitine are red meat, fish, and dairy products. In meat eaters, approximately 75% of body carnitine comes from the diet and 25% from de novo biosynthesis.[32] Omnivorous humans ingest 2 to 12 μmol of carnitine per kg of body weight per day,[32] and unabsorbed L-carnitine is mostly degraded by microorganisms in the large intestine.[33] Strict vegetarians obtain very little carnitine from their diet, and endogenous biosynthesis is the main source of their body carnitine.[34]

Free and acylcarnitines are in dynamic balance, and the normal acyl to fee carnitine ratio is ≤ 0.4. Acetyl-L-carnitine is the principal acylcarnitine ester in plasma.[35]

The carnitine cycle is a well-coordinated system for the transfer of long-chain FAs from the cytosol for their oxidation in the intramitochondrial matrix (Figure 7.1). The transfer, activation, and oxidation of short- and medium-chain FAs occur independently of carnitine within the mitochondria. FFAs and long-chain acyl-CoA will not penetrate the permeability barrier in the inner mitochondrial membrane and become oxidized unless they form acylcarnitines. CPT I (MIM 600528), located on the inner side of the outer mitochondrial membrane, converts long-chain acyl CoA to fatty acylcarnitine, which is able to penetrate mitochondria and gain access to the enzymes of β-oxidation. Fatty acylcarnitine are transported by CACT (MIM 613698) through the inner mitochondrial membrane. This translocase acts as a membrane carnitine exchange transporter; the transport of acylcarnitine into the mitochondrial matrix is coupled by the transport out of one molecule of carnitine. The acylcarnitine then reacts with CoA, catalyzed by CPT II (MIM 600650), which is attached to the inside of the inner mitochondrial membrane. Acyl-CoA ester is reformed in the mitochondrial matrix and becomes the substrate for the β-oxidation cycle, and carnitine is released to start a second cycle.

Carnitine is also important in the transfer of peroxisomal oxidation products, including acetyl-CoA, proprionyl-CoA, and medium-chain acyl-CoA esters, to the mitochondria.[36] However, there is no clear evidence for the presence of a carnitine/acylcarnitine carrier in the peroxisomal membrane. In addition, carnitine is involved in the excretion of toxic, poorly metabolized acyl groups as carnitine esters.

CPT I plays a pivotal role in the regulation of the carnitine cycle and FA oxidation. This regulatory function is mediated through the potent inhibitory action of malonyl-CoA, the first committed intermediate in FA synthesis (lipogenesis), on CPT I.[37] In hyperketotic states such as starvation and uncontrolled diabetes, low levels of insulin along with increased glucagon/insulin ratio stimulate mobilization of FFAs from peripheral fat stores, inhibit FA esterification, and enhance their intramitochondrial oxidation. In feeding states, high insulin and low glucagon/insulin ratio stimulate hepatic synthesis of FAs and consequently the levels of malonyl-CoA rise causing suppression of CPT I.

Acetyl-CoA carboxylase 1 (ACC1; MIM 200350) and (acetyl-CoA carboxylase 2 ACC2; MIM 601557) are biotin-containing multifunctional enzymes that catalyze the carboxylation of acetyl-CoA, the product of pyruvate dehydrogenase, to yield malonyl-CoA. Malonyl-CoA is the building block of long-chain FA synthesis and, as indicated above, a regulator of FA oxidation through the inhibition of CPT I; hence function of these carboxylases interrelate three metabolic pathways: FA synthesis, FA oxidation, and carbohydrate metabolism.[38] In animals and human, there are two major acetyl-CoA carboxylase isoforms—ACC1 (M_r 265,000) and ACC2 (M_r 280,000)—which are encoded by separate genes and are localized onto different chromosomes, 17q12 and 12q24.11, respectively.[39,40] ACC1 is abundant in lipogenic tissues such as liver and adipose tissue while ACC2 is highly expressed in the heart, skeletal muscle, and the liver.[39,40] ACC1 is a cytosolic enzyme, which catalyzes the synthesis of malonyl-CoA, a key substrate for the synthesis of palmitate by fatty acid synthase. ACC2 is localized to the mitochondria, and the malonyl-CoA it generates regulates the carnitine shuttle system, hence the β-oxidation of FAs.[38] Therefore, ACC1 and ACC2 play major roles in regulating the rates of FA synthesis and oxidation, respectively, as they relate to energy homeostasis.

By using knockout studies, it has been shown that mice lacking ACC1 were embryonically lethal[41]; however, deletion of the ACC2 gene in mice resulted in higher FA oxidation in heart, liver, muscle, and adipose tissue.[42–45] As a result, ACC2 mutant mice are leaner; resistant to diet inducing obesity, and protected against fatty liver compared to the wild type mice. Hence, ACC2 is a promising target against diseases that comprise the metabolic syndrome.

Malonyl-CoA is also regulated by its decarboxylation to acetyl-CoA by malonyl-CoA decarboxylase (MIM 606761). The balance of malonyl-CoA synthesis and degradation is thought to have a significant regulatory role in FA metabolism. Malonyl-CoA decarboxylase deficiency (MIM 248360) is a rare autosomal recessive disorder characterized by malonic aciduria and the diagnostic metabolite, malonylcarnitine (C_3DC), and a variable presentation of developmental delay, epilepsy, hypoglycemia, acidosis, short stature, abnormal genitalia, renal dysplasia, brain abnormalities, hypotonia, and cardiomyopathy.[46,47] Treatment with a low-fat, high medium-chain triglycerides (MCT)/carbohydrate diet seems to improve some of the clinical findings if diet is modified before significant disease symptoms.[48]

ACC1 and ACC2 activities are regulated also by covalent modification mediated through phosphorylation/dephosphorylation mechanisms. Adenosine monophosphate-activated protein kinase (AMPK) phosphorylates ACC1 and ACC2 and reduces their activities.[49] When metabolic fuel is low and ATP is needed in situations of increased energy demand, AMPK is activated, where it then phosphorylates and turns off ACC1 and ACC2 and subsequently causes reduction in the levels of malonyl-CoA. ACC inhibition leads to an increase in FA oxidation and a decrease in FA biosynthesis, causing increased generation and decreased consumption of ATP.[50,51]

Carnitine Cycle Defects

Carnitine is synthesized from lysine and methionine in the liver, kidney, and brain.[31,32] Recently, a deficiency of the X-linked 6-N-trimethyllysine dioxygenase (also known as trimethyllysine hydroxylase, epsilon; MIM 300777), the first enzyme of the carnitine biosynthesis pathway, was described (MIM 300872) in ~1 in 350 control males of European descent.[52,53] However, the clinical significance of this finding is still debated.

Most tissues, except for kidney, liver, and brain, do not have the complete set of enzymes to synthesize carnitine, and therefore they depend on active transport of carnitine from blood mediated by carnitine transporter (OCTN2; MIM 603377). OCTN2 is expressed in the proximal and distal renal tubules, myocardium, skeletal muscle, placenta, and different parts of the brain.[54] The result of the active uptake is 20- to 50-fold higher concentrations of carnitine in tissues as compared to blood.[55] This high-affinity, sodium-dependent carnitine transport system is also involved in efficient renal tubular carnitine reabsorption,[54] which is enhanced if body stores of carnitine are low.[33] OCTN1 (MIM 604190), a homologue of OCTN2, is a low-affinity transporter of carnitine, which is expressed predominantly in the liver, kidney, and small intestine.[56]

Patients with primary systemic carnitine deficiency (PSCD; MIM 212140), an autosomal recessive disorder caused by mutations in the *SLC22A5* gene that encodes the carnitine transporter OCTN2,[57] exhibit very low plasma and tissue carnitine concentrations due to excessive renal and intestinal carnitine wasting. If untreated with L-carnitine supplementation, patients show symptoms of recurrent episodes of hypoketotic hypoglycemic encephalopathy, cardiomyopathy, hepatomegaly, myopathy, hyperammonaemia, and failure to thrive. Plasma free, acyl, and total carnitine levels in affected individuals are usually below 10% of controls.[58] Newborn screening (NBS) can identify infants with PSCD by the detection of low levels of free carnitine (C_0) using tandem mass spectrometry. Confirmation of the diagnosis usually requires postnatal measurement of free and total carnitine and sequence analysis of the *SLC22A5* gene.[59] Carnitine is transferred in utero across the placenta, and carnitine levels in neonates reflect those of their mothers.[60] In fact, there are many reports now of maternal PSCD uncovered by the detection of low carnitine levels in NBS.[61,62] These cases illustrate that the phenotype of PSCD can be very mild or asymptomatic. Such milder phenotypes are expected to be underdiagnosed; therefore, it is difficult to determine the relative prevalence of different phenotypes associated with PSCD. A recent study found that 15 of 42 adult reported cases (35.7%) ascertained through NBS were symptomatic; five patients (12%) had cardiac arrhythmias. This phenotypic variability among patients with PSCD remains unexplained.[63] Heterozygous individuals lose two to three times the normal amount of filtered carnitine in their urine, explaining their mildly reduced plasma carnitine levels.[60] One study showed that heterozygotes for *SLC22A5* mutations were predisposed to late-onset benign cardiac hypertrophy.[64] However, another study found that heterozygosity for PSCD is not more frequent in patients with cardiomyopathy, and therefore this association has been questioned.[65]

Secondary carnitine deficiency can be seen in organic aciduria and fatty acid oxidation defects and is characterized by increased acyl carnitine excretion in urine due to accumulation of organic acids.[31] It can also be associated with poor diet, renal tubular disorders, dialysis, liver disease, pharmacological therapy such as pivampicillin, cyclosporin, or valproic acid, and prematurity.

Carnitine palmitoyltransferase I was found to exist in tissue-specific isoforms.[37] The liver isoform, CPT 1A, is expressed in liver, kidney, white adipose tissue, testis, ovary, pancreatic islet, lung, spleen, brain, intestine, and at much lower levels in heart.[66] The muscle isoform, CPT 1B, is expressed in brown adipose tissue, testis, heart, and skeletal muscle.[67] The isoform CPT 1C is expressed mainly in the brain. Homozygous Cpt1b deficiency in mice is embryonically lethal, and heterozygous showed decreased cold tolerance and increased fatal hypothermia after a cold-challenge test compared to the wild type.[67] There are no confirmed reports of CPT1B deficiency in humans. On the other hand, mutations in the *CPT1A* gene, which encodes CPT IA, cause an autosomal recessive condition (MIM 255120) characterized by severe episodes of hypoketotic hypoglycemia precipitated by fasting or acute illnesses. Isolated elevation of free carnitine (C_0) (> 140 micromol/L) in the NBS in an apparently healthy term neonate warrants further investigation to rule out CPT I deficiency.[68] Avoidance of fasting and diet enriched with MCT are the mainstay of therapy. MCT are made up of C_6-C_{12} medium-chain FAs bound to glycerol and the metabolism of which is independent of CPT I, CACT, CPT II, very-long-chain acyl-CoA dehydrogenase

(VLCAD; MIM 609575), trifunctional protein (TFP; MIM 600890 and 143450), and long-chain hydroxy-acyl-CoA dehydrogenase deficiency (LCHAD; MIM 600890) enzyme activities. MCT cross the mitochondrial membrane very rapidly, and, unlike long chain FA, they do not require carnitine.

CACT deficiency (MIM 212138) is associated with multiple biochemical abnormalities, including hypoketotic hypoglycemia, secondary to hepatic glycogen depletion and impaired gluconeogenesis, and hyperammonemia due to low levels of N-acetylglutamate secondary to low acetyl-CoA concentration.[36] The hypoketosis is due to impaired FA transport and oxidation. In addition, increased levels of muscle enzymes and transaminases are common findings. Elevated concentrations of long-chain FA acylcarnitine esters (C_{16-18}) are found in CACT and CPT II deficiency. Secondary carnitine deficiency, with extremely low free carnitine concentrations, is common among patients with CACT due to renal clearance of increased levels of acylcarnitines that also inhibit the carnitine transporter responsible for extensive renal tubular carnitine reabsorption.[69] Dicarboxylic aciduria, commonly observed in FA oxidation defects, can be detected by urine organic acid or acylglycine analyses and reflects microsomal ω-oxidation of the circulating FAs that are present in high concentrations due to the original defect. The clinical findings in CACT deficiency include neurologic abnormalities, cardiomyopathy, arrhythmias, skeletal muscle damage, and liver dysfunction.[36] The mortality is high due to rapid deterioration during neonatal period. The pathogenesis of the clinical abnormalities in CACT deficiency is related to a combination of energy depletion (hypoglycemia, hypoketonemia, and impaired β oxidation) and toxicity of accumulating chemicals (hyperammonemia and long-chain acylcarnitines).[70] The management of CACT deficiency is similar to other long-chain FA disorders. Treatment of hyperammonemia, if present, is essential to avoid any neurologic insults. The long-term management plan includes avoidance of fasting and restriction of long-chain FAs intake. Since patients with CACT deficiency usually have severe carnitine deficiency, supplementation with carnitine is often necessary.

CPT II deficiency has three clinical presentations: lethal neonatal form, severe infantile hepatocardiomuscular form, and myopathic form. The lethal neonatal form (MIM 608836) is characterized by hypoketotic hypoglycemia, cardiomyopathy, arrhythmias, encephalopathy, seizures, and facial, renal, and brain malformations. The infantile CPT II deficiency (MIM 600649) is characterized by hepatopathy, cardiomyopathy, seizures, hypoketotic hypoglycemia, and myopathy. The myopathic form of CPT II (MIM 255110), the most common inherited disorder of lipid metabolism affecting skeletal muscle,[71] is characterized by exercise-induced myalgia and weakness and sometimes is associated with rhabdomyolysis and myoglobinuria. This presentation should be differentiated from other metabolic causes of rhabdomyolysis and myoglobinuria, including VLCAD deficiency (VLCADD), glycogen storage disease type V (McArdle disease), glycogen storage disease type VII (Tarui disease), and respiratory chain defects. Tandem mass spectrometry of serum/plasma acylcarnitine profile detects an elevation of C_{12} to C_{18} acylcarnitines, notably of C_{16} and $C_{18:1}$ and elevated $(C_{16:0}+C_{18:1})/C_2$ ratio.[72] Confirmation of the diagnosis can be performed by the measurement of CPT II enzyme activity in muscle or by molecular testing. Symptomatic heterozygotes for CPT II deficiency have been reported in several studies, and the influence of polymorphisms in the second allele, epigenetic factors, and the dominant negative effect of some mutations on the tetrameric structure of the CPT II complex have all been suggested as possible explanations.[73] The treatment plan of this condition includes limiting the amount of long-chain dietary fat, providing a large fraction of calories as carbohydrates and fat as MCT. Exercise restriction is recommended for all patients to avoid episodes of muscle pain and rhabdomyolysis. During rhabdomyolytic episodes, acute therapy includes glucose infusion to reduce lipid mobilization and large volumes of fluid and alkalinization to enhance renal excretion of myoglobin. A pilot trial to evaluate the therapeutic effect of the hypolipidemic drug bezafibrate for the mild form of CPT II deficiency showed promising results. After bezafibrate treatment, the palmitoyl-carnitine oxidation levels, CPT2 messenger RNA in skeletal muscle, CPT2 protein level, physical functioning, and quality of life score increased significantly in all treated patients.[74] Encouraging results were obtained also with the triheptanoin (anaplerotic) diet in patients with adult-onset CPT II deficiency.[75] It is hypothesized that energy metabolism is seriously impaired in long-chain FA oxidation defects by the inability to fuel the citric acid cycle by β-oxidation, and triheptanoin can be a source for intramitochondrial acetyl-CoA and oxaloacetate.[75]

Fatty Acid Oxidation

FAs are important for energy production once glycogen stores are depleted during fasting or during prolonged aerobic exercise or in acute illnesses when energy demands are significantly increased. FAs are catabolized in the mitochondrial matrix via the β-oxidation cycle, but a small part of them is metabolized in the peroxisomes. Long-chain FAs, released from adipose tissue or fat in the diet, are the main substrates for the mitochondrial β-oxidation pathway, which provides up to 80% of energy to the heart and liver. Each cycle of acyl-CoA ester oxidation results in the production of a shortened acyl-CoA molecule and one molecule of 2-carbon unit of acetyl-CoA. Acetyl-CoA then can enter the Krebs cycle or be used to generate ketone bodies (Figure 7.1).

Each cycle of the FA β-oxidation spiral requires the sequential action of four enzymes: acyl-CoA dehydrogenase, 2-enoyl-CoA hydratase, 3-hydroxyacyl-CoA dehydrogenase (HADH), and 3-ketoacyl-CoA thiolase (Figure 7.1). The first step is catalyzed by acyl-CoA dehydrogenase enzymes specific for different acyl-CoA substrates: VLCAD (MIM 609575) acts on C_{14}-C_{20} substrates, medium-chain acyl-CoA dehydrogenase (MCAD; MIM 607008) acts on C_6-C_{12} substrates, and short-chain acyl-CoA dehydrogenase (SCAD; MIM 606885) acts on C_4-C_6 substrates. The reactions catalyzed by acyl-CoA dehydrogenase produce two reducing equivalents that convert flavin adenine dinucleotide (FAD), the coenzyme of the acyl-CoA dehydrogenases, to FADH2. FADH2 is reoxidized by electron transfer flavoprotein, which is oxidized by electron transfer flavoprotein dehydrogenase and the released reducing equivalents are then transferred by coenzyme Q to complex III of the mitochondrial electron transport chain. Step 3 of the β-oxidation spiral is catalyzed by two different forms of HADH: LCHAD and the short- to medium-chain hydroxyacyl-CoA dehydrogenase (MIM 601609). TFP (also known as mitochondrial trifunctional protein [MTP]) has three enzyme activities: LCHAD, long-chain enoyl-CoA hydratase, and long-chain 3-keto acyl-CoA thiolase. VLCAD and TFP are inner mitochondrial membrane-associated enzymes. At a length of 12 to 14 carbons, the acyl-CoAs are released into the mitochondrial matrix where they are further metabolized by MCAD and SCAD. The reducing equivalents from the oxidation of 3-hydroxyacyl-CoAs are transferred to NAD^+, which is reduced to NADH and reoxidized by complex I of the respiratory chain.

The activity of the enzymes of FA β-oxidation can be allosterically regulated by the ratios of $NADH/NAD^+$ and acetyl-CoA/CoA and by the level of the products of their reactions.[76] An increase in the levels of these products or in the $NADH/NAD^+$ or acetyl-CoA/CoA ratios results in inhibition of FA β-oxidation. In addition, there is a transcriptional regulation of proteins involved in FA β-oxidation mediated through a number of transcription factors. Peroxisome proliferator-activated receptors (PPARs) act by binding to gene promoters containing the PPAR response elements. PPARs serve as lipid sensors that can be activated by FAs and their derivatives.[77] PPARs heterodimerize with members of the retinoid X receptor family and bind to promoters of genes encoding proteins involved in FA β-oxidation including FATP, acyl-CoA synthetase, CD36/FAT, CPT I, and MCAD.[77,78] The PPARγ coactivator-1 (PGC-1α) regulates genes involved in the cellular uptake and mitochondrial oxidation of FAs through direct coactivation of PPARs and estrogen-related receptors.[79,80]

Fatty acid β-oxidation defects are associated with impaired production of ketone bodies causing nonketotic or hypoketotic hypoglycemic encephalopathy, and life-threatening cardiac events may occur. Clinical symptoms and serious metabolic derangement are triggered by prolonged fasting, which usually occurs in the context of intercurrent infections or febrile illness, when the body mostly relies on fatty acid β-oxidation as a main source of energy. The clinical abnormalities in these defects result from either toxicity due to accumulation of acyl-CoA esters that cause cardiomyopathy and cardiac arrhythmias or from energy deficiency due to inability to synthesize ketone bodies and/or ATP. The clinical presentations of β-oxidation defects may include fasting hypoketotic hypoglycemia, rhabdomyolysis, hypotonia, myalgia, cardiomyopathy, peripheral neuropathy, retinopathy, and/or nonfasting hypoglycemia due to hyperinsulinism.

Fatty Acid Oxidation Defects

Short-Chain Acyl-CoA Dehydrogenase Deficiency

SCAD deficiency (SCADD; MIM# 201470) is an autosomal recessive FA oxidation defect associated with variable clinical manifestations. SCAD catalyzes the dehydrogenation of butyryl-CoA (C_4-CoA) during the first step of the short-chain β-oxidation spiral. SCADD results in accumulation of its substrate (C_4-CoA), butyryl carnitine (C_4), butyryl glycine, butyrate, and ethylmalonic acid.[81]

The spectrum of the clinical phenotype ranges from asymptomatic to severe; the latter can be associated with metabolic acidosis, hypoglycemia, neurologic impairment, and feeding difficulties/failure to thrive.[82,83] Neurologic findings include lethargy, developmental delay, seizures, hypotonia, dystonia, and myopathy. SCADD can also present with failure to thrive and hypotonia without developmental delay, and a smaller group may have dysmorphic features.[82,83] Today, the majority of patients with SCADD are detected through expanded NBS, and most of them remain asymptomatic. These observations raised questions regarding the clinical relevance of SCADD, and it has been suggested that the association between the reported clinical findings and the genotypes of the *ACADS* gene could be coincidental.[81]

There are two common susceptibility variants in the SCAD gene (*ACADS*): p.R171W (c.511C>T) and p.G209S (c.625G>A). The prevalence of homozygosity for the c.511C>T variant is approximately 0.3% and 5.5% for the c.625G > A variant.[84,85] Homozygosity for these variants is considered to confer susceptibility to clinical disease. Patients with abnormal NBS results can be homozygous for a mutation on both alleles or compound heterozygous for a mutation on one allele and a common susceptibility variant on the other allele or rarely, depending on the NBS cutoff for butyrylcarnitine, homozygous/compound heterozygous for the susceptibility variants.

Medium-Chain Acyl-CoA Dehydrogenase Deficiency

MCAD deficiency (MCADD; MIM# 201450) is the most common autosomal recessive disorder of mitochondrial β-oxidation. Affected patients have impaired ability to break down medium-chain FAs during fasting. Heterozygotes commonly present with residual activities of >50% of normal and do not present clinical manifestations. It affects between 1:10,000 and 1:30,000 newborns in the United States.[86] It typically presents at three months to two years of age as a metabolic decompensation triggered by common febrile illnesses, recurrent episodes of emesis, or decreased oral intake. The classic presentation is hypoketotic hypoglycemia associated with lethargy or seizures. The hepatic involvement can be in the form of hepatomegaly and acute liver disease. If not diagnosed and timely treated, the condition can quickly progress to coma and death. Patients who experience several episodes of metabolic crises may develop brain injury and muscle weakness.[87] MCADD can be a cause of sudden and unexplained death, including sudden infant death syndrome.[88,89] When undetected, approximately 20% to 25% of infants will die or suffer permanent neurologic impairment during their first acute presentation.[86,90] They may also die or suffer permanent brain damage from cerebral edema. The central nervous system effects in MCADD are believed to be partly due to hypoglycemia, but accumulation of toxic medium-chain FAs and their intermediates and by-products was postulated to be a prominent contributing factor.[91] During acute metabolic decompensation, many patients have metabolic acidosis with increased anion gap, hyperuricemia, elevated liver transaminases, and mild hyperammonemia. The biochemical abnormalities can be detected by acylcarnitine profile analysis, which is characterized by elevation of C_6 to C_{10} species, with prominent octanoylcarnitine (C_8). Urine organic acid analysis is often unremarkable in patients with MCADD who are stable and are not decompensated. However, in symptomatic patients, medium-chain dicarboxylic acids are elevated with a characteristic pattern ($C_6 > C_8 > C_{10}$). Ketones are inappropriately low even during hypoglycemia. Urine acylglycine analysis detects elevation of hexanoylglycine (C_6), 3-phenylpropionylglycine (C_8), and suberylglycine (C_{10}) even when patients are stable.

Currently, MCADD is detected in many countries through the NBS programs. While early intervention after NBS has improved outcome, it has not been completely successful, and there are reports of deaths and life-threatening episodes of metabolic decompensation in screened infants.[92]

c.985A>G (p.K304E; Lys304Glu) is the most prevalent MCAD mutation among individuals of Northern European descent. The prevalence of the c.985A>G mutation is very high in clinical cases but is lower in cases ascertained by NBS, suggesting a more severe phenotype for this mutation.[93] The most severely affected patients with MCADD have either one or two copies of this mutation.[94] Other missense mutations and null-mutations have been identified in asymptomatic patients detected through NBS or mildly affected patients.

Homozygosity for the c.985A>G mutation, having nonsense or splice site mutations or having a more severe elevation of C_8 on the NBS can be indicative for increased susceptibility to catabolic stress.[95,96] However, no genotype or biochemical phenotype was found to be protective from symptoms, suggesting that other factors may also contribute to outcome (e.g., synergistic heterozygosity in FA oxidation or other related pathways). Newborns who are homozygous for the c.985A>G mutation have very low residual enzyme activities ranging from 0% to 8%.[97] Homozygosity for other missense mutations or small deletions is also associated with low residual activities ranging from 3% to 16%.[97] The NBS also detects asymptomatic newborns with less severe mutations. For example, the c.199T>C (p.Y42H) mutation is found with allele frequency of approximately 6%. However, this mutation has never been conclusively linked to clinical symptoms.[97,98]

The c.985A>G mutation affects protein folding and oligomer assembly and stability due to elimination of the positively charged lysine and its replacement with the negatively charged glutamic acid.[99] In vitro studies showed the thermostability of the c.199T>C (p.Y42H) variant was decreased at high temperatures but not to the same extent as that of the c.985A>G mutation. This mild mutation only slightly affects the substrate binding, interaction with the natural electron acceptor, and the binding of the prosthetic group, FAD.[100] Several MCAD mutations showed by thermal inactivation experiments a 50% loss of function at temperatures <40°C, as compared to 44.5°C for wild type, probably explaining metabolic decompensations occurring during febrile illnesses.[98] Mutations located in the N-terminal α-domain, such as c.155C>T (p.A27V) and c.199T>C, showed moderate effects on tetramer assembly and thermal stability with variable catalytic activity.[97,100] Mutations in the C-terminal α-domain (c.985A>G, c.1001G>A, c.1067T>C) often affect helix-helix interactions crucial for tetramer assembly leading to aggregation.[98,99] Mutations mapping to the β-domain of the protein predispose to severe destabilization.[98]

Reversal of catabolic states is needed in symptomatic patients to avoid neurologic deterioration. The maximal duration of tolerable fasting in children with MCADD is eight hours between six months and one year of age, 10 hours in the second year of life, and 12 hours thereafter.[101] Intravenous glucose solutions to maintain a glucose infusion rate of 8 to 12 mg/kg/min is required if the patient is unable to maintain oral intake.[102] Patients with MCADD may develop secondary carnitine deficiency. Previous studies suggested that L-carnitine supplementation may enhance the elimination of toxic metabolites and improve exercise tolerance.[103]

Very-Long-Chain Acyl-CoA Dehydrogenase Deficiency

VLCAD deficiency (VLCADD; MIM 609575) is the most common long-chain FA oxidation disorder, with an estimated incidence between 1:30,000 and 1:100,000.[104] VLCADD is an autosomal recessive condition characterized by impaired mitochondrial β-oxidation of FAs with a chain length of 14 and 20 carbons. Typical phenotypes associated with VLCADD are cardiomyopathy, hypoketotic hypoglycemia, hepatopathy, muscle weakness, and episodic rhabdomyolysis.[105]

The clinical manifestations are heterogeneous with variable age of onset ranging from infancy to adulthood.[106] In general, severe neonatal disease is associated with null mutations and no residual enzyme activity, and milder phenotypes are often associated with some residual enzyme activity due to missense mutations.[106] The cardiomyopathic presentation is an infant-onset phenotype usually presents before eight months of age with hypertrophic/dilated cardiomyopathy, arrhythmias, hypotonia, severe hypoglycemia, and sudden infant death syndrome. The hepatic phenotype presents with hypoketotic hypoglycemia or a Reye-like episode triggered by metabolic stress and is rarely associated with cardiomyopathy. The myopathic phenotype is characterized by episodic muscle weakness, muscle cramps, and rhabdomyolysis triggered by strenuous exercise or severe catabolic states.[106] It was suggested that the residual VLCAD activity in patients with the myopathic phenotype becomes insufficient to sustain the increasing demands of exercising muscle in adults.[106,107] Seizures reported in patients with β-oxidation defects may be the result of cerebral bioenergetic failure associated with acute episodes of hypoglycemic encephalopathy or hypoxic-ischemic encephalopathy in the context of cardiac arrhythmias and/or cardiomyopathy.[108] Furthermore, long-chain acyl-CoAs that accumulate in VLCADD are toxic metabolites since they impair the citric acid cycle, gluconeogenesis, the urea cycle, and fatty-acid oxidation.[109]

The biochemical hallmark of the disease is elevation of $C_{14:1}$-carnitine in blood, but $C_{12:1}$, C_{14}, $C_{14:2}$, $C_{16:2}$, and $C_{18:1}$ acylcarnitines may also be elevated.[110] Medium- and long-chain dicarboxylic acidurias are detected especially during acute metabolic decompensation by urine organic acid assay. Mutation analysis of the *ACADVL* gene, enzyme assay, or in vitro FA oxidation in cultured fibroblasts is frequently needed to confirm the diagnosis.

VLCADD mice (VLCAD$^{-/-}$) hearts demonstrated microvesicular lipid accumulation and marked mitochondrial proliferation, exhibited facilitated induction of polymorphic ventricular tachycardia, and had altered expression of a variety of genes in the FA metabolic pathway from birth.[111] Fasting in these mice is associated with hepatopathy due to excessive accumulation of liver lipids, strong upregulation of peroxisomal and microsomal oxidation pathways, as well as antioxidant enzyme activities.[112] Interestingly, a diet enriched with MCT does not prevent hepatic damage.[112] VLCAD$^{-/-}$ mice compensate for VLCADD either by induction of other mitochondrial acyl-CoA dehydrogenases (LCAD and MCAD) or by enhancement of glucose oxidation, explaining why these mice are asymptomatic during normal life and develop symptoms mainly under catabolic situations. However, MCT diet does not improve these strategies long term.[113]

The mainstay of therapy in severe VLCADD includes restriction of fat, MCT supplementation, and avoidance of fasting and excessive physical exertion. However, recent mice data raised questions regarding the long-term efficacy of a low fat, carbohydrate-enriched diet in the treatment of VLCADD patients. This dietary intervention reverses endogenous compensatory mechanisms in muscles that have evolved in VLCAD$^{-/-}$ mice, resulting in pronounced energy deficiency.[114,115] It also causes impaired lipid metabolism and induces hepatic steatosis.[116] In addition, a marked accumulation of C_{16}-C_{18} acylcarnitines in skeletal and cardiac muscle of VLCAD$^{-/-}$ was observed, probably caused by chronic energy deficiency in this tissue.[115] There is no consensus regarding the treatment of patients with milder forms of VLCADD detected through NBS.[104]

Carnitine supplementation in VLCADD has been controversial, and there has been no consensus regarding the use of carnitine during acute illness.[104] There is some evidence suggesting that high levels of long chain acylcarnitine esters may be responsible for arrhythmias.[117]

Trifunctional Protein and Long-Chain 3-Hydroxyacyl-CoA Dehydrogenase Deficiencies

The mitochondrial TFP is a multienzyme complex bound to the inner mitochondrial membrane that catalyzes the last three steps of FA β-oxidation through long-chain enoyl-CoA hydratase, LCHAD, and long-chain 3-ketoacyl-CoA thiolase activities. It is a hetero-octamer composed of four α subunits and four β subunits encoded by the *HADHA* and *HADHB* genes, respectively. The four α subunits mediate the long-chain enoyl-CoA hydratase and LCHAD activities, and the four β subunits harbor the long-chain 3-ketoacyl-CoA thiolase activity.

Different mutations in the mitochondrial TFP cause isolated LCHAD deficiency (LCHADD; MIM 609016) or general TFP deficiency (TFPD, MIM 609015). TFPD is characterized by loss of both subunits and reduced activity of all three TFP enzymes, and isolated LCHADD is associated with reduced LCHAD activity only with normal expression of both subunits enzymes.[118]

The main presentation of isolated LCHADD is hypoketotic hypoglycemia that can cause sudden unexpected death, but one-quarter of patients present with chronic problems, including failure to thrive, feeding difficulties, cholestatic liver disease, and/or hypotonia.[119] Isolated LCHADD leads to irreversible retinopathy in 30% to 50% of patients and irreversible peripheral neuropathy in 5% to 10% of patients.[120,121] All symptoms are reversible with sufficient energy supply, but neuropathy and retinopathy are progressive and irreversible despite current treatment measures.[120] The common α-subunit mutation, c.1528G>C (p.E474Q), which directly affects the catalytic region of the LCHAD domain, is found in at least 60% abnormal alleles associated with isolated LCHADD.[122,123] It has a minor effect on the association of α- and β-subunits, and therefore the stability of the TFP is less severely affected.

Mutations in either subunit can cause TFP deficiency. Three clinical phenotypes were described with TFP deficiency due to β-subunit mutations: a severe neonatal presentation with cardiomyopathy, Reye-like symptoms, and early death; a hepatic form with recurrent hypoketotic hypoglycemia; and a milder, later-onset form with progressive peripheral neuropathy and episodic myoglobinuria, which is the presentation in the majority of patients.[123,124] Outer loop missense mutations do not alter the structure of the protein as much as mutations in regions that are part of the dimerization domains. Therefore, they are less expected to alter protein stability and were found only among patients with milder phenotypes.[123]

The biochemical markers of TFP deficiency include 3-hydroxy dicarboxylic aciduria and accumulation in blood of 3-hydroxy C16:0-, C16:1-, C18:0-, and C18:1-acylcarnitines.[125] NBS can detect asymptomatic cases of TFPD and LCHADD, but these remain life-threatening disorders.[126]

Initial studies showed that women carrying fetuses with LCHADD, specifically due to the p.Glu474Gln mutation, have an increased risk hemolysis, elevated liver enzymes and low platelets(HELLP) syndrome and acute fatty liver of pregnancy.[127] Subsequent studies showed that all classifications of FA oxidation defects were at high risk of developing maternal liver disease and found maternal liver disease in 16% of all FA oxidation defect pregnancies (an 18.1-fold increase) compared with 0.88% in the general population.[128]

Mice with MTP α-subunit null allele (Mtpa(-/-)) develop neonatal hypoglycemia and sudden death six to 36 hours after birth. Mtpa(-/-) fetuses accumulate long-chain fatty acid metabolites and have low birthweight. Histopathological analysis of these mice revealed moderate to severe hepatic steatosis.[129]

3-Hydroxyacyl-CoA Dehydrogenase Deficiency

The matrix HADH is a dimeric enzyme that plays major parts in catalyzing the third reaction of the FA β-oxidation spiral. This enzyme catalyzes the NAD$^+$ dependent conversion of L-3-hydroxyacyl-CoA to 3-ketoacyl-CoA of medium- and short-chain acyl-CoA intermediates (C_4–C_{12}).[130] Mutations in the *HADH* gene encoding the HADH cause diazoxide-responsive familial hyperinsulinemic hypoglycemia-4 (MIM 60997).[131] Mutations in *GLUD1* encoding glutamate dehydrogenase (GDH) cause leucine sensitive hyperinsulinemic hypoglycemia and hyperammonemia. Recent data suggest that GDH and HADH have direct protein-protein interaction, which is lost in patients with *HADH* mutations.[132] GDH enzyme kinetic studies in pancreatic islets of knock-out mice for the HADH gene [hadh(-/-)] showed an increase in GDH affinity for its substrate, α-ketoglutarate, indicating that hyperinsulinism in HADH deficiency is caused by activation of GDH via loss of inhibitory regulation of GDH by HADH.[59] A subset of patients with HADH deficiency (MIM# 231530) present with hypoglycemia, hypotonia, cardiomyopathy, hepatic steatosis, and even sudden death.[133,134] The disease referred to as SCHAD deficiency in the literature is actually caused by a deficiency of HADH.[135] HADH deficiency can now be diagnosed presymptomatically through NBS by analysis of blood spot acylcarnitines which showed C_4-OH elevation.[130] The condition is also characterized by increased 3-hydroxyglutaric acid in urine organic acids.[130]

Acyl-CoA Dehydrogenase 9 Deficiency

Acyl-CoA dehydrogenase 9 (ACAD9; MIM# 611103) is active predominantly against unsaturated long-chain acyl-CoA substrates but also has activity against saturated substrates.[136] There is a high degree of homology between ACAD9 and VLCAD, but they do not complement each other's functions when either is deficient.[137] ACAD9 deficiency (MIM 611126) presents in humans with episodic liver dysfunction during otherwise mild illnesses, Reye-like episodes, or cardiomyopathy, along with chronic neurologic dysfunction.[137] Interestingly, mitochondrial complex I deficiency characterized by infantile onset of acute metabolic acidosis, hypertrophic cardiomyopathy, and muscle weakness was found to be associated with mutations in *ACAD9*.[138] One patient with this form of complex I deficiency received vigorous treatment with riboflavin, which resulted in a favorable clinical response; he had no cognitive impairment and normal psychomotor development at five years of age.[138] Recently, two additional ACADs with long chain acyl-CoA activity, ACAD10 and ACAD11, were characterized and found to predominantly localize, in contrast to the localization of other acyl-CoA dehydrogenases to energy-generating tissues, in the human brain. It was hypothesized that these enzymes are involved in serving novel physiologic functions in the central nervous system such as controlling FA composition of cellular lipids and metabolizing aromatic amino acids intermediates.[139] This observation raises speculation about the significance of mitochondrial β-oxidation in human brain.

Ketone Bodies Production and Utilization

Ketone bodies are seen as major shuttles for transferring energy from the liver to extrahepatic tissues and are the main source of FA-derived energy for the brain. They become major body fuels during prolonged fasting and consumption of a ketogenic (high-fat, low-carbohydrate) diet.[3] During fasting, ketone bodies serve as an important source of energy for many tissues, including heart, skeletal muscle, and liver.

The transition from an intrauterine (continuous transplacental supply of glucose) to an extrauterine, high-fat nutritional environment is associated with major metabolic changes. High energy-demanding organs, like skeletal muscle and the heart, can generate energy from oxidative metabolism of FAs and lactate since they have the enzymatic machinery required to perform these processes.[140] On the other hand, neurons are dependent on hepatic gluconeogenesis to support their energy needs because they do not oxidize FAs efficiently.[141] Alternatively, ketone bodies serve as another energy substrate for the neonatal brain. In fact, the rate of ketone body extraction and utilization in the newborn brain is about five- to 40-fold greater than that of an infant or adult brain.[142]

Ketone bodies diffuse to the circulation for use in extrahepatic tissues.[143] The circulating levels of ketone bodies are determined by their rates of production and utilization. In addition, the rate of utilization of ketone bodies is proportional to their circulating levels.[3] When the concentration of circulating FAs is high, the synthesis of hepatic intramitochondrial acetyl-CoA can exceed cellular energy requirements, leading to ketogenesis. Circulating plasma ketone body levels exhibit inter-individual and sampling-time variations. These levels can be below 0.1 mM if the sample was drawn postprandially but can reach 6 mM after prolonged fasting and can go up to 25 mM during episodes of diabetic ketoacidosis.[3]

The primary ketogenic substrates are acetoacetyl-CoA and acetyl-CoA, predominantly products of mitochondrial FA beta-oxidation but also derived from certain amino acids, such as leucine. Ketogenesis (ketone body synthesis) occurs in mitochondria of different tissues

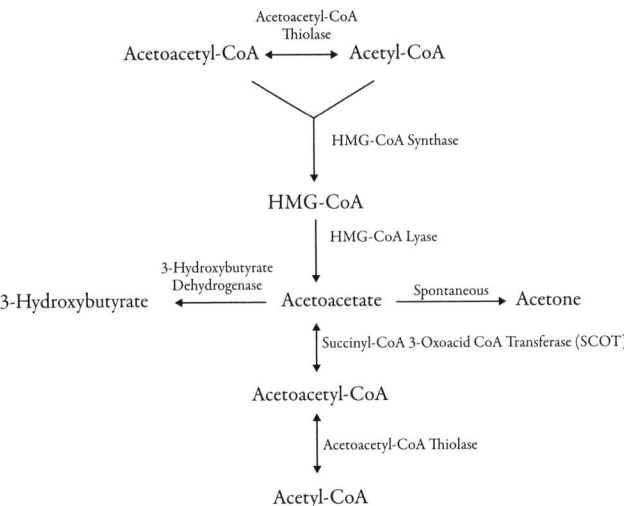

FIGURE 7.2 Biochemical pathways of ketogenesis and ketolysis.

but predominantly in the liver to generate 3-hydroxybutyrate (3OHB) and acetoacetate (AcAc; Figure 7.2). Mitochondrial HMG-CoA synthase, encoded by the *HMGCS2* gene, catalyzes the condensation of acetoacetyl-CoA and acetyl-CoA to form HMG-CoA, which is cleaved by HMG-CoA lyase to release acetyl-CoA and acetoacetate; the latter can undergo nonenzymatic degradation to acetone, which can be eliminated in breath. The cytoplasmic HMG-CoA synthase, encoded by *HMGCS1* gene, mediates an early step in cholesterol synthesis. There are two isoforms of HMGA-CoA lyase, which are both encoded by *HMGCL* gene on chromosome 1. The main isoform comprises 298 amino acids and is located in the mitochondria, where it catalyzes the conversion of HMG-CoA into AcAc and acetyl-CoA. The peroxisomal isoform comprises 325 amino acids, and it may be involved in cholesterol synthesis or degradation of long-chain FAs but its precise role is still unknown.[144,145] AcAc is converted to 3OHB via 3OHB dehydrogenase in an NAD$^+$/NADH-coupled redox reaction. The ratio of 3OHB to AcAc reflects the redox state within the mitochondrial matrix.[146] Ketone bodies are utilized as a source of energy in a process called ketolysis by their conversion to acetyl-CoA in the mitochondria of extrahepatic tissues, predominantly in the brain. In ketolytic tissues, 3OHB dehydrogenase is used to oxidize 3OHB back to AcAc. Succinyl-CoA 3-oxoacid CoA transferase, encoded by *OXCT1* (*SCOT*) gene, catalyzes the first step of ketone body utilization by reversibly transferring CoA from succinyl-CoA to acetoacetate to generate acetoacetyl-CoA. Acetoacetyl-CoA is converted to acetyl-CoA by the mitochondrial acetoacetyl-CoA thiolase (T2), which is encoded by the *ACAT1* gene. The cytosolic acetoacetyl-CoA thiolase, encoded by *ACAT2* gene, is not involved in ketone body metabolism but is essential for the synthesis of isoprenoid compounds.

Ketogenesis/Ketolysis Defects

Patients with ketogenesis and ketolysis defects tend to be asymptomatic, but severe disturbances of energy metabolism can arise with fasting, infection, or other catabolic states.

Genetic defects in ketogenesis include mitochondrial HMG-CoA synthase and HMG-CoA lyase deficiencies. Patients with mitochondrial HMG-CoA synthase (MIM 605911) and HMG-CoA lyase (MIM 246450) deficiency present, like FA oxidation disorders, with episodes of hypoketotic or nonketotic encephalopathic hypoglycemia with massive elevation of plasma FFAs and hepatomegaly.[147] Urinary organic acids demonstrate increased dicarboxylic and 3-hydroxydicarboxylic acids in the absence of significant ketonuria. Free carnitine can be low, and supplementation of L-carnitine is accompanied by a large and unexpected increase in acetylcarnitine (C_2) due to accumulation of acetyl-CoA, the final product of FA oxidation.[148] 3-Hydroxy-3-methylglutaryl-CoA lyase deficiency or 3-hydroxy-3-methylglutaric aciduria causes metabolic acidosis without ketonuria, hypoglycemia, and elevation of urinary 3-hydroxy-3-methylglutaric, 3-methylglutaric, and 3-hydroxyisovaleric acids. Other findings include hepatomegaly, hyperammonemia, macro/microcephaly, global developmental delay, acute pancreatitis, and dilated cardiomyopathy with arrhythmia.[145] Abnormal cerebral white matter changes have been described[148] and probably reflect the role of ketone bodies as substrates for the synthesis of lipids such as cholesterol in myelin.[149] This disorder is frequent in Saudi Arabia and the Iberian Peninsula (Portugal and Spain), where two mutations (c.122G>A and c.109G>A) have been identified in majority of cases. The hypoglycemia seen in these defects is attributed to impaired gluconeogenesis or to excessive glucose consumption due to the lack of ketone body production.

On the other hand, the biochemical features in ketolysis defects are dominated by severe ketoacidosis. Succinyl-CoA 3-oxoacid CoA transferase (SCOT) deficiency (MIM 245050), caused by mutations in the *OXCT1* gene, is characterized by recurrent episodes of severe ketoacidosis that can also be associated with emesis and altered neurologic status. Persistent ketosis in postprandial state or with normoglycemia should alert the physician to the possibility of SCOT deficiency.[150] SCOT is not expressed in liver and has no role other than ketolysis explaining the restriction of biochemical abnormalities to episodic ketoacidosis. In addition, SCOT-deficient mice exhibit adaptive energy mechanisms such as increased oxidation of glucose in the brain and increased lactate oxidation in skeletal muscle.[146] *Oxct1* -/-mice exhibit intact oxidation of 3OHB to AcAc, but the latter was not incorporated into the tricarboxylic acid metabolites. Instead, the accumulation of AcAc yields a reverse of the normal (3:1) 3OHB:AcAc ratio to 1:3.[146] In addition to its ketolytic activity, T2 participates in ketogenesis by converting acetyl-CoA to acetoacetyl-CoA and in catabolism of isoleucine by converting methylacetoacetyl-CoA plus CoA into acetyl-CoA and propionyl-CoA. Although patients with T2 deficiency (β-ketothiolase deficiency) (MIM 203750) excrete intermediates of isoleucine catabolism, their main presentation is intermittent ketoacidotic episodes,[151] suggesting that T2 is more essential for the ketolytic process. In general, T2 deficiency has a favorable outcome, and 23 of 26 patients in one study developed normally; one died during the first ketoacidotic episode and two have developmental delay.[152]

New Therapeutic Developments

We indicated above that PPARs serve as lipid sensors that can be activated by FAs and their derivatives and subsequently regulate the transcription of proteins involved in FA

TABLE 7.1 **Fatty Acid Metabolism Defects**

Gene	Protein	Locus	Phenotype
Fatty Acid Transport Defects			
PNPLA2	ATGL	11p15.5	Neutral lipid storage disease with myopathy (MIM 610717)
ABHD5	Coactivator of ATGL	3p21.33	Chanarin-Dorfman syndrome (MIM 275630)
PLIN1	Perilipin 1	15q26.1	Partial lipodystrophy, type 4 (MIM 613877)
SLC27A4	Fatty acid transport protein 4	9q34.11	Ichthyosis prematurity syndrome (MIM 608649)
Carnitine Cycle Defects			
TMLHE	Trimethyllysine hydroxylase, epsilon	Xq28	Carnitine biosynthesis defect (MIM 300872)
SLC22A5	Organic cation/carnitine transporter	5q31.1	Systemic (primary) carnitine deficiency (MIM 212140)
CPT1A	Carnitine palmitoyltransferase IA	11q13.3	Hypoketotic hypoglycemia and hepatic dysfunction; ↑free carnitine (MIM 255120)
SLC25A20	Carnitine-acylcarnitine translocase	3p21.31	Hypoketotic hypoglycemia,↑NH3, ↑CK, secondary carnitine deficiency;↑long-chain acylcarnitines (MIM 212138)
CPT2	Carnitine palmitoyltransferase 2	1p32.3	Lethal neonatal (MIM 608836), infantile (MIM 600649) and myopathic (adult) (MIM 255110)
Fatty Acid Oxidation Defects			
ACADS	Short-chain acyl-CoA dehydrogenase	12q24.31	Asymptomatic to severe; metabolic acidosis, hypoglycemia, neurologic impairment, and feeding difficulties/failure to thrive; ↑C_4, ↑ethylmalonic acid (MIM# 201450)
ACADM	Medium chain Acyl-CoA dehydrogenase	1p31.1	Hypoketotic hypoglycemia, lethargy, seizures, SIDS, liver involvement; ↑C_6, C_{10} (MIM# 201450)
ACADVL	Very long chain acyl-CoA dehydrogenase	17p13.1	Cardiomyopathic phenotype: hypertrophic/dilated cardiomyopathy, arrhythmias, hypotonia, severe hypoglycemia, and SIDS; hepatic phenotype with hypoketotic hypoglycemia and Reye-like episodes; myopathic phenotype: episodic muscle weakness, muscle cramps, and rhabdomyolysis (MIM 609575). ↑ long-chain acylcarnitines
HADHA	α subunit of trifunctional protein (3-hydroxyacyl-CoA dehydrogenase and enoyl-CoA hydratase activities)	2p23.3	Trifunctional protein deficiency (see below); acute fatty liver of pregnancy, maternal HELLP syndrome; LCHAD deficiency (MIM 609016): common mutation, c.G1528C, hypoketotic hypoglycemia, FTT, feeding difficulties, cholestatic liver disease, retinopathy, peripheral neuropathy, hypotonia. ↑ long-chain OHacylcarnitines
HADHB	β subunit of trifunctional protein (3-ketoacyl-CoA thiolase activity)	2p23.3	Trifunctional protein deficiency (MIM 609015): severe neonatal form with cardiomyopathy, Reye-like symptoms, and early death; a hepatic form with recurrent hypoketotic hypoglycemia; majority have a milder later-onset progressive peripheral neuropathy and episodic myoglobinuria; ↑ long-chain OHacylcarnitines
HADH	3-hydroxyacyl-CoA dehydrogenase	4q25	Familial hyperinsulinemic hypoglycemia-4 (MIM 60997); HADH deficiency (MIM# 231530): hypoglycemia, hypotonia, cardiomyopathy, hepatic steatosis.

(continued)

TABLE 7.1 Continued

Gene	Protein	Locus	Phenotype
ACAD9	Acyl-CoA dehydrogenase 9	3q21.3	Episodic liver dysfunction, cardiomyopathy, chronic neurologic dysfunction (MIM 611126); mitochondrial complex I deficiency
Ketogenesis and Ketolysis Defects			
HMGCS2	3-hydroxy-3-methylglutaryl-CoA synthase 2	1p12	Ketogenesis defect (MIM 605911): hypoketotic hypoglycemia, hepatomegaly, macro/microcephaly, global developmental delay, pancreatitis, and dilated cardiomyopathy
HMGCL	3-Hydroxy-3-methylglutaryl-CoA lyase	1p36.11	Ketogenesis defect (MIM 246450): early-onset hypoketotic hypoglycemia, hepatomegaly metabolic/lactic acidosis, pancreatitis, abnormal brain MRI abnormalities
OXCT1	3-oxoacid CoA transferase 1	5p13.1	Ketolysis defect: SCOT deficiency (MIM 245050); Recurrent ketoacidosis, hypotonia and lethargy, ±cardiomegaly, hypo- or hyperglycemia
ACAT1	Mitochondrial acetoacetyl-CoA thiolase	11q22.3	Ketolysis defect (thiolase) or β-ketothiolase deficiency (MIM 203750); intermittent ketoacidotic episodes, seizures, ±CNS involvement, ataxia, dystonia, abnormalities in the basal ganglia

Note. ATGL = adipose triglyceride lipase; SIDS = sudden infant death syndrome; HELLP = elevated liver enzymes and low platelets; LCHAD = long-chain hydroxy-acyl-CoA dehydrogenase deficiency; FTT = failure to thrive; HADH = 3-hydroxyacyl-CoA dehydrogenase; SCOT = succinyl-CoA 3-oxoacid CoA transferase; CNS = central nervous system.

β-oxidation.[77] They bind to promoters of genes encoding proteins involved in FA β-oxidation, including FATP, acyl-CoA synthetase, CD36/FAT, CPT1, and MCAD. Because of their crucial role in energy homeostasis, PPARs were targets for therapeutic intervention. The hypolipidemic drug fibrate is a PPAR agonist and was shown to be a potent pharmaceutical tool to stimulate FA oxidation in different tissues and animal models.[153] The addition of bezafibrate or fenofibric acid in the culture medium of cells from patients with the myopathic form of VLCADD induced a dose-dependent increase in palmitate oxidation due to drug-induced increases in VLCAD mRNA, protein, and residual enzyme activity.[154] Interestingly, bezafibrate induced no changes in FA oxidation capacities in fibroblasts from patients with severe neonatal or infantile VLCAD phenotypes. A pilot trial to evaluate the therapeutic effect of bezafibrate for the mild form of CPT II deficiency showed promising results. After bezafibrate treatment, the palmitoyl L-carnitine oxidation levels, CPT2 messenger RNA in skeletal muscle, CPT2 protein level, physical functioning, and quality of life score increased significantly in all treated patients.[74] A recent study showed that incubation of SCADD fibroblasts with antioxidants (Vitamins C and E or N-acetylcysteine) and bezafibrate significantly increased their viability and decreased their vulnerability to menadione-induced oxidative stress.[155]

In aerobic metabolism, ATP production is largely dependent on the TCA cycle, and therefore a decrease in the availability of its intermediates can impair energy production. Anaplerotic (refilling) reactions are needed to continuously replenish these metabolites in order to attain high rates of TCA cycle flux. It is hypothesized that energy metabolism is seriously affected in long-chain FA oxidation defects by the inability to fuel the TCA by β-oxidation.[75] Triheptanoin is a medium-chain triglyceride containing three odd chain fatty acid heptanoate molecules. Its catabolism yields propionyl-CoA, which can be used for anaplerosis in most tissues, and C_5 ketone bodies in liver that are also converted to propionyl-CoA, which can be transported and used for anaplerosis in peripheral tissues. Through these pathways, triheptanoin can be a source for intramitochondrial acetyl-CoA and oxaloacetate.[75] Using triheptanoin as an anaplerotic molecule in patients with adult-onset CPT II deficiency caused an improvement of muscle pain with exercise and a reduction in rhabdomyolysis.[75]

Summary

In this chapter, we presented an overview of the fatty acid metabolism and its associated metabolic defects. Beta-oxidation is a complex multistep pathway by which FAs are catabolised to produce energy. Membrane uptake of long-chain FAs is a highly regulated process that is mediated by different transport mechanisms. Once inside the cell, FAs are convertd to fatty acylCoA before they are transferred into the mitochondrial matrix through the carnitine cycle. In the mitochondrial matrix, the long-chain acyl-CoA enters the FA β-oxidation spiral reactions to produce acetyl-CoA, NADH, and FADH2. Acetyl-CoA can be fully oxidized in the TCA cycle to produce NADH and FADH2, which are used to generate ATP or utilized for ketone body production. Our understanding of the overall regulation of these processes has improved but is still incomplete. The concepts of intramitochondrial channelling of specific metabolites to their targets and the structural organization of the enzymatic machinery mediating FA metabolism are being thoroughly investigated. In this chaper, we reviewed our current knowledge on inborn errors of FA metabolism (Table 7.1). The mainstay of treatment is avoidance of fasting and diet modifications, in addition to aggressive measures to avoid catabolism, especially during common illnesses. The introduction of the expanded NBS enabled early detection and intervention, which improved the clinical outcome for many of these disorders. However, the increasing number of identified milder phenotypes in NBS poses significant challenges to the clinician in regard to treatment and genetic counseling. The clinical significance of many of these "hypomorphic" phenotypes is unknown at this time. It is also unclear if the cut-offs used in screening laboratories should be changed to avoid these "false positives" or if we should treat all patients with these "clinically underdiagnosed" phenotypes.

References

1. Simard JR, Pillai BK, Hamilton JA. Fatty acid flip-flop in a model membrane is faster than desorption into the aqueous phase. *Biochemistry*. 2008; 47(35): 9081–9089.
2. Su X, Abumrad NA. Cellular fatty acid uptake: a pathway under construction. *Trends Endocrinol Metab*. 2009; 20(2): 72–77.
3. Fukao T, Lopaschuk GD, Mitchell GA. Pathways and control of ketone body metabolism: on the fringe of lipid biochemistry. *Prostaglandins Leukot Essent Fatty Acids* 2004; 70(3): 243–251.
4. Holm C. Molecular mechanisms regulating hormone-sensitive lipase and lipolysis. *Biochem Soc Trans*. 2003;31 (Pt 6): 1120–1124.

5. Anthonsen MW, Rönnstrand L, Wernstedt C, Degerman E, Holm C. Identification of novel phosphorylation sites in hormone-sensitive lipase that are phosphorylated in response to isoproterenol and govern activation properties in vitro. *J Biol Chem*. 1998; 273(1): 215–221.
6. Wang SP, Laurin N, Himms-Hagen J, et al. The adipose tissue phenotype of hormone-sensitive lipase deficiency in mice. *Obes Res* 2001; 9(2): 119–128.
7. Zimmermann R, Strauss JG, Haemmerle G, et al. Fat mobilization in adipose tissue is promoted by adipose triglyceride lipase. *Science*. 2004; 306(5700): 1383–1386.
8. Haemmerle G, Lass A, Zimmermann R, et al. Defective lipolysis and altered energy metabolism in mice lacking adipose triglyceride lipase. *Science*. 2006; 312(5774): 734–737.
9. Das SK, Eder S, Schauer S, et al. Adipose triglyceride lipase contributes to cancer-associated cachexia. *Science*. 2011; (6039): 233–238.
10. Fischer J, Lefèvre C, Morava E, et al. The gene encoding adipose triglyceride lipase (PNPLA2) is mutated in neutral lipid storage disease with myopathy. *Nat Genet*. 2007; 39(1): 28–30.
11. Ghosh AK, Ramakrishnan G, Chandramohan C, Rajasekharan R. CGI-58, the causative gene for Chanarin-Dorfman syndrome, mediates acylation of lysophosphatidic acid. *J Biol Chem* 2008; 283: 24525–24533.
12. Brasaemle DL, Subramanian V, Garcia A, Marcinkiewicz A, Rothenberg A. Perilipin A and the control of triacylglycerol metabolism. *Mol Cell Biochem*. 2009; 326: 15–21.
13. Granneman JG, Kimler VA, Moore HP. Cell Biology Symposium: imaging the organization and trafficking of lipolytic effectors in adipocytes. *J Anim Sci*. 2011; 89: 701–710.
14. Wang H, Hu L, Dalen K, et al. Activation of hormone-sensitive lipase requires two steps, protein phosphorylation and binding to the PAT-1 domain of lipid droplet coat proteins. *J Biol Chem*. 2009; 284(46): 32116–32125.
15. Wang H, Sreenevasan U, Hu H, et al. Perilipin 5, a lipid droplet-associated protein, provides physical and metabolic linkage to mitochondria. *J Lipid Res*. 2011; 52(12): 2159–2168.
16. Gandotra S, Le Dour C, Bottomley W, et al. Perilipin deficiency and autosomal dominant partial lipodystrophy. *N Engl J Med*. 2011; 364(8): 740–748.
17. Boutet E, El Mourabit H, Prot M, et al. Seipin deficiency alters fatty acid Delta9 desaturation and lipid droplet formation in Berardinelli-Seip congenital lipodystrophy. *Biochimie*. 2009; 91: 796–803.
18. Doege H, Stahl A. Protein-mediated fatty acid uptake: novel insights from in vivo models. *Physiology* (Bethesda). 2006; 21: 259–268.
19. Mashek DG, Coleman RA. Cellular fatty acid uptake: the contribution of metabolism. *Curr Opin Lipidol*. 2006; 17: 274–278.
20. Malhotra KT, Malhotra K, Lubin BH, Kuypers FA. Identification and molecular characterization of acyl-CoA synthetase in human erythrocytes and erythroid precursors. Biochem J. 1999; 344(Pt 1): 135–143.
21. Watkins PA, Maiguel D, Jia Z, Pevsner J. Evidence for 26 distinct acyl-coenzyme A synthetase genes in the human genome. *J Lipid Res*. 2007; 48(12): 2736–2750.
22. Watkins PA. Very-long-chain acyl-CoA synthetases. *J Biol Chem*. 2008; 283(4): 1773–1777.
23. Ellis JM, Frahm JL, Li LO, Coleman RA. Acyl-coenzyme A synthetases in metabolic control. *Curr Opin Lipidol*. 2010; 21(3): 212–217.
24. Black PN, DiRusso CC. Vectorial acylation: linking fatty acid transport and activation to metabolic trafficking. *Novartis Found Symp*. 2007; 286: 127–138.
25. Pohl J, Ring A, Ehehalt R, Herrmann T, Stremmel W. New concepts of cellular fatty acid uptake: role of fatty acid transport proteins and of caveolae. *Proc Nutr Soc*. 2004; 63(2): 259–262.
26. Gimeno RE. Fatty acid transport proteins. *Curr Opin Lipidol*. 2007; 18: 271–276.
27. Richards MR, Harp JD, Ory DS, Schaffer JE. Fatty acid transport protein 1 and long-chain acyl coenzyme A synthetase 1 interact in adipocytes. *J Lipid Res*. 2006; 47(3): 665–672.
28. Melton EM, Cerny RL, Watkins PA, DiRusso CC, Black PN. Human fatty acid transport protein 2a/very long chain acyl-CoA synthetase 1 (FATP2a/Acsvl1) has a preference in mediating the channeling of exogenous n-3 fatty acids into phosphatidylinositol. *J Biol Chem*. 2011; 286(35): 30670–30679.
29. Klar J, Schweiger M, Zimmerman R, et al. Mutations in the fatty acid transport protein 4 gene cause the ichthyosis prematurity syndrome. *Am J Hum Genet*. 2009; 85(2): 248–253.
30. Li H, Vahlquist A, Törmä H. Interactions between FATP4 and ichthyin in epidermal lipid processing may provide clues to the pathogenesis of autosomal recessive congenital ichthyosis. *J Dermatol Sci*. 2012; 69:195–201.

31. Flanagan JL, Simmons PA, Vehige J, Willcox MD, Garrett Q. Role of carnitine in disease. *Nutr Metab (Lond)*. 2010; 7: 30.
32. Vaz FM, Wanders RJ.Carnitine biosynthesis in mammals. *Biochem J*. 2002; 361(Pt 3): 417–429.
33. Rebouche CJ: Kinetics, pharmacokinetics, and regulation of L-carnitine and acetyl-L-carnitine metabolism. *Ann NY Acad Sci* 2004, 1033: 30–41.
34. Krajcovicová-Kudláčková M, Simoncic R, Béderová A, Babinská K, Béder I. Correlation of carnitine levels to methionine and lysine intake. *Physiol Res*. 2000; 49(3): 399–402.
35. Rebouche CJ, Seim H: Carnitine metabolism and its regulation in microorganisms and mammals. *Annu Rev Nutr* 1998, 18: 39–61.
36. Rubio-Gozalbo ME, Bakker JA, Waterham HR, Wanders RJ. Carnitine-acylcarnitine translocase deficiency, clinical, biochemical and genetic aspects. *Mol Aspects Med*. 2004; 25(5-6): 521–532.
37. McGarry JD, Brown NF. The mitochondrial carnitine palmitoyltransferase system. From concept to molecular analysis. *Eur J Biochem*. 1997; 244(1): 1–14.
38. Wakil SJ, Abu-Elheiga L. Fatty acid metabolism: target for metabolic syndrome. *J Lipid Res*. 2009; 50(Suppl): S138–S143.
39. Abu-Elheiga L, Jayakumar A, Baldini A, Chirala SS, Wakil SJ. Human acetyl-CoA carboxylase: characterization, molecular cloning, and evidence for two isoforms. *Proc Natl Acad Sci USA*. 1995; 92(9): 4011–4015.
40. Abu-Elheiga L, Almarza-Ortega DB, Baldini A, Wakil SJ. Human acetyl-CoA carboxylase 2: molecular cloning, characterization, chromosomal mapping, and evidence for two isoforms. *J Biol Chem*. 1997; 272(16): 10669–10677.
41. Abu-Elheiga L, Matzuk MM, Kordari P, et al. Mutant mice lacking acetyl-CoA carboxylase 1 are embryonically lethal. *Proc Natl Acad Sci USA*. 2005; 102(34): 12011–12016.
42. Abu-Elheiga L, Matzuk MM, Abo-Hashema KA, Wakil SJ. Continuous fatty acid oxidation and reduced fat storage in mice lacking acetyl-CoA carboxylase 2. *Science*. 2001; 291: 2613–1616.
43. Abu-Elheiga L, Oh W, Kordari P, Wakil SJ. Acetyl-CoA carboxylase 2 mutant mice are protected against obesity and diabetes induced by high-fat/high-carbohydrate diets. *Proc Natl Acad Sci USA*. 2003; 100: 10207–10212.
44. Oh W, Abu-Elheiga L, Kordari P, Gu Z, Shaikenov T, Chirala SS, Wakil SJ. Glucose and fat metabolism in adipose tissue of acetyl-CoA carboxylase 2 knockout mice. *Proc Natl Acad Sci USA*. 2005; 102(5): 1384–1389.
45. Essop MF, Camp HS, Choi CS, et al. Reduced heart size and increased myocardial fuel substrate oxidation in ACC2 mutant mice.*Am J Physiol Heart Circ Physiol*. 2008; 295(1): H256–H265.
46. Wightman PJ, Santer R, Ribes A, et al. MLYCD mutation analysis: evidence for protein mistargeting as a cause of MLYCD deficiency.*Hum Mutat*. 2003; 22(4): 288–300.
47. Salomons GS, Jakobs C, Pope LL, et al. Clinical, enzymatic and molecular characterization of nine new patients with malonyl-coenzyme A decarboxylase deficiency. *J Inherit Metab Dis*. 2007; 30: 23–28.
48. Footitt EJ, Stafford J, Dixon M, et al. Use of a long-chain triglyceride-restricted/medium-chain triglyceride-supplemented diet in a case of malonyl-CoA decarboxylase deficiency with cardiomyopathy. *J Inherit Metab Dis*. 2010 Jun 15.
49. Hardie DG, Pan DA. Regulation of fatty acid synthesis and oxidation by the AMP-activated protein kinase. *Biochem Soc Trans* 2002; 30: 1064–1070.
50. Wakil SJ, Abu-Elheiga LA. Fatty acid metabolism: target for metabolic syndrome. *J lipid Res*. 2008; 50: S138–S143.
51. Lopaschuk GD, Ussher JR, Folmes CD, Jaswal JS, Stanley WC. Myocardial fatty acid metabolism in health and disease. *Physiol Rev* 2010; 90: 207–258.
52. Celestino-Soper PB, Shaw CA, Sanders SJ, et al. Use of array CGH to detect exonic copy number variants throughout the genome in autism families detects a novel deletion in TMLHE. *Hum Mol Genet*. 2011; (22): 4360–4370.
53. Celestino-Soper PB, Violante S, Crawford EL, et al. A common X-linked inborn error of carnitine biosynthesis may be a risk factor for nondysmorphic autism. *Proc Natl Acad Sci USA*. 2012; 109(21): 7974–7981.
54. Wu X, Huang W, Prasad PD, et al. Functional characteristics and tissue distribution pattern of organic cation transporter 2 (OCTN2), an organic cation/carnitine transporter. *J Pharmacol Exp Ther*. 1999; 290(3): 1482–1492.
55. Stanley CA.Carnitine deficiency disorders in children. *Ann NY Acad Sci*. 2004; 1033: 42–51.

56. Wu X, George RL, Huang W, et al. Structural and functional characteristics and tissue distribution pattern of rat OCTN1, an organic cation transporter, cloned from placenta. *Biochim Biophys Acta*. 2000; 1466(1-2): 315–327.
57. Nezu J, Tamai I, Oku A et al. Primary systemic carnitine deficiency is caused by mutations in a gene encoding sodium iondependent carnitine transporter. *Nat Genet* 1999, 21: 91–94.
58. Longo N, Amat di San Filippo N, Pasquali M. Disorders of carnitine transport and the carnitine cycle. *Am J Med Genet C Semin Med Genet*. 2006; 142C: 77–85.
59. Li C, Chen P, Palladino A, et al. Mechanism of hyperinsulinism in short-chain 3-hydroxyacyl-CoA dehydrogenase deficiency involves activation of glutamate dehydrogenase. *J Biol Chem* 2010; 285: 31806–31818.
60. Scaglia F, Longo N. Primary and secondary alterations of neonatal carnitine metabolism. *Semin Perinatol*. 1999; 23: 152–61.
61. El-Hattab AW, Li FY, Shen J, et al. Maternal systemic primary carnitine deficiency uncovered by newborn screening: clinical, biochemical, and molecular aspects. *Genet Med*. 2010; 12: 19–24.
62. Lee NC, Tang NL, Chien YH, Chen CA, Lin SJ, Chiu PC, Huang AC, Hwu WL. Diagnoses of newborns and mothers with carnitine uptake defects through newborn screening. *Mol Genet Metab*. 2010; 100: 46–50.
63. Spiekerkoetter U, Huener G, Baykal T, et al. Silent and symptomatic primary carnitine deficiency within the same family due to identical mutations in the organic cation/carnitine transporter OCTN2. *J Inherit Metab Dis*. 2003; 26: 613–615.
64. Koizumi A, Nozaki J, Ohura T, et al. Genetic epidemiology of the carnitine transporter OCTN2 gene in a Japanese population and phenotypic characterization in Japanese pedigrees with primary systemic carnitine deficiency. *Hum Mol Genet*. 1999; 8: 2247–2254.
65. Amat di San Filippo C, Taylor MR, Mestroni L, Botto LD, Longo N. Cardiomyopathy and carnitine deficiency. *Mol Genet Metab*. 2008; 94: 162–166.
66. Nyman LR, Cox KB, Hoppel CL, et al. Homozygous carnitine palmitoyltransferase 1a (liver isoform) deficiency is lethal in the mouse. *Mol Genet Metab*. 2005; 86(1-2): 179–187.
67. Ji S, You Y, Kerner J, Hoppel CL, Schoeb TR, Chick WS, Hamm DA, Sharer JD, Wood PA. Homozygous carnitine palmitoyltransferase 1b (muscle isoform) deficiency is lethal in the mouse. *Mol Genet Metab*. 2008 ; 93(3): 314–322.
68. Sim KG, Wiley V, Carpenter K, Wilcken B. Carnitine palmitoyltransferase I deficiency in neonate identified by dried blood spot free carnitine and acylcarnitine profile. *J Inherit Metab Dis*. 2001; 24(1): 51–59.
69. Stanley CA, Hale DE, Berry GT, Deleeuw S, Boxer J, Bonnefont JP. Brief report: a deficiency of carnitine acylcarnitine translocase in the inner mitochondrial membrane. *N Engl J Med*. 1992; 327: 19–23.
70. Yamada KA, Kanter EM, Newatia A. Long-chain acylcarnitine induces Ca2+ efflux from the sarcoplasmic reticulum. *J Cardiovasc Pharmacol*. 2000; 36(1): 14–21.
71. Taroni F, Verderio E, Dworzak F, Willems PJ, Cavadini P, DiDonato S. Identification of a common mutation in the carnitine palmitoyltransferase II gene in familial recurrent myoglobinuria patients. *Nat Genet* 1993; 4: 314–320.
72. Gempel K, Kiechl S, Hofmann S, et al. Screening for carnitine palmitoyltransferase II deficiency by tandem mass spectrometry. *J Inherit Metab Dis*. 2002; 25: 17–27.
73. Anichini A, Fanin M, Vianey-Saban C, et al. Genotype–phenotype correlations in a large series of patients with muscle type CPT II deficiency. *Neurol Res*. 2011; 33: 24–32.
74. Bonnefont JP, Bastin J, Behin A, Djouadi F. Bezafibrate for an inborn mitochondrial beta-oxidation defect. *N Engl J Med*. 2009; 360: 838–840.
75. Roe CR, Yang BZ, Brunengraber H, Roe DS, Wallace M, Garritson BK. Carnitine palmitoyltransferase II deficiency: successful anaplerotic diet therapy. *Neurology*. 2008; 71: 260–264.
76. Schulz H. Regulation of fatty acid oxidation in heart. *J Nutr* 1994; 124: 165–171.
77. Poulsen Ll, Siersbæk M, Mandrup S. PPARs: fatty acid sensors controlling metabolism. *Semin Cell Dev Biol* 2012; 23: 631–639.
78. Huss JM, Kelly DP. Nuclear receptor signaling and cardiac energetics. *Circ Res*. 2004; 95: 568–578.
79. Lin J, Handschin C, Spiegelman BM. Metabolic control through the PGC-1 family of transcription coactivators. Cell Metabolism. 2005;1: 361–370.
80. Scarpulla RC. Metabolic control of mitochondrial biogenesis through the PGC-1 family regulatory network. *Biochim Biophys Acta* 2011; 1813: 1269–1278.

81. van Maldegem BT, Wanders JA, Wijburg FA. Clinical aspects of short-chain acyl-CoA dehydrogenase deficiency. *J Inherit Metab Dis.* 2010; 33: 507–511.
82. Pedersen CB, Kølvraa S, Kølvraa A, et al. The ACADS gene variation spectrum in 114 patients with short-chain acyl-CoA dehydrogenase (SCAD) deficiency is dominated by missense variations leading to protein misfolding at the cellular level. *Hum Genet* 2008; 124: 43–56.
83. Waisbren SE, Levy HL, Noble M, et al. Short-chain acyl-CoA dehydrogenase (SCAD) deficiency: an examination of the medical and neurodevelopmental characteristics of 14 cases identified through newborn screening or clinical symptoms. *Mol Genet Metab* 2008; 95: 39–45.
84. Nagan N, Kruckeberg KE, Tauscher AL, Bailey KS, Rinaldo P, Matern D. The frequency of short-chain acyl-CoA dehydrogenase gene variants in the US population and correlation with the C(4)-acylcarnitine concentration in newborn blood spots. *Mol Genet Metab.* 2003; 78: 239–246.
85. van Maldegem BT, Waterham HR, Duran M, et al. The 625G>A SCAD gene variant is common but not associated with increased C4-carnitine in newborn blood spots. *J Inherit Metab Dis.* 2005; 28: 557–562.
86. Grosse SD, Khoury MJ, Greene CL, Crider KS, Pollitt RJ. The epidemiology of medium chain acyl-CoA dehydrogenase deficiency: an update. *Genet Med.* 2006; 8(4): 205–212.
87. Iafolla AK, Thompson RJ Jr, Roe CR. Medium-chain acyl-coenzyme A dehydrogenase deficiency: clinical course in 120 affected children. *J Pediatr.* 1994;124:409-415.
88. Boles RG, Buck EA, Blitzer MG, et al. Retrospective biochemical screening of fatty acid oxidation disorders in postmortem livers of 418 cases of sudden death in the first year of life. *J Pediatr.* 1998;132:924–933.
89. Chace DH, DiPerna JC, Mitchell BL, et al. Electrospray tandem mass spectrometry for analysis of acylcarnitines in dried postmortem blood specimens collected at autopsy from infants with unexplained cause of death. *Clin Chem.* 2001;47:1166-1182.
90. Derks TG, Reijngoud DJ, Waterham HR, et al. The natural history of medium-chain acyl CoA dehydrogenase deficiency in the Netherlands: clinical presentation and outcome. *J Pediatr* 2006; 148(5): 665–670.
91. Gregersen N, Andresen BS, Pedersen CB, Olsen RK, Corydon TJ, Bross P. Mitochondrial fatty acid oxidation defects—remaining challenges. *J Inherit Metab Dis.* 2008; 31(5): 643–657.
92. Hsu HW, Zytkovicz TH, Comeau AM, et al. Spectrum of medium-chain acyl-CoA dehydrogenase deficiency detected by newborn screening. *Pediatrics* 2008; 121(5): e1108–e1114.
93. Rhead WJ. Newborn screening for medium-chain acyl-CoA dehydrogenase deficiency: a global perspective. *J Inherit Metab Dis.* 2006; 29(2-3): 370–377.
94. Andresen BS, Bross P, Udvari S, et al. The molecular basis of medium-chain acyl-CoA dehydrogenase (MCAD) deficiency in compound heterozygous patients: is there correlation between genotype and phenotype? *Hum Mol Genet.* 1997; 6(5): 695–707.
95. Arnold GL, Saavedra-Matiz CA, Galvin-Parton PA, et al. Lack of genotype–phenotype correlations and outcome in MCAD deficiency diagnosed by newborn screening in New York State. *Mol Genet Metab.* 2010; 99(3): 263–268.
96. Waddell L, Wiley V, Carpenter K, et al. Medium-chain acyl-CoA dehydrogenase deficiency: genotype-biochemical phenotype correlations. *Mol Genet Metab.* 2006; 87: 32–39.
97. Maier EM, Gersting SW, Kemter KF, et al. Protein misfolding is the molecular mechanism underlying MCADD identified in newborn screening. *Hum Mol Genet* 2009; 18: 1612–1623.
98. Sturm M, Herebian D, Mueller M, Laryea MD, Spiekerkoetter U. Functional effects of different medium-chain acyl-CoA dehydrogenase genotypes and identification of asymptomatic variants. *PLoS One* 2012; 7(9): e45110.
99. Bross P, Jespersen C, Jensen TG, et al. Effects of two mutations detected in medium chain acyl-CoA dehydrogenase (MCAD)-deficient patients on folding, oligomer assembly, and stability of MCAD enzyme. *J Biol Chem.* 1995; 270(17): 10284–10290.
100. O'Reilly L, Bross P, Corydon TJ, et al. The Y42H mutation in medium-chain acyl-CoA dehydrogenase, which is prevalent in babies identified by MS/MS-based newborn screening, is temperature sensitive. *Eur J Biochem* 2004; 271(20): 4053–4063.
101. Derks TG, van Spronsen FJ, Rake JP, van der Hilst CS, Span MM, Smit GP. Safe and unsafe duration of fasting for children with MCAD deficiency. *Eur J Pediatr.* 2007; 166(1): 5–11.
102. Saudubray JM, Martin D, de Lonlay P, et al. Recognition and management of fatty acid oxidation defects: a series of 107 patients. *J Inherit Metab Dis* 1999; 22(4): 488–502.
103. Huidekoper HH, Schneider J, Westphal T, Vaz FM, Duran M, Wijburg FA. Prolonged moderate-intensity exercise without and with L-carnitine supplementation in patients with MCAD deficiency. *J Inherit Metab Dis.* 2006; 29(5): 631–636.

104. Arnold GL, Van Hove J, Freedenberg D, et al. A Delphi clinical practice protocol for the management of very long chain acyl-CoA dehydrogenase deficiency. *Mol Genet Metab.* 2009; 96: 85–90.
105. Kompare M, Rizzo WB. Mitochondrial fatty-acid oxidation disorders. *Semin Pediatr Neurol* 2008; 15: 140–149.
106. Andresen BS, Olpin S, Poorthuis BJ, et al. Clear correlation of genotype with disease phenotype in very-long-chain acyl-CoA dehydrogenase deficiency. *Am J Hum Genet.* 1999; 64: 479–494.
107. Shchelochkov O, Wong LJ, Shaibani A, Shinawi M. Atypical presentation of VLCAD deficiency associated with a novel ACADVL splicing mutation. *Muscle Nerve.* 2009; 39: 374–82.
108. Tein I. Role of carnitine and fatty acid oxidation and its defects in infantile epilepsy. *J Child Neurol* 2002; 17: S57–S82.
109. Primassin S, Ter Veld F, Mayatepek E, Spiekerkoetter U. Carnitine supplementation induces acylcarnitine production in tissues of very-long-chain acyl-CoA dehydrogenase-deficient mice, without replenishing low free carnitine. *Pediatr Res* 2008; 63: 632–637.
110. Schymik I, Liebig M, Mueller M, et al. Pitfalls of neonatal screening for very-long chain acyl-CoA dehydrogenase deficiency using tandem mass spectrometry. *J Pediatr* 2006; 149: 128–130.
111. Exil VJ, Roberts RL, Sims H, et al. Very-long-chain acyl-coenzyme a dehydrogenase deficiency in mice. *Circ Res.* 2003; 93: 448–455.
112. Tucci S, Primassin S, Spiekerkoetter U. Fasting-induced oxidative stress in very long chain acyl-CoA dehydrogenase-deficient mice. *FEBS J.* 2010; 277: 4699–4708.
113. Tucci S, Herebian D, Sturm M, Seibt A, Spiekerkoetter U. Tissue-specific strategies of the very-long chain acyl-CoA dehydrogenase-deficient (VLCAD-/-) mouse to compensate a defective fatty acid β-oxidation. *PLoS One.* 2012; 7: e45429.
114. Primassin S, Tucci S, Spiekerkoetter U. Hepatic and muscular effects of different dietary fat content in VLCAD deficient mice. *Mol Genet Metab.* 2011; 104: 546–551.
115. Tucci S, Pearson S, Herebian D, Spiekerkoetter U. Long-term dietary effects on substrate selection and muscle fiber type in very-long-chain acyl-CoA dehydrogenase deficient (VLCAD (-/-)) mice. *Biochim Biophys Acta.* 2013 Jan 9.
116. Tucci S, Primassin S, Ter Veld F, Spiekerkoetter U. Medium-chain triglycerides impair lipid metabolism and induce hepatic steatosis in very-long-chain acyl-CoA dehydrogenase (VLCAD)-deficient mice. *Mol Genet Metab.* 2010;101: 40–47.
117. Bonnet D, Martin D, de Lonlay P, et al. Arrhythmias and conduction defects as presenting symptoms of fatty acid oxidation disorders in children. *Circulation.* 1999; 100: 2248–2253.
118. Ushikubo S, Aoyama T, Kamijo T, et al. Molecular characterization of mitochondrial trifunctional protein deficiency: formation of the enzyme complex is important for stabilization of both a- and b-subunits. *Am J Hum Genet* 1996; 58: 979–988.
119. den Boer ME, Wanders RJ, Morris AA, IJlst L, Heymans HS, Wijburg FA. Long-chain 3-hydroxyacyl-CoA dehydrogenase deficiency: clinical presentation and follow-up of 50 patients. *Pediatrics.* 2002; 109: 99–104.
120. Spiekerkoetter U. Mitochondrial fatty acid oxidation disorders: clinical presentation of long-chain fatty acid oxidation defects before and after newborn screening. *J Inherit Metab Dis.* 2010; 33: 527–532.
121. Fletcher AL, Pennesi ME, Harding CO, Weleber RG, Gillingham MB. Observations regarding retinopathy in mitochondrial trifunctional protein deficiencies. *Mol Genet Metab* 2012; 106: 18–24.
122. IJlst L, Ruiter JP, Hoovers JM, Jakobs ME, Wanders RJ. Common missense mutation G1528C in long-chain 3-hydroxyacyl-CoA dehydrogenase deficiency. Characterization and expression of the mutant protein, mutation analysis on genomic DNA and chromosomal localization of the mitochondrial trifunctional protein alpha subunit gene. *J Clin Invest* 1996; 98: 1028–33.
123. Spiekerkoetter U, Sun B, Khuchua Z, Bennett MJ, Strauss AW. Molecular and phenotypic heterogeneity in mitochondrial trifunctional protein deficiency due to beta-subunit mutations. *Hum Mutat.* 2003; 21: 598–607.
124. Schaefer J, Jackson S, Dick DJ, Turnbull DM. Trifunctional enzyme deficiency: adult presentation of a usually fatal beta-oxidation defect. *Ann Neurol.* 1996; 40: 597–602.
125. den Boer ME, Dionisi-Vici C, Chakrapani A, van Thuijl AO, Wanders RJ, Wijburg FA. Mitochondrial trifunctional protein deficiency: a severe fatty acid oxidation disorder with cardiac and neurologic involvement. *J Pediatr.* 2003; 142: 684–689.
126. Sperk A, Mueller M, Spiekerkoetter U. Outcome in six patients with mitochondrial trifunctional protein disorders identified by newborn screening. *Mol Genet Metab* 2010; 101: 205–207.

127. Ibdah JA, Bennett MJ, Rinaldo P, et al. 1999. A fetal fatty-acid oxidation disorder as a cause of liver disease in pregnant women. *N Engl J Med.* 1999; 340: 1723–1731.
128. Browning MF, Levy HL, Wilkins-Haug LE, Larson C, Shih VE. Fetal fatty acid oxidation defects and maternal liver disease in pregnancy. *Obstet Gynecol.* 2006; 107: 115–120.
129. Ibdah JA, Paul H, Zhao Y, Binford S, et al. Lack of mitochondrial trifunctional protein in mice causes neonatal hypoglycemia and sudden death. *J Clin Invest.* 2001; 107: 1403–1409.
130. Vilarinho L, Marques JS, Rocha H, et al. Diagnosis of a patient with a kinetic variant of medium and short-chain 3-hydroxyacyl-CoA dehydrogenase deficiency by newborn screening. *Mol Genet Metab* 2012; 106: 277–280.
131. Flanagan SE, Patch AM, Locke JM, et al. Genome-wide homozygosity analysis reveals HADH mutations as a common cause of diazoxide-responsive hyperinsulinemic-hypoglycemia in consanguineous pedigrees. *J Clin Endocrinol Metab.* 2011; 96: E498–E502.
132. Heslegrave AJ, Kapoor RR, Eaton S, et al. Leucine-sensitive hyperinsulinaemic hypoglycaemia in patients with loss of function mutations in 3-Hydroxyacyl-CoA Dehydrogenase. *Orphanet J Rare Dis.* 2012; 7: 25.
133. Bennett MJ, Weinberger MJ, Kobori JA, Rinaldo P, Burlina AB. Mitochondrial short-chain l-3-hydroxyacyl-coenzyme A dehydrogenase deficiency: a new defect of fatty acid oxidation. *Pediatr Res.* 1996; 39: 185–188.
134. Yang SY, He XY, Schulz H. 3-Hydroxyacyl-CoA dehydrogenase and short chain 3-hydroxyacyl-CoA dehydrogenase in human health and disease. *FEBS J.* 2005; 272: 4874–4883.
135. He XY, Yang SY. 3-hydroxyacyl-CoA dehydrogenase (HAD) deficiency replaces short-chain hydroxyacyl-CoA dehydrogenase (SCHAD) deficiency as well as medium- and short-chain hydroxyacyl-CoA dehydrogenase (M/SCHAD) deficiency as the consensus name of this fatty acid oxidation disorder. *Mol Genet Metab.* 2007; 91: 205–206.
136. Ensenauer R, He M, Willard JM, et al. Human acyl-CoA dehydrogenase-9 plays a novel role in the mitochondrial beta-oxidation of unsaturated fatty acids. *J Biol Chem.* 2005; 280: 32309–32316.
137. He M, Rutledge SL, Kelly DR, et al. A new genetic disorder in mitochondrial fatty acid beta-oxidation: ACAD9 deficiency. *Am J Hum Genet* 2007; 8: 87–103.
138. Haack,TB, Danhauser K, Haberberger B, et al. Exome sequencing identifies ACAD9 mutations as a cause of complex I deficiency. *Nature Genet* 2010; 42: 1131–1134.
139. He M, Pei Z, Mohsen AW, Watkins P, Murdoch G, Van Veldhoven PP, Ensenauer R, Vockley J. Identification and characterization of new long chain acyl-CoA dehydrogenases. *Mol Genet Metab.* 2011; 102: 418–429.
140. Alaynick WA, Kondo RP, Xie W, et al. ERRgamma directs and maintains the transition to oxidative metabolism in the postnatal heart. *Cell Metab.* 2007; 6: 13–24.
141. Hertz L, Dienel GA. Energy metabolism in the brain. *Int Rev Neurobiol.* 2002; 51: 1–102.
142. Ward Platt M, Deshpande S. Metabolic adaptation at birth. *Semin Fetal Neonatal Med* 2005; 10: 341–350.
143. Sato K, Kashiwaya Y, Keon CA, et al. Insulin, ketone bodies, and mitochondrial energy transduction. *FASEB J.* 1995; 9: 651–658.
144. Ashmarina LI, Robert MF, Elsliger MA, Mitchell GA. Characterization of the hydroxymethylglutaryl-CoA lyase precursor, a protein targeted to peroxisomes and mitochondria. *Biochem J.* 1996; 315(Pt 1): 71–75.
145. Pié J, López-Viñas E, Puisac B, et al. Molecular genetics of HMG-CoA lyase deficiency. *Mol Genet Metab* 2007; 92: 198–209.
146. Cotter DG, d'Avignon DA, Wentz AE, Weber ML, Crawford PA. Obligate role for ketone body oxidation in neonatal metabolic homeostasis. *J Biol Chem* 2011; 286: 6902–6910.
147. Aledo R, Mir C, Dalton RN, et al. Refining the diagnosis of mitochondrial HMG-CoA synthase deficiency. *J Inherit Metab Dis.* 2006; 29: 207–211.
148. Yalçinkaya C, Dinçer A, Gündüz E, Fiçicioğlu C, Koçer N, Aydin A. MRI and MRS in HMG-CoA lyase deficiency. Pediatr Neurol 1999;20:375–380.
149. Morris AA. Cerebral ketone body metabolism. *J Inherit Metab Dis.* 2005; 28: 109–121.
150. Kayer MA. Disorders of ketone production and utilization. *Mol Genet Metab.* 2006; 87: 281–283.

151. Fukao T, Nguyen HT, Nguyen NT, et al. A common mutation, R208X, identified in Vietnamese patients with mitochondrial acetoacetyl-CoA thiolase (T2) deficiency. *Mol Genet Metab* 2010; 100: 37–41.
152. Fukao T, Scriver CR, Kondo N; T2 Collaborative Working Group. The clinical phenotype and outcome of mitochondrial acetoacetyl-CoA thiolase deficiency (beta-ketothiolase or T2 deficiency) in 26 enzymatically proved and mutation-defined patients. *Mol Genet Metab.* 2001; 72: 109–114.
153. Berger J, Moller DE. The mechanisms of action of PPARs. *Annu Rev Med.* 2002; 53: 409–435.
154. Djouadi F, Aubey F, Schlemmer D, et al. Bezafibrate increases very-long-chain acyl-CoA dehydrogenase protein and mRNA expression in deficient fibroblasts and is a potential therapy for fatty acid oxidation disorders. *Hum Mol Genet.* 2005; 14(18): 2695–2703.
155. Zolkipli Z, Pedersen CB, Lamhonwah AM, Gregersen N, Tein I. Vulnerability to oxidative stress in vitro in pathophysiology of mitochondrial short-chain acyl-CoA dehydrogenase deficiency: response to antioxidants. *PLoS One* 2011; 6: e17534.

8

Mitochondrial Disorders

AYMAN W. EL-HATTAB AND FERNANDO SCAGLIA

Introduction

Mitochondria are double membrane organelles found in all nucleated human cells that generate most of the cellular energy. The electron transport chain (ETC) complexes that transfer electrons and produce adenosine triphosphate (ATP) are embedded in the inner mitochondrial membrane. Mitochondria contain extrachromosomal DNA (mitochondrial DNA, mtDNA). However, only a very small proportion of mitochondrial proteins are encoded by that DNA; whereas the majority of mitochondrial proteins are encoded by the nuclear DNA (nDNA).

Mutations in mtDNA or mitochondria-related nDNA genes can result in mitochondrial dysfunction and mitochondrial diseases that arise as a result of inadequate ATP production required to meet the energy needs of various organs, particularly those with high energy demand. Disturbed mitochondrial function in various tissues and organs explains the multiorgan manifestations of mitochondrial diseases, including epilepsy, intellectual disability, skeletal and cardiac myopathy, hepatopathy, diabetes, sensorineural hearing loss, and renal impairment. Some patients with mitochondrial diseases display a cluster of clinical features that fall into a discrete clinical syndrome. However, there is often considerable clinical variability, and many affected individuals do not fit into one particular syndrome.

Defects in nDNA genes are inherited in an autosomal recessive, autosomal dominant, or X-linked manner; whereas mtDNA is maternally inherited. Mitochondrial diseases can result from mutations of nDNA genes encoding subunits of the ETC complexes or their assembly factors, proteins associated with the mitochondrial import machinery, mitochondrial translation factors, or proteins involved in mtDNA maintenance. MtDNA defects can be either point mutations or rearrangements.

The diagnosis of mitochondrial disorders is based on clinical recognition, biochemical screening, assessment of the multiorgan involvement, histopathological studies, ETC activity assays, and molecular genetic testing. The diagnosis of mitochondrial diseases remains challenging in many cases.

Currently, there are no satisfactory therapies available for mitochondrial disorders. Treatment remains largely symptomatic and does not significantly alter the course of the disease.

Biology and Genetics of Mitochondria

Mitochondria are found in all nucleated human cells. Each of those cells typically contains several hundreds of cytoplasmic mitochondria, which generate most of the cellular energy in the form of ATP. Mitochondria have their characteristic double membrane structure with the outer being smooth and inner being highly folded, forming structures called cristae. The large surface area of the inner mitochondrial membrane accommodate energy-generating multipolypeptide enzyme complexes called respiratory chain or ETC complexes that produce ATP via a process called oxidative phosphorylation (OXPHOS). Mitochondria contain mtDNA, and they are under dual genetic control of both nDNA and mtDNA.

Mitochondrial Genetics

It has been estimated that approximately 1,500 genes are involved in maintaining mitochondrial structure and function. Only 37 are encoded by mtDNA, while the remainder are encoded by nuclear genes. Each mitochondrion contains mtDNA in the form of multicopy, 16.6 kb circular double-stranded DNA. MtDNA encodes 13 essential polypeptides for the ETC complexes and 24 different RNAs, including two rRNAs and 22 tRNAs. The remaining ETC complexes subunits, as well as hundreds of proteins needed to assemble the ETC complexes (assembly factors), maintain mtDNA, and transport molecules across the mitochondrial membranes, are encoded by nDNA, synthesized on cytoplasmic ribosomes, and imported to mitochondria.[1]

Unlike nDNA, which replicates with each cell division, mtDNA replicates continuously and independently of cell division. Two nDNA-encoded enzymes play major roles in mtDNA replication: DNA polymerase gamma and twinkle protein. DNA polymerase gamma is required for mtDNA synthesis as it is the only DNA polymerase in humans that allows for replication and repair of mtDNA. The twinkle protein serves the important function of a DNA helicase that is required for mtDNA replication.[2,3]

Transcription of mtDNA produces a polycistronic precursor RNA that is then processed to produce individual mRNA, tRNA, and rRNA molecules. The nDNA-encoded mitochondrial RNA polymerase and mitochondrial transcriptions factors are needed for the mitochondrial transcription process.[4,5]

The mRNAs for the 13 mtDNA proteins are translated on mitochondrial ribosomes. Mitochondrial tRNAs and rRNAs are required for this process in addition to several nDNA-encoded proteins, including mitochondrial ribosomal proteins and mitochondrial translation factors.[6]

Energy Generation in Mitochondria

Mitochondria produces most of the energy needed by cells via the process of OXPHOS that incorporates five multipolypeptide enzyme complexes. Complexes I, II, III, and IV make up the ETC, whereas complex V is the ATP synthase. Carbohydrates and fatty acids are transported to the mitochondria, where they are metabolized by glycolysis and β-oxidation pathways, respectively. Acetyl-CoA is generated and oxidized via the tricarboxylic acid (TCA) cycle to generate CO_2 and hydrogen atoms. Hydrogen atoms generated from different catabolic pathways bind to nicotinamide adenine dinucleotide (NAD^+) and flavin adenine dinucleotide (FAD) to yield NADH+H and $FADH_2$, respectively. NADH+H is oxidized by complex I (NADH dehydrogenase), and the electrons are transported through flavin mononucleotide and multiple iron-sulfur (Fe-S) centers in complex I until they are transferred to coenzyme Q_{10} (CoQ_{10}). CoQ_{10} also accepts hydrogen atoms from $FADH_2$ generated by β-oxidation and the TCA enzyme succinate dehydrogenase, which is considered complex II in the ETC. Electrons are subsequently transferred from CoQ_{10} to complex III (bc1 complex) within which the electrons move through cytochrome b, cytochrome c1, and the Fe-S components. The electrons are then transferred from complex III to cytochrome c, which transfers the electrons to complex IV (cytochrome c oxidase). Within this complex, the electrons are transferred through copper centers and cytochrome a and a3 and ultimately combine with O_2 to generate H_2O. The energy that is released during electron transfer is used to pump protons from inside the mitochondrial matrix across the inner mitochondrial membrane into the inter-membrane space through complexes I, III, and IV. The resulting electrochemical gradient forces protons to move back through proton channel in complex V (ATP synthase), which utilizes this energy in synthesizing ATP.[7]

The ETC complexes are multipolypeptides encoded by both mtDNA and nDNA except for complex II, which is encoded entirely by nDNA. Complex I is composed of 46 polypeptides, only seven of which are encoded by mtDNA. Complex II is part of the TCA cycle and is composed of four subunits, all of which are encoded by nDNA. Complex III is composed of 11 polypeptides, and only one is encoded by mtDNA. Thirteen polypeptides compose complex IV, three of which are encoded by mtDNA. Finally, complex V is composed of 16 polypeptides, two of which are encoded by mtDNA. In addition to these complexes subunits, a group of nDNA-encoded assembly factors are needed to construct the functional complexes. Defects in either the complex subunits or assembly factors can interfere with the formation of functional complexes and impair mitochondrial energy production.

Mitochondrial Protein Import

The mitochondrion contains 13 mtDNA-encoded and ~1,500 nDNA-encoded polypeptides. The latter are synthesized on cytosolic ribosomes and transported into the mitochondria via mitochondrial protein import systems, including the TOM (translocase of the outer membrane) and TIM (translocase of the inner membrane) complexes.

The proteins that are imported into the mitochondria have amino-terminal mitochondrial targeting sequences that are cleaved during the import process. While in the cytosol, these proteins interact with cytosolic chaperones until they interact with the TOM complexes that recognize the targeting sequences and transport these proteins across the outer mitochondrial membrane. Once proteins are transported across the outer mitochondrial membrane, they can either be inserted into the inner mitochondrial membrane or transported to the mitochondrial matrix via TIM complexes that recognize the targeting sequences and transport these proteins across the inner mitochondrial membrane. Once proteins are in the mitochondrial matrix, the targeting sequences are cleaved off by mitochondrial processing peptides and the proteins are folded by mitochondrial chaperone complexes.[8]

Mitochondrial Dysfunction

Defects in mtDNA- or nDNA-encoded mitochondrial proteins result in mitochondrial dysfunction and impaired energy production. Mitochondrial diseases arise as a result of dysfunctional mitochondria, leading to inadequate ATP production required to meet the energy needs of various organs, particularly those with high energy demands such as the central nervous system, skeletal and cardiac muscles, kidneys, liver, and endocrine systems. Disturbed mitochondrial function in various tissues and organs explains the multiorgan manifestations of mitochondrial diseases such as epilepsy, intellectual disability, skeletal and cardiac myopathy, hepatopathy, diabetes, sensorineural hearing loss, and renal impairment.[9,10]

Mitochondrial disorders are not uncommon. Combing the results of different epidemiological studies on childhood and adult mitochondrial disease suggests that the minimum prevalence of mitochondrial diseases is 1 in 5,000 and could be much higher.[10]

Basic Principles of Mitochondrial Diseases: Inheritance, Heteroplasmy, Segregation, and Threshold Effect

Mitochondrial diseases can be caused by defects of mtDNA or nDNA. Mutations in nDNA genes are inherited in an autosomal recessive, autosomal dominant, or X-linked manner. Defects in mtDNA are inherited maternally due to the fact that the mammalian oocyte contains about 100,000 mitochondria while the sperm contains in the order of 100 mitochondria, which are selectively destroyed and eliminated after fertilization.[11] Although the general role for mtDNA is to be maternally inherited, a patient with mitochondrial myopathy was reported to have a mutation in the mtDNA gene *MT-ND2* that was paternally inherited.[12]

Each human cell contains up to thousands of copies of mtDNA. The term "homoplasmy" means that all the mtDNA copies are identical, whereas "heteroplasmy" indicates the presence of a mixture of two or more types of mtDNA within each cell. Some mutations affect all copies of the mtDNA (homoplasmic mutations), while most of the mutations are present in only some copies of mtDNA and cells harbor a mixture of mutant and normal mtDNA (heteroplasmic mutations).[13]

When a cell harboring a heteroplasmic mtDNA mutation divides, it is a matter of chance whether the mutant mtDNAs will be partitioned into one daughter cell or another. Therefore, over time, the percentage of mutant mtDNAs can differ in different tissues and organs. This process, which is called replicative segregation, explains why the percentage level of mutant mtDNA may vary among patients within the same family and also among organs and tissues within the same individual.[14]

The different tissues and organs rely on mitochondrial energy to different extents. As the percentage of mutated mtDNA increases, energy production declines. When the proportion of mutant mtDNA crosses a critical threshold level, the impaired energy production will result in organ dysfunction and clinical manifestations. The threshold level varies among different organs and tissues depending on their energy requirement. It is suggested that the thresholds of human organs are, in decreasing order, the central nervous system, cardiac and skeletal muscles, renal system, endocrine system, and liver.[15] The replicative segregation and variety of different organ threshold levels can explain in part the varied clinical phenotypes observed in patients with mtDNA mutations.

Clinical Manifestations of Mitochondrial Diseases

Mitochondria are essential components of all nucleated cells. Therefore, mitochondrial dysfunction affects many organs, particularly those with high energy requirements, including the central nervous system, skeletal and cardiac muscles, kidneys, liver, and endocrine systems. Although the vast majority of mitochondrial diseases involve multiple organ systems, some mitochondrial diseases affect a single organ (e.g., Leber hereditary optic neuropathy and nonsyndromic hearing loss). Mitochondrial diseases can begin at any age. Table 8.1 summarizes the most frequent manifestations of mitochondrial diseases at different age groups.[16-24]

Many patients with mitochondrial diseases display a cluster of clinical features that fall into a discrete clinical syndrome such as Kearns-Sayre syndrome (KSS), mitochondrial encephalomyopathy with lactic acidosis and stroke-like episodes (MELAS), myoclonic epilepsy with ragged-red fibers (MERRF), neurogenic weakness with ataxia and retinitis pigmentosa (NARP), or mitochondrial neurogastrointestinal encephalopathy (MNGIE) (Table 8.2).[25,26] However, there is often considerable clinical variability, and many affected individuals do not fit into one particular syndrome.

Categorization of Mitochondrial Diseases

Mitochondrial dysfunction results from defects in either mtDNA or mitochondria-related nDNA genes (Table 8.3).

Mutations in nDNA genes encoding ETC complexes subunits or their assembly factors result in impaired ETC complexes and mitochondrial energy failure. Examples are listed in Table 8.3. Furthermore, the mitochondrial protein import system is encoded by nDNA genes and is essential to import nDNA-encoded mitochondrial proteins into the mitochondria. Defective import of mitochondrial proteins can arise from mutations in the targeting signals within precursor proteins, from mutations that disrupt components of the mitochondrial import complexes, or from deficiencies in the chaperones involved in the proper folding of proteins once they are imported. Errors in these events can result in a protein not reaching its final destination, ultimately leading to mitochondrial dysfunction and energy failure. Examples are listed in Table 8.3. Defect in mitochondrial protein translation is another mechanism of mitochondrial dysfunction. Several nDNA-encoded proteins, including mitochondrial ribosomal proteins and mitochondrial translational factors, are required for this process. Therefore, defects of these proteins result in impaired

TABLE 8.1 Common Features of Mitochondrial Diseases

Fetal Period
- Intrauterine growth restriction
- Polyhydraminos or oligohydraminos
- Arthrogryposis
- Hypertrophic cardiomyopathy
- Hydrops fetalis

Neonatal Period
- Central nervous system
  - Apnea
  - Lethargy and coma
  - Epilepsy
  - Peripheral and truncal hypotonia
  - Spasticity
- Cardiac and skeletal muscle
  - Skeletal myopathy (weakness, hypotonia, atrophy)
  - Hypertrophic cardiomyopathy
- Renal system
  - Tubulopathy
- Liver
  - Hepatomegaly
  - Hepatic dysfunction
  - Hepatic failure
- Metabolic derangements
  - Lactic acidosis
  - Hypoglycemia
- Hematologic
  - Anemia
  - Neutropenia
  - Pancytopenia

Infancy
- Central nervous system
  - Apnea
  - Truncal hypotonia
  - Spasticity
  - Stroke-like episodes
  - Epilepsy
  - Encephalopathy and leukodystrophy
  - Developmental delay and psychomotor regression
  - Ataxia
  - Sensorineural hearing loss
  - Optic atrophy
  - Ophthalmoplegia
  - Pigmentary retinopathy
  - Ptosis
  - Cataract
- Cardiac and skeletal muscles
  - Cardiomyopathy (hypertrophic, dilated, and left ventricular noncompaction)
  - Skeletal myopathy (weakness, hypotonia, atrophy)
- Renal system
  - Tubulopathy
  - Nephrotic syndrome
  - Renal impairment
  - Renal failure
- Liver
  - Hepatomegaly
  - Hepatic dysfunction
  - Hepatic failure
- Gastrointestinal system
  - Recurrent vomiting
  - Chronic diarrhea
  - Villous atrophy
  - Exocrine pancreatic insufficiency
  - Intestinal pseudo-obstruction

(continued)

TABLE 8.1 **Continued**

Infancy (*cont.*)
- Metabolic derangements
  - Lactic acidosis
  - Hypoglycemia
- Growth
  - Failure to thrive
  - Short stature
- Hematologic
  - Anemia
  - Neutropenia
  - Pancytopenia

Childhood
- Central nervous system
  - Epilepsy
  - Intellectual disability
  - Ataxia
  - Spasticity
  - Dystonia
  - Stroke-like episodes
  - Leukodystrophy
  - Cortical atrophy
  - Cerebellar atrophy
  - Ophthalmoplegia
  - Optic atrophy
  - Ptosis
  - Pigmentary retinopathy
  - Sensorineural hearing loss
- Cardiac and skeletal muscles
  - Myopathy
  - Cardiomyopathy
  - Arrhythmia
- Renal system
  - Tubulopathy
- Endocrine
  - Growth hormone deficiency
  - Diabetes mellitus
  - Hypothyroidism
  - Hypoparathyroidism
  - Adrenal insufficiency
- Respiratory
  - Hypoventilation
  - Apnea
- Liver
  - Hepatic dysfunction
  - Hepatic failure
- Gastrointestinal system
  - Vomiting
  - Dysphagia
  - Failure to thrive
- Metabolic derangements
  - Lactic acidosis
- Growth
  - Failure to thrive
- Hematologic
  - Anemia
  - Pancytopenia

Adulthood
- Central nervous system
  - Migraine
  - Strokes-like episodes
  - Epilepsy
  - Dementia
  - Ataxia
  - Peripheral neuropathy
  - Ophthalmoplegia
  - Optic atrophy

(*continued*)

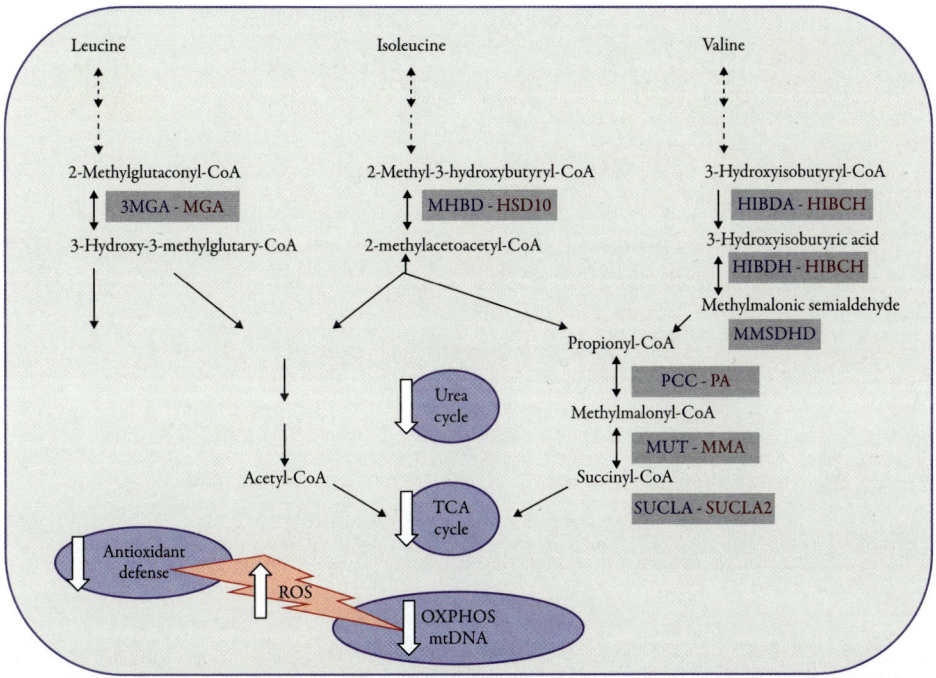

FIGURE 4.3 **Secondary Mitochondrial Dysfunction is Associated with Enzymatic Defects in the Terminal Steps of Branched Chain Amino Acid Metabolism.** Dysfunction of the urea or Krebs cycle and the oxidative phosphorylation or mtDNA maintenance, as well as increased reactive oxygen species (ROS) formation with depletion of antioxidant pools (glutathione), have been observed in disorders caused by defects in distant steps of BCAA metabolic pathways.

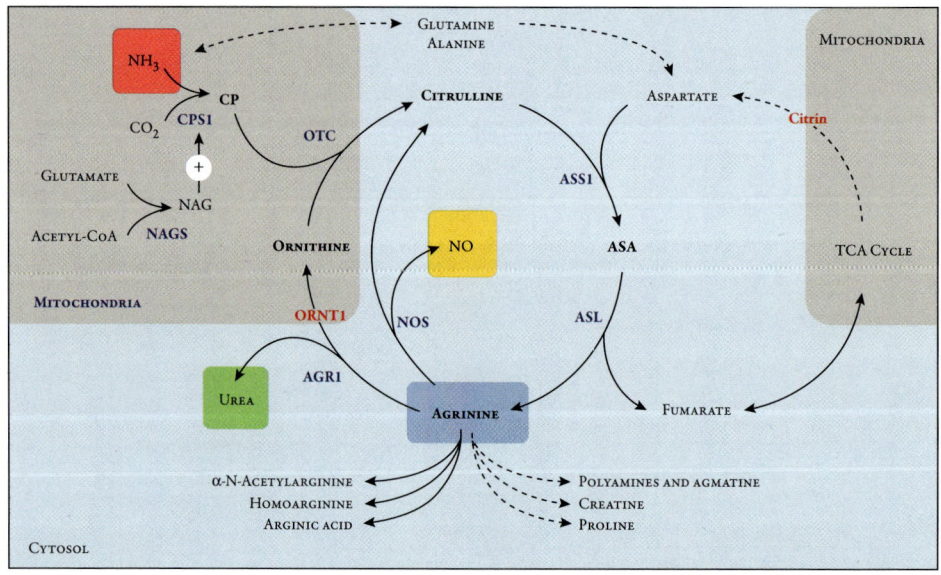

FIGURE 6.1 Urea Cycle and Its Nitrogen Exchange with Other Pathways. *Abbreviations:* ASA = argininosuccinic acid; ASL = argininosuccinate lyase; ASS1 = argininosuccinate synthase 1; ARG1 = arginase 1; CP = carbamoyl phosphate; CPS1 = carbamoyl-phosphate synthase 1; NAG = N-acetylglutamate; NAGS = N-acetylglutamate synthase; NO = nitric oxide; NOS = nitric oxide synthase; OTC = ornithine transcarbamylase; ORNT1 = ornithine transporter 1; TCA cycle = tricarboxylic acid cycle.

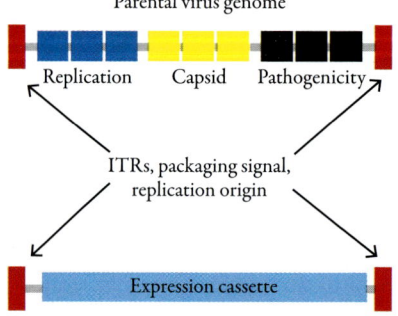

FIGURE 13.1 Schematic of a viral genome containing genes involved in replication, virion structure (capsid), and pathogenicity. The viral genome is flanked by cis-acting sequences providing the viral origin of replication and the packaging signal. Minimally, gene therapy vectors contain the essential *cis*-acting elements and the expression cassette with the transcriptional regulatory elements replacing the viral coding sequences. *Abbreviations: ITRs= inverted terminal repeats.*

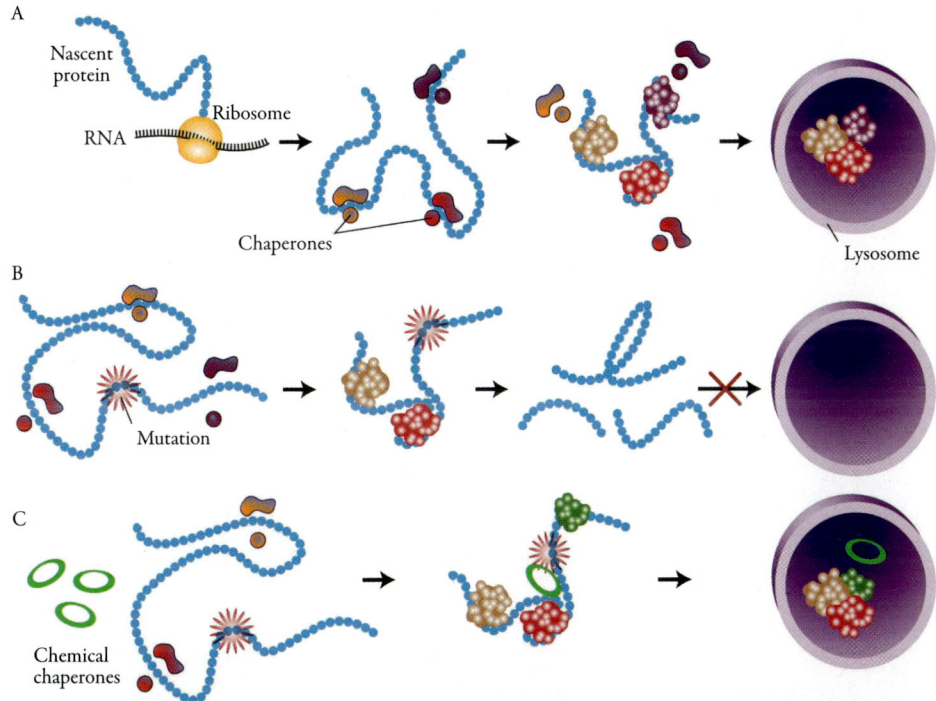

FIGURE 15.1 (A) Wild type enzyme: The normal protein folding process is shown. The enzyme is synthesized and folded with the assistance of cellular chaperones. After post-synthesis modification, the folded enzyme is transported into the lysosome. (B) Mutant enzyme: The mutant enzyme is synthesized but cannot fold properly due to the mutation. The protein is subsequently degraded or aggregates into an aberrant protein; the enzyme is not transported to the lysosome. (C) Mutant enzyme corrected with a pharmacologic chaperone: As in (B), the mutant enzyme is synthesized but cannot fold properly. However, the pharmacological chaperone binds to the active site of the misfolded enzyme, preventing its premature degradation and facilitating its trafficking into the lysosome.

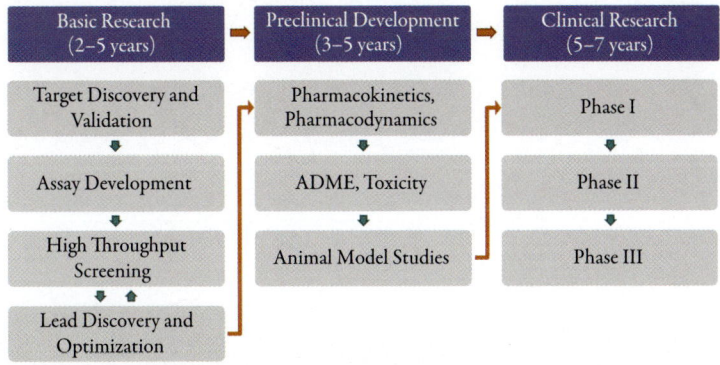

FIGURE 15.2 Timeline of drug discovery and development.

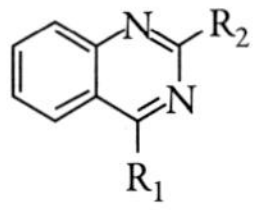

Compound number	R1	R2	AC$_{50}$ (µM)
1	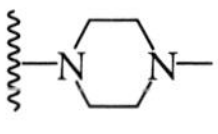 -N(piperazine)N-CH$_3$	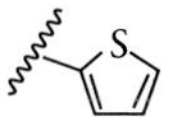 thiophene	Inactive
2	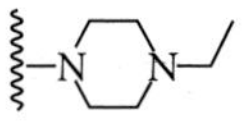 -N(piperazine)N-ethyl	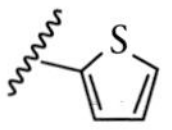 thiophene	Inactive
3	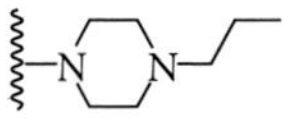 -N(piperazine)N-propyl	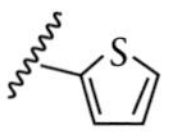 thiophene	Inactive
4	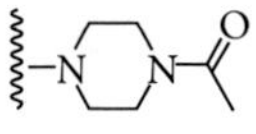 -N(piperazine)N-C(=O)CH$_3$	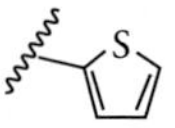 thiophene	79.97
5	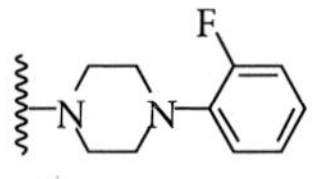 -N(piperazine)N-(2-fluorophenyl)	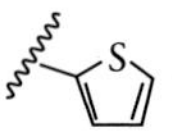 thiophene	63.52
6	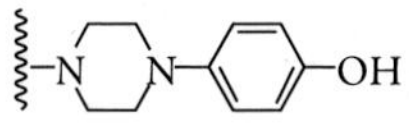 -N(piperazine)N-(4-hydroxyphenyl)	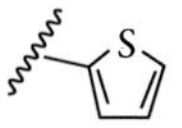 thiophene	63.52
7	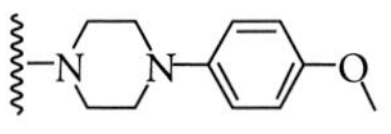 -N(piperazine)N-(4-methoxyphenyl)	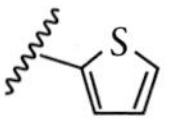 thiophene	79.97

FIGURE 15.3 An example of structure-activity relationship (SAR) of a pharmacological chaperone. The different R1 and R2 groups result in chemicals with differing AC50 values.

TABLE 8.1 **Continued**

Adulthood (*cont.*)
- Ptosis
- Pigmentary retinopathy
- Cataracts
- Sensorineural hearing loss
- Cardiac and skeletal muscles
  - Skeletal myopathy
  - Myalgia
  - Exercise intolerance
  - Recurrent myoglubinuria
  - Cardiomyopathy and heart failure
  - Heart block
- Endocrine
  - Diabetes mellitus
  - Hypothyroidism
  - Hypoparathyroidism
  - Ovarian failure
- Respiratory
  - Respiratory failure
  - Nocturnal hypoventilation
  - Aspiration pneumonia
- Gastrointestinal system
  - Constipation
  - Dysphagia
  - Irritable bowel

mtDNA-encoded protein synthesis and mitochondrial dysfunction. Examples are listed in Table 8.3.[8,27,28]

The mtDNA is maintained by a group of nDNA-encoded proteins that function either in mitochondrial deoxyribonucleoside triphosphate (dNTP) synthesis or mtDNA replication. Mutations in any of these genes result in depletion of the mitochondrial dNTP pool or impaired mtDNA replication, leading to severe reduction in mtDNA content (mtDNA depletion) in affected tissues and organs. An adequate amount of mtDNA is required for the production of key subunits of ETC complexes and energy production. Therefore, mtDNA depletion results in organ dysfunction that is due to insufficient synthesis of ETC components needed for adequate energy production. Examples are listed in Table 8.3.[29]

CoQ_{10} is an essential component of the ETC and is synthesized *de novo* in human cells *via* a group of nDNA-encoded enzymes. Mutations in genes involved in CoQ_{10} biosynthesis result in primary CoQ_{10} deficiency leading to impaired ETC activity and mitochondrial dysfunction. Examples are listed in Table 8.3.[30,31]

Fe-S clusters are ubiquitous cofactors composed of iron and inorganic sulfur. These clusters are important prosthetic groups that are required for the function of proteins involved in a wide range of activities, including electron transport in ETC complexes. Fe-S clusters are incorporated into the TCA enzymes aconitase and succinate dehydrogenase (ETC complex II), and into ETC complexes I and III. Defects in the process of Fe-S clusters can result in impaired ETC activity and mitochondrial diseases. Fe-S clusters biosynthesis defects can also result in the impairment of lipoic acid synthase, which is involved in lipoic

TABLE 8.2 Common Syndromes of Mitochondrial Diseases

Myoclonic Epilepsy With Ragged-Red Fibers (MERRF)
- Myoclonus
- Epilepsy
- Ataxia
- Dementia
- Myopathy
- Peripheral neuropathy
- Spasticity
- Optic atrophy
- Sensorineural deafness
- Cardiomyopathy
- Pigmentary retinopathy
- Lipomatosis

Leigh Syndrome
- Motor and intellectual developmental delay or regression
- Brain stem symptoms (apnea, swallowing difficulty, and thermoregulation dysfunction).
- Basal ganglia symptoms (dystonia, chorea)
- Bilateral symmetric signal abnormality in the brain stem and/or basal ganglia in neuroimaging
- Raised lactate in blood and cerebrospinal fluid (CSF)
- Hypotonia
- Spasticity
- Ataxia
- Peripheral neuropathy
- Hypertrophic cardiomyopathy
- Hepatomegaly or liver failure
- Renal tubulopathy or diffuse glomerulocystic kidney damage

Neurogenic Weakness With Ataxia and Retinitis Pigmentosa (NARP)
- Peripheral motor and sensory neuropathy
- Ataxia
- Pigmentary retinopathy
- Epilepsy
- Intellectual disability
- Cerebral and cerebellar atrophy in neuroimmaging

Mitochondrial Encephalomyopathy With Lactic Acidosis and Stroke-Like Episodes (MELAS)
- Stroke-like episodes
- Epilepsy
- Intellectual disability/dementia
- Ragged-red fibers
- Lactic acidosis
- Diabetes mellitus
- Cardiomyopathy
- Sensorineural hearing loss
- Ataxia
- Migraine

Kearns-Sayre Syndrome (KSS)
- Ophthalmoplegia
- Pigmentary retinopathy
- Ataxia
- Heart block
- Sensorineural hearing loss
- Myopathy
- Dysphagia
- Diabetes mellitus
- Hypoparathyroidism
- Dementia
- Increased CSF protein

Pearson Syndrome
- Sideroblastic anemia of childhood
- Pancytopenia
- Exocrine pancreatic failure
- Renal tubular defects

(*continued*)

TABLE 8.2 **Continued**

Alpers-Huttenlocher Syndrome
- Developmental delay and regression
- Epilepsy
- Myoclonus
- Hypotonia
- Choreoathetosis
- Nystagmus
- Neuropathy and ataxia
- Hepatic dysfunction or failure
- Renal tubulopathy

Chronic Progressive External Ophthalmoplegia (CPEO)
- External ophthalmoplegia
- Bilateral ptosis
- Mild proximal myopathy

Leber Hereditary Optic Neuropathy (LHON)
- Visual loss, optic atrophy
- Dystonia
- Peripheral neuropathy

acid synthesis and requires the function of Fe-S clusters. Lipoic acid is an essential prosthetic group of four mitochondrial enzymes involved in the oxidative decarboxylation of pyruvate, α-ketoglutarate, and branched chain amino acids and in the glycine cleavage. Biosynthetic defects of Fe-S clusters or lipoic acid synthase can result in lipoic acid deficiency, leading to the impairment of lipoic acid-dependent enzymes.[32–34] Recently, mutations in the *SERAC1* gene were found to be the cause of MEGDEL syndrome (3-methylglutaconic aciduria with deafness, encephalopathy, and Leigh-like syndrome). SERAC1 is key player in the phosphatidylglycerol remodeling that is essential for mitochondrial function.[35]

MtDNA defects can be either point mutations or rearrangements. Point mutations in mtDNA can affect protein-encoding genes or genes encoding tRNA or rRNA. These mutations are maternally inherited, typically heteroplasmic, and associated with very variable phenotypes. Rearrangements of mtDNA include deletions and duplications that differ in size and position but typically encompass several genes. These rearrangements are usually heteroplasmic and sporadic arising *de novo* but can be maternally inherited. Examples are listed in Table 8.3. Occasionally, mtDNA rearrangement can result from mutations in nDNA-encoded proteins that function in mtDNA replication, including *POLG* and *C10orf2*.[36]

Mechanisms of Mitochondrial Diseases

A central function of mitochondria is the production of the cellular energy currency ATP through OXPHOS, which is carried out by the ETC complexes in the inner mitochondrial membrane. Apart from energy production, mitochondria take part in a number of other processes, including heme and steroid hormone biosynthesis, calcium homeostasis, and apoptosis. Mitochondrial diseases occur where one or more of the ETC complexes are defective, resulting in OXPHOS dysfunction and ATP production impairment.

TABLE 8.3 Categorization of Mitochondrial Disorders According to Genetic Defect

A. Mitochondrial Diseases due to nDNA Defects

1. **Mutations in subunits of ETC complexes**
   a. Mitochondrial complex I deficiency due to mutations in nDNA-encoded subunit genes (*NDUFV1, NDUFV2, NDUFS1, NDUFS2, NDUFS3, NDUFS4, NDUFS6, NDUFS7, NDUFS8, NDUFA2, NDUFA11, NDUFAF3, NDUFA10, and NDUFB3*)
   b. Mitochondrial complex II deficiency due to mutations in a nDNA-encoded subunit gene (*SDHA*)
   c. Mitochondrial complex III deficiency due to mutations in nDNA-encoded subunit genes (*TTC19, UQCRB, UQCRQ, UQCRC2*).
   d. Mitochondrial complex IV deficiency due to mutations in a nDNA-encoded subunit gene (*COX6B1*)

2. **Mutations in assembly factors of ETC complexes**
   a. Mitochondrial complex I deficiency due to mutations in nDNA-encoded assembly factor genes (*NDUFAF1, NDUFAF2, NDUFAF4, NDUFAF5, and NUBPL*).
   b. Mitochondrial complex II deficiency due to mutations in a nDNA-encoded assembly factor gene (*SDHAF1*)
   c. Mitochondrial complex III deficiency due to mutations in a nDNA-encoded assembly factor gene (*BCS1L*).
   d. Mitochondrial complex IV deficiency due to mutations in nDNA-encoded assembly factor genes (*SCO1, SCO2, COA5, COX10, COX15, and SURF1*)

3. **Defects in the mitochondrial import**
   a. Deafness-dystonia (Mohr-Tranebjaerg) syndrome (*TIMM8A* encodes a component of the translocase of inner mitochondrial membrane complex)
   b. Dilated cardiomyopathy with ataxia (*DNAJC19* encodes a component of the translocase of inner mitochondrial membrane complex)
   c. Spastic paraplegia 13 (*HSPD1* encodes a mitochondrial chaperone)

4. **Defect in mitochondrial translation**
   a. Combined oxidative phosphorylation deficiency 1 (*GFM1* encodes a mitochondrial translation elongation factor)
   b. Combined oxidative phosphorylation deficiency 2 (*MRPS16* encodes a mitochondrial ribosomal protein)
   c. Combined oxidative phosphorylation deficiency 3 (*TSFM* encodes a mitochondrial translation elongation factor)
   d. Combined oxidative phosphorylation deficiency 4 (*TUFM* encodes a mitochondrial translation elongation factor)
   e. Combined oxidative phosphorylation deficiency 5 (*MRPS22* encodes a mitochondrial ribosomal protein)

5. **Defect in mtDNA maintenance (mtDNA depletion syndromes)**
   a. Myopathic mtDNA depletion syndrome (*TK2* functions in maintaining mitochondrial dNTP pool; and *MGME1* encodes a mitochondrial exonuclease that is essential for mtDNA maintenance)
   b. Encephalomyopathic mtDNA depletion syndromes (*SUCLA2, SUCLG1*, and *RRM2B* all function in maintaining mitochondrial dNTP pool; and *FBXL4* which functions in controlling bioenergetic homeostasis and mtDNA maintenance)
   c. Hepatocerebral mtDNA depletion syndromes (*DGUOK* functions in maintaining mitochondrial dNTP pool; *POLG* and *C10orf2* both function in mtDNA replication; and *MPV17*)
   d. Neurogastrointestinal mtDNA depletion syndromes (*TYMP* functions in maintaining mitochondrial dNTP pool)
   e. Cardiomyopathic mtDNA depletion syndrome (*SLC25A4* encodes the mitochondrial adenine nucleotide translocator)

6. **Primary coenzyme Q_{10} deficiency**
   a. Primary CoQ_{10} deficiency 1 (*COQ2* encodes parahydroxybenzoid-polyprenyltransferase which is one CoQ_{10} biosynthetic enzymes).
   b. Primary CoQ_{10} deficiency 2 (*PDSS1* encodes a subunit of prenyldiphosphate synthase which is one CoQ_{10} biosynthetic enzymes).
   c. Primary CoQ_{10} deficiency 3 (*PDSS2* encodes a subunit of prenyldiphosphate synthase which is one CoQ_{10} biosynthetic enzymes).
   d. Primary CoQ_{10} deficiency 4 (*ADCK3* encodes the yeast homolog of COQ8 which is involved in CoQ_{10} biosynthesis).
   e. Primary CoQ_{10} deficiency 5 (*COQ9* encodes COQ10 which is involved in CoQ_{10} biosynthesis).
   f. Primary CoQ_{10} deficiency 6 (*COQ6* encodes coenzyme Q6 monooxygenase which is one CoQ_{10} biosynthetic enzymes).

7. **Other metabolic defects affecting mitochondrial function**
   a. Friedreich ataxia (*FXN* encodes Frataxin which is an iron chaperone involved in Fe-S biogenesis)
   b. Pyridoxine-refractory sideroblastic anemia (*GLRX5* encodes a glutaredoxin that might act as an intermediate scaffold in Fe-S biogenesis)
   c. Myopathy with lactic acidosis (*ISCU* encodes iron-sulfur cluster assembly enzyme that is a scaffold protein functioning in assembly of Fe-S for aconitase and SDH).
   d. Mitochondrial complex I deficiency (*NUBPL* encodes a protein that is responsible for transfer of Fe-S cluster to complex I).
   e. Multiple mitochondrial dysfunctions syndrome 1 (*NFU1* encodes a protein responsible for delivering Fe-S cluster to lipoic acid synthase)
   f. Multiple mitochondrial dysfunctions syndrome 2 (*BOLA3* encodes a protein that plays an essential role in Fe-S cluster biogenesis)
   g. Lipoic acid synthetase deficiency (*LIAS* encodes lipoic acid synthetase).
   h. Phosphatidylglycerol remodeling defects (*SERAC1* functions in transacylation reaction)

(continued)

TABLE 8.3 **Continued**

B. Mitochondrial Diseases due to mtDNA Defects

1. **Rearrangement (deletions and duplications)**
   a. Kearns-Sayre Syndrome
   b. Pearson Syndrome
   c. Progressive external ophthalmoplegia
2. **Point mutations in protein encoding genes**
   a. Leber hereditary optic neuropathy (*MTND1, MTND4, and MTND6*)
   b. Leigh syndrome (*MTATP6, MTTL1, MTTK, MTTW, MTTV, MTND1, MTND2, MTND3, MTND4, MTND5, MTND6, and MTCO3*)
   c. NARP (*MTATP6*)
3. **Point mutations in tRNA genes**
   a. MELAS syndrome (*MTTL1*)
   b. MERRF syndrome (*MTTK*)
   c. Mitochondrial encephalopathy (*MTTL2*)
   d. Familial hypertrophic cardiomyopathy (*MTTI*)
   e. Nonsyndromic sensorineural hearing loss (*MTTS1*)
4. **Point mutations in rRNA genes**
   a. Aminoglycoside-induced nonsyndromic hearing loss (*MTRNR1*)
   b. Nonsyndromic sensorineural hearing loss (*MTRNR1*)

Note. ETC = electron transport chain; MELAS = mitochondrial encephalomyopathy with lactic acidosis and stroke-like episodes; MERRF = myoclonic epilepsy with ragged-red fibers.

OXPHOS dysfunction can result from (a) structural defects in ETC complexes due to mutations in mtDNA or nDNA genes encoding ETC complexes subunits, (b) defects in the assembly factors that are encoded by nDNA and required for the assembly of functional ETC complexes, (c) defects in mtDNA maintenance that are nDNA encoded and function in mitochondrial dNTP synthesis and mtDNA replication, (d) disordered mitochondrial protein synthesis resulting from defects in nDNA-encoded mitochondrial translation factors and ribosomal proteins, and mitochondrial tRNA and rRNA mutations and mtDNA deletions, (e) defective mitochondrial import, and (f) Fe-S clusters and CoQ_{10} deficiencies (see Table 8.3).

In addition to deficiency of ATP, consequences of OXPHOS impairment include calcium handling dysfunction, metabolite buildup, and reactive oxygen species (ROS) production, all of which contribute to the pathogenesis of mitochondrial diseases.[37]

ATP deficiency is a major consequence of OXPHOS impairment. Decreased ATP production can result in ATP deficiency, leading to cellular dysfunction in mitochondrial disorders. However, energy deficiency is not the sole underlying factor in mitochondrial diseases. An aberrant calcium signaling can also lead to cell dysfunction in mitochondrial disease. One of the mitochondrial functions is calcium buffering; in addition, mitochondrial ATP production is needed to fuel calcium pumps in the endoplasmic reticulum. Therefore, OXPHOS impairment can result in aberrant calcium handling.[38] This model could contribute to the frequent involvement of muscle and nerve tissues in mitochondrial diseases, since these cells rely heavily on ATP and on fluctuating levels of intracellular calcium.[37]

Mitochondria produce ROS as a side product of OXPHOS. These compounds can irreversibly modify many cellular macromolecules; therefore, they are considered toxic for cells. ROS are detoxified by various systems, including the glutathione system, which provides the main protection against oxidative damage. Increased ROS production in mitochondrial diseases can result in the depletion of intracellular antioxidant stores, including glutathione, which was found to be low in blood samples of patients with mitochondrial diseases.[39] Depletion of antioxidant stores leads to the accumulation of ROS, resulting in protein, lipid, and DNA damage. Furthermore, ROS can further inhibit respiratory chain function, thus initiating a vicious cycle that ultimately increases the chances of accumulation of new mutations in mtDNA.[39,40]

Mitochondria are also a major regulator of apoptosis. In response to several intracellular stress conditions, apoptosis is initiated when the inner mitochondrial membrane loses its integrity and becomes permeable, leading to the release of several toxic mitochondrial proteins into the cytosol, including cytochrome c. These proteins activate latent forms of caspases, resulting in the execution of apoptosis.[41] Excessive ROS production in mitochondrial diseases can act as stressor that initiates apoptosis, leading to cell death and contributing to the pathogenesis of mitochondrial diseases.

Another consequence of OXPHOS dysfunction is that NADH produced by the TCA cycle cannot be utilized, leading to elevation of the NADH:NAD ratio, which results in the inhibition of the TCA cycle. Pyruvate, produced through glycolysis, is increased due to the TCA cycle inhibition. Both elevated pyruvate and NADH:NAD ratio can result in shifting the equilibrium of lactate dehydrogenase toward the production of lactate from pyruvate. Lactate can accumulate, causing systemic acidosis. Lactic acidosis is one of the most common biochemical features of mitochondrial disorders.[9]

Energy depletion due to mitochondrial dysfunction can explain the multiorgan manifestations of mitochondrial disease, including myopathy, epilepsy, and diabetes. In addition to reduced energy production, there is growing evidence that nitric oxide (NO) deficiency occurs in mitochondrial diseases and can play a major role in the pathogenesis of several complications observed in mitochondrial diseases, including stroke-like episodes, myopathy, diabetes, and lactic acidosis.[42-45] NO deficiency in mitochondrial disorders is believed to be multifactorial in origin, including impaired NO production and postproduction sequestration. Impaired NO production can result from endothelial dysfunction, decreased availability of NO precursors arginine and citrulline, and impaired NO synthase activity. NO deficiency in mitochondrial diseases can also result from postproduction NO sequestration by increased cytochrome c oxidase and shunting NO into reactive nitrogen species formation.[45]

Diagnosis of Mitochondrial Diseases

The diagnosis of mitochondrial diseases remains challenging in many cases. The difficulties in recognizing and diagnosing mitochondrial diseases can be due to:

1. The multiorgan involvement of mitochondrial diseases that are nonspecific and can be mimicked by other genetic diseases.
2. The different mode of inheritance in mitochondrial disease.
3. The heteroplasmy of mtDNA defects that can lead to failure in detecting the abnormality if an unaffected tissue was tested.

4. The fact that the majority of mitochondrial-related nDNA genes are yet to be discovered and clinical testing is available for only a small proportion of these genes.

The diagnosis of mitochondrial disorders is based on clinical recognition, biochemical screening, assessment of the extent of multiorgan involvement, histopathological studies, ETC activity assays, measurement of mtDNA content, and molecular genetic testing.

Clinical Recognition of Mitochondrial Disorders

Although there is no consensus on clinical criteria for when to suspect mitochondrial diseases, evaluation of mitochondrial diseases is suggested to be initiated in the following clinical situations[22,46]:

1. Family history consistent with maternal inheritance
2. Multiorgan involvement
3. Complex neurologic picture or specific combination of neurological symptoms (e.g., epilepsy and ataxia)
4. Presence of characteristic clinical features (e.g., biventricular cardiac hypertrophy)
5. Clinical manifestations consistent with a recognizable phenotype (e.g., MELAS syndrome)

If the clinical features are consistent with a recognizable syndrome, molecular testing by sequencing the suspected mtDNA or nDNA gene need to be performed to confirm the diagnosis. If one organ is involved or the clinical picture is not consistent with a specific syndrome, further evaluation is needed, as explained in the following sections.

Biochemical Screening Tests

Screening tests for mitochondrial disorders include the determination of plasma lactate, blood glucose, urine organic acids, and plasma amino acids. Lactic acidemia results from an inability of dysfunctional mitochondria to generate sufficient ATP, leading to shifting to anaerobic glycolysis and increased lactate production. Although lactic acidemia is a common feature of many mitochondrial disorders, it is neither specific nor sensitive. Lactate level can be normal in some mitochondrial disorders. On the other hand, elevated lactate can be seen in conditions associated with hypoperfusion. Other technical factors can also affect lactate level measurements, including difficulties with specimen collection, improper specimen handling, and delays in plasma separation and sample processing that may lead to spurious elevations of lactate.[47]

Hypoglycemia can be seen in patients with mtDNA depletion syndrome and can be measured during the screening process. Urine organic acid analysis can show nonspecific findings, including elevated lactate, ketone bodies, and TCA intermediates. Furthermore, urine organic acids analysis consistently shows elevated methylmalonic acid in *SUCLA2* and *SUCLG1*-related encephalomyopathic mtDNA depletion syndromes.[29] A plasma amino acid profile may show alterations suggestive of mitochondrial diseases; an elevated plasma alanine level can be a reflection of lactic acidemia. The metabolism of branched-chain amino acids takes place in mitochondria via the branched-chain ketoacid dehydrogenase complex.[48] Elevated branched-chain amino acids may reflect another aspect of mitochondrial dysfunction. The glycine cleavage system is a lipoic acid-dependent enzyme; therefore, glycine elevation can be observed in lipoic acid deficiency.[34]

Recent molecular studies have found that serum fibroblast growth factor 21 (FGF21) is increased in the serum of patients with mitochondrial myopathy. Therefore, FGF21 may have the potential to be a sensitive and specific biomarker for this group of mitochondrial diseases.[49]

Assessment of Multiorgan Involvement Extent

Due to the multiorgan nature of the majority of mitochondrial diseases, evaluation of these diseases should include a systematic screening for all the targeted organs.

For central nervous system involvement, a computerized tomography (CT scan) of the head may show basal ganglia calcification and diffuse brain atrophy. Brain magnetic resonance imaging (MRI) can show leukodystrophy, signal intensity changes in cerebrum and cerebellum, basal ganglia and brain stem lesions, and focal atrophy of cortex or cerebellum.[50] Magnetic resonance spectroscopy (MRS) can show increased lactate in basal ganglia. An electroencephalogram (EEG) is needed when epilepsy is suspected. The assessment of the peripheral nervous system can include nerve conduction velocity (NCV) studies to assess peripheral neuropathy. Hearing assessment and ophthalmologic examination are needed to evaluate for hearing loss and optic atrophy and retinal degeneration, respectively.

An echocardiogram should be performed to screen for cardiomyopathy and assess the cardiac function. An electrocardiogram (ECG) is needed to evaluate for heart block when suspected. Skeletal muscle involvement can be assessed by measuring serum creatinine phosphokinase (CPK) levels and performing an electromyogram (EMG), which can show myopathic changes.

Measuring blood urea nitrogen and creatinine is necessary to assess renal function. Urine analysis may show proteinuria. To screen for renal tubular dysfunction, measuring urine amino acids and electrolytes is needed. Serum transaminases, bilirubin, albumin, and coagulation profile screenings are needed to assess liver dysfunction. Hematological system involvement can be assessed by doing a complete blood count to screen for anemia, thrombocytopenia, and neutropenia. A growth hormone stimulation test can be performed, and thyroid function tests, and parathyroid hormone can be measured to evaluate for endocrine involvement.

Histopathology

The histology of affected muscles typically shows ragged red fibers, which can be demonstrated using the modified Gomori tricrome stains and contains peripheral and intermyofibrillar accumulation of abnormal mitochondria. Although ragged red fibers are considered a histological hallmark of mitochondrial myopathy, their absence does not rule out the diagnosis of mitochondrial disease. Examining the muscle under an electron microscopy can demonstrate mitochondrial proliferation and abnormal mitochondrial morphology in mitochondrial myopathies. Histochemical staining for different ETC complexes can be used to estimate the severity and heterogeneity of ETC complex deficiencies in the muscle tissue.[24]

Assessment of Electron Transport Chain Activity

The enzymatic activity of different ETC complexes can be assessed using a spectrophotometric methodology that consists of measuring the ETC complexes enzymatic activities separately or in groups using specific electron acceptors and donors. This assessment is usually carried out on skeletal muscle, skin fibroblast, or liver tissue. While interpreting the ETC activity results, it is important to keep in mind that a normal ETC activity does not preclude mitochondrial dysfunction even when the tissue tested clinically expresses the disease. Heteroplasmy can provide one explanation for that. On the other hand, ETC activity can be impaired in other conditions, including other inborn errors of metabolisms (e.g., propionic acidemia and fatty acid oxidation defects) and chromosomal abnormalities (e.g., 1p36 deletion).[7]

Mitochondrial ETC activity can also be assessed by the more recently developed methodology using extracellular flux analyzers, which can simultaneously measure the two major energy-producing pathways of the cell (mitochondrial respiration and glycolysis) in a microplate, in real time. Determining the rate of oxygen consumption, which is a measure of mitochondrial respiration, and rate of extracellular acidification, which is measure of glycolysis, can provide data that can identify mitochondrial dysfunction.[51-53]

Measurement of mtDNA Content

Alteration in mtDNA copy number is an indication of mitochondrial disorder. Increased mtDNA content suggests a compensatory mechanism due to deficient mitochondrial function, while reduced mtDNA content implies defects in mtDNA biosynthesis, leading to mtDNA depletion syndromes. Measurement of mtDNA copy number is performed by real-time quantitative polymerase chain reaction using an mtDNA probe and a unique nuclear gene reference. The copy number ratio of mtDNA/nDNA is a measure of mtDNA content. Measurement of mtDNA content in an affected tissue may assist with narrowing the cause of the disease to a group of nuclear genes for sequence analysis. Therefore, assessment of mtDNA copy number in affected tissues such as muscle and liver is a screening method for the identification of mtDNA depletion syndromes or mtDNA compensatory overamplification.[54-56]

Molecular Testing

If the clinical features of a mitochondrial disease are consistent with a recognizable syndrome, the mtDNA or nDNA gene known to be responsible for that syndrome can be tested to confirm the diagnosis. For example, one might test for the m.3243 A>G mutation in a patient with stroke-like episodes, lactic acidosis, and myopathy who is suspected to have MELAS syndrome.

If a maternally inherited mitochondrial disease is suspected in a patient with clinical features that do not fit with a recognizable syndrome, whole mtDNA sequencing can be performed. This test is available clinically.

The newly developed next-generation massively parallel sequencing allows simultaneous sequencing of multiple genes at high coverage and low cost.[57] Next-generation sequencing has allowed the development of panel tests that include several related genes and can be used in situations where the patient is suspected to have a genetically heterogeneous mitochondrial disease (e.g., Leigh disease). Panels can also be helpful in cases where there is a specific ETC complex deficiency (e.g., a panel includes complex IV subunits and assembly factors for patients with complex IV deficiency) or evidence of mtDNA depletion (e.g., a panel includes the known genes associated with mtDNA depletion for patients with mtDNA depletion syndromes). Several panels are available for clinical testing.

In many situations, neither the clinical manifestations nor the biochemical testing offers enough information to help direct the investigation toward a specific gene or a group of genes. In such a situation, if the suspicion of a mitochondrial diseases remains high, a more extensive panel that includes all the known mitochondrial genes can be considered. Currently, fewer than 200 nDNA genes have been found to play a role in mitochondrial structure and function. Clinical testing, including sequencing the mtDNA and all the known mitochondrial-related nDNA genes, is currently available for clinical testing. However, it has been estimated that ~1,500 genes are involved in maintaining mitochondrial structure and function; therefore, the larger portion of mitochondrial-related nDNA genes are not yet discovered. Sequencing the whole exome or genome using next-generation sequencing methodology can be considered in cases where all the previous testing has failed to define the diagnosis molecularly.

Therapeutic Options for Mitochondrial Diseases

Currently, there are no satisfactory therapies available for mitochondrial disorders. Treatment remains largely symptomatic and does not significantly alter the course of the disease. Treatment for mitochondrial disorders includes symptomatic treatment, cofactor supplementations, NO donors, and exercise.

Symptomatic Treatment

Treatment for mitochondrial disorders remains largely symptomatic. Examples of symptomatic treatment includes physical therapy for hypotonia and motor delays; hearing aids or cochlear implant for hearing loss; slow infusion of sodium bicarbonate during acute exacerbation of lactic acidosis; pancreatic enzymes for exocrine pancreatic dysfunction; and diet, sulfonylurea, and insulin for diabetes mellitus.

Cofactor Supplementation

Several cofactor supplementations have been tried. The data supporting the beneficiary effect of most of these supplementations are limited to a small number of clinical trials that are not randomized or blinded and include only small number of subjects. In addition, the results are often inconsistent among these studies. An exception is ubiquinone (coenzyme Q_{10}, CoQ_{10}) supplementation for patients with CoQ_{10} deficiency. CoQ_{10} acts as electron shuttle between ETC complexes and is deficient in CoQ_{10} biosynthetic defects. Large-dose

CoQ_{10} supplementation results in restoring the electron flow and a dramatic improvement in clinical manifestations associated with CoQ_{10} deficiency.[58-60] Apart from this rare situation, CoQ_{10} supplementation has limited benefits.

EPI-743 is a *para*-benzoquinone analog for CoQ_{10} that is more potent than CoQ_{10}. Recent studies have shown results suggesting that EPI-743 can modify disease progression in patients with mitochondrial diseases. EPI-743 was found to improve clinical outcomes in children with genetically confirmed Leigh syndrome. The mechanism of action may rely on increasing the glutathione pools in these subjects.[61,62]

Some studies have shown that creatine monohydrate supplementation can improve exercise capacity in some patients with mitochondrial myopathies.[63] Supplementation with riboflavin has been associated with improvement in a few patients with complex I deficiency myopathy. Carnitine supplementation can be used in patients with secondary carnitine deficiency. B vitamins and antioxidants such as alpha lipoic acid, vitamin E, and vitamin C all have been used in mitochondrial disorders; however, there is very limited evidence for their effect.[64,65]

Nitric Oxide Donors

NO deficiency occurs in mitochondrial diseases and can play a major role in the pathogenesis of several complications observed in mitochondrial diseases. The amino acids arginine and citrulline act as NO precursors and can be used to restore NO production and may be of therapeutic utility in treating NO deficiency-related manifestations of mitochondrial diseases.[66] Arginine supplementation to individuals with MELAS syndrome resulted in an improvement in clinical symptoms associated with stroke-like episodes and a decrease in the frequency and severity of these episodes.[43] However, there are no clinical studies evaluating the effect of arginine or citrulline supplementation on other mitochondrial diseases.

Exercise

Lack of exercise in healthy individuals leads to an overall reduction in mitochondrial ETC activity, whereas endurance training improves ETC activity. Resistance training can stimulate the incorporation of satellite cells into existing muscle fibers. It has been suggested that for patients with mtDNA mutations, resistance training can lead to an overall reduction in the proportion of mutated mtDNA, as satellite cells contain a low or negligible amount of mutated mtDNA. Endurance training might therefore improve the mitochondrial function.[67-69] Furthermore, exercise can result in mitochondrial proliferation through inducing PGC-1α, which is the master transcription regulator that stimulates mitochondrial biogenesis.[70]

Diet Management in Mitochondrial Diseases

No specific dietary manipulation has shown consistent benefit for patients with mitochondrial disorders, though a high-lipid, low-carbohydrate diet has been suggested because glucose oxidation is largely aerobic and a high-carbohydrate diet can be metabolically challenging in patients with impaired OXPHOS.[24] Although hypoglycemia is not common in mitochondrial disorders, it has been observed in the hepatocerebral mtDNA depletion syndromes. Patients with hypoglycemia must avoid fasting by frequent or continuous feedings. In addition, uncooked cornstarch may reduce symptomatic hypoglycemia in mtDNA depletion syndromes such as MPV17 deficiency.[29]

Drugs and Anesthesia

It is advisable to avoid sodium valproate and barbiturates, which inhibit the ETC and have occasionally been shown to precipitate and/or accelerate liver disease in children with mitochondrial disorders.[71,72] Tetracyclines and chloramphenicol should also be avoided, as they inhibit mitochondrial protein synthesis. The oral hypoglycemic agent metformin should be avoided in mitochondrial diseases because it may aggravate lactate acidosis.[73]

One of the known side effects of aminoglycosides is ototoxicity, which is typically related to the dose and/or plasma concentration of aminoglycosides. On the other hand, the homoplasmic 1555A>G mutation in the mtDNA gene *MT-RNR1* predisposes to hearing loss caused by aminoglycoside exposure. Hearing loss occurs within a few days to weeks after administration of any amount of aminoglycoside antibiotic, such as gentamycin, tobramycin, amikacin, kanamycin, or streptomycin.[74,75] Therefore, aminoglycosides should be avoided in children with a maternal family history of aminoglycoside-induced hearing loss.

Patients with mitochondrial diseases often require general anesthesia as part of their diagnostic workup and subsequent management. Open muscle biopsy under general anesthesia is preferred to ensure suitability of biopsy material for ETC enzyme analysis. General anesthesia is therefore a common requirement for these patients, both for diagnosis and for ongoing disease management such as gastrostomy or central line insertion.[76] Mitochondria are a potential site of action for general anesthetic agents, and it is feasible that children with mitochondrial disease will respond abnormally to anesthetic drugs.[77] There are various concerns with regard to general anesthesia in this patient group. These concerns in part relate to the general stress response to surgery and to the use of the anesthetic agents themselves. Several complications have been reported in patients with mitochondrial diseases who underwent general anesthesia using different anesthetic agents, including lactic acidemia, respiratory failure, prolonged recovery, and malignant hyperthermia.[76] Although uncommon, mitochondrial diseases can pose many challenges for the anesthesiologist. It has been suggested that there is no "safest" anesthetic technique, but the choice of anesthetic should be individualized to the patient's needs. On the other hand, consultation with experts in the field and the subspecialists in a multidisciplinary approach can provide excellent assistance with comorbid issues and allow for a good prognosis even in complex patients with multiorgan mitochondrial disease.[78]

Future Directions

Although it has been estimated that 1,500 genes are involved in maintaining mitochondrial structure and function, only a small fraction of those genes have been identified. The utilization of next-generation sequencing to sequence the whole exome/genome in patients with different genetic and metabolic disorders has allowed the discovery of several novel genes.

The application of this methodology in patients with mitochondrial diseases has led to the discovery of several novel mitochondrial-related nDNA genes.[79–81] This field is an evolving one, and further discoveries are expected over the coming years. Identifying the mitochondrial-related genes would not only help in diagnosis but aid in a better understanding of normal mitochondrial functions and the derangements that occur due to defects of proteins encoded by these genes.

There is no satisfactory therapy for mitochondrial disorders. The current treatment is largely symptomatic and does not significantly alter the course of the disease. Clinical research is currently being conducted to evaluate the effect of different supplementations on mitochondrial diseases, including the CoQ_{10} analogue EPI-743,[61,62] the NO donors arginine and citrulline,[66] and the energy-storing compound creatine.[63]

Summary

Mitochondria generate most of the cellular energy. MtDNA encodes only a very small proportion of mitochondrial proteins, whereas the majority of mitochondrial proteins are encoded by nDNA. Mutations in mtDNA or mitochondria-related nDNA genes can result in mitochondrial dysfunction and mitochondrial diseases, which arise as a result of inadequate ATP production required to meet the energy needs of various organs, particularly those with high energy demands. MtDNA is typically maternally inherited, while defects in nDNA genes are inherited in an autosomal recessive, autosomal dominant, or X-linked manner. The diagnosis of mitochondrial diseases remains challenging in many cases and is based on clinical recognition, biochemical screening, assessment of the multiorgan involvement, histopathological studies, ETC activity assays, and molecular genetic testing. The use of whole exome sequencing has resulted in the discovery of several novel mitochondrial-related nDNA genes. Currently, there are no therapies with proven efficacy available for mitochondrial disorders. Several clinical trials are currently being conducted to evaluate the effect of novel and existing compounds on mitochondrial diseases. However, further clinical studies are needed to evaluate the currently used supplementation to determine their efficacy and utility in mitochondrial diseases.

References

1. Lang BF, Gray MW, Burger G. Mitochondrial genome evolution and the origin of eukaryotes. *Annu Rev Genet*. 1999; 33: 351–397.
2. Carrodeguas JA, Theis K, Bogenhagen DF, Kisker C. Crystal structure and deletion analysis show that the accessory subunit of mammalian DNA polymerase-γ, Pol-γB, functions as a homodimer. *Mol Cell*. 2001; 7: 43–54.
3. Spelbrink JN, Li FY, Tiranti V, et al. Human mitochondrial DNA deletions associated with mutations in the gene encoding Twinkle, a phage T7 gene 4-like protein localized in mitochondria. *Nature Genet*. 2001; 28: 223–231.
4. Clayton DA. Replication and transcription of vertebrate mitochondrial DNA. *Annu Rev Cell Biol*. 1991; 7: 453–478.
5. Ojala D, Montoya J, Attardi G. tRNA punctuation model of RNA processing in human mitochondria. *Nature*. 1981; 290: 470–474.

6. Jacobs HT. Disorders of mitochondrial protein synthesis. *Hum Mol Genet.* 2003; 12: R293–R301.
7. Thorburn DR, Sugiana C, Salemi R, et al. Biochemical and molecular diagnosis of mitochondrial respiratory chain disorders. *Biochim Biophys Acta.* 2004; 1659: 121–128.
8. MacKenzie JA, Payne RM. Mitochondrial protein import and human health and disease. *Biochim Biophys Acta.* 2007; 1772: 509–523.
9. Wallace DC. Mitochondrial diseases in man and mouse. *Science.* 1999; 283; 1482–1488.
10. Schaefer AM, Taylor RW, Turnbull DM, Chinnery PF. The epidemiology of mitochondrial disorders-past, present and future. *Biochim Biophys Acta.* 2004; 1659: 115–120.
11. Shitara H, Hayashi JI, Takahama S, Kaneda H, Yonekawa H. Maternal inheritance of mouse mtDNA in interspecific hybrids: segregation of the leaked paternal mtDNA followed by the prevention of subsequent paternal leakage. *Genetics.* 1998; 148: 851–857.
12. Schwartz M, Vissing J. Paternal inheritance of mitochondrial DNA. *N Engl J Med.* 2002; 347: 576–580.
13. Holt IJ, Harding AE, Petty RKH, Morgan-Hugues JA. A new mitochondrial disease associated with mitochondrial DNA heteroplasmy. *Am J Hum Genet* 1990; 46: 428–433.
14. Macmillan C, Lach B, Shoubridge EA. Variable distribution of mutant mitochondrial DNAs (tRNA(Leu[3243])) in tissues of symptomatic relatives with MELAS: the role of mitotic segregation. *Neurology.* 1993; 43: 1586–1590.
15. Schon EA, Bonilla E, DiMauro S. Mitochondrial DNA mutations and pathogenesis. *J Bioenerg Biomembr.* 1997; 29: 131–149.
16. Rötig A, Cormier V, Blanche S, et al. Pearson's marrow-pancreas syndrome. A multisystem mitochondrial disorder in infancy. *J Clin Invest.* 1990; 86: 1601–1608.
17. Cormier V, Rustin P, Bonnefont JP, et al. Hepatic failure in disorders of oxidative phosphorylation with neonatal onset. *J Pediatr.* 1991; 119: 951–954.
18. Rötig A, Bessis JL, Romero N, et al. Maternally inherited duplication of the mitochondrial genome in a syndrome of proximal tubulopathy, diabetes mellitus, and cerebellar ataxia. *Am J Hum Genet.* 1992; 50: 364–370.
19. Rustin P, Lebidois J, Chretien D, et al. Endomyocardial biopsies for early detection of mitochondrial disorders in hypertrophic cardiomyopathies. *J Pediatr.* 1994; 124: 224–228.
20. Cormier-Daire V, Bonnefont JP, Rustin P, et al. Mitochondrial DNA rearrangements with onset as chronic diarrhea with villous atrophy. *J Pediatr.* 1994; 124: 63–70.
21. von Kleist-Retzow JC, Cormier-Daire V, Viot G, et al. Antenatal manifestations of mitochondrial respiratory chain deficiency. *J Pediatr.* 2003; 143: 208–212.
22. Taylor RW, Turnbull DM. Mitochondrial DNA mutations in human disease. *Nat Rev Genet.* 2005; 6: 389–402.
23. Delettre C, Lenaers G, Griffoin JM, et al. Nuclear gene OPA1, encoding a mitochondrial dynamin-related protein, is mutated in dominant optic atrophy. *Nat Genet.* 2000; 26: 207–210.
24. Munnich A. Defects of the respiratory chain. In: Fernandes J, Saudubray J-M, van den Berghe G, Walter JH, eds. *Inborn Metabolic Diseases Diagnosis and Treatment*, 4th ed. Berlin: Springer; 2006: 197–209.
25. DiMauro S, Schon EA. Mitochondrial DNA mutations in human disease. *Am J Med Genet.* 2001; 106: 18–26.
26. Munnich A, Rustin P. Clinical spectrum and diagnosis of mitochondrial disorders. *Am J Med Genet.* 2001; 106: 4–17.
27. Miller C, Saada A, Shaul N, et al. Defective mitochondrial translation caused by a ribosomal protein (MRPS16) mutation. *Ann Neurol.* 2004; 56: 734–738.
28. Coenen MJ, Antonicka H, Ugalde C, et al. Mutant mitochondrial elongation factor G1 and combined oxidative phosphorylation deficiency. *N Engl J Med.* 2004; 351: 2080–2086.
29. El-Hattab AW, Scaglia F. Mitochondrial DNA depletion syndromes: review and updates of genetic basis, manifestations, and therapeutic options. *Neurotherapeutics.* 2013; 10: 186–198.
30. Potgieter M, Pretorius E, Pepper MS. Primary and secondary coenzyme Q10 deficiency: the role of therapeutic supplementation. *Nutr Rev.* 2013; 71: 180–188.
31. Emmanuele V, López LC, Berardo A, et al. Heterogeneity of coenzyme Q10 deficiency: patient study and literature review. *Arch Neurol.* 2012; 69: 978–983.
32. Rouault TA. Biogenesis of iron-sulfur clusters in mammalian cells: new insights and relevance to human disease. *Dis Model Mech.* 2012; 5: 155–164.
33. Lill R, Hoffmann B, Molik S, et al. The role of mitochondria in cellular iron-sulfur protein biogenesis and iron metabolism. *Biochim Biophys Acta.* 2012; 1823: 1491–1508.

34. Mayr JA, Zimmermann FA, Fauth C, et al. Lipoic acid synthetase deficiency causes neonatal-onset epilepsy, defective mitochondrial energy metabolism, and glycine elevation. *Am J Hum Genet*. 2011; 89: 792–797.
35. Wortmann SB, Vaz FM, Gardeitchik T, et al. Mutations in the phospholipid remodeling gene SERAC1 impair mitochondrial function and intracellular cholesterol trafficking and cause dystonia and deafness. *Nat Genet*. 2012; 44: 797–802.
36. Brandon MC, Lott MT, Nguyen KC, et al. MITOMAP: a human mitochondrial genome database-2004 update. *Nucleic Acids Res*. 2005; 33: D611–D613.
37. Ylikallio E, Suomalainen A. Mechanisms of mitochondrial diseases. *Ann Med*. 2012; 44: 41–59.
38. Willems PH, Valsecchi F, Distelmaier F, et al. Mitochondrial Ca2+ homeostasis in human NADH:ubiquinone oxidoreductase deficiency. *Cell Calcium*. 2008; 44: 123–133.
39. Atkuri KR, Cowan TM, Kwan T, et al. Inherited disorders affecting mitochondrial function are associated with glutathione deficiency and hypocitrullinemia. *Proc Natl Acad Sci USA*. 2009; 106: 3941–3945.
40. Balaban RS, Nemoto S, Finkel T. Mitochondria, oxidants, and aging. *Cell* 2005; 120: 483–495.
41. Galluzzi L, Kepp O, Trojel-Hansen C, Kroemer G. Mitochondrial control of cellular life, stress, and death. *Circ Res*. 2012; 111: 1198–1207.
42. Tengan CH, Kiyomoto BH, Godinho RO, et al. The role of nitric oxide in muscle fibers with oxidative phosphorylation defects. *Biochem Biophys Res Commun*. 2007; 359: 771–777.
43. Koga Y, Akita Y, Nishioka J, et al. MELAS and L-arginine therapy. *Mitochondrion*. 2007; 7: 133–139.
44. Vattemi G, Mechref Y, Marini M, et al. Increased protein nitration in mitochondrial diseases: evidence for vessel wall involvement. *Mol Cell Proteomics*. 2011; 10: M110.002964.
45. El-Hattab AW, Hsu JW, Emrick LT, et al. Restoration of impaired nitric oxide production in MELAS syndrome with citrulline and arginine supplementation. *Mol Genet Metab*. 2012; 105: 607–614.
46. Chinnery PF. Mitochondrial disorders overview. In: Pagon RA, Bird TD, Dolan CR, et al., eds. *GeneReviews*™ [Internet]. Seattle: University of Washington; 1993–. Published June 8, 2000. Updated September 16, 2010.
47. Sacks DB. Carbohydrates. In: Burtis CA and Ashwood ER, eds. *Tietz Textbook of Clinical Chemistry*, 2nd ed. Philadelphia: W.B. Saunders Company; 1994: 928–1001.
48. Harris RA, Joshi M, Jeoung NH, Obayashi M. Overview of the molecular and biochemical basis of branched-chain amino acid catabolism. *J Nutr*. 2005; 135: 1527S–1530S.
49. Suomalainen A. Fibroblast growth factor 21: a novel biomarker for human muscle-manifesting mitochondrial disorders. *Expert Opin Med Diagn*. 2013; 7: 313–317.
50. Scaglia F, Wong LJ, Vladutiu GD, Hunter JV. Predominant cerebellar volume loss as a neuroradiologic feature of pediatric respiratory chain defects. *AJNR Am J Neuroradiol*. 2005; 26: 1675–1680.
51. Bonnen PE, Yarham JW, Besse A, et al. Mutations in FBXL4 cause mitochondrial encephalopathy and a disorder of mitochondrial DNA maintenance. *Am J Hum Genet*; 2013: 93: 471–481.
52. Haack T B, Rolinski B, Haberberger B, et al. Homozygous missense mutation in BOLA3 causes multiple mitochondrial dysfunctions syndrome in two siblings. *J Inherit Metab Dis*; 2013: 36: 55–62.
53. Ghezzi D, Baruffini E, Haack TB, et al. Mutations of the mitochondrial-tRNA modifier MTO1 cause hypertrophic cardiomyopathy and lactic acidosis. *Am J Hum Genet*; 2012: 90: 1079–1087.
54. Bai RK, Wong LJ. Simultaneous detection and quantification of mitochondrial DNA deletion(s), depletion, and over-replication in patients with mitochondrial disease. *J Mol Diagn*. 2005; 7: 613–622.
55. Wong LJ. Molecular genetics of mitochondrial disorders. *Dev Disabil Res Rev*. 2010; 16: 154–162.
56. Wong LJ, Perng CL, Hsu CH, et al. Compensatory amplification of mtDNA in a patient with a novel deletion/duplication and high mutant load. *J Med Genet*. 2003; 40: e125.
57. Metzker ML. Sequencing technologies—the next generation. *Nat Rev Genet*. 2010; 11: 31–46.
58. Di Giovanni S, Mirabella M, Spinazzola A, et al. Coenzyme Q10 reverses pathological phenotype and reduces apoptosis in familial CoQ10 deficiency. *Neurology*. 2001; 57: 515–518.
59. Musumeci O, Naini A, Slonim AE, et al. Familial cerebellar ataxia with muscle coenzyme Q10 deficiency. *Neurology*. 2001; 56: 849–855.
60. Rötig A, Appelkvist EL, Geromel V, et al. Quinone-responsive multiple respiratory-chain dysfunction due to widespread coenzyme Q10 deficiency. *Lancet*. 2000; 356: 391–395.
61. Martinelli D, Catteruccia M, Piemonte F, et al. EPI-743 reverses the progression of the pediatric mitochondrial disease-genetically defined Leigh syndrome. *Mol Genet Metab*. 2012; 107: 383–388.
62. Enns GM, Kinsman SL, Perlman SL, et al. Initial experience in the treatment of inherited mitochondrial disease with EPI-743. *Mol Genet Metab*. 2012; 105: 91–102.

63. Tarnopolsky MA. Creatine as a therapeutic strategy for myopathies. *Amino Acids*. 2011; 40: 1397–1407.
64. Gold DR, Cohen BH. Treatment of mitochondrial cytopathies. *Semin Neurol* 2001; 21: 309–325.
65. Rodriguez MC, MacDonald JR, Mahoney DJ, Parise G, Beal MF, Tarnopolsky MA. Beneficial effects of creatine, CoQ10, and lipoic acid in mitochondrial disorders. *Muscle Nerve*. 2007; 35: 235–242.
66. El-Hattab AW, Emrick LT, Craigen WJ, Scaglia F. Citrulline and arginine utility in treating nitric oxide deficiency in mitochondrial disorders. *Mol. Genet. Metab*. 2012; 107: 247–252.
67. Taivassalo T, Fu K, Johns T, Arnold D, Karpati G, Shoubridge EA. Gene shifting: a novel therapy for mitochondrial myopathy. *Hum Mol Genet*. 1999; 8: 1047–1052.
68. Clark KM, Bindoff LA, Lightowlers RN, et al. Reversal of a mitochondrial DNA defect in human skeletal muscle. *Nat Genet*. 1997; 16: 222–224.
69. Taivassalo T, Shoubridge EA, Chen J, et al. Aerobic conditioning in patients with mitochondrial myopathies: physiological, biochemical, and genetic effects. *Ann Neurol*. 2001; 50: 133–141.
70. Kang C, Li Ji L. Role of PGC-1α signaling in skeletal muscle health and disease. *Ann N Y Acad Sci*. 2012;1271:110–117.
71. Bicknese AR, May W, Hickey WF, Dodson WE. Early childhood hepatocerebral degeneration misdiagnosed as valproate hepatotoxicity. *Ann Neurol* 1992; 32: 767–775.
72. Saneto RP, Lee IC, Koenig MK, et al. POLG DNA testing as an emerging standard of care before instituting valproic acid therapy for pediatric seizure disorders. *Seizure*. 2010; 19: 140–146.
73. Maassen JA, Hart LM, Van Essen E, et al. Mitochondrial diabetes: molecular mechanisms and clinical presentation. *Diabetes*. 2004; 53: S103–S109.
74. Bates DE. Aminoglycoside ototoxicity. *Drugs Today (Barc)*. 2003; 39: 277–285.
75. Bravo O, Ballana E, Estivill X. Cochlear alterations in deaf and unaffected subjects carrying the deafness-associated A1555G mutation in the mitochondrial 12S rRNA gene. *Biochem Biophys Res Commun*. 2006; 344: 511–516.
76. Footitt EJ, Sinha MD, Raiman JA, Dhawan A, Moganasundram S, Champion MP. Mitochondrial disorders and general anaesthesia: a case series and review. *Br J Anaesth*. 2008; 100: 436–441.
77. Shipton EA, Prosser DO. Mitochondrial myopathies and anaesthesia. *Eur J Anaesthesiol* 2004; 21: 173–178.
78. Ellinas H, Frost EA. Mitochondrial disorders–a review of anesthetic considerations. *Middle East J Anesthesiol*. 2011; 21: 235–242.
79. Craigen WJ, Graham BH, Wong LJ, Scaglia F, Lewis RA, Bonnen PE. Exome sequencing of a patient with suspected mitochondrial disease reveals a likely multigenic etiology. *BMC Med Genet*. 2013; 14: 83.
80. Jonckheere AI, Renkema GH, Bras M, et al. A complex V ATP5A1 defect causes fatal neonatal mitochondrial encephalopathy. *Brain*. 2013; 136: 1544–1554.
81. Kevelam SH, Bugiani M, Salomons GS, et al. Exome sequencing reveals mutated SLC19A3 in patients with an early-infantile, lethal encephalopathy. *Brain*. 2013; 136: 1534–1543.

9

Cholesterol, Sterols, and Isoprenoids

YASEMEN EROGLU, JEAN-BAPTISTE ROULLET,
AND ROBERT D. STEINER

Introduction

Cholesterol is a steroid lipid synthesized de novo primarily by the liver, intestine and adrenal glands from mevalonic acid (MVA) and is also obtained from dietary sources. Cholesterol is the major lipid component of mammalian cellular membranes. It maintains plasma membrane fluidity and concentrates in plasma membrane microdomains (caveolae), thereby having an effect on several essential cellular functions such as ion transport and G-protein coupled receptor mediated signaling. Cholesterol is also implicated in embryomorphogenesis via the Hedgehog (Hh) protein signal transduction pathways[1] and as the precursor for bile acid and steroid hormone synthesis. A cholesterol precursor, 7-dehydrocholesterol is also the precursor of vitamin D and thus contributes to bone and mineral homeostasis.

Cholesterol biosynthesis is a complex multistep process starting with the production of MVA from acetyl-CoA. MVA is phosphorylated by mevalonate kinase (MK) and decarboxylated into isoprentenyl pyrophosphate (PP), the building block for cellular isoprenoids (e.g., farnesyl-PP, geranylgeranyl-PP, dolichol, heme A, and ubiquinone). Cholesterol is then formed after condensation of two farnesyl-PP molecules and a well-orchestrated series of reductions, hydroxylations, and demethylations (Figure 9.1). Inborn errors of cholesterol biosynthesis comprise a heterogeneous group of disorders, each associated with multiple congenital malformations and most with mental retardation. At least nine disorders are presently recognized, with more likely to be identified. Currently, the list of cholesterol synthesis disorders includes Smith-Lemli-Opitz syndrome (SLOS), congenital hemidysplasia with ichthyosiform erythroderma and limb defects (CHILD syndrome), chondrodysplasia punctata 2, lathosterolosis, desmosterolosis, sterol C4 methyl oxidase deficiency, autosomal recessive Antley–Bixler syndrome, and possibly hydrops-ectopic calcification-moth-eaten (HEM) skeletal dysplasia (Figure 9.1). SLOS is the most common and best characterized inborn error of cholesterol biosynthesis. Related to the disorders of cholesterol biosynthesis is cerebrotendinous xanthomatosis (CTX), an inborn error of bile acid synthesis due to impaired conversion of cholesterol to chenodeoxycholic acid.

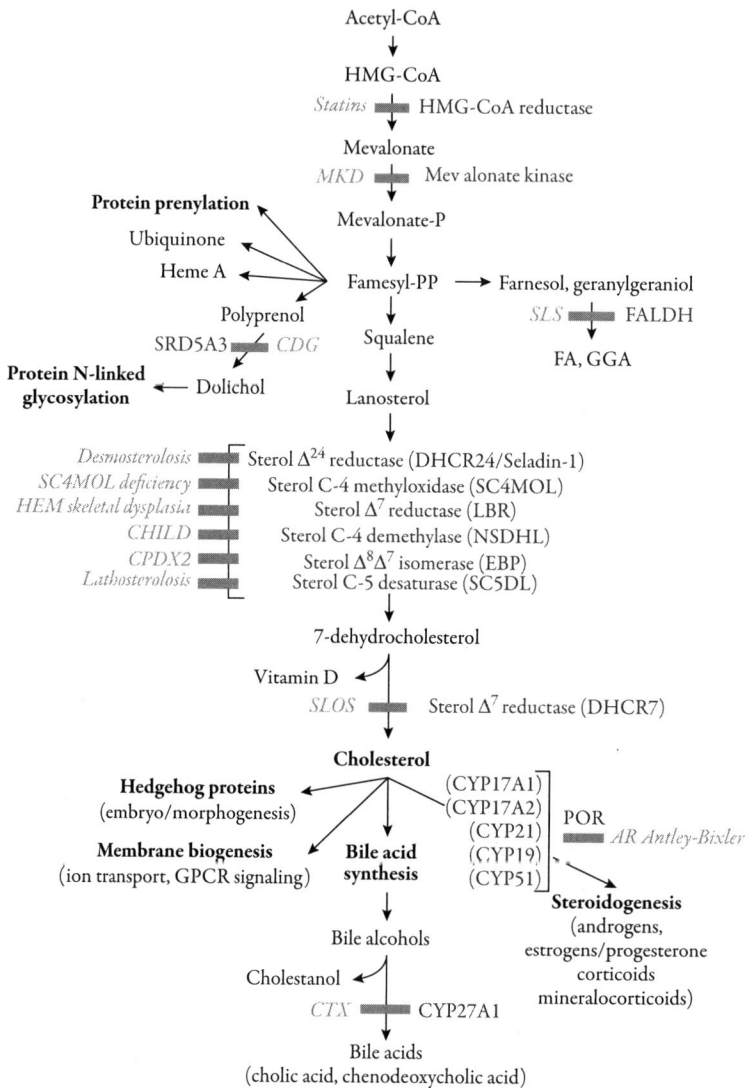

FIGURE 9.1 Metabolic pathways of cholesterol and isoprenoid synthesis with corresponding sterol and isoprenoid disorders. *Abbreviations:* *MKD* = mevalonate kinase deficiency; *SLS* = Sjögren-Larsson syndrome; *CDG* = congenital disorders of glycosylation; *HEM skeletal dysplasia* = hydrops-ectopic calcification-moth-eaten skeletal dysplasia; *CHILD* = congenital hemidysplasia with ichthyosiform erythroderma and limb defects; *CPDX2* = X-linked dominant chondrodysplasia punctata type 2; *CTX* = cerebrotendinous xanthomatosis; *SLOS* = Smith-Lemli-Opitz syndrome; *FA* = farnesoic acid; *GGA* = geranylgeranoic acid; *GPCR* = G-protein coupled receptors; *POR* = P450 (cytochrome) oxidoreductase.

Finally, the initial and intermediate steps in the cholesterol synthetic pathway are also involved in the synthesis of isoprenoids. Isoprenoids are implicated in a variety of cell functions such as mitochondrial respiration, signaling, apoptosis, and protein posttranslational modifications (glycosylation and prenylation), and genetic disorders affecting their metabolism have been identified: mevalonate kinase deficiency (MKD), SRD5A3 deficiency (a congenital disorder of glycosylation [CDG] caused by impaired dolichol synthesis), and the Sjögren-Larsson syndrome (SLS) caused by deficiency in fatty aldehyde dehydrogenase, an enzyme recently implicated in the metabolism of isoprenols. This chapter discusses the disorders of the cholesterol and isoprenoid biosynthesis pathways, their clinical and laboratory features, diagnosis, management, pathogenesis, and areas of future research. Disorders caused by defects in the biosynthesis of other isoprenoids such as heme A (cytochrome oxidase deficiency),[2] ubiquinone (coenzyme Q_{10} deficiency),[3] and prenylated proteins (choroideremia, MIM 303100[4]; Griscelli syndrome type 2[5]; X-linked form of Charcot-Marie-Tooth disease[6,7]) are treated elsewhere in this book.

Smith-Lemli-Opitz Syndrome

Clinical Presentation, Diagnosis, Treatment, and Pathways

SLOS (OMIM 270400) was first described by David Smith, Luc Lemli, and John Opitz in 1964.[8] It is a multiple congenital malformation/mental retardation syndrome with microcephaly; dysmorphism; growth and developmental retardation; limb anomalies; photosensitivity; and eye, heart, genitourinary, and other anomalies.[9–15] There is great variability in expression, with some individuals exhibiting only subtle dysmorphic facial features and toe syndactyly (Figure 9.2), while others have malformations in virtually every organ system. SLOS is one of the most common autosomal recessive genetic disorders. Its incidence

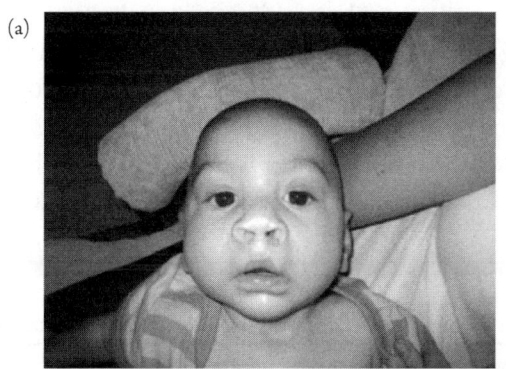

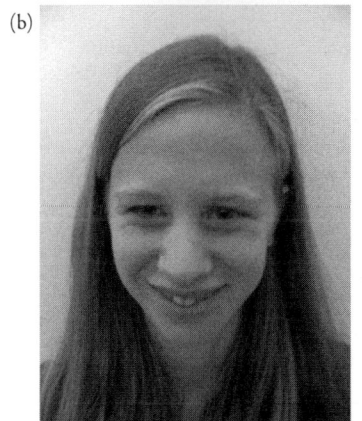
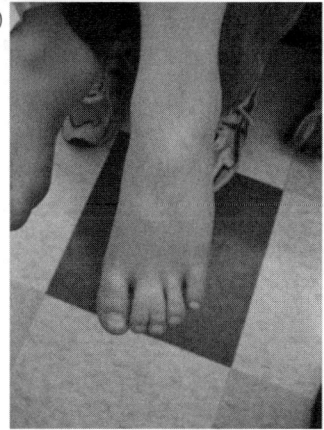

FIGURE 9.2 Typical features of children with Smith-Lemli-Opitz syndrome. (a) microcephaly, broad nose with anteverted nares, ptosis, low-set ears; (b) Subtle dysmorphic facial features in Smith-Lemli-Opitz syndrome; (c) toe syndactyly.

is predicted to be 1:13,500 with a carrier frequency of 1% to 2% in Caucasians, but the observed incidence seems to be closer to 1:20,000 maximum.[16–19]

The phenotypic spectrum of SLOS is very wide. Severely affected infants with major malformations often die in the perinatal period. Mildly affected patients may demonstrate subtle dysmorphic facial features, syndactyly, and learning disabilities.[20,21] Intellectual disability is typical, while autism and behavioral disturbances are common.[10,12,22–25] Tierney et al. found that 53% patients with SLOS met the diagnostic criteria for autistic disorder,[26] while Steiner et al. reported an even higher (71% to 86%) percentage.[22] Moreover, about 20% of children with autism spectrum disorder have cholesterol levels below the fifth percentile, indicating an association between sterol metabolism and autism.[25] Feeding problems, failure to thrive, and short stature are frequently seen in SLOS. The spectrum of clinical features in SLOS patients is illustrated in Table 9.1.

SLOS is due to deficient sterol Δ^7-reductase (7-dehydrocholesterol Δ^7-reductase or DHCR7) activity. This enzyme reduces 7DHC to yield cholesterol in the final step of cholesterol biosynthesis (Figure 9.1).[27,28] Both 7DHC and its isomer, 8DHC, accumulate in serum and tissues of patients.[29–34] SLOS patients can have reduced or normal cholesterol levels. SLOS diagnosis is confirmed in the proper clinical context with sterol analysis typically by gas-chromatography/mass spectrometry showing elevated 7DHC (8DHC), and diagnosis can also be confirmed by *DHCR7* mutation analysis. In cases where there is strong clinical suspicion but sterol analysis is equivocal or nondiagnostic and mutation results are not readily available or showing only a single mutation, measurement of 7DHC in cell media with patient cells incubated in cholesterol free media can be useful. *DHCR7* maps to human chromosome 11q12-13, and is encoded by nine exons. Over 130 different mutations have been identified.[35–38] The most common mutation is c.964-1G>C, a splice acceptor mutation. This mutation is responsible for one-third of mutant alleles in SLOS patients. Other common mutations are p.T93M, p.W151X, p.R404C and p.V326L accounting for

TABLE 9.1 **Clinical Features and Congenital Anomalies in Smith-Lemli-Opitz Syndrome**

General	Failure to thrive, developmental delay, mental retardation, hypotonia,
	Insomnia, self-injurious/aggressive behaviors, autism
Skin	Photosensitivity, eczema
Head	Microcephaly, bitemporal narrowing, broad nose with anteverted nares, micrognathia, arched palate, cleft palate/uvula, holoprosencephaly
Eyes	Ptosis, epicanthal folds, strabismus, cataracts, optic nerve hypoplasia/atrophy
Cardiac	Atrial septal defect, ventricular septal defect, patent ductus arteriosus, atrioventricular canal, hypertension
Gastrointestinal	Pyloric stenosis, Hirschprung's disease, malrotation, constipation, reflux, feeding problems, cholestatic liver disease
Urogenital	Sexual ambiguity, hypospadias, cryptorchidism, renal malformations
Limbs	Rhizomelia, 2-3 toe syndactyly, polydactyly, short thumbs

10%, 6%, 5%, and 5% of mutations, respectively. Prenatal diagnosis of SLOS can be made by sterol analysis on amniotic fluid or chorionic villus sample or by molecular genetic testing. During pregnancy, the fetal cholesterol synthesis defect can cause decreased unconjugated estriol levels in maternal serum and a resulting abnormal triple or quad screen, but this is not a sensitive or specific indicator for SLOS.[39] Measurement of desaturated steroids in maternal urine during pregnancy has been proposed as a potential prenatal diagnostic test for SLOS.[40]

Pathogenesis

The precise cause of the malformations, intellectual disability, and other features of SLOS remains unclear. Cholesterol is a major lipid component of the plasma membrane of all cells, including brain cells. It is a precursor of bile acids, steroid hormones, neuroactive steroids, and oxysterols. Cholesterol is a major component of myelin in the nervous system. Cholesterol deficiency, generalized sterol deficiency, and accumulation of precholesterol sterol intermediates (e.g., 7DHC, 8DHC) likely play a role in the pathogenesis of SLOS. 7DHC and its metabolites may have toxic effects. Accumulation of 7DHC in fibroblasts causes impairment of intracellular cholesterol transport similar to that seen in Niemann-Pick type C.[41] 7DHC appears to increase the degradation rate of HMG-CoA reductase (HMGR), resulting in decreased sterol synthesis in SLOS patients.[42]

The deficiency of cholesterol and substitution of 7DHC for cholesterol affects cellular membranes, altering their lipid raft stability, rigidity, and membrane fluidity.[43–45] SLOS cells are transcriptionally deficient in the cholesterol-binding, scaffolding, and cellular signaling caveolar protein caveolin-1, which may be a direct result of altered bilayer organization. This may eventually lead to globally impaired membrane electrophysiology.[45] Studies have shown that, beyond the cholesterol biosynthesis defect, global metabolic alterations in the interaction between cholesterol and other metabolic pathways as well as lipid and protein oxidation likely contribute to retinal disease in a pharmacologic rat model of SLOS.[46] Supporting this study, ophthalmologic evaluations from SLOS patients revealed abnormalities, with some of these patients showing abnormal electroretinograms, abnormal optic nerves, retinal pigmentary deposits, early nuclear cataracts, and reduction in visual acuity.[47,48] What happens in the retinas of affected patients may be recapulated in other organ systems.

Some of the malformations in SLOS appear to be related to impaired Hh functioning. Hh proteins are a family of signaling proteins important in patterning during embryogenesis and activated by covalent binding of cholesterol.[49] Since 7DHC can substitute for cholesterol in activating Hh proteins, it is likely that defective signaling downstream of Hh in SLOS rather than impaired Hh covalent modification per se is at least partially responsible for malformations in SLOS.[50,51]

Oxidative stress may play a role in SLOS pathogenesis.[52,53] When keratinocytes enriched in 7DHC and deficient in cholesterol are exposed to ultraviolet radiation, eightfold greater reactive oxygen species are produced than in normal keratinocytes, and cell death occurs at 24 hours; antioxidants inhibit these responses.[52] High levels of 7DHC are associated with exaggerated photosensitivity to ultraviolet radiation in SLOS patients. These findings support an apoptotic mechanism due to reactive oxygen species.

Areas of Research

Much has been learned about SLOS in the 15 years that have elapsed since discovery of the biochemical defect. However, our understanding of the pathogenesis is still incomplete, and there is no proven treatment.

Several rodent models are available for SLOS, but none of them are optimal for study. A genetic knock-out mouse is not viable.[54,55] Porter et al. developed a viable hypomorphic mouse model by introducing a mutation equivalent to the human T93M mutation; however, biochemical defects normalize with age.[56] The pharmacologic agent AY9944 produces a rat model mimicking key features of the human disease. Better animal models are needed to understand the pathogenesis and to test treatments.

The effects of deficient cholesterol synthesis and excess 7DHC on brain metabolism and function are not well characterized. Until the discovery of 24-S hydroxycholesterol (24S), there was no practical method for evaluating cholesterol metabolism in human brain. 24S hydroxylation represents the major pathway for turnover of brain cholesterol.[57] There seems to be a continuous flux of 24S from the brain into plasma that parallels brain cholesterol synthesis.[58] 24S in human plasma also originates from the brain.[59] Thus plasma 24S level is a surrogate marker of brain cholesterol synthesis. As a result of generally reduced cholesterol content in SLOS, one expects low plasma 24S levels. Plasma 24S has been measured in a small number of SLOS subjects and appears reduced.[60] These data need to be confirmed in larger studies and 24S levels validated as a useful biomarker for clinical trials.

SLOS is one of the most common autosomal recessive genetic disorders. Xiong et al. reported a colorimetric assay for 7DHC with potential application to screen SLOS.[61] There have been reports of targeted screening for most common *DHCR7* mutations. However, newborn screening is not yet available, another target for research.

Potential Therapies

Cholesterol supplementation: Dietary cholesterol supplementation is now widely used in SLOS, from 20 mg/kg/day to 300 mg/kg/day. In addition to providing cholesterol to tissues, cholesterol supplementation down-regulates HMGR activity and presumably suppresses 7DHC synthesis.[14,62] Animal studies suggest that cholesterol supplementation might be beneficial in preventing malformations[63,64] and 7DHC-induced learning impairment,[65] increasing the cholesterol to 7DHC ratio.[66] A few uncontrolled early human studies showed that cholesterol supplementation results in increased plasma cholesterol concentration[67–69] and positive behavioral and affective changes in SLOS patients.[23,26,70,71] These reports need to be confirmed in controlled longitudinal studies. Steiner et al reported that cholesterol supplementation does not improve developmental progress in SLOS.[22] Cholesterol does not likely cross the blood–brain barrier; however, its use may ameliorate the extra-CNS phenotype of SLOS, perhaps even affecting neuroactive steroid production so that its use, which has become standard in SLOS, is justified until more effective treatment options are developed.

Statins: Statin medications, routinely used to treat hypercholesterolemia, inhibit HMGR. It might be beneficial to inhibit HMGR in SLOS to reduce the accumulation of potentially toxic 7DHC and 8DHC while whole-body cholesterol is preserved by cholesterol supplementation.[72-74] Studies suggest that statins can reduce oxidative stress by reducing cell superoxide production and by decreasing low density lipoproteins cholesterol available for oxidation.[75-77] Therefore, statins could be useful in SLOS treatment by multiple mechanisms.

Lipid-soluble statins like simvastatin cross the blood–brain barrier to reduce brain 7DHC and 8DHC and could improve neurological and cognitive outcomes. In the $T^{93M}/\Delta 3-5$ hypomorphic mouse, combined treatment with cholesterol and simvastatin resulted in decreased 7DHC levels in both peripheral tissues and brain and upregulated expression of a *Dhcr7* allele with residual enzymatic activity.[56] Similar findings were reported with human SLOS fibroblasts.[78] Finally, long-term treatment of two SLOS patients with simvastatin was associated with long-lasting improvement of the 7DHC to cholesterol ratio in plasma and in cerebrospinal fluid. In that very small study, cholesterol concentration normalized with simvastatin and growth, and mental, motor, and social development improved.[79,80] However, a retrospective study of simvastatin in 39 SLOS patients revealed that cholesterol supplementation plus simvastatin decreased the plasma (7DHC + 8DHC)/(cholesterol) ratio, a ratio considered as a severity index of the disease, but improvements in growth and behavior were not confirmed.[74]

Caution is advised when administering statins in SLOS, as statins are inhibitors of HMGR, the rate-limiting enzyme of cholesterol synthesis. Statins have been found to reduce plasma 24S levels in non-SLOS subjects[81] suggesting a reduction in brain cholesterol synthesis. Whether they cause more profound reductions in cholesterol synthesis in SLOS subjects needs to be confirmed with further studies. Marked elevations in transaminases and creatine kinase have been reported in patients more severely affected with SLOS given statins.[7] Controlled, long-term studies in SLOS patients are needed to confirm the efficacy and safety of simvastatin.

Bile acids: Dietary cholesterol absorption in SLOS is reduced.[74] Bile acids are natural enhancers of cholesterol absorption. Ursodeoxycholic acid and chenodeoxycholic acid have been used in early trials of cholesterol supplementation in SLOS to ameliorate potential bile acid deficiency and improve cholesterol absorption and are still used in certain situations.[78] Recently, tauroursodeoxycholic acid (TUDCA), a taurine-conjugated bile acid with antioxidant, antiapoptotic, and neuroprotective properties appears to be a potential therapy. In animals, TUDCA prevents bile-acid induced hepatocyte damage and has cytoprotective effects.[79-82] There is evidence that TUDCA crosses the blood–brain barrier.[83] Unfortunately, TUDCA has high critical micellar concentration; therefore, its effect in increasing cholesterol absorption may be limited.

Antioxidants: Oxidative stress may be implicated in the pathogenesis of SLOS, and it is likely the consequence of 7DHC or other oxysterols accumulation associated with secondary stimulation of reactive oxygen species production and general reduction in oxidant buffering capacity of SLOS cells and tissues. Dietary cholesterol itself induces oxidative stress as well. Therefore a combination of cholesterol and antioxidants is proposed as potentially superior to dietary cholesterol alone. However, long-term, controlled studies are lacking.

Vitamins and minerals: Feeding difficulties, slow growth, and short stature are hallmarks of SLOS. Supplements with antioxidant vitamins and minerals may potentially be useful for SLOS patients not only for attenuation of cellular oxidative stress but also for deficiencies related to poor nutritional status.

Novel Treatments

Gene therapy: Watson et al. reported on restoring DHCR7 activity in mice liver by adenovirus-associated viral vector containing the DHCR7 gene.[84] Preliminary data showed improved DHC/cholesterol ratio. If effective in humans, it might offer a possible alternative to exogenous cholesterol therapy; however, a complete cure is not possible as some consequences of the defect are already established during prenatal development.

Molecular chaperones: Accumulation of 7DHC in SLOS fibroblasts alters intracellular transport of cholesterol similar to that seen in Niemann-Pick type C.[41] In vitro treatment of SLOS cells with an inhibitor of glycosphingolipid biosynthesis, miglustat, reversed the defect in the intracellular transport of cholesterol.[85] Inhibition of glycosphingolipid synthesis appears to be a potential novel treatment by increasing the bioavailability of cholesterol.

Neurosteroids: In contrast to cholesterol, neuroactive steroids do cross the blood–brain barrier and may provide insight to novel treatments that could potentially affect SLOS behavioral type.

Prenatal treatment: Irons et al. hypothesized that prenatal supplementation of cholesterol could potentially interrupt adverse consequences of cholesterol deficiency in fetal development.[86] They demonstrated that fetal cholesterol could be increased by supplementing cholesterol via fetal intravenous or intraperitoneal transfusions of fresh frozen plasma. In hamsters, fetal cholesterol was shown to increase when maternal cholesterol concentration elevated with diet.[87] Woollett et al. demonstrated that the efflux of cholesterol from placental cells and secretion of cholesterol from endodermal yolk sac cells to the fetal circulation can be regulated.[88] Increased exogenous cholesterol supply early in gestation, such as during the first trimester when the blood–brain barrier has not yet formed, could potentially improve SLOS phenotype.

Sterol-Related Disorders

Cerebrotendinous Xanthomatosis

CTX (MIM# 213700) is a rare autosomal recessive disorder caused by a defect in bile acid synthesis.[89] Often, the disorder first presents in infancy with chronic diarrhea, although this is frequently noted in retrospect. Because of the rarity of the disorder and the nonspecific nature of diarrhea, CTX is usually not diagnosed until additional signs or symptoms become evident. Cataracts become evident in childhood or adolescence, and tendon and brain xanthomas may develop in the second and third decades of life. Premature atherosclerosis is a characteristic feature in older individuals with CTX. Significant neurologic impairment also occurs, often including seizures, dementia, and extrapyramidal dysfunction. They typically begin in the third decade of life and in the absence of treatment progressing until death, often in the sixth decade of life if the condition goes untreated. The presentation and course vary widely, and treatment can dramatically alter the natural history, especially with early initiation. The first case of CTX was reported in 1937 by van

Bogaert.[90] Since then the disorder has been characterized clinically biochemically and genetically, and several hundred patients have been diagnosed.[91]

The disorder is caused by inactivating mutations (missense, nonsense, frameshift, and splice junction) of the gene coding for mitochondrial sterol 27-hydroxylase (CYP27A1).[92,93] CYP27A1 is involved in the normal oxidation of the steroid side-chain, a key step in the conversion of cholesterol to the primary bile acid chenodeoxycholic acid. In unaffected individuals, cholesterol is first converted to 7α-hydroxycholesterol, then to 7α-hydroxy-4-cholesten-3-one. 7α-hydroxy-4-cholesten-3-one is converted to bile alcohol CYP27A1 substrates, the precursors of cholic and chenodeoxycholic acids (classical bile acid synthesis pathway).[91] In CTX, cholesterol 7α-hydroxylase (CYP7A1, the rate-limiting enzyme in bile acid synthesis) is upregulated to compensate for defective sterol 27-hydroxylase. Bile acid precursors accumulate in the plasma and liver[94] and are shunted into the 5α-cholestanol pathway, causing tissue accumulation of cholestanol.[95,96] The precursors are also shunted into the 25-hydroxylase pathway, the microsomal pathway initially described by Shefer et al.,[97] leading to urinary and fecal excretion of complex bile alcohols.[98]

Treatment with oral chenodeoxycholic acid down regulates CYP7A1, resulting in the normalization of the biochemical abnormalities, possible disappearance of peripheral xanthomas, and improvement of the neurological symptoms.[99] Importantly, treatment with chenodeoxycholic acid started in infancy in asymptomatic patients may completely prevent the CTX phenotype,[100] whereas only moderate symptomatic improvements may be achieved if treatment is starts during adulthood.[100,101] Combined treatment with HMGR inhibitors (statins) may further decrease plasma cholestanol levels in CTX and improve therapeutic outcomes, but there is no solid evidence of increased efficacy, and statins are not widely used in the treatment of CTX.

CTX should be suspected in all patients with tendon xanthomas and normal or mildly elevated serum cholesterol, or in all patients with unexplained juvenile cataracts. Indeed, CTX should probably be considered in all patients with xanthomas, since the treatment is so different from the common cause of xanthoma, familial hypercholesterolemia. CTX should be considered in cases of chronic diarrhea in which no other etiology can be found. Diagnosis of CTX is by quantitation of cholestanol in serum by gas chromatography or gas chromatography mass spectrometry.[102] Screening methods have been proposed including the identification of 7α-hydroxylated bile alcohols in urine[103] and, more recently, the measurement of 7α-hydroxy-4-cholesten-3-one.[104] Further diagnostic confirmation may be obtained by measurement of enzyme activity in cultured fibroblasts, but this testing is not routinely available. *CYP27A1* DNA mutation analysis is more widely available for further diagnostic confirmation.

Because an effective treatment is available, early diagnosis is important in preventing irreversible CNS consequences of the disease.

CHILD Syndrome, Chondrodysplasia Punctata 2, Desmosterolosis, Lathosterolosis, Sterol C4 Methyl Oxidase Deficiency, and Autosomal Recessive Antley–Bixler Syndrome

Other rare genetic disorders affecting distal steps of the cholesterol synthetic pathway have been identified.[105-109] These include CHILD syndrome (MIM 308050),[110] chondrodysplasia punctata 2 syndrome (MIM 302960),[111] desmosterolosis (MIM 602398),[112,113] lathosterolosis (MIM 607330),[114–116] the autosomal recessive Antley–Bixler syndrome (MIM 201750),[117] and the recently reported sterol C4 methyl oxidase deficiency.[118,119] Many of these disorders present with congenital malformations, a multisystemic phenotype, and skin manifestations. The phenotypes may be caused by a lack of cholesterol or other sterols downstream of the enzymatic block, leading to impaired Hh signaling pathway,[1] by accumulation of upstream precursors, and/or by shunting into alternative pathways for example with production of toxic oxysterols.

CHILD syndrome (MIM 308050) is an X-linked dominant, male lethal, multisystemic disease characterized by an inflammatory nevus with lateralization and strict midline demarcation and ispilateral hypoplasia of the body.[110] It is caused by mutations of the *NSDHL* gene coding for (NAD(P)H) steroid-dehydrogenase-like protein, an enzyme that removes the C-4 methyl group from lanosterol.[120]

X-linked dominant chondrodysplasia punctata type 2 (MIM 302960; formerly Conradi-Hünermann-Happle syndrome) is one of several forms of chondrodysplasia punctata (the others have not proven to be cholesterol disorders) characterized by skeletal dysplasia, stippled epiphyses, cataracts, transient ichthyosis, and atrophoderma in a mosaic pattern.[111] It is caused by mutations in emopamil-binding protein that encodes 3β-hydroxysterol-Δ^8, Δ^7-isomerase, which catalyzes the conversion of 8(9)-cholestenol to lathosterol, resulting in diagnostic elevations in serum 8-dehydrocholesterol and 8(9) cholestenol.[121,122] At least 60 different mutations have been described.[123] The disease affects primarily females, but several cases of affected males have been reported.[124]

Desmosterolosis (MIM 602398) is an autosomal recessive disease characterized by prominent congenital malformations, abnormalities in brain development, and severe developmental and neurological dysfunction, with low cholesterol and high desmosterol levels.[112,113] It is caused by mutations in the gene coding for 3β-hydroxy-steroid-Δ^{24}-reductase (DHCR24/seladin-1), a multifunctional protein with antiapoptotic, antioxidant, and neuroprotective activity.[125–127] It is premature to describe the phenotypic spectrum, with only two cases reported.

Lathosterolosis (MIM 607330) is an extremely rare autosomal recessive disease. To date only four cases have been reported.[114–116] The phenotype associates congenital multisystem malformations and signs of lysosomal storage. It is caused by a deficiency in sterol C_5 desaturase (SC5DL), the enzyme immediately upstream of DHCR7 that converts lathosterol into 7-dehydrocholesterol. As with desmosterolosis, it is premature to describe the phenotypic spectrum. Statins and liver transplantation have been tried in two patients. Both treatment showed encouraging results.[116,128]

Autosomal recessive ABS is caused by homozygous or compound heterozygous mutation of the POR gene encoding nicotinamide adenine dinucleotide phosphate-oxidase-cytochrome P450 oxidoreductase, an enzyme involved in steroid biosynthesis.[129–131] The phenotype includes congenital malformations with characteristic pear-shaped nose and simple ears, adrenal failure, and ambiguous genitalia.[132,133] The pathogenesis is thought to be related to the decreased activity of POR, an electron donor for all microsomal P450 enzymes, including steroidogenic enzymes (CYP17A1/17α-hydroxylase, CYP17A2/17,20-lyase,

CYP21/21-hydroxylase, and CYP19/aromatase) and enzymes involved in cholesterol biosynthesis (CYP51 lanosterol 14α-demethylase).[134]

HEM skeletal dysplasia (MIM 215140) is a very rare autosomal recessive chondrodystrophy characterized by early in utero lethality.[135–137] Only nine cases have been reported to date.[138] The disorder is caused by inactivating mutations of the gene encoding for the lamin B receptor, a multifunctional protein with sterol Δ^{14} reductase activity.[139] Elevated levels of cholesta-8,14-dien-3β-ol were found in cultured fibroblasts isolated from a fetus with HEM, and initially it appeared that HEM skeletal dysplasia was a cholesterol synthesis disorder. However, recently data have been published showing that the disorder is not likely caused by a defect in cholesterol synthesis because in HEM skeletal dysplasia patients another gene (*TM7SF2*) with DHCR14 activity provides enzymatic redundancy.[140]

Sterol C4 methyl oxidase deficiency: Recently, four cases caused by a mutation in the *SC4MOL* gene were reported.[118,119] The patients presented with congenital cataracts, developmental delay, microcephaly, and severe psoriasiform dermatitis, together with elevated serum levels of methylsterols and altered immune function. Treatment with statins in combination with cholesterol supplementation and bile acids normalized methylsterol levels and improved the clinical phenotype.[119] However, more cases need to be identified to fully characterize disease phenotype, pathogenesis, and response to treatment.

Isoprenoid Disorders

Mevalonate Kinase Deficiency

Clinical Presentation, Diagnosis, Treatment, and Pathways

MKD (MIMs 251170, 260920) is an autosomal recessive metabolic disorder caused by mutations of *MVK* (12q24; MIM# 251170). MK phosphorylates mevalonate produced by HMGR, one of the rate-limiting steps of the mevalonate pathway.[140] The complexity of the mevalonate pathway and its role in regulating cell functions such as growth, signaling, apoptosis, and respiration, has been extensively reviewed by others.[141–146] Because MK controls an early step of the cholesterol and isoprenoid synthesis pathway, MKD has the potential to impact all cell functions regulated by downstream metabolites in the pathway.

Initially, two separate syndromes were reported: mevalonic aciduria (MA; MIM 251170)[147] and hyperimmunoglobulinemia D with periodic fever syndrome (HIDS; MIM 260920).[148] However, it was later recognized that both are caused by mutations in the same gene, *MVK*,[149,150] and represent the severe (MA) and mild (HIDS) ends of the clinical spectrum of the same disorder.[151] MKD is a rare disorder. Approximately 30 patients with MA have been reported.[152,153] The number of patients with HIDS worldwide is not known, but HIDS is rare. A study by van der Hilst et al. compiled clinical data for 103 HIDS patients,[154] and by 2010 only 134 MVK mutation-positive patients had signed up in the HIDS International registry (http://www.hids.net/index_files/HIDSregistry.htm).

Both MA and HIDS are characterized by recurrent episodes of high fever, but they primarily differ in the presence of neurological defects in MA and prognosis (MA is often fatal during childhood). Most MA patients show failure to thrive, mild to severe intellectual disability, recurrent febrile crises, hypotonia, and myopathy. Crises occur as often as 25 times per year and last on average four to five days with associated fever, vomiting, diarrhea, and, in some patients, arthralgia, subcutaneous edema, and morbilliform rash. Laboratory investigations show elevated erythrocyte sedimentation rate, C-reactive protein and leukocytosis, elevated immunoglobulins (classically IgD but also IgA and IgE),[155] and increased urinary excretion of inflammatory cytokine leukotriene E4.[156,157]

HIDS is generally considered a relatively benign condition, though young children may have frequent febrile episodes with significant discomfort. HIDS was recently categorized as an autoinflammatory disease characterized by systemic inflammation without apparent infectious etiology.[158,159] In HIDS, febrile attacks usually start before the end of the first year of life, occur every two to six weeks and last three to seven days. They are very similar to attacks in MA.[154] Between episodes, patients are free of symptoms. Symptomatic episodes are associated with increased concentrations of inflammatory cytokines such as TNF-α, IL-6, IFN-γ and anti-inflammatory molecules such as IL-ra and soluble TNF receptor p55 and p75.[160] Leukotriene E4 excretion is also increased in HIDS but only during febrile episodes.[161] Most but not all HIDS patients have continuously elevated IgD and high IgA.[150,155,162,163]

MKD diagnosis relies on DNA testing, urine and blood analysis of MVA, immunoglobulins, and enzyme activity. Typically, MVA urinary excretion is massive in MA (1-56 mol/mol creatinine) and correlates with the severity of the clinical presentation.[147] In HIDS the excretion is often 10-fold higher than normal between episodes[164] and increases 100- to 500-fold above normal during febrile episodes. Mevalonate concentration in urine, plasma, or cerebrospinal fluid may be elevated in HIDS especially during a febrile episode, but, unlike MA, lack of MVA elevation does not rule out MKD. IgD can be a useful initial screening test in the evaluation of recurrent fever. HIDS should be suspected in such cases when IgD is elevated (typically >100 U/ml or 141 mg/L). Assay of MK activity in white blood cells or cultured fibroblasts can be a useful adjunct in diagnosis, but activity in affected patients with HIDS may be close to the carrier range. Molecular genetic testing (*MVK* DNA mutation analysis) is now routinely available and is the diagnostic method of choice for HIDS. Prenatal diagnosis is possible for MA based on elevated levels of MVA and metabolites in maternal urine,[165,166] decreased MK activity in cultured aminocytes, or biopsied chorionic villus, or for MA or HIDS most reliably by DNA mutation analysis.

Treatment of MKD with dietary supplementation of cholesterol has shown no efficacy. Administration of ursodeoxycholic acid, ubiquinone, and vitamin E did not translate into measurable clinical or biochemical improvement in MA.[147] Statin treatment of MA improved inflammatory attacks in one study[151] but worsened the clinical presentation in another.[147] Conventional anti-inflammatory drugs such as thalidomide and nonsteroidal anti-inflammatory drugs have shown variable therapeutic benefit.[147,154,167] prednisone at high dose was effective in reducing severity and duration of crises but is not used routinely.[147,154] Targeted treatment of the inflammatory response seems more promising. Etanercept has shown efficacy in HIDS,[168–170] and treatment with anakinra, an interleukin-1 receptor antagonist significantly and rapidly improved disease manifestations.[154,168,171]

Pathogenesis

The pathogenesis of MKD is incompletely understood. The biochemical defect in MVA was described in 1986 by Hoffmann et al.[172] The gene defect causing MA was identified in

1992 by Schafer et al.[173] whereas the relationship between HIDS and *MVK* mutations was reported more than a decade ago.[149] A number of mutations of *MVK* have been reported, affecting the catalytic site of the enzyme, protein maturation, stability, and thermal inactivation.[174-176] Importantly, almost all characterized mutations result in MVK protein with decreased enzymatic activity. Overall, enzyme activity correlates with the severity of the disease, with no detectable activity in the cultured fibroblasts or lymphoblasts of patients with severe MA,[147,164] and a measurable activity (up to 28% of control) in the cells of HIDS patients.[177,178]

The metabolic consequences of MKD have been investigated in the hopes of identifying the precise pathways implicated in the pathogenesis of the disease. However, to date no satisfactory explanation of the clinical phenotype has been proposed. As expected, studies focused on the impact of MKD on the synthesis of downstream metabolites of the mevalonate pathway. Cellular cholesterol synthesis was reported as decreased or normal depending on culture conditions, but blood cholesterol, bile acid, and steroid hormone levels were normal in patients, suggesting that overall cholesterol homeostasis is not significantly impaired in MKD.[179,180] Small G protein prenylation also seems to be preserved, suggesting that MKD does not significantly impair the synthesis of nonsterol isoprenoids farnesyl-PP and geranylgeranyl-PP.[181] In contrast, the synthesis of other isoprenoids may be compromised. Most but not all studies with MA patients' skin fibroblasts and lymphoblasts have shown impaired synthesis of dolichol, coenzyme Q_{10}, and glycosylated macromolecules.[180,182,183] The deficiency in coenzyme Q_{10} seems more prevalent in MKD than the deficiency in dolichol. The concentration of dolichyl-P was found to be normal in the liver of a severely affected MA abortus.[184] In contrast, coenzyme Q_{10} deficiency was observed in the brain and liver of an aborted fetus with MKD and in MA patients' plasma.[147,182] However, in the absence of overt lactic acidosis, such deficiency is not thought to have a significant consequence on electron transport in the respiratory chain.[147]

Areas of Research

Great progress has been made in understanding the genetic, metabolic, and clinical presentation of MKD. However, the pathogenesis of the disease is still elusive, and there is no cure. The origin of the periodicity of the febrile episodes and its connection with a potential periodicity in isoprenoid deficiency, the molecular cause of hyperthermia, and the pathways implicated in selective IgD and IgA expression have not been identified. It has been proposed that the lack of mevalonate-derived isoprenoids may cause oxidative stress and lead to inflammation.[181,185] Studies showing that natural isoprenols (geraniol, farnesol, geranylgeraniol) prevent inflammation in a mouse model of MKD induced by alendronate-muramyldipeptide,[186] and others showing that drugs like statins and aminobiphosphonates that block the production of cellular isoprenoids can lead in vitro and in vivo to inflammation reactions[187,188] have been cited in support of this hypothesis. A recent study further showed that blocking protein farnesyltransferase with specific protein farnesyltransferase inhibitors to increase the production of geranylgeranyl-PP from farnesyl-PP in alendronate-treated mice and in monocytes isolated from MKD patients reduce the expression of inflammatory markers, suggesting that compounds that restore intracellular isoprenoid homeostasis may be beneficial in patients with MKD.[189] However, direct evidence for decreased levels of anti-inflammatory isoprenoids in MKD is lacking, and the alendronate mouse model does not fully reproduce the metabolic and clinical MKD phenotype. Further, most clinical and laboratory studies have shown that statins *inhibit* the activation of the immune response and have significant anti-inflammatory and antioxidant properties.[190-192] Thus a direct causal relationship between isoprenoid biosynthesis and inflammation in MKD remains largely unproven, and the development of relevant cellular and animal models (e.g., conditional KO mice) will be critical to further our understanding of the disease and help test new therapeutic strategies.

There have been only a few controlled trials in HIDS and MA patients. This is often the case with rare diseases, but it is perhaps also related to the absence of quantifiable surrogate biomarkers to gauge treatment efficacy. Studies that carefully monitor metabolic and inflammatory markers during the course of the disease may help identify such markers. Newer anti-inflammatory treatments (anti-TNF and IL-6 receptor antagonist) hold the promise of significant improvement in the quality of life of patients with MKD. However, multicenter trials will likely need to be designed to fully evaluate the benefits of these therapeutic options.

Steroid 5α-Reductase Type 3 Deficiency

A recent report describes a new type of congenital glycosylation disorder caused by mutations in the steroid 5α-reductase type 3 (*SRD5A3*) gene.[193] Patients present with a multisystemic syndrome that include mental retardation and ophthalmic and cerebellar defects. The gene was found to code not for a steroid reductase but for a protein with polyprenol reductase activity and key regulatory role in dolichol biosynthesis. It is too early to fully understand the pathogenesis of the disease. However, the study suggests that in affected patients, impaired dolichol synthesis alters posttranslational N-linked protein glycosylation and affects cell growth and differentiation, ultimately resulting in widespread tissue malformation and functional deficiencies.

Sjögren-Larsson Syndrome

Sjögren-Larsson syndrome is caused by inactivating mutations of the *ALDH3A2* gene coding for ER-bound fatty aldehyde dehydrogenase. The clinical presentation (mental retardation, seizures, congenital ichthyosis) and the molecular and metabolic basis of the disease are comprehensively treated in another chapter of this book. However, it is worth mentioning here the possibility that impaired isoprenoid biosynthesis is implicated in SLS pathogenesis. In a preliminary report by Roullet et al.,[194] the authors suggest that in SLS, the metabolism of short-chain isoprenols (farnesol and geranylgeraniol) into farnesoic and geranylgeranoic acids is compromised (Figure 9.1). Because isoprenols and related acids are implicated in cell growth and apoptosis, skin differentiation, and neuronal signaling, it is possible that impaired isoprenoid metabolism contributes to the SLS phenotype. More studies are needed to explore the relationship between fatty aldehyde dehydrogenase deficiency, isoprenoids, and disease symptoms.

References

1. Cooper MK, Wassif CA, Krakowiak PA, et al. A defective response to Hedgehog signaling in disorders of cholesterol biosynthesis. *Nature Genetics.* 2003; 33: 508–513.
2. Valnot I, von Kleist-Retzow JC, Barrientos A, et al. A mutation in the human heme A: farnesyltransferase gene (COX10) causes cytochrome c oxidase deficiency. *Hum Mol Gen.* 2000; 9: 1245–1249.
3. Rotig A, Appelkvist E-L, Geromel V, et al. Quinone-responsive multiple respiratory-chain dysfunction due to widespread coenzyme Q10 deficiency. *Lancet.* 2000; 356: 391–395.
4. Seabra MC, Ho YK, Anant JS. Deficient geranylgeranylation of Ram/Rab27 in choroideremia. *J Biol Chem.* 1995; 270: 24420–24427.
5. Menasche G, Pastural E, Feldman J, et al. Mutations in RAB27A cause Griscelli syndrome associated with haemophagocytic syndrome. *Nat Genet.* 2000; 25: 173–176.
6. Bergoffen J, Scherer SS, Wang S, et al. Connexin mutations in X-linked Charcot-Marie-Tooth disease. *Science.* 1993; 262: 2039–2042.
7. Huang Y, Sirkowski EE, Stickney JT, Scherer SS. Prenylation-defective human connexin 32 are normally localized and function equivalently to wild-type connexin 32 in myelinating Schwann cells. *J Neurosci.* 2005; 25(31): 7111–7120.
8. Smith DW, Lemli L, Opitz JM. A newly recognized syndrome of multiple congenital anomalies. *J Pediatr.* 1964; 64: 210–217.
9. Cunniff C, Kratz LE, Moser A, Natowicz MR, Kelley RI. Clinical and biochemical spectrum of patients with RSH/Smith-Lemli-Opitz syndrome and abnormal cholesterol metabolism. *Am J Med Genet.* 1997; 68: 263–269.
10. Ryan, AK, Bartlett K, Clayton P, et al. Smith-Lemli-Opitz syndrome: a variable clinical and biochemical phenotype. *J Med Genet.* 1998; 35: 558–565.
11. Battaile KP, Steiner RD. Smith-Lemli-Opitz syndrome: the first malformation syndrome associated with defective cholesterol synthesis. *Mol Genet Metab.* 2000; 71: 154–162.
12. Kelley RI, Hennekam RC. The Smith-Lemli-Opitz syndrome. *J Med Genet.* 2000; 37: 321–335.
13. Porter FD. RSH/Smith-Lemli-Opitz syndrome: a multiple congenital anomaly/mental retardation syndrome due to an inborn error of cholesterol biosynthesis. *Mol Genet Metab.* 2000; 71: 163–174.
14. Ginat S, Maslen CL, Connor WE, Porter FD, Steiner RD. Smith-Lemli-Opitz syndrome: a multiple malformation/ mental retardation syndrome caused by cholesterol synthesis. *Endocrinologist.* 2000; 10: 300–301.
15. Nwokoro NA, Wassif CA, Porter FD. Genetic disorders of cholesterol biosynthesis in mice and humans. *Mol Genet Metab.* 2001; 74: 105–119.
16. Waye JS, Nakamura LM, Eng B, et al. Smith-Lemli-Opitz syndrome: carrier frequency and spectrum of DHCR7 mutations in Canada. *J Med Genet.* 2002; 39: E31.
17. Battaile KP, Battaile BC, Merkens LS, Maslen CL, Steiner RD. Carrier frequency of the common mutation IVS8-1G>C in DHCR7 and estimate of the expected incidence of Smith-Lemli-Opitz syndrome. *Mol Genet Metab.* 2001; 72: 67–71.
18. Nowaczyk,MJ, McCaughey D, Whelan DT, Porter FD. Incidence of Smith-Lemli-Opitz syndrome in Ontario, Canada. *Am J Med Genet.* 2001; 102: 18–20.
19. Nowaczyk MJ, Nakamura LM, Eng B, Porter FD, Waye JS. Frequency and ethnic distribution of the common DHCR7 mutation in Smith-Lemli-Opitz syndrome. *Am J Med Genet.* 2001; 102: 383–386.
20. Mueller C, Patel S, Irons M, et al. Normal cognition and behavior in a Smith-Lemli-Opitz syndrome patient who presented with Hirschsprung disease. *Am J Med Genet, Part A.* 2003; 123: 100–106.
21. Langius FA, Waterham HR, Romeijn GJ, et al. Identification of three patients with a very mild form of Smith-Lemli-Opitz syndrome. *Am J Med Genet, Part A.* 2003; 122: 24–29.
22. Sikora DM, Ruggiero M, Pettit-Kekel K, Merkens LS, Connor WE, Steiner RD. Cholesterol supplementation does not improve developmental progress in Smith-Lemli- Opitz syndrome. *J Pediatr.* 2004; 144: 783–791.
23. Tierney E, Nwokoro NA, Kelley RI. Behavioral phenotype of RSH/Smith-Lemli- Opitz syndrome. *Ment Retard Dev Disabil Res Rev.* 2000; 6: 131–134.
24. Sikora DM, Pettit-Kekel K, Penfield J, Merkens LS, Steiner RD. The near universal presence of autism spectrum disorders in children with Smith-Lemli-Opitz syndrome. *Am J Med Genet, Part A.* 2006; 140: 1511–1518.
25. Tierney E, Bukelis I, Thompson RE, et al. Abnormalities of cholesterol metabolism in autism spectrum disorders. *Am J Med Genet, Part B.* 2006; 141: 666–668.

26. Tierney E, Nwokoro NA, Porter FD, Freund LS, Ghuman JK, Kelley RI. Behavior phenotype in the RSH/Smith-Lemli-Opitz syndrome. *Am J Med Genet*. 2001; 98:191–200.
27. Honda A, Tint GS, Salen G, Batta AK, Chen TS, Shefer S. Defective conversion of 7-dehydrocholesterol to cholesterol in cultured skin fibroblasts from Smith-Lemli-Opitz syndrome homozygotes. *J Lipid Res*. 1995; 36: 1595–1601.
28. Shefer S, Salen G, Batta AK, et al. Markedly inhibited 7-dehydrocholesterol-delta 7-reductase activity in liver microsomes from Smith-Lemli-Opitz homozygotes. *J Clin Invest*. 1995; 96: 1779–1785.
29. Irons M, Elias ER, Salen G, Tint GS, Batta AK. Defective cholesterol biosynthesis in Smith-Lemli-Opitz syndrome. *Lancet*. 1993; 341: 1414.
30. Tint GS. Cholesterol defect in Smith-Lemli-Opitz syndrome. *Am J Med Genet*. 1993; 47: 573–574.
31. Batta AK, Salen G, Tint GS, Shefer S. Identification of 19-nor-5,7,9(10)- cholestatrien-3 beta-ol in patients with Smith-Lemli-Opitz syndrome. *J Lipid Res*. 1995; 36: 2413–2418.
32. Batta AK, Tint GS, Shefer S, Abuelo D, Salen G. Identification of 8- dehydrocholesterol (cholesta-5,8-dien-3 beta-ol) in patients with Smith-Lemli-Opitz syndrome. *J Lipid Res*. 1995; 36: 705–713.
33. Ruan B, Wilson WK, Pang J, et al. Sterols in blood of normal and Smith-Lemli-Opitz subjects. *J Lipid Res*. 2001; 42: 799–812.
34. Tint GS, Irons M, Elias ER, et al. Defective cholesterol biosynthesis associated with the Smith-Lemli- Opitz syndrome. *N Engl J Med*. 1994; 330: 107–113.
35. Fitzky BU, Witsch-Baumgartner M, Erdel M, et al. Mutations in the Delta7-sterol reductase gene in patients with the Smith-Lemli-Opitz syndrome. *Proc Natl Acad Sci USA*. 1998; 95: 8181–8186.
36. Wassif CA, Maslen C, Kachilele-Linjewile S, et al. Mutations in the human sterol delta7-reductase gene at 11q12–13 cause Smith-Lemli-Opitz syndrome. *Am J Hum Genet*. 1998; 63: 55–62.
37. Waterham HR, Wijburg FA, Hennekam RC, et al. Smith-Lemli-Opitz syndrome is caused by mutations in the 7- dehydrocholesterol reductase gene. *Am J Hum Genet*. 1998; 63: 329–338.
38. Correa-Cerro LS, Porter FD. 3beta-hydroxysterol Delta7-reductase and the Smith-Lemli-Opitz syndrome. *Mol Genet Metab*. 2005; 84: 112–126.
39. Bradley LA, Palomaki GE, Knight GJ, et al. Levels of unconjugated estriol and other maternal serum markers in pregnancies with Smith-Lemli-Opitz (RSH) syndrome fetuses. *Am J Med Genet*. 1999; 82: 355–358.
40. Shackleton CH, Marcos J, Palomaki GE, et al. Dehydrosteroid measurements in maternal urine or serum for the prenatal diagnosis of Smith-Lemli-Opitz syndrome (SLOS). *Am J Med Genet, Part A*. 2007; 143: 2129–2136.
41. Wassif CA, Vied D, Tsokos M, Connor WE, Steiner RD, Porter FD. Cholesterol storage defect in RSH/Smith-Lemli-Opitz syndrome fibroblasts. *Mol Genet Metab*. 2002; 75: 325–334.
42. Fitzky BU, Moebius FF, Asaoka H, et al. 7-Dehydrocholesterol-dependent proteolysis of HMG-CoA reductase suppresses sterol biosynthesis in a mouse model of Smith-Lemli-Opitz/RSH syndrome. *J Clin Invest*. 2001; 108(6): 905–915.
43. Megha, Bakht O, London E. Cholesterol precursors stabilize ordinary and ceramide-rich ordered lipid domains (lipid rafts) to different degrees: implications for the Bloch hypothesis and sterol biosynthesis disorders. *J Biol Chem*. 2006; 281: 21903–21913.
44. Gondre-Lewis MC, Petrache HI, Wassif CA, et al. Abnormal sterols in cholesterol-deficiency diseases cause secretory granule malformation and decreased membrane curvature. *J Cell Sci*. 2006; 119: 1876–1885.
45. Tulenko TN, Boeze-Battaglia K, Mason RP, et al. A membrane defect in the pathogenesis of the Smith-Lemli-Opitz syndrome. *J Lipid Res*. 2006; 47: 134–143.
46. Fliesler SJ, Peachey NS, Richards MJ, Nagel BA, Vaughan DK. Retinal degeneration in a rodent model of Smith-Lemli-Opitz syndrome: electrophysiologic, biochemical, and morphologic features. *Arch Ophthalmol*. 2004; 122: 1190–1200.
47. Elias ER, Fulton A, Mayer DL, Hansen RM. Retinal dysfunction in patients with the Smith-Lemli-Opitz syndrome. *A J Hum Gen*. 2000; 67(4 Suppl. 2): 36 A132.
48. Elias ER, Hansen RM, Irons M, Quinn NB, Fulton AB. Rod photoreceptor responses in children with Smith-Lemli-Opitz syndrome. *Arch Ophthalmol*. 2003; 121: 1738–1743.
49. Porter JA, Young KE, Beachy PA. Cholesterol modification of hedgehog signaling proteins in animal development. *Science*. 1996; 274(5285): 255–259.
50. Mann RK, Beachy PA. Cholesterol modification of proteins. *Biochim Biophys Acta*. 2000; 1529: 188–202.

51. Cooper MK, Wassif CA, Krakowiak PA, et al. A defective response to Hedgehog signaling in disorders of cholesterol biosynthesis. *Nat Genet.* 2003; 33: 508–513.
52. Valencia A, Rajadurai A, Carle AB, Kochevar IE. 7-Dehydrocholesterol enhances ultraviolet A-induced oxidative stress in keratinocytes: roles of NADPH oxidase, mitochondria, and lipid rafts. *Free Rad Biol Med.* 2006; 41: 1704–1718.
53. Chignell CF, Kukielczak BM, Sik RH, Bilski PJ, He YY. Ultraviolet A sensitivity in Smith-Lemli-Opitz syndrome: possible involvement of cholesta-5,7,9(11)-trien-3beta-ol. *Free Radical Bio Med.* 2006; 41: 339–346.
54. Wassif CA, Zhu P, Kratz L, et al. Biochemical, phenotypic and neurophysiological characterization of a genetic mouse model of RSH/Smith-Lemli-Opitz syndrome. *Hum Mol Genet.* 2001; 10: 555–564.
55. Yu H, Li M, Tint GS, Chen J, Xu G, Patel SB. Selective reconstitution of liver cholesterol biosynthesis promotes lung maturation but does not prevent neonatal lethality in Dhcr7 null mice. *BMC Dev Biol.* 2007; 7: 27–42.
56. Correa-Cerro LS, Wassif CA, Kratz L, et al. Development and characterization of a hypomorphic Smith-Lemli-Opitz syndrome mouse model and efficacy of simvastatin therapy. *Hum Mol Genet.* 2006; 15: 839–851.
57. Lutjohann D, von Bergmann K. 24S-hydroxycholesterol: a marker of brain cholesterol metabolism. *Pharmacopsychiatry.* 2003; 36(Suppl. 2): S102–S106.
58. Björkhem I, Lutjohann D, Breuer O, Sakinis A, Wennmalm A. Importance of a novel oxidative mechanism for elimination of brain cholesterol: turnover of cholesterol and 24(S)-hydroxycholesterol in rat brain as measured with $^{18}O_2$ techniques in vivo and in vitro. *J Biol Chem.* 1997; 272: 30178–30184.
59. Björkhem I, Lutjohann D, Diczfalusy U, Stahle L, Ahlborg G, Wahren J. Cholesterol homeostasis in human brain: turnover of 24S- hydroxycholesterol and evidence for a cerebral origin of most of this oxysterol in the circulation. *J Lipid Res.* 1998; 39: 1594–1600.
60. Björkhem I, Starck L, Andersson U, et al. Oxysterols in the circulation of patients with the Smith-Lemli-Opitz syndrome: abnormal levels of 24S- and 27-hydroxycholesterol. *J Lipid Res.* 2001; 42: 366–371.
61. Xiong Q, Ruan B, Whitby FG, et al. A colorimetric assay for 7-dehydrocholesterol with potential application for Smith-Lemli-Opitz syndrome. *Chem Phys Lipids.* 2002; 115: 1–15.
62. Linck LM, Lin DS, Flavell D, Connor WE, Steiner RD. Cholesterol supplementation with egg yolk increases plasma cholesterol and decreases plasma 7-dehydrocholesterol in Smith-Lemli-Opitz syndrome. *Am J Med Genet.* 2000; 93: 360–365.
63. Gofflot F, Gaoua W, Bourguignon L, Roux C, Picard JP. Expression of Sonic Hedgehog downstream genes is modified in rat embryos exposed in utero to a distal inhibitor of cholesterol biosynthesis. *Dev Dyn.* 2001; 220: 99–111.
64. Gaoua W, Wolf C, Chevy F, Ilien F, Roux C. Cholesterol deficit but not accumulation of aberrant sterols is the major cause of the teratogenic activity in the Smith-Lemli-Opitz syndrome animal model. *J Lipid Res.* 2000; 41: 637–646.
65. Xu G, Servatius RJ, Shefer S, et al. Relationship between abnormal choesterol synthesis and retarded learning in rats. *Metabolism.* 1998; 47: 878–882.
66. Xu G, Salen G, Shefer S, et al. Treatment of the cholesterol biosynthetic defect in Smith-Lemli-Opitz syndrome reproduced in rats by BM 15.766. *Gastroenterology.* 1995; 109: 1301–1307.
67. Irons M, Elias ER, Tint GS, et al. Abnormal cholesterol metabolism in the Smith-Lemli-Opitz syndrome: report of clinical and biochemical findings in four patients and treatment in one patient. *Am J Med Genet.* 1994; 50: 347–352.
68. Elias ER, Irons MB, Hurley AD, Tint GS, Salen G. Clinical effects of cholesterol supplementation in six patients with the Smith-Lemli-Opitz syndrome (SLOS). *Am J Med Genet.* 1997; 68: 305–310.
69. Nwokoro NA, Mulvihill JJ. Cholesterol and bile acid replacement therapy in children and adults with Smith-Lemli-Opitz (SLO/RSH) syndrome. *Am J Med Genet.* 1997; 68: 315–321.
70. Martin A, Koenig K, Scahill L, Tierney E, Porter FD, Nwokoro NA. Smith-Lemli-Opitz syndrome. *J Am Acad Child Adolesc Psychiatry.* 2001; 40: 506–507.
71. Kelley RI. RSH/Smilth-Lemli-Opitz syndrome: mutations and metabolic morphogenesis. *Am J Hum Genet.* 1998; 63: 322–326.
72. Jira PE, Wevers RA, de Long J, et al. A new therapeutic approach for Smith-Lemli-Opitz syndrome. *J Lipid Res.* 2000; 41: 1339–1346.
73. Starck L, Lovgren-Sandblom A, Björkhem I. Simvastatin treatment in the SLOS syndrome: a safe approach? *Am J Med Genet.* 2002; 113: 183–189.

74. Haas D, Garbade SF, Vohwinkel C, et al. Effects of cholesterol and simvastatin treatment in patients with Smith-Lemli-Opitz syndrome (SLOS). *J Inherit Metab Dis*. 2007; 30: 375–387.
75. Wagner AH, Kohler T, Ruckschloss U, Just I, Hecker, M. Improvement of nitric oxide-dependent vasodilatation by HMG-CoA reductase inhibitors through attenuation of endothelial superoxide anion formation. *Arterioscler Thromb Vasc Biol*. 2000; 20: 61–69.
76. Delbosc S, Morena M, Djouad F, Ledoucen C, Descomps B, Cristol JP. Statins, 3-hydroxy-3-methylglutaryl coenzyme A reductase inhibitors, are able to reduce superoxide anion production by NADPH oxidase in THP-1-derived monocytes. *J Cardiovasc Pharmacol*. 2002; 40: 611–617.
77. Norata GD, Pirillo A, Catapano AL. Statins and oxidative stress during atherogenesis. *J Cardiovasc Risk*. 2003; 10: 181–189.
78. Wassif CA, Krakowiak PA, Wright BS, et al. Residual cholesterol synthesis and simvastatin induction of cholesterol synthesis in Smith-Lemli-Opitz syndrome fibroblasts. *Mol Genet Metab*. 2005; 85: 96–107.
79. Jira P, Wevers R, de Jong J, Rubio-Gozalbo E, Smeitink J. New treatment strategy for Smith-Lemli-Opitz syndrome. *Lancet*. 1997; 349: 1222.
80. Lin DS, Steiner RD, Flavell DP, Connor WE. Intestinal absorption of cholesterol by patients with Smith-Lemli-Opitz syndrome. *Pediatr Res*. 2005; 57: 765–770.
81. Vega GL, Weiner MF, Lipton AM, et al. Reduction in levels of 24S-hydroxycholesterol by statin treatment in patients with Alzheimer disease. *Arch Neurol*. 2003; 60(4): 510–515.
82. Rossi M, Vajro P, Iorio R, et al. Characterization of liver involvement in defects of cholesterol biosynthesis: long-term follow-up and review. *Am J Med Genet. Part A*. 2005; 132: 144–151.
83. Heuman DM, Pandak WM, Hylemon PB, Vlahcevic ZR. Conjugates of ursodeoxycholate protect against cytotoxicity of more hydrophobic bile salts: in vitro studies in rat hepatocytes and human erythrocytes. *Hepatology*. 1991; 14: 920–926.
84. Matabosch X, Ying L, Serra M, et al. Increasing cholesterol synthesis in 7-dehydrosterol reductase (DHCR7) deficient mouse models through gene transfer. *J Steroid Biochem Mol Biol*. 2010; 122: 303–309.
85. Merkens LS, Wassif C, Healy K, et al. Smith-Lemli-Opitz syndrome and inborn errors of cholesterol synthesis: summary of the 2007 SLO/RSH Foundation scientific conference sponsored by the National Institutes of Health. *Genet Med*. 2009; 11(5): 359–364.
86. Irons MB, Nores J, Stewart TL, et al. Antenatal therapy of Smith-Lemli-Opitz syndrome. *Fetal Diagn Ther*. 1999; 14: 133–137.
87. McConihay JA, Horn PS, Woollett LA. Effect of maternal hypercholesterolemia on fetal sterol metabolism in the Golden Syrian hamster. *J Lipid Res*. 2001; 42: 1111–1119.
88. Woollett LA. Maternal cholesterol in fetal development: transport of cholesterol from maternal to fetal circulation. *Am J Clin Nutr*. 2005; 82: 1155–1161.
89. Setogushi T, Salen G, Tint GS, Mosbach EH. A biochemical abnormality in cerebrotendinous xanthomatosis: impairment of bile acid biosynthesis associated with incomplete degradation of the cholesterol side chain. *J Clin Invest*. 1974; 531: 1393–1401.
90. Van Bogaert L, Scherer HJ, Epstein E. *Une forme cérébrale de cholestérinose généralisée*. Paris: Masson & Cie; 1937.
91. Björkhem I, Hansson M. Cerebrotendinous xanthomatosis: an inborn error in bile acid synthesis with defined mutations but still a challenge. *Biochem Biophys Res Commun*. 2010; 396: 46–49.
92. Calli JJ, Hsieh CL, Franke U, Russell DW. Mutations in the bile acid biosynthetic enzyme sterol 27-hydroxylase underlie cerebrotendinous xanthomatosis. *J Biol Chem*. 1991; 266: 7779–7783.
93. Gallus GN, Dotti MT, Federico A. Clinical and molecular diagnosis of cerebrotendinous xanthomatosis with a review of the mutations in the CYP27A1 gene. *Neurol Sci*. 2006; 27: 143–149.
94. Björkhem I, Skrede S, Buchmann MS, East C, Grundy S. Accumulation of 7α-hydroxy-4-cholesten-3-one and cholesta-4,6-dien-3-one in patients with CTX: effect of treatment with chenodeoxycholic acid. *Hepatology*. 1997; 7: 266–271.
95. Menkes JH, Schimschock JR, Swanson PD. Cerebrotendinous xanthomatosis: the storage of cholestanol within the nervous system. *Arch Neurol*. 1968; 19: 47–53.
96. Salen G. Cholestanol deposition in cerebrotendinous xanthomatosis: a possible mechanism. *Ann Intern Med*. 1971; 75: 843–851.
97. Shefer S, Cheng FW, Dayal B, et al. A 25-hydroxylase pathway of cholic acid biosynthesis in man and rat. *J Clin Invest*. 1976; 57: 897–903.

98. Björkhem I, Oftebro H, Skrede S, Pedersen JI. Assay of intermediates in bile acid biosynthesis using isotope dilution-mass spectrometry: hepatic levels in the normal state and in cerebrotendinous xanthomatosis. *J. Lipid Res*. 1981; 22: 191–200.
99. Berginer VM, Salen G, Shefer S. Long term reatment of cerebrotendinous xanthomatosis with chenodeoxycholic acid. *NEJM*. 1984; 311(26): 1649–1652.
100. Berginer VM, Gross B, Morad K, et al. Chronic diarrhea and juvenile cataracts: think cerebrotendinous xanthomatosis and treat. *Pediatrics*. 2009;123: 143-147
101. Ginanneschi F, Mignarri A, Mondelli M,et al. Polyneuropathy in cerebrotendinous xanthomatosis and response to treatment with chenodeoxycholic acid. *J Neurol*. 2013;260: 268-274
102. Seyama Y, Ichikawa K, Yamakawa T. Quantitative determination of cholestanol in plasma with mass fragmentography: biochemical diagnosis of cerebrotendinous xanthomatosis. *J Biochem*. 1976; 80: 223–228.
103. Koopman BJ, Molen JC, Wolthers BG, Waterrreus RJ. Screening for CTX by using an enzymatic assay for 7α-hydroxylated steroids in urine. *Clin Chem*. 1987; 33: 142–143.
104. DeBarber AE, Connor WE, Pappu AS, Merkens LS, Steiner RD. ESI-MS/MS quantification of 7α-hydroxy-4-cholesten-3-one facilitates rapid, convenient diagnostic testing for cerebrotendinous xanthomatosis. *Clin Chim Acta*. 2009; 411: 43–48.
105. Moebius FF, Fitzky BU, Glossmann H. Genetic defects in postsqualene cholesterol biosynthesis. *Trends Endocrinol Metab*. 2000; 11: 106–114.
106. Kelley, RI, Herman GE. Inborn errors of sterol biosynthesis. *Annu Rev Genomics Hum Genet*. 2001; 2: 299–341.
107. Haas D, Kelley RI, Hoffmann GF. Inherited disorders of cholesterol biosynthesis. *Neuropediatrics*. 2001; 32: 113–122.
108. Porter, FD. Human malformation syndromes due to inborn errors of cholesterol synthesis. *Curr Opin Pediatr*. 2003; 15: 607–613.
109. Herman GE. Disorders of cholesterol biosynthesis: prototypic metabolic malformation syndromes. *Hum Mol Genet*. 2003; 12: 75–88.
110. König A, Happle R, Bornholdt D, Engel H, Grzeschik KH. Mutations in the NSDHL gene, encoding a 3beta-hydroxysteroid dehydrogenase, cause CHILD syndrome. *Am J Med Genet*. 2000; 90: 339–346.
111. Happle R. X-linked dominant chondrodysplasia punctata. *Hum Genet*. 1979; 53: 65–73.
112. Andersson HC, Kratz L, Kelley R. Desmosterolosis presenting with multiple congenital anomalies and profound developmental delay. *Am J Med Genet*. 2002; 113: 315–319.
113. Waterham HR, Koster J, Romeijn GJ, et al. Mutations in the 3β-hydroxysterol Δ^{24}-reductase gene cause desmosterolosis, an autosomal recessive disorder of cholesterol biosynthesis. *Am J Hum Genet*. 2001; 69: 685–694.
114. Brunetti-Pierri N, Corso G, Rossi M, et al. Lathosterolosis, a novel multiple-malformation/mental retardation syndrome due to deficiency of 3beta-hydroxysteroiddelta5-desaturase. *Am J Hum Genet*. 2002; 71: 952–958.
115. Rossi M, D'Armiento M, Parisi I, et al. Clinical phenotype of lathosterolosis. *Am J Med Genet*. 2007; 143A: 2371–2381.
116. Ho AC, Fung CW, Siu TS, et al. Lathosterolosis: a disorder of cholesterol biosynthesis resembling Smith-Lemli-Opitz syndrome. *JIMD Rep*. 2014; 12: 129–134.
117. Flück CE, Tajima T, Pandey AV, et al. Mutant P450 oxidoreductase causes disordered steroidogenesis with and without Antley–Bixler syndrome. *Nat Genet*. 2004; 36: 228–230.
118. He M, Kratz LE, Michel JJ, et al. Mutations in the human SC4MOL gene encoding a methyl sterol oxidase cause psoriasiform dermatitis, microcephaly, and developmental delay. *J Clin Invest*. 2011; 121: 976–984.
119. He M, Smith LD, Chang R, Li X, Vockley J. The role of sterol-C4-methyl oxidase in epidermal biology. *Biochim Biophys Acta*. 2014; 1841: 331–335.
120. Bornholdt D, König A, Happle R, et al. Mutational spectrum of NSDHL in CHILD syndrome. *J Med Genet*. 2005; 42: e17. http://www.jmedgent.com/cgi/content/full/42/2/e17
121. Grange DK, Kratz LE, Braverman NE, Kelley RI. CHILD syndrome caused by deficiency of 3β-hydroxysteroid-Δ^8, Δ^7-isomerase. *Am J Med Genet* 2000; 90; 328–335.
122. Kolb-Maurer A, Grzeschick KH, Haas D, Brocker EB, Hamm H. Conradi-Hunermann-Happle syndrome (X-linked dominant chondrodysplasia punctata) confirmed by plasma sterol and mutation analysis. *Acta Dermato-Venereol*. 2008; 88: 47–51.

123. Ausavarat S, Tanpaiboon P, Tongkobpetch S, Suphapeetiporn K, Shotelersuk V. Two novel EBP mutations in Conradi-Hunermann-Happle syndrome. *Eur J Dermatol* 2008; 18: 391–393.
124. Milunsky JM, Maher TA, Metzenberg AB. Molecular, biochemical, and phenotypic analysis of a hemizygous male with a severe atypical phenotype for X-linked Dominant Conradi-Hunermann-Happle syndrome and a mutation in EBP. *Am J Hum Gen*. 2003; 116: 249–254.
125. Wu C, Miloslavskaya I, Demontis S, Maestro R, Galaktionov K. Regulation of cellular response to oncogenic and oxidative stress by Seladin-1. *Nature*. 2004; 432: 640–645.
126. Lu X, Kambe F, Cao X, et al. DHCR24 is a hydrogen peroxide scavenger, protecting cells from oxidative-stress-induced apoptosis. *Endocrinology*. 2008; 149: 3267–3273.
127. Batistat M-C, Roberge C, Matinez A, Gallo-Payet N. 24-Dehydrocholesterol reductase/Seladin-1: a key protein differentially involved in adrenocorticotropin effects observed in human and rat adrenal cortex. *Endocrinology*. 2009; 150: 4180–4190.
128. Calvo PL, Brunati A, Spada M, et al. Liver transplantation in defects of cholesterol biosynthesis: the case of lathosterolosis. *Am. J. Transplant*. 2014;14: 960–965.
129. Arlt W, Walker EA, Draper N, et al. Congenital adrenal hyperplasia caused by mutant P450 oxidoreductase and human androgen synthesis: analytical study. *Lancet*. 2004; 363: 2128–2135.
130. Adachi M, Tachibana K, Asakura Y, Yamamoto T, Hanaki K, Oka A. Compound heterozygous mutations of cytochrome P450 oxidoreductase gene (POR) in two patients with Antley–Bixler syndrome. *Am J Med Genet, Part A*. 2004; 128: 333–339.
131. Ko JM, Cheon CK, Kim GH, Yoo HW. A case of Antley–Bixler syndrome caused by compound heterozygous mutations of the cytochrome P450 oxidoreductase gene. *Eur J Pediatr*. 2009; 168: 877–880.
132. Lijima S, Ohishi A, Ohzeki T. Cytochrome P450 oxidoreductase deficiency with Antley–Bixler syndrome: steroidogenic capacities. *J Pediatr Endocrinol*. 2009; 22: 469–475.
133. But WM, Lo IF, Shek CC, Tse WY, Lam ST. Ambiguous genitalia, impaired steroidogenesis, and Antley–Bixler syndrome in a patient with P450 oxidoreductase deficiency. *Hong Kong Med J*. 2010; 16: 59–62.
134. Kelley RI, Kratz LE, Glaser RL, Netzloff ML, Wolf LM, Jabs EW. Abnormal sterol metabolism in a patient with Antley–Bixler syndrome and ambiguous genitalia. *Am J Med Genet*. 2002; 110: 95–102.
135. Greenberg CR, Rimoin DL, Gruber HE, DeSa DJ, Reed M, Lachman RS. A new autosomal recessive lethal chondrodystrophy with congenital hydrops. *Am J Med Genet*. 1988; 29: 623–632.
136. Chitayat D, Gruber H, Mullen BJ, et al. Hydrops-ectopic calcification-moth-eaten skeletal dysplasia (Greenberg dysplasia): prenatal diagnosis and further delineation of a rare genetic disorder. *Am J Med Genet*. 1993; 47: 272–277.
137. Horn LC, Faber R, Meiner A, Piskazeck U, Spranger J. Greenberg dysplasia: first reported case with additional nonskeletal malformations and without consanguinity. *Prenat Diagn*. 2000; 20: 1008–1011.
138. Konstantinidou A, Karadimas C, Waterham HR, et al. Pathologic, radiographic and molecular findings in three fetuses diagnosed with HEM/Greenberg skeletal dysplasia. *Prenat. Diagn*. 2008;28: 309-312
139. Waterham HR, Koster J, Mooyer P, et al. Autosomal recessive HEM/Greenberg skeletal dysplasia is caused by 3β-hydroxysterol Δ^{14}-reductase deficiency due to mutations in the lamin B receptor gene. *Am J Hum Genet*. 2003; 72: 1013–1017.
140. Wassif CA, Brownson KE, Sterner AL, et al. HEM dysplasia and ichthyosis are likely laminopathies and not due to 3betahydroxysterol Δ^{14}-reductase deficiency. *Hum Mol Genet*. 2007; 16: 1176–1187.
141. Goldstein JL, Brown MS. Regulation of the mevalonate pathway. *Nature*. 1990; 343: 425–430.
142. Ericsson J, Dallner G. Distribution, biosynthesis, and function of the mevalonate pathway lipids. *SubCell Biochem*. 1993; 21: 229–272.
143. Buhaescu I, Izzedine H. Mevalonate pathway: a review of clinical and therapeutical implications. *Clin Biochem*. 2007; 40: 575–584.
144. Fritz G. Targeting the mevalonate pathway for improved cancer therapy. *Curr. Cancer Drug Targets*. 2009; 9: 626–638.
145. Zeiser R, Maas K, Youssef S, Durr C, Steinman L, Negrin RS. Regulation of different inflammatory diseases by impacting the mevalonate pathway. *Immunology*. 2009; 127: 18–25.
146. Joo JH, Jetten AM. Molecular mechanisms involved in farnesol-induced apoptosis. *Cancer Lett*. 2010; 287: 123–135.
147. Hoffmann GF, Charpentier C, Mayatepek E, et al. Clinical and biochemical phenotype in 11 patients with mevalonic aciduria. *Pediatrics*. 1993; 91: 915–921.

148. van der Meer JW, Vossen JM, Radl J, et al. Hyperimmunoglobulinaemia D and periodic fever: a new syndrome. *Lancet.* 1984;1:1087-1090.
149. Drenth JP, Cuisset L, Grateau G, et al. Mutations in the gene encoding mevalonate kinase cause hyper-IgD and periodic fever syndrome: International Hyper-IgD Study Group. *Nat Genet.* 1999; 22: 178–181.
150. Houten SM, Kuis W, Duran M, et al. Mutations in MVK, encoding mevalonate kinase, cause hyperimmunoglobulinaemia D and periodic fever syndrome. *Nat Genet.* 1999; 22: 175–177.
151. Simon A, Drewe E, van der Meer JWM, et al. Simvastatin treatment for inflammatory attacks of the hyperimmunoglobulinemia D and periodic fever syndrome. *Clin Pharmacol Ther.* 2004; 75: 476–483.
152. Bretón Martínez JR, Cánovas Martínez A, Casaña Pérez S, Escribá Alepuz J, Giménez Vázquez F. Mevalonic aciduria: report of two cases. *J Inherit Metab Dis.* 2007; 30: 829.
153. Neven B, Valayannopoulos V, Quartier P, et al. Allogeneic bone marrow transplantation in mevalonic aciduria. *N Engl J Med.* 2007; 26: 2700–2703.
154. van der Hilst JC, Bodar EJ, Barron KS, et al. Long-term follow-up, clinical features, and quality of life in a series of 103 patients with hyperimmunoglobulinemia D syndrome. *Medicine.* 2008; 87: 301–310.
155. Haas D, Hoffman GF. Mevalonate kinase deficiencies: from mevalonic aciduria to hyperimmunoglobulinemia D syndrome. *Orphanet J Rare Dis.* 2006; 1: 13.
156. Mayatepek E, Hoffmann GF, Bremer HJ. Enhanced urinary excretion of leukotriene E_4 in patients with mevalonate kinase deficiency. *J Pediatr.* 1993; 123: 96–98.
157. Mayatepek E, Tiepelmann B, Hoffmann GF. Enhanced excretion of urinary leukotriene E4 in mevalonic aciduria is not caused by an impaired peroxisomal degradation of cysteinyl leukotrienes. *J Inherit Metab Dis.* 1997; 20: 721–722.
158. Mandey SH, Schneiders MS, Koster J, Waterham HR. Mutational spectrum and genotype-phenotype correlations in mevalonate kinase deficiency. *Hum Mutat.* 2006; 27: 796–802.
159. Goldsmith DP. Periodic fever syndromes. *Pediatrics in Review.* 2009; 30: e34–e41
160. Drenth JP, van Deuren M, van der Ven-Jongekrijg J, Schalkwijk CG, van der Meer JW. Cytokine activation during attacks of the hyperimmunoglobulinemia D and periodic fever syndrome. *Blood.* 1995; 85: 3586–3593.
161. Frenkel J, Willemsen MA, Weemaes CM, Dorland L, Mayatepek E. Increased urinary leukotriene E(4) during febrile attacks in the hyperimmunoglobulinaemia D and periodic fever syndrome. *Arch Dis Child.* 2001; 85: 158–159.
162. Haraldsson A, Weemaes CM, De Boer AW, Bakkeren JA, Stoelinga GB Immunological studies in the hyper-immunoglobulin D syndrome. *J Clin Immunol.* 1992; 12: 424–428.
163. Klasen IS, Goertz JH, van de Weil GA, Weemaes CM, van der Meer JW, Drenth JP. Hyper-immunoglubulin A in the hyperimmunoglobulinemia D syndrome. *Clin Diagn Lab Immunol.* 2001; 8: 58–61.
164. Houten SM, Romeijn GJ, Koster J, et al. Identification and characterization of three novel missense mutations in mevalonate kinase cDNA causing mevalonic aciduria, a disorder of isoprene biosynthesis. *Hum Mol Genet.* 1999; 8: 1523–1528.
165. Hoffmann G, Sweetman L, Bremer HJ, et al. Facts and artefacts in mevalonic aciduria: development of a stable isotope dilution GCMS assay for mevalonic acid and its application to physiological fluids, tissue samples, prenatal diagnosis and carrier detection. *Clin Chim Acta.* 1991; 198: 209–227.
166. Mancini J, Philip N, Chabrol B, Divry P, Rolland MO, Pinsard N. Mevalonic aciduria in 3 siblings: a new recognizable metabolic encephalopathy. *Pediatr Neurol.* 1993; 9: 243–246.
167. Drenth JP, Vonk AG, Simon A, Powell R, van der Meer JW. Limited efficacy of thalidomide in the treatment of febrile attacks of the hyper-IgD and periodic fever syndrome: a randomized, double-blind, placebo-controlled trial. *J Pharmacol Exp Ther.* 2001; 298: 1221–1226.
168. Bodar EJ, van der Hilst JC, Drenth JP, van der Meer JW, Simon A. Effect of etanercept and anakinra on inflammatory attacks in the hyper-IgD syndrome: introducing a vaccination provocation model. *Neth J Med.* 2005; 63: 260–264.
169. Demirkaya E, Caglar MK, Waterham HR, Topaloglu R, Ozen S. A patient with hyper-IgD syndrome responding to anti-TNF treatment. *Clin Rheumatol.* 2007; 26: 1757–1759.
170. Topaloglu R, Ayaz NA, Waterham HR, Yuce A, Gumruk F, Sanal O. Hyperimmunoglobulinemia D and periodic fever syndrome; treatment with etanercept and follow-up. *Clin Rheumatol.* 2008; 27: 1317–1320.
171. Lequerré T, Vittecoq O, Pouplin S, et al. Mevalonate kinase deficiency syndrome with structural damage responsive to anikinra. *Rheumatol.* 2007; 46: 1862–1863.

172. Hoffmann G, Gibson KM, Brandt IK, Bader PI, Wappner RS, Sweetman L. Mevalonic aciduria—an inborn error of cholesterol and nonsterol isoprene biosynthesis. *N Engl J Med.* 1986; 314: 1610–1614.
173. Schafer BL, Bishop RW, Kratunis VJ, et al. Molecular cloning of human mevalonate kinase and identification of a missense mutation in the genetic disease mevalonic aciduria. *J Biol Chem.* 1992; 267: 13229–13238.
174. Houten SM, Wanders RJA, Waterham HR. Biochemical and genetic aspects of mevalonate kinase and its deficiency. *Biochim Biophys Acta.* 2000; 1529: 19–32.
175. Houten SM, Schneiders MS, Wanders RJA, Waterham HR. Regulation of isoprenoid/cholesterol biosynthesis in cells from mevalonate kinase-deficient patients. *J Biol Chem.* 2003; 278: 5736–5743.
176. Hager EJ, Tse HM, Piganelli JD, et al. Deletion of a single mevalonate kinase (Mvk) allele yields a murine model of hyper-IgD syndrome. *J Inherit Metab Dis.* 2007; 30: 888–895.
177. Houten SM, Koster J, Romeijn GJ, et al. Organization of the mevalonate kinase (MVK) gene and identification of novel mutations causing mevalonic aciduria and hyperimmunoglobulinaemia D and periodic fever syndrome. *Eur J Hum Genet.* 2001; 9: 253–259.
178. Cuisset L, Drenth JP, Simon A, et al. Molecular analysis of MVK mutations and enzymatic activity in hyper-IgD and periodic fever syndrome. *Eur J Hum Genet.* 2001; 9: 260–266.
179. Gibson KM, Hoffmann G, Schwall A, et al. 3-Hydroxy-3-methylglutaryl coenzyme A reductase activity in cultured fibroblasts from patients with mevalonate kinase deficiency: differential response to lipid supplied by fetal bovine serum in tissue culture medium. *J Lipid Res.* 1990; 31: 515–521.
180. Hoffmann GF, Wiesmann UN, Brendel S, Keller RK, Gibson KM. Regulatory adaptation of isoprenoid biosynthesis and the LDL receptor pathway in fibroblasts from patients with mevalonate kinase deficiency. *Pediatr Res.* 1997; 41: 541–546.
181. Houten SM, Frenkel J, Waterham HR. Isoprenoid biosynthesis in hereditary periodic fever syndromes and inflammation. *Cell Mol Life Sci.* 2003; 60: 1118–1134.
182. Hubner C, Hoffmann GF, Charpentier C, et al. Decreased plasma ubiquinone-10 concentration in patients with mevalonate kinase deficiency. *Pediatr Res.* 1993; 34: 129–133.
183. Haas D, Niklowitz P, Hörster F, et al. Coenzyme Q10 is decreased in fibroblasts of patients with methylmalonic aciduria but not in mevalonic aciduria. *J Inherit Metab Dis.* 2009; 32: 570–575.
184. Keller RK, Simonet WS. Near normal levels of isoprenoid lipids in severe mevalonic aciduria. *Biochem Biophys Res Commun.* 1988; 152: 857–861.
185. Celec P, Behuliak M. The lack of non-steroid isoprenoids causes oxidative stress in patients with mevalonic aciduria. *Med. Hypotheses.* 2008;70: 938-940
186. Marcuzzi A, Pontillo A, De Leo L, et al. Natural isoprenoids are able to reduce inflammation in a mouse model of mevalonate kinase deficiency. *Pediatr Res.* 2008; 64: 177–182.
187. Kiener PA, Davis PM, Murray JL, Youssef S, Rankin BM, Kowala M. Stimulation of inflammatory responses in vitro and in vivo by lipophilic HMG-CoA reductase inhibitors. *Int Immunopharmacol.* 2001; 1: 105–108.
188. Hewitt RE, Lissina A, Green AE, Slay ES, Price DA, Sewell AK. The biphosphonate acute phase response: rapid and copious production of proinflammatory cytokines by peripheral blood gd T cells in response to aminophosphonates is inhibited by statins. *Clin Exp Immunol.* 2005; 139: 101–111.
189. De Leo L, Marcuzzi A, Decorti G, et al. Targeting farnesyl-transferase as a novel therapeutic strategy for mevalonate kinase deficiency: in vitro and in vivo approaches. *Pharmacol. Res.* 2010;61: 506-510
190. Greenwood J, Steinman L, Zamvil SS. Statin therapy and autoimmune disease: from protein prenylation to immunomodulation. *Nat Rev Immunol.* 2006; 6: 358–370.
191. Guasti L, Marino F, Cosentino M, et al. Prolonged statin-associated reduction in neutrophil reactive oxygen species and angiotensin II type 1 receptor expression: 1-year follow-up. *Eur Heart J.* 2008; 29: 1118–1126.
192. Van der Most PJ, Dolga AM, Nijholt IM, Luiten PG, Eisel UL. Statins: mechanisms of neuroprotection. *Prog. Neurobiol.* 2009;88: 64-75
193. Cantagel V, Lefeber DJ, Ng BG, et al. SRD5A3 is required for converting polyprenol to dolichol and is mutated in a congenital glycosylation disorder. *Cell.* 2010; 142: 1–15.
194. Roullet J-B, Steiner R, Rizzo W. Sjögren-Larsson & Isoprenoids. *International Congress of Inborn Errors in Metabolism.* October 13–16, 2006. Tokyo, Japan. (Abstract)

10

Disorders of One-Carbon Metabolism

Luis Umaña and William J. Craigen

Introduction

One-carbon metabolism refers to the formation of methyl groups derived from substrates that can be demethylated and subsequently remethylated through a complex series of steps that involve two different cycles: the folate and methionine cycles. Both of these cycles have been extensively studied in the past, and excellent descriptions of the different enzymatic steps required for each cycle are widely available.[1–12]

The methyl groups formed through these two cycles are needed for a multitude of other metabolic processes, with disruption in one-carbon metabolism having important consequences for a number of other metabolic pathways. In light of the role of demethylation and remethylation in a variety of metabolic pathways, the clinical presentation of methylation disorders is quite heterogeneous and can include apparently unconnected physiological events such as closure of the neural tube during embryogenesis, intermediary metabolism, and carcinogenesis.[8,13–17]

One-carbon metabolism has been the subject of study for many years, beginning with pioneering work describing the intramitochondrial oxidation of one-carbon donors such as serine, sarcosine, glycine, and methylglycine. In the dissection of these pathways, folates were found to play an essential role.[10,18] Folate or folic acid consists of a p-aminobenzoic molecule attached to a pteridine ring and one molecule of glutamic acid and is essential for the synthesis of nucleic acids (DNA and RNA) and in the metabolism of amino acids. Reduced folate acts as a carrier of methyl groups from one-carbon donors such as serine, glycine, and methylglycine. The methylated folate then acts as a cofactor in the *de novo* synthesis of purines and thymidylates. An additional pathway involves the methionine cycle, where homocysteine is methylated into methionine. After conversion to S-adenosyl methionine (SAM), the methyl group of methionine is a cofactor in multiple biological processes, including neurotransmitter and creatine synthesis, protein and DNA methylation, and RNA capping.[15]

The mitochondrion is the primary site for the oxidation of one-carbon donors, and, although there are parallel cytoplasmic and mitochondrial pathways, the flux between the folate pools in each compartment is limited. This flux of tetrahydrofolate (THF) is not enough to supply the mitochondrial demand for one-carbon units, underscoring the role of one-carbon donors in meeting the intramitochondrial demand; this has led to the concept of separate mitochondrial transport systems for folates and for individual one-carbon donors.[2,10]

Along with folate, another water soluble vitamin, cobalamin or B12, is also essential for one-carbon metabolism, and disorders associated with the metabolism of cobalamin, including its enteral absorption, transport bound to plasma proteins, intracellular trafficking, and final modifications to its active forms adenosylcobalamin and methylcobalamin, have been described. The clinical consequences of these disorders are increasingly known and a matter of ongoing research.[19-23]

The second cycle in one-carbon metabolism is the methionine cycle. Methionine is the immediate source of methyl groups used for methylation of lipids, proteins, and DNA. The folate cycle will in turn provide the methyl group used in the methionine cycle during a process of remethylation of homocysteine to methionine.[1,4,7]

Studies in animal models on the effect of disruptions in one-carbon metabolism have been difficult given that the consequence to most vertebrate models is a very high rate of embryonic lethality. While invertebrate models are considered to be too great of an evolutionary distance to be relevant to mammalian biology, the Zebrafish has been proposed as a valuable tool since embryogenesis is very rapid, the embryo is easier to visualize due to its early transparency, and Zebrafish are easier to genetically manipulate and breed. Zebrafish with disruptions of the folate cycle exhibit early embryonic lethality, as has been seen in other organisms, but the defects are more readily definable and involve defects in somitogenesis, cardiovascular development, and neurulation. The proposed mechanism involves disruption in the cell cycle secondary to depletion in the folate substrate for thymidylate synthase, with subsequent depletion of deoxythymidylate triphosphates (dTTPs) necessary for DNA synthesis.[15]

The One-Carbon Metabolism Pathways

One-carbon metabolism comprises the interaction of two different but inherently interdependent metabolic pathways the folate and the methionine cycles. The methionine cycle is in turn part of the larger cobalamin cycle (the folate and methionine cycles will be described further in specific sections for each compound). The step that links the 2 cycles is the action of methionine synthase that converts homocysteine into methionine through a transmethylation process utilizing reduced THF (5-methyltetrahydrofolate) as a source for the methyl group. This process will generate both methionine for protein synthesis and methionine to serve as a source of methyl groups. Tetrahydrofolate is generated by this process and, following further modification by serine hydroxymethyltransferase to 5-10-methylenetetrahydrofolate, is used in DNA and RNA synthesis.[24,25]

Methionine is activated by ATP into S-adenosylmethionine (SAM) by methionine adenosyltransferases. SAM is then transmethylated to S-adenosylhomocysteine (SAH) via a variety of methyltransferases (more than 40 exist in mammals), leading to a methyl group being transferred to an acceptor such as protein, lipids, nucleic acids, guanidinoacetate, myo-inositol, neurotransmitters, or phosphatidylethanolamine. The resulting SAH is then converted back to homocysteine by S-adenosylhomocysteine hydrolase, where it can undergo two fates. Homocysteine can be methylated into methionine by betaine homocysteine methyltransferase in a folate independent mechanism or by methionine synthase with cobalamin as a cofactor. Alternatively, homocysteine can enter a second metabolic pathway in which it is trans-sulfurated into cysteine and taurine through a series of irreversible reactions in which pyridoxine (Vitamin B6) is a cofactor.[24,26,27]

One-carbon donors enter into these pathways in the form of choline, glycine, sarcosine, or serine, and through a series of transmethylation reactions that form several cyclical processes. Choline is demethylated into dimethylglycine, which in turn is demethylated into sarcosine by the action of dimethylglycine dehydrogenase. Sarcosine is also demethylated into glycine by the action of sarcosine dehydrogenase, and each of the released methyl groups is added to THF to form 5-10 methylenetetrahydrofolate, which is one of the active forms of folate.[5,28–32] Choline is mainly derived from phosphatidylcholine, which is synthesized by SAM–dependent phosphatidylethanolamine S-methyltransferase. The synthesis of each molecule of phosphatidylcholine consumes 3 molecules of SAM, generating 3 molecules of SAH. Choline can subsequently be converted to betaine, which will act as a carbon donor for the enzyme betaine homocysteine methyltransferase.[28,33]

Folate

Folate is a water soluble vitamin (B9) closely related to the more basic pterins. Folates are ubiquitously present in eukaryotic cells and contain 3 distinct moieties; a fully reduced pterin ring, a p-aminobenzoyl group, and glutamate.[9]

Dietary folates can be obtained as naturally occurring THF or as folic acid, which is a synthetic biochemically stable form of folate added to fortified foods. Folates are transported via two widely expressed facilitative transporters the reduced folate carrier and the proton-coupled folate transporter. In addition, there is a family of glycosyl-phosphatidylinositol-anchored receptors with tissue-restricted expression profiles that are typically described as folate receptors. Both THF and folic acid are absorbed across the intestinal epithelium through the proton-coupled folate transporter. Folates are transported in the serum as monoglutamates, which are imported into cells by the reduced folate carrier or by endocytosis via glycosyl-phosphatidylinositol-linked folate receptors.[9]

The different forms of intracellular folates are sequentially reduced to dihydrofolate and finally to THF (the active form of the cofactor) by dihydrofolate reductase (DHFR) and undergo polyglutamation, with the addition of up to nine glutamate residues. These polyglutamated folates are then modified with one-carbon groups at their N5 or N10 positions.[9,10] The conversion into polyglutamates is brought about by folylpolyglutamate synthase. This polyglutamylation of cellular folates leads to metabolic trapping and allows for the retention of folates that would otherwise be lost from cells. In the cytoplasm, THF can undergo several fates: formylation by 10-formyl-THF synthase and methylation by serine hydroxymethyltransferase to 5,10-methylene-THF. The interconversion of 5,10-methylene-THF and 5,10-methenyl-THF, interconversion of 5,10-methenyl-THF and 10-formyl-THF, and condensation of THF with formate to synthesize 10-formyl-THF are mediated by a trifunctional protein 5,10-methylenetetrahydrofolate dehydrogenase (MTHFD1). The metabolism of 5,10-methylene-THF to 5-methyl-THF in the liver is catalyzed by methylene-THF reductase (MTHFR). 5-methyl-THF is then widely distributed via the bloodstream to target organs. Folates are transported into mitochondria by the mitochondrial folate transporter as a reduced folate, likely as 5-methyl THF or 5-formyl THF, and one carbon is then removed in order to form a stable THF pool.[10] Both intracytoplasmatic and intramitochondrial folates follow almost identical pathways, providing one-carbon units in both compartments.

Pathologic States

Folate deficiency states are characterized by a deficiency of methylation substrates with accumulation of one-carbon donors such as methylglycine and serine and downstream accumulations of homocysteine due to the lack of methyl groups to be supplied for the remethylation of homocysteine into methionine. The main manifestations are hematological (megaloblastic anemia), as well as progressive and severe neurocognitive involvement.

Hereditary Folate Malabsorption

Autosomal recessive mutations affecting the *SLC46A1* gene encoding the proton-coupled folate transporter (OMIM: 193090) are associated with infantile onset of megaloblastic anemia, seizures, diarrhea, and progressive neurological impairment associated with low blood and cerebrospinal fluid folate levels, reflecting both impaired intestinal transport and central nervous system uptake.[17,34-36] Hypogammaglobulinemia with increased predisposition to *Pneumocystis jiroveci* infection is a characteristic finding in this disorder that may lead clinicians to misidentify it as severe combined immunodeficiency, delaying the correct diagnosis and management.[34] Although this disorder occurs in all populations, with most mutations being described as private, there is a high incidence of a common splice site mutation in Puerto Rico. The carrier frequency of this mutation is estimated to be 0.2% island-wide and 6.3% in the region of Villalba.[35]

Treatment

Oral folic acid at high doses has not been shown to correct all of the clinical features of this condition, in particular the central nervous system manifestations, and there is concern that folic acid may compete with 5MTHF for transport at the level of the choroid plexus.[34,37,38]

Cerebral Folate Deficiency

This autosomal recessive disorder resulting from brain-specific folate deficiency is typically characterized by normal development until age four to six months, followed by agitation, dyskinesias, psychomotor delay and deceleration of head growth, and seizures.[39] The biochemical findings in this disorder include low levels of 5-MTHF in cerebrospinal fluid, while plasma levels are normal, indicating a defect in the transport of folate across the blood–brain barrier.[37] Mutations in the high-affinity, low-capacity folate receptor *FOLR1* (OMIM: 613068), which encodes FRα, have been identified as the principle genetic basis in the cerebral folate deficiencies.[37] The folate receptor FRα is located on the epithelial surface of the choroid plexus together with proton coupled folate carriers and reduced folate carriers. Alterations in transport can come from mutations in *FOLR1* or due to the presence of autoantibodies against the receptor.[37,38,40] Due to unknown mechanisms, cerebral folate deficiency has also been observed in other syndromes, including Aicardi-Goutières syndrome, Rett syndrome, and mitochondrial disorders with altered respiratory chain function.[38,40]

Treatment

The treatment for cerebral folate deficiency is based on supplementation with oral folinic acid. The administration of folic acid should be avoided in this condition since it has high affinity for the folate receptor and competes with 5-MTHF, therefore potentially increasing the cerebral folate deficiency. A secondary concern is that folic acid might correct the hematologic abnormalities, giving a false sense of therapeutic success without having any significant effect on the central nervous system manifestations.[38] Treatment with folinic acid has led to different responses in patients with this condition; in some patients the neurological response to folinic acid can be rapid and dramatic while in others it may be years before any benefits are seen.[40]

Methylene-Tetrahydrofolate Reductase Deficiency

MTHFR deficiency is one of the more common and controversial of the disorders of folate metabolism, as common DNA polymorphisms in the *MTHFR* gene have been examined for potential associations with multiple pathologic processes, including increased fetal loss, aneuploidies, neural tube defects, carcinogenesis, psychiatric conditions, and cardiovascular disease. Common polymorphisms in *MTHFR* include the c.677C>T (pA233G) and 1298A>C (p.E429A). Variants have been identified in many populations with varying prevalence rates and confer mild effects on enzyme function. When homozygous or compound heterozygous, these variants can be associated with modest elevations of homocysteine in the face of decreased folate levels in some individuals. While numerous studies have associated or refuted the risks of these polymorphisms in a wide variety of diseases, including neural tube defects, cancers such as colon, breast, head/neck, and prostate, and mental illness a widely accepted view is that, with the exception of risk for neural tube defects in the face of low folate intake, they are mostly benign variants with no unequivocal evidence of disease association.[41,42] In contrast, bonafide MTHFR enzyme deficiency (OMIM: 236250) has been described in patients varying from infants to adults with homocystinuria and homocysteinemia with low methionine levels but not megaloblastic anemia. Other manifestations include thromboembolic events, psychiatric symptoms, and progressive intellectual disability, in addition to severe infantile forms with early death. Included in the phenotypic spectrum are clinically asymptomatic adults with only biochemical findings who have been identified through ascertainment of an affected sibling. This condition can lead to symptoms of cerebral folate deficiency due to an insufficient amount of MTHF available to cross the blood–brain barrier, rather than an uptake defect by mutations in folate receptors as described above. The treatment of MTHFR deficiency consists of suspplementation with betaine, which is a substrate for betaine homocysteine methyltransferase, leading to an increase in methionine and a reduction of homocysteine. Other treatments include folic or folinic acid supplementation and possibly methionine supplementation. With early diagnosis and initiation of betaine treatment, the outcome can be good and suggests there would be benefits to including homocysteine in newborn screening programs.

Dihydrofolate Reductase Deficiency

DHFR deficiency (OMIM: 613839) is a recently described inborn error of folate metabolism.[43,44] DHFR is a key enzyme in folate metabolism, reducing dihydrofolate into THF via NADPH, and is an important target of several pharmacological compounds, including methotrexate and trimethoprim. Three patients reported by Banka et al.[44] had profound psychomotor developmental delay, generalized seizures, and cerebral and cerebellar atrophy, with cerebrospinal fluid studies demonstrating markedly decreased 5-methyltetrahydrofolate (5MTHF) and low tetrahydrobiopterin. In contrast, the three siblings reported by Cario et al.[43] were either asymptomatic or had childhood absence epilepsy with eyelid myoclonus and mild learning disabilities. In the reported families, molecular studies demonstrated missense mutations in *DHFR* associated with enzymatic deficiency. Cerebral folate levels, anemia, and pancytopenia were corrected by treatment with folinic acid.

5,10-Methylenetetrahydrofolate Dehydrogenase Deficiency

5,10-MTHFD1 is a cytoplasmic trifunctional protein composed of 5,10-methylenetetrahydrofolate dehydrogenase/5,10-methenyl-tetrahydrofolate cyclohydrolase/formyltetrahydrofolate synthase activities needed for the interconversion of 5,10-methylene-THF, 5,10-methenyl-THF, 10-formyl-THF, and formylation of THF. MTHFD1 deficiency was recently reported in an infant exhibiting severe combined immunodeficiency complicated by *Pneumocystis jiroveci* infection, along with megaloblastic anemia, leukopenia, atypical hemolytic uremic syndrome, and neurologic abnormalities, and in whom methylcobalamin and 5MTHF therapy provided partial immune reconstitution and resolution of the biochemical findings.[45,46]

Cobalamin

Cobalamin (vitamin B12) is a tetrapyrrole with a corrin ring enclosing a central cobalt ion via four nitrogen bonds in the corrin ion, a fifth bond to a dimethylbenzimidazole group, and has a sixth position that can be occupied by either a cyano group (–CN), a hydroxyl group (–OH), a methyl group (–CH3), or a 5'-deoxyadenosyl group. This latter position defines the form of cobalamin as cyanocobalamin, OH-cobalamin, methylcobalamin, or adenosylcobalamin.[23] Cobalamin is widely distributed in nature, but the complex, multistep synthesis pathway required to form B12 is present only in certain prokaryotes, making it an essential nutrient for higher organisms. After ingestion, the absorption and activation of cobalamin is not any less complex. It requires the functional integrity of multiple receptors, transporters, and modifying enzymes that will take cobalamin from the intestinal lumen into its final intracellular destination, where it is a cofactor for two metabolic processes the methylation of homocysteine to methionine, through methionine synthase (5-methyltetrahydrofolate homocysteine methyltransferase), and the conversion of methylmalonyl-CoA into succinyl-CoA through the action of methylmalonyl-CoA mutase.[23]

Cobalamin requires an elaborate absorption and transport system within humans. Cobalamin is released from dietary protein in the stomach by peptidases and binds to the salivary glycoprotein haptocorrin (also known as transcobalamin I [TCNI]) to protect from degradation. Intrinsic factor secreted by the gastric parietal cells then replaces haptocorrin as the cobalamin-binding protein in the duodenum. The intrinsic factor-cobalamin complex is then recognized by a receptor on the surface of enterocytes of the terminal ileum, cubilin. Cobalamin is endocytosed through the apical surface of the enterocyte, and intrinsic factor is degraded in the lysosome, releasing cobalamin. The ATP-dependent transporter ABCC1 (also known as multidrug resistance protein 1) that is within the basolateral membrane of intestinal epithelial cells exports cobalamin bound to transcobalamin II to the portal system. In the blood, cobalamin is bound to transcobalamin II (TCN2) or haptocorrin. It has been estimated that about 20% of circulating cobalamin is bound to transcobalamin II, while the remainder, including incomplete B12 derivatives and other corrinoid compounds, is bound to haptocorrin to be exported via the biliary system, possibly to avoid interfering with binding of intact cobalamin. The transcobalamin-cobalamin complex enters peripheral cells via the transcobalamin II receptor (also known as CD320) and is internalized to the lysosome. Prior to the identification of the genes involved in cobalamin metabolism, cell complementation assays done by fusing cell lines derived from patients exhibiting increased homocysteine and/or methylmalonic acid diagnosed and defined the underlying defect in cobalamin metabolism as complementation groups A to G.[23] Transport of cobalamin across the lysosomal membrane requires two membrane proteins: LMBD1 and ABCD4. Mutations in the genes encoding these two transporters result in accumulation of cobalamin in lysosomes and are classified as cblF (LMBD1) and the recently discovered cblJ (ABCD4) complementation groups.

Following cobalamin export from the lysosome, MMACHC (cobalamin C [cblC]), carries out the decyanation and dealkylation of C1–C6 alkyl, adenosyl, cyano, and hydroxyl group modified cobalamins. MMACHD (cblD) appears to define the destination of cobalamin to either the cytosol or the mitochondrion. While cblD does not bind cobalamin directly, the ability of cblC and cblD to form a complex suggests that CblD may assist in delivering cobalamin from cblC to downstream targets within the cytoplasm and mitochondria. In the cytoplasm methionine synthase, responsible for the cblG complementation group, catalyzes the methyl transfer from 5-methyltetrahydrofolate to homocysteine in a two-step process. First, the methyl group is transferred from MeCbl to homocysteine to generate methionine and cob(I)alamin. Second, the cob(I)alamin removes the methyl group from 5-methyltetrahydrofolate to reform MeCbl and generate THF. Occasional oxidation of the bound cob(I)alamin to the inactive cob(II)alamin state would eventually render cobalamin inactive, hence there is a repair system using a reductive methylation reaction where the methyl group of SAM is transferred to cobalamin in the presence of NADPH and methionine synthase reductase, which is encoded by the cblE locus.

Cobalamin directed to the mitochondrion is converted into 5'-deoxyadenosylcobalamin via modification by the ATP-dependent cob(I)alamin adenosyltransferase encoded by the cblB locus, producing the essential cofactor for methylmalonyl mutase (MUT) activity. Loss of the 5'-deoxyadenosine intermediate during MUT catalysis requires the removal of oxidized cobalt to reestablish its reactivity, and this is performed by a G-protein chaperone (encoded by the cblA locus) bound to MUT, which uses the binding energy of guanosine triphosphate to drive the expulsion of inactive cob(II)alamin from the active site of MUT, allowing for the reinsertion of Ado-Cbl into MUT by adenosyltransferase. Several aspects of these biological transformations remain to be resolved, including how cblD functions in targeting cobalamin to different intracellular compartments and how cobalamins enter mitochondria.[19,23]

Pathologic States

Numerous defects in the transport and metabolism of cobalamin have been described, and their main signs and symptoms depend on which of the two final metabolic fates of cobalamin is affected. The biochemical perturbations include either isolated methylmalonic acidemia associated with defects in AdoCbl formation (cblA and cblB), isolated homocysteinemia due to loss of methylcobalamin (cblE and cblG), or combined homocystinuria and methylmalonic acidemia in deficiencies of both AdoCbl and MeCbl (cblC, cblD, cblF, cblJ). Similarly, defects in the uptake and transport of cobalamin can exhibit the same biochemical findings. Clinical problems associated with cobalamin disorders are quite varied and include megaloblastic anemia, metabolic acidosis, hyperammonemia, progressive renal disease, optic atrophy, retinal dystrophy, intellectual disability, and pancreatitis. With one exception, the disorders described here are inherited in an autosomal recessive fashion.

Absorption and Transport Disorders

Hereditary forms of cobalamin deficiency can be due to genetically abnormal intrinsic factor, abnormal synthesis of transcobalamin, a defect of the intestinal uptake of IF-cobalamin (Imerslund-Grasbeck disease or megaloblastic anemia-1), or defective uptake of transcobalamin II-cobalamin. In contrast, the autoimmune disorder pernicious anemia is associated with plasma autoantibodies to gastric parietal cells or gastric intrinsic factor. Typically, there is gastric atrophy, and pernicious anemia is commonly associated with thyroiditis and myxedema. The markedly higher frequency of pernicious anemia in adults with multiple myeloma or immunoglobulin deficiency points to immune dysfunction as the underlying cause.

Haptocorrin (transcobalamin I) deficiency (OMIM: 193090) is associated with reduced serum cobalamin levels but appears to be a benign condition in light of the continued presence of TCNII. Mutations in the gene encoding the gastric intrinsic factor cause congenital pernicious anemia (OMIM: 261000), leading to early-onset megaloblastic anemia and cobalamin deficiency. Onset of anemia is typically observed by one year of age but can be delayed, and there is considerable variability in neurologic manifestations. Defects in intestinal uptake can be due to defects in the receptor cubilin (OMIM: 602997) or its coreceptor Megalin (AMN, LRP2, OMIM: 605799); the latter is associated with proteinuria and is common in Norway, and the former is found more commonly in Finland. Transcobalamin II deficiency (OMIM: 275350) typically comes to attention in infancy with megaloblastic anemia, thrombocytopenia, and neutropenia in association with gastrointestinal and immunologic manifestations. Untreated, neurologic decline is common, and biochemical features include homocystinuria and methylmalonic aciduria. Serum cobalamin levels are generally normal since haptocorrin is still present, but cellular uptake is impaired.

Finally, deficiency of the TCNII-Cbl receptor (TCblR/CD320; OMIM: 613646) was recently identified by newborn screening based on increased propionylcarnitine (C3; a surrogate for methylmalonic acid). Two of four cases also exhibited increased homocysteine, and treatment with cobalamin normalized the biochemical abnormalities.

Intracellular Processing Disorders

As previously stated, the disorders of intracellular cobalamin processing have been defined by complementation studies and can be divided into those causing isolated homocystinuria, isolated methylmalonic aciduria, or both. Structural similarities to bacterial proteins, linkage mapping, and/or whole genome sequencing strategies have been used to identify the relevant genes. Here we provide a brief discussion of each disorder that affects methylation.

Cobalamin C

Deficiency of cblC (OMIM: 277400) is the most common of the complementation groups and causes combined methylmalonic acidemia and homocystinuria. The gene associated with cblC is *MMACHC*, and more than 50 mutations have been identified, including founder mutations in restricted populations.[19,47,48] The clinical picture of this disorder is quite variable, from a neonatal presentation with acute metabolic decompensation to adult-onset neurodegeneration not unlike pernicious anemia. Prenatal onset of disease may include intrauterine growth restriction, microcephaly, congenital heart disease, and facial dysmorphisms.[19,22] The most common presentation is during infancy, including hypotonia, failure to thrive, megaloblastic anemia with hemolytic-uremic syndrome, developmental delay and seizures, and macular degeneration. Nonetheless, initial presentations at later ages have been documented and are associated mainly with neurological symptoms that can include progressive leukoencephalopathy and subacute spinal degeneration. Older patients can exhibit a pigmentary retinopathy. A second subset of symptoms is associated to homocystinuria and include chronic thrombotic microangiopathy and thromboembolic events.[19,20,22,48,49] Newborn screening using the analyte C3 can detect affected individuals, but milder forms of the disease may be missed by screening.

CblD

MMADHC forms a complex with MMACHC and directs cobalamin to the methylcobalamin or adenosylcobalamin pathway. This locus is unique in that it can present either as a combined methylmalonic aciduria/homocystinuria or as isolated methylmalonic aciduria or isolated homocystinuria (OMIM: 277410). Identification of different mutations in the gene provide some insight into the genotype-phenotype relationship, where mutations in the N-terminal domain are associated with isolated methylmalonic aciduria due to abnormal adenosylcobalamin synthesis and missense mutations in the C terminal domain associated with isolated homocystinuria. In the former case, downstream methionine residues can still direct protein synthesis of a shorter protein that can participate in methylcobalamin synthesis; however, nonsense or splice site mutations near the C terminal domain are seen in patients with the combined phenotype, indicative of disruption of both pathways.[50,51] The clinical features depend on the variant form within the group but parallel that of other complementation groups.

CblF

LMBRD1 (OMIM: 277380) encodes LMBD1 (Lmbr1 domain-containing protein 1), which has been characterized as a lysosomal export protein. Defects associated with this protein cause a combined methylmalonic acidemia/homocysteinemia syndrome with high levels of intracellular free cobalamin. In the patients identified to date, the clinical phenotype is variable, ranging from intrauterine growth restriction and developmental delay to asymptomatic long-term survival.

CblJ

Mutations in *ABCD4* encoding ABCD4 (ATP-binding cassette, subfamily D, member 4) have been identified in two subjects with combined methylmalonic aciduria and homocysteinemia (OMIM: 614857) with accumulation of free cobalamin similar to that seen in cblF. ABCD4 has been shown to colocalize with LMBD1 to the lysosome, although the complete function of the protein in cobalamin metabolism still remains to be fully described.[52] Patients have developed symptoms in infancy, including hypotonia, blood marrow failure, and biochemical evidence of cobalamin deficiency.

CblX

The most recent addition to cobalamin disorders was the identification of mutations in the gene encoding the transcriptional co-regulator HCFC1. The locus had previously been identified as causing nonsyndromic X-linked intellectual disability (MRX3),[53] but in children with biochemical findings of methylmalonic acidemia and homocysteinemia, whole exoe sequencing demonstrated mutations in *HCFC1* and further studies showed a reduction in MMACHC transcription. In 14 unrelated patients reported by Yu and colleagues five different hemizygous missense mutations were identified.[54] Most patients had combined methylmalonic acidemia and homocysteinemia, although five had normal plasma homocysteine, findings suggestive of a mild cblC disorder. Prior complementation analysis in most of the patients suggested cblC, but molecular analysis excluded mutations in the *MMACHC* locus. All patients showed moderate to severe intellectual disability, suggesting that additional gene targets of HCFC1 action contribute to the clinical phenotype. Other problems included failure to thrive, microcephaly, movement disorders, and intractable epilepsy.

Diagnosis

As with the other combined methylmalonic acidemia and homocystinuria disorders, the main findings of newborn screening include an elevation in C3 as well as variable increases in total homocysteine. Further analysis of plasma amino acids reveal low methionine with elevated homocysteine. It is worth noting that routine plasma amino acid analysis does not measure total homocysteine in that homocysteine is mainly bound to serum proteins and the sample must be treated with a reducing agent to be quantitatively analyzed. The levels of methylmalonic acid, methionine, and total plasma homocysteine also serve as the monitoring parameters for the efficiency of treatment. To further differentiate the underlying genetic disorders, both cultured cell complementation studies and gene sequencing are clinically available, although complementation studies are increasingly less commonly used on a clinical basis in light of more widely available DNA testing.

Treatment

As with other inborn errors of metabolism characterized by deficiency of a product and increases in substrate(s), treatment is aimed toward supplementation of cofactors or products, reduction in substrate, or provision of alternative substrates for the affected reactions.

In the case of the combined methylmalonic acidemia and homocystinuria syndromes, this can be accomplished in part by the administration of parenteral hydroxycobalamin. Other forms of cobalamin such as methylcobalamin and cyanocobalamin, as well as oral administration of hydroxycobalamin, have proven to be ineffective in the treatment of these disorders. It is important to monitor the metabolic parameters periodically since dose requirements vary not only as the patient grows but also between the different disorders.[55, 56] A second compound that has proven to improve biochemical parameters is the concurrent administration of oral betaine. This compound is essential for a cobalamin-independent transmethylation of homocysteine and in conjunction with hydroxycobalamin improves the levels of homocysteine.[56]

Other agents have been proposed for the management of these conditions, but at this moment their efficacy has not been clearly established and therefore they do not yet form part of the current management for these conditions. These agents include levocarnitine, since some patients might develop secondary carnitine deficiency, and folinic acid, with the rationale that this will provide substrate for the folate cycle in the face of loss of 5-methyltetrahydrofolate secondary to a decrease in methionine synthase activity.[19] While dietary restriction of protein could theoretically reduce amino acid flux to methylmalonic acid, there is little evidence that this strategy is effective or necessary.

Effects of One-Carbon Metabolism on Other Biological Processes

A variety of complex phenomena, including epigenetic changes, embryologic development, and the genesis of complex diseases such as cancer, cardiovascular disease, and neurodegenerative disorders, have been associated to one-carbon metabolism.[57,58] These effects might be secondary to the interactions of one-carbon metabolism with multiple other cycles to which it provides substrates either in the form of methyl groups or by production of new intermediates such as cystathionine. Cystathionine is produced via cystathionine beta synthase (CBS) by the condensation of homocysteine with serine and is then converted into cysteine, α-ketobutyrate and ammonia by cysteine γ lyase (cystathionase). α-ketobutyrate can enter the TCA cycle as propionyl-CoA, and cysteine will be the precursor of both taurine and glutathione, which is the major intracellular antioxidant.[6]

Homocysteine is considered a risk factor for vascular wall injury as suggested by both the finding of elevated homocysteine levels in patients with vascular disease as well as by the development of prominent vascular disease in patients with homocystinuria due to cystathionine beta synthase deficiency. It is not completely clear at this moment if there is a causal relationship, but there is evidence of an interaction between homocysteine and the atherogenic lipoprotein Lp(a).[59] Furthermore, recent studies have shown that homocysteine-lowering therapies might not decrease the risk of fatal myocardial infarction and stroke.[57]

The role of one-carbon metabolism in cancer risk has also been explored extensively, but a definite link has not yet been demonstrated.[16,60] Common variants in a number of folate metabolizing genes, including *MTHFR, DHFR, MTR, MTRR, SHMT1, MTHFD1*, thymidylate synthetase, and *CBS*, have been studied in numerous case control studies in search of associations for cancers ranging from leukemia to breast cancer.[61] Since the DNA methyltransferases involved in DNA methylation use SAM as the methyl donor, it is not surprising that epigenetic changes in DNA methylation patterns may be related to variants in methylation pathways, but the confounding nature of gene–diet and gene–gene interactions makes these analyses challenging. At a more cellular level, the shift in one-carbon metabolism observed in certain cancer cells continues to provide fodder for the exploration of perturbed methylation pathways in cancer.[62,63] The importance of folate on embryogenesis, specially regarding closure of the neural tube is more clear, but the mechanism by which folate deficiency or defects in folate metabolism cause neural tube defects is not well understood and association studies with the common folate pathway polymorphisms appear to be population specific.[13,57,60,64]

Newborn Screening for Disorders of Folate and Cobalamin Metabolism

Currently newborn screening programs in the United States do not screen for disorders of intracellular folate metabolism, and these are not included in the American College of Medical Genetics uniform testing panel.[65] In contrast, methylmalonic acidemia is included in the uniform panel. This includes those cases of isolated methylmalonic acidemia associated MUT, cblA, and cblB but may also identify disorders leading to combined methylmalonic acidemia and homocysteinemia. Screening is accomplished by detection of elevated C3 by tandem mass spectrometry. Elevated C3 is not specific to any one disorder; it can detect propionic acidemia, methylmalonic acidemia secondary to methylmalonyl-CoA mutase deficiency, and defects in cobalamin metabolism. Urine organic acid analysis differentiates propionic acidemia from methylmalonic acidemia but does not distinguish the various causes of methylmalonic acidemia in these patients. This differentiation can be made only by molecular or functional analysis.[66-69]

Isolated homocystinuria associated cystathione b synthase deficiency, which is associated with classic homocystinuria, can be detected by newborn screening through the finding of increased blood methionine, unlike patients with homocystinuria due to cblG or cblE where methionine is low and thus does not lead to detection by the newborn screening methods used by most states. These patients are identified by finding markedly elevated levels of total homocysteine associated hematological manifestations of megaloblastic anemia but by definition will be symptomatic.[69,70]

Another limitation of newborn screening for disorders of cobalamin metabolism is the detection of asymptomatic mothers or dietary deficiencies in the mother that might have initial biochemical manifestations in the newborn but are not necessarily due to an inborn error of metabolism. Further investigation will be required in order to institute the most appropriate treatment for these cases.[67,71]

Although in cases of nutritional deficiency children may have elevations in methylmalonic acid, total homocysteine, and low methionine, the levels of C3 might not be high enough to cross the threshold for newborn screening, and these children may remain undiagnosed and untreated, putting them at considerable risk of neurological sequelae secondary to vitamin B12 deficiency.[72]

References

1. Albers E. Metabolic characteristics and importance of the universal methionine salvage pathway recycling methionine from 5'-methylthioadenosine. *IUBMB Life*. 2009; 61(12): 1132–1142.
2. Appling DR. Compartmentation of folate-mediated one-carbon metabolism in eukaryotes. *FASEB J*. 1991; 5(12): 2645–2651.
3. Carmel R, Green R, Rosenblatt DS, Watkins D. Update on cobalamin, folate, and homocysteine. *Hematology*. 2003; 1: 62–81.
4. Chen Z, Chakraborty S, Banerjee R. Demonstration that mammalian methionine synthases are predominantly cobalamin-loaded. *J Biol Chem*. 1995; 270(33): 19246–19249.
5. Kalhan SC, Hanson RW. Resurgence of serine: an often neglected but indispensable amino acid. *J Biol Chem*. 2012; 287(24): 19786–19791.

6. Kalhan SC, Marczewski SE. Methionine, homocysteine, one carbon metabolism and fetal growth. *Rev Endocr Metab Disord*. 2012; 13(2): 109–119.
7. Martinov MV, Vitvitsky VM, Banerjee R, Ataullakhanov FI. The logic of the hepatic methionine metabolic cycle. *Biochim Biophys Acta*. 2010; 1804(1): 89–96.
8. Stover PJ. Physiology of folate and vitamin B12 in health and disease. *Nutr Rev*. 2004; 62(6 Pt 2): S3–S12; discussion S13.
9. Stover PJ, Field MS. Trafficking of intracellular folates. *Adv Nutr*. 2011; 2(4): 325–331.
10. Tibbetts AS, Appling DR. Compartmentalization of mammalian folate-mediated one-carbon metabolism. *Annu Rev Nutr*. 2010; 30: 57–81.
11. Ulrich CM, Reed MC, Nijhout HF. Modeling folate, one-carbon metabolism, and DNA methylation. *Nutr Rev*. 2008; 66(Suppl. 1): S27–S30.
12. Woodard JC. Study of one-carbon metabolism in neonatal vitamin B12-deficient rats. *J Nutr*. 1969; 98(2): 139 146.
13. Greene ND, Stanier P, Copp AJ. Genetics of human neural tube defects. *Hum Mol Genet*. 2009; 18(R2): R113–R129.
14. Ikeda S, Koyama H, Sugimoto M, Kume S. Roles of one-carbon metabolism in preimplantation period—effects on short-term development and long-term programming. *J Reprod Dev*. 2012; 58(1): 38–43.
15. Lee MS, Bonner JR, Bernard DJ, et al. Disruption of the folate pathway in zebrafish causes developmental defects. *BMC Dev Biol*. 2012; 12: 12.
16. Martinelli M, Scapoli L, Mattei G, et al. A candidate gene study of one-carbon metabolism pathway genes and colorectal cancer risk. *Br J Nutr*. 2012; 109(6): 984–989.
17. Watkins D, Rosenblatt DS. Update and new concepts in vitamin responsive disorders of folate transport and metabolism. *J Inherit Metab Dis*. 2012; 35(4): 665–670.
18. Goodwin LD, Kinney JM. Studies of one-carbon metabolism in man. *J Biol Chem*. 1958; 230(1): 487–496.
19. Carrillo-Carrasco N, Chandler RJ, Venditti CP. Combined methylmalonic acidemia and homocystinuria, cblC type I: clinical presentations, diagnosis and management. *J Inherit Metab Dis*. 2012; 35(1): 91–102.
20. Carrillo-Carrasco N, Venditti CP. Combined methylmalonic acidemia and homocystinuria, cblC type II: complications, pathophysiology, and outcomes. *J Inherit Metab Dis*. 2012; 35(1): 103–114.
21. Depeint F, Bruce WR, Shangari N, Mehta R, O'Brien PJ. Mitochondrial function and toxicity: role of B vitamins on the one-carbon transfer pathways. *Chem Biol Interact*. 2006; 163(1–2): 113–132.
22. Martinelli D, Deodato F, Dionisi-Vici C. Cobalamin C defect: natural history, pathophysiology, and treatment. *J Inherit Metab Dis*. 2011; 34(1): 127–135.
23. Nielsen MJ, Rasmussen MR, Andersen CB, Nexo E, Moestrup SK. Vitamin B12 transport from food to the body's cells—a sophisticated, multistep pathway. *Nat Rev Gastroenterol Hepatol*. 2012; 9(6): 345–354.
24. Finkelstein JD. Inborn errors of sulfur-containing amino acid metabolism. *J Nutr*. 2006; 136(Suppl. 6): 1750S–1754S.
25. Ho V, Massey TE, King WD. Thymidylate synthase gene polymorphisms and markers of DNA methylation capacity. *Mol Genet Metab*. 2011; 102(4): 481–487.
26. Parveen N, Cornell KA. Methylthioadenosine/S-adenosylhomocysteine nucleosidase, a critical enzyme for bacterial metabolism. *Mol Microbiol*. 2011; 79(1): 7–20.
27. Elmore CL, Matthews RG. The many flavors of hyperhomocyst(e)inemia: insights from transgenic and inhibitor-based mouse models of disrupted one-carbon metabolism. *Antioxid Redox Signal*. 2007; 9(11): 1911–1921.
28. Ueland PM. Choline and betaine in health and disease. *J Inherit Metab Dis*. 2011; 34(1): 3–15.
29. Binzak BA, Wevers RA, Moolenaar SH, Lee YM, Hwu WL, Poggi-Bach J, Engelke UF, Hoard HM, Vockley JG, Vockley J. Cloning of dimethylglycine dehydrogenase and a new human inborn error of metabolism, dimethylglycine dehydrogenase deficiency. *Am J Hum Genet*. 2001; 68(4): 839–847.
30. McAndrew RP, Vockley J, Kim JJ. Molecular basis of dimethylglycine dehydrogenase deficiency associated with pathogenic variant H109R. *J Inherit Metab Dis*. 2008; 31(6): 761–768.
31. Snell K. Enzymes of serine metabolism in normal, developing and neoplastic rat tissues. *Adv Enzyme Regul*. 1984; 22: 325–400.
32. Wagner C, Briggs WT, Cook RJ. Covalent binding of folic acid to dimethylglycine dehydrogenase. *Arch Biochem Biophys*. 1984; 233(2): 457–461.

33. Pajares MA, Perez-Sala D. Betaine homocysteine S-methyltransferase: just a regulator of homocysteine metabolism? *Cell Mol Life Sci*. 2006; 63(23):2792–2803.
34. Atabay B, Turker M, Ozer EA, Mahadeo K, Diop-Bove N, Goldman ID. Mutation of the proton-coupled folate transporter gene (PCFT-SLC46A1) in Turkish siblings with hereditary folate malabsorption. *Pediatr Hematol Oncol*. 2010; 27(8): 614–619.
35. Mahadeo KM, Diop-Bove N, Ramirez SI, et al. Prevalence of a loss-of-function mutation in the proton-coupled folate transporter gene (PCFT-SLC46A1) causing hereditary folate malabsorption in Puerto Rico. *J Pediatr*. 2011; 159(4): 623–627 e1.
36. Zhao R, Min SH, Qiu A, et al. The spectrum of mutations in the PCFT gene, coding for an intestinal folate transporter, that are the basis for hereditary folate malabsorption. *Blood*. 2007; 110(4): 1147–1152.
37. Perez-Duenas B, Ormazabal A, Toma C, et al. Cerebral folate deficiency syndromes in childhood: clinical, analytical, and etiologic aspects. *Arch Neurol*. 2011; 68(5): 615–621.
38. Serrano M, Perez-Duenas B, Montoya J, Ormazabal A, Artuch R. Genetic causes of cerebral folate deficiency: clinical, biochemical and therapeutic aspects. *Drug Discov Today*. 2012; 17(23–24): 1299–1230.
39. Mangold S, Blau N, Opladen T, et al. Cerebral folate deficiency: a neurometabolic syndrome? *Mol Genet Metab*. 2011; 104(3): 369–372.
40. Hyland K, Shoffner J, Heales SJ. Cerebral folate deficiency. *J Inherit Metab Dis*. 2010; 33(5): 563–570.
41. Carr DF, Whiteley G, Alfirevic A, Pirmohamed M, FolATED. Investigation of inter-individual variability of the one-carbon folate pathway: a bioinformatic and genetic review. *Pharmacogenomics J*. 2009; 9(5): 291–305.
42. Marini NJ, Gin J, Ziegle J, et al. The prevalence of folate-remedial MTHFR enzyme variants in humans. *Proc Natl Acad Sci USA*. 2008; 105(23): 8055–8060.
43. Cario, Smith DE, Bloom H, et al. Dihydrofolate reductase deficiency due to a homozygous DHFR mutation causes megaloblastic anemia and cerebral folate deficiency leading to severe neurologic disease. *Am J Hum Genet*. 2011; 88(2): 226–231.
44. Banka S, Ryan K, Thompson W, Newman WG. Pernicious anemia - genetic insights. *Autoimmun Rev*. 2011; 10(8): 455–459.
45. Watkins D, Schwartzentruber JA, Ganesh J, et al. Novel inborn error of folate metabolism: identification by exome capture and sequencing of mutations in the MTHFD1 gene in a single proband. *J Med Genet*. 2011; 48: 590–592.
46. Keller MD, Ganesh J, Heltzer M, et al. Severe combined immunodeficiency resulting from mutations in MTHFD1. *Pediatrics*. 2013; 131(2): e629–e634.
47. Hannibal L, DiBello PM, Yu M, et al. The MMACHC proteome: hallmarks of functional cobalamin deficiency in humans. *Mol Genet Metab*. 2011; 103(3): 226–239.
48. Morel CF, Lerner-Ellis JP, Rosenblatt DS. Combined methylmalonic aciduria and homocystinuria (cblC): phenotype-genotype correlations and ethnic-specific observations. *Mol Genet Metab*. 2006; 88(4): 315–321.
49. Reynolds E. Vitamin B12, folic acid, and the nervous system. *Lancet Neurol*. 2006; 5(11): 949–960.
50. Coelho D, Suormala T, Stucki M, et al. Gene identification for the cblD defect of vitamin B12 metabolism. *N Engl J Med*. 2008; 358(14): 1454–1464.
51. Watkins D, Rosenblatt DS. Inborn errors of cobalamin absorption and metabolism. *Am J Med Genet C Semin Med Genet*. 2011; 157(1): 33–44.
52. Coelho D, Kim JC, Miousse IR, et al. Mutations in ABCD4 cause a new inborn error of vitamin B(12) metabolism. *Nat Genet*. 2012; 44(10): 1152–1155.
53. Huang L, Jolly LA, Willis-Owen S, et al. A noncoding, regulatory mutation implicates HCFC1 in nonsyndromic intellectual disability. *Am J Hum Genet*. 2012; 91: 694–702.
54. Yu H-C, Sloan JL, Scharer G, et al. An X-linked cobalamin disorder caused by mutations in transcriptional coregulator HCFC1. *Am J Hum Genet*. 2013; 93: 506–514.
55. Carrillo-Carrasco N, Sloan J, Valle D, Hamosh A, Venditti CP. Hydroxocobalamin dose escalation improves metabolic control in cblC. *J Inherit Metab Dis*. 2009; 32(6): 728–731.
56. Ribes A, Briones P, Vilaseca MA, et al. Methylmalonic aciduria with homocystinuria: biochemical studies, treatment, and clinical course of a Cbl-C patient. *Eur J Pediatr*. 1990; 149(6): 412–415.
57. Blom HJ, Smulders Y. Overview of homocysteine and folate metabolism. With special references to cardiovascular disease and neural tube defects. *J Inherit Metab Dis*. 2011; 34(1): 75–81.

58. Zhu H, Yang W, Lu W, et al. Gene variants in the folate-mediated one-carbon metabolism (FOCM) pathway as risk factors for conotruncal heart defects. *Am J Med Genet A*. 2012; 158A(5): 1124–1134.
59. Baños-González MA, Anglés-Cano E, Cardoso-Saldaña G, et al. Lipoprotein(a) and homocysteine potentiate the risk of coronary artery disease in male subjects. *Circ J*. 2012; 76(8): 1953–1957.
60. Stover PJ. One-carbon metabolism-genome interactions in folate-associated pathologies. *J Nutr*. 2009; 139(12): 2402–2405.
61. Nazki FH, Sameer AS, Ganaie BA. Folate: metabolism, genes, polymorphisms and the associated diseases. *Gene*. 2014; 533(1): 11–20.
62. Vander Heiden MG, Lunt SY, Dayton TL, et al. Metabolic pathway alterations that support cell proliferation. *Cold Spring Harb Symp Quant Biol*. 2011; 76: 325–334.
63. Tedeschi PM, Markert EK, Gounder M, et al. Contribution of serine, folate and glycine metabolism to the ATP, NADPH and purine requirements of cancer cells. *Cell Death Dis*. 2013; 4: e877.
64. Benevenga NJ. Consideration of betaine and one-carbon sources of N5-methyltetrahydrofolate for use in homocystinuria and neural tube defects. *Am J Clin Nutr*. 2007; 85(4): 946–949.
65. American College of Medical Genetics Newborn Screening Expert G. Newborn screening: toward a uniform screening panel and system—executive summary. *Pediatrics*. 2006; 117(5 Pt 2): S296–S307.
66. Fletcher J. Disorders of vitamin B12 metabolism presenting through newborn screening. *Ann Acad Med Singapore*. 2008; 37(Suppl. 12): 79–72.
67. Hinton CF, Ojodu JA, Fernhoff PM, Rasmussen SA, Scanlon KS, Hannon WH. Maternal and neonatal vitamin B12 deficiency detected through expanded newborn screening—United States, 2003–2007. *J Pediatr*. 2010; 157(1): 162–163.
68. Quadros EV, Lai SC, Nakayama Y, et al. Positive newborn screen for methylmalonic aciduria identifies the first mutation in TCblR/CD320, the gene for cellular uptake of transcobalamin-bound vitamin B(12). *Hum Mutat*. 2010; 31(8): 924–929.
69. Weisfeld-Adams JD, Morrissey MA, Kirmse BM, et al. Newborn screening and early biochemical follow-up in combined methylmalonic aciduria and homocystinuria, cblC type, and utility of methionine as a secondary screening analyte. *Mol Genet Metab*. 2010; 99(2): 116–123.
70. Refsum H, Grindflek AW, Ueland PM, et al. Screening for serum total homocysteine in newborn children. *Clin Chem*. 2004; 50(10): 1769–1784.
71. Marble M, Copeland S, Khanfar N, Rosenblatt DS. Neonatal vitamin B12 deficiency secondary to maternal subclinical pernicious anemia: identification by expanded newborn screening. *J Pediatr*. 2008; 152(5): 731–733.
72. Sarafoglou K, Rodgers J, Hietala A, Matern D, Bentler K. Expanded newborn screening for detection of vitamin B12 deficiency. *JAMA;* 2011. 305(12): 1198–1200.

11

Neurotransmission and Neurotoxicity (Phenylketonuria and Dopamine)

Uta Lichter-Konecki

Neurotransmitters have been conceived as chemical messengers that are released by neurons at synapses and elicit an immediate response from a postsynaptic cell (e.g., another neuron). We are not accustomed to thinking of them as being involved in the development of the brain and its connectivity and as having long-term effects on cognition and intellectual ability.

The major neurotransmitters in brain are acetylcholine; the biogenic amines dopamine, norepinephrine, and epinephrine synthesized from tyrosine (Tyr); serotonin synthesized from tryptophan; and the amino acid neurotransmitters, namely glutamate, gamma-aminobutyric acid (synthesized from glutamate), glycine, and D-serine.[1–3]

Well-studied and delineated classic metabolic diseases of amino acid metabolism such as phenylketonuria (PKU) are very familiar to us with regard to the metabolic pathway that is interrupted and the biochemical consequences of the disease. However, we are only beginning to understand or have not yet understood the causes of the gravest consequence of these diseases, namely the severe brain damage that ensues when the patient is not treated or poorly treated. While other classic metabolic diseases such as nonketotic hyperglycinemia have been recognized as members "of the growing class of inborn errors of neurotransmission"[4]; PKU has not, and we have not yet adapted our views on PKU to regard it as a disorder of disturbed neurotransmission and brain development affecting specific brain areas at crucial times of development.

Phenylketonuria and the Hyperphenylalaninemias and Dopamine
Clinical Presentation, Diagnosis, Treatment, and Basic Biochemical Pathways
Background

PKU is a disorder of amino acid metabolism, which is inherited in an autosomal recessive mode and leads to severe brain damage unless treated by a rigorous low-phenylalanine diet from the newborn period on. Classic PKU and its variants are caused by a deficiency of the enzyme phenylalanine hydroxylase (PAH), which catalyzes the hydroxylation of phenylalanine to Tyr[5] and is mainly expressed in the human liver and kidney.[6] PAH deficiency leads to elevated plasma phenylalanine (Phe) levels and low Tyr levels and in a patient with a complete enzyme block Tyr becomes an essential amino acid. The diet limits Phe intake to the absolute minimum needed for normal growth and development and supplements protein intake with Phe-free medical formula.

The paradigm that a metabolic disease can be treated by eliminating the offending molecule, in this case the amino acid Phe, from the diet was proven for the first time in 1954 on the example of PKU when the ability to treat PKU using a Phe-free formula was first demonstrated.[7] Because it was immediately clear that this treatment could be successful in preventing brain damage only if it was implemented as soon after birth as possible, PKU also served as the paradigm for the development of newborn screening (NBS) for metabolic diseases. A blood spot collected on a filter paper card by pricking the heel of a newborn was used to look for elevated blood Phe levels in a bacterial inhibition assay pioneered and first implemented by Robert Guthrie in the United States.[8] After initiation of population-wide NBS for PKU in 1963 in Massachusetts and in 1964 in Germany, it became obvious that in addition to the children with very high Phe levels (>1,200 μM or 20 mg/dl) previously seen in intellectually disabled patients, there were other children with any degree of Phe elevation (hyperphenylalaninemia). NBS detected a continuum of elevated Phe levels.

Children with classic untreated PKU have a plasma Phe level > 20 mg/dl or 1,200 μM and severe intellectual disability, are hypopigmented (if they are Caucasian children they have blue eyes and are blond), and have eczema; their urine has a mousy odor from phenyl ketones; and they may develop neurological symptoms (spasticity, epilepsy, and psychoses). Patients with Phe levels below 20 mg/dl or 1,200 μM but above 10 mg/dl or 600 μM have mild PKU and less or no intellectual disability, and patients with levels below 10 mg/dl or 600 μM do not have intellectual disability and are said to have mild hyperphenylalaninemia. Another commonly used classification scheme defines four types: classical PKU (Phe >1,200 μM), moderate PKU (Phe levels 900–1,200 μM), mild PKU (Phe levels 600–900 μM), and hyperphenylalaninemia (Phe levels <600 μM).[9] In countries where NBS has been established for decades, the classical clinical presentation is not seen anymore unless a child was missed by NBS. Besides patients with elevated plasma Phe levels due to PAH deficiency, NBS also detects patients with elevated Phe levels due to tetrahydrobiopterin (BH4) deficiency. BH4 is the cofactor of PAH needed for the enzyme to reach its full catalytic potential.

PAH (E.C. 1.14.16.1) is one of three aromatic amino acid hydroxylases that emerged from the same ancestral gene, and all use the same cofactor, BH4. The other two aromatic amino acid hydroxylases are Tyr hydroxylase (TH; E.C. 1.14.16.2) and tryptophan hydroxylase (TPH; E.C. 1.14.16.4), both essential for neurotransmitter synthesis. In addition, dopamine β-hydroxylase (DβH; EC 1.14.17.1), nitric oxide synthase (E.C. 1.14.23), and glyceryl-ether monooxygenase (E.C. 1.14.16.5) also use BH4 as cofactor. A defect in BH4 synthesis or regeneration thus affects many more pathways besides the Phe metabolic pathway.[9] Most patients with these rarer defects have a movement disorder in addition to variable degrees of hyperphenylalaninemia and often require neurotransmitter substitution. If left untreated, they also develop intellectual disability and die. The extent of treatment efficacy in achieving normal intellectual ability and function in BH4 deficient patients remains unclear.

Diagnostic Workup / Differential Diagnosis of an Elevated Phenylalanine Level

An elevated Phe level detected on NBS in the United States of America is followed up by quantitative plasma amino acid analysis. To assess for cofactor deficiency measurement of dihydropteridine reductase activity in a blood spot and urine pterin analysis for the percentage of biopterin detected are obtained (1% to 2% of patients with elevated plasma Phe levels have cofactor deficiency). In some countries, patients will also undergo an oral BH4-loading test after diagnosis (using 10 to 20 mg/kg of BH4 at Phe levels above 400 μmol/l) to assess for response to cofactor supplementation.[9] PAH activity measurement for classification would require a liver biopsy and is not done anymore. Phenotyping can be performed (i) by assessing the maximum Phe level reached before treatment was initiated or during a decompensation, (ii) by a standardized protein loading test, and (iii) by assessing Phe tolerance. However, except for the standardized protein loading test, these are inaccurate clinical parameters as they are not measured under standardized conditions, and the ranges of pretreatment Phe level elevations that are associated with the different types of PKU and hyperphenylalaninemia will have to be redefined now that NBS is performed in the first 24 to 72 hr of life when there is much less of a Phe level elevation than previously observed when NBS was performed later. In other words, the currently used pretreatment Phe level ranges that were established as classification criteria when NBS was performed later are not valid anymore. The standardized protein loading test has been abandoned because it exposes the infant to high amounts of Phe and is most reliable when performed on an inpatient basis (i.e., during a three- to four-day hospitalization). Genotyping has thus become a valuable additional tool for patient classification if DNA analysis for PAH-gene mutations detects both mutations in a patient and especially if the combination of these two mutations was previously observed and the associated biochemical phenotype and the response to BH4 is known (BIOPKU database).[10,11] Correct classification of a patient is important for day-to-day clinical management because a good characterization of the patient allows the treating team of metabolic specialists to gauge from the beginning what the likely Phe tolerance of the patient will be rather than determining it by careful diet titration over the course of many months or even years.

Patients with elevated Phe on NBS and abnormal dihydropteridine reductase activity or percentage of biopterin in urine (the NBS follow-up test used in the United States) are evaluated further for a disorder of BH4 synthesis or regeneration.

Disorders of BH4 synthesis are guanosine triphosphate (GTP) cyclohydrolase I (GTPCH) deficiency, which causes very low urinary neopterin and biopterin levels (with a normal ratio) and 6-pyruvoyl-tetrahydropterin synthase deficiency which is the most common cofactor deficiency disorder. 6-pyruvoyl-tetrahydropterin synthase deficiency causes elevated neopterin levels and low biopterin levels and thus an increased neopterin/biopterin ratio.

Dihydropteridine reductase deficiency is a disorder of BH4 regeneration. It causes elevated total biopterin levels in urine. Rare cases of pterin-4-carbinolamin dehydratase deficiency have also been described. Pterin-4-carbinolamin dehydratase is the first enzyme in the BH4 regeneration pathway.

GTPCH deficiency in its autosomal recessive form constitutes a BH4 synthesis defect with variably elevated Phe levels and very low urinary neopterin and biopterin levels. Cerebrospinal fluid neopterin, biopterin, and neurotransmitter metabolite levels are also very low. The autosomal dominant form of GTPCH deficiency causes dopa-responsive dystonia, a disease that has the neurological phenotype of BH4 deficiency but lacks the biochemical block in Phe metabolism. Sepiapterin reductase deficiency is another condition related to BH4 deficiency. Like the autosomal dominant form of GTPCH deficiency, it is not associated with elevated Phe levels.

Treatment

Treatment Initiation, and Treatment Goals—Current Practice

The mainstay of therapy has been dietary restriction of Phe intake since the inception of this treatment by Horst Bickel in 1954.[7] Historically dietary therapy was begun immediately after confirmation of an elevated plasma Phe level above 10 mg/dl or 600 μM. The Phe level at which diet should be implemented has been a subject of controversy. A survey conducted at the beginning of 2011 among 60 centers in the United States and Canada showed that 21% of these centers start treatment at 600 μmol/L or higher, 10% at 480 μmol/L or higher, 63% at 360 μmol/L, and 9% at 240 μmol/L (survey and results described in Blau et al.[9]).[12] An international survey conducted among 23 countries subsequently showed that >50% of PKU clinics worldwide initiate treatment at a Phe level of 360 and another >17% at 480 μM. Only 19% start at a level of 600 μM or higher while 10% even started at a level above 240 μM.[9]

The current goal of therapy is a Phe level between 120 μM and 360 μM or 2 and 6 mg/dl. Previously, centers that performed life-long treatment relaxed the treatment range above 12 years of age to between 120 μM and 600 μM or 2 and 10 mg/dl. However, now a treatment range of 120 μM to 360 μM throughout life is recommended.

A "Comparative Effectiveness Review of Adjuvant Treatment for Phenylketonuria (PKU)," based on research conducted by the Evidence-based Practice Center (under contract to the Agency for Healthcare Research and Quality,[13] concluded that there is moderate evidence for a "threshold effect of a phe level of 400 μmol/L associated with IQ

<85. . . . Increased phe is associated with decreased IQ, with a probability of IQ less than 85 exceeding the population probability (approximately 15%) at phe over 400 μmol/L and leveling off at about 80% at 2,000 μmol/L. This supports the typical target goal for phe level in individuals with PKU (120 to 360 μmol/L). . . . The strongest associations are seen in the group for which historical measurements were taken during the critical period (<6 years old), . . . Hence, control of phe levels during the critical period is particularly important, and there is no evidence that control can be relaxed after early childhood. Current clinical practice is to maintain phe control even in adulthood, which is supported by this analysis."

Chaperone Therapy

A Phe restricted diet is no longer the only means of lowering Phe levels. In December of 2007, sapropterin dihydrochloride, a synthetic form of the natural cofactor BH4, was approved for adjuvant therapy of hyperphenylalaninemia in the United States. Enzyme cofactors can function as chaperones, meaning they can stabilize a defective enzyme sufficiently to increase residual enzyme function and improve flux through the respective metabolic pathway. This, however, requires that a defective enzyme be produced that can be stabilized before being degraded by cellular mechanisms. Most mutations of the *PAH* gene are missense mutations theoretically allowing for a mutant enzyme to be produced; however, for those missense mutations associated with severe classical PKU no residual enzyme activity has been detected.[10]

When testing patients for cofactor deficiency during routine diagnostic workup, it was discovered that higher doses of BH4 supplementation led to a positive response not only in cofactor deficient patients but also in some patients with PAH deficiency. These results indicated that BH4 not only is beneficial for patients with a block in cofactor synthesis or regeneration but (at increased doses) can also serve as a chaperone for an unstable apo-enzyme (PAH). This observation led to the development of BH4-chaperone therapy for PKU.[9] Lindegren et al. reviewed clinical trials of cofactor treatment and concluded, "Phe levels were reduced by at least 30% (the level used in studies submitted to the FDA to support responsiveness) in up to half of treated participants (32 to 50%) at dosages of 5 to 20 mg/kg/day and for up to 22 weeks of observation in comparative studies. . . phe tolerance improved over time."[13]

Treatment Goals During Pregnancy

The fact that elevated Phe levels in a pregnant mother cause a severe embryo fetopathy was recognized as early as 1963.[14,15] The maternal PKU (MPKU) syndrome consists of microcephaly, intrauterine growth retardation, congenital heart defects, impaired cognition, intellectual disability, and dysmorphic features such as flat nasal bridge, long palpebral fissures, wide outer canthus, and long smooth philtrum.[16]

The "Comparative Effectiveness Review" of the literature by Lindegren et al. confirmed "that the relationship between maternal blood phe and offspring cognitive outcomes was not linear, that a threshold of 360 μmol/L is the level at which cognitive impairment was significantly more common in offspring of mothers with PKU than in controls, and that a linear relationship between Phe levels and impaired cognitive outcomes occurred after this threshold. Importantly, while other factors, including maternal characteristics, severity of mutations, and offspring head circumference, contributed strongly to outcomes at 1 year of age, by age 2, maternal Phe strongly overtook other factors in predicting cognitive impairment."[13]

Although lifelong dietary treatment is now recommended, when a young woman who is on diet wants to become pregnant, the dietary control must be reassessed. Typically, a more rigorous diet has to be implemented to reach the treatment goal of Phe levels between 2 and 6 mg/dl for pregnant women as set forth by the Maternal PKU Collaborative Study or 1 to 4 mg/dl as recommended in Britain and Germany. The safety of cofactor therapy during pregnancy is currently being assessed via a patient registry that is sponsored by the pharmaceutical industry.

Outcomes With Emphasis on Emerging Questions and Variant Phenotypes

PKU/hyperphenylalaninemia was the first inborn error of metabolism detected by NBS, and we now have 50 years of experience with PKU screening, treatment, and outcome.

Large national collaborative studies followed patients detected by NBS and treated with a low-Phe diet longitudinally and measured treatment outcome. The "Collaborative Study of Children Treated for Phenylketonuria" of the United States published in 1977[17] and in 1981[18] showed that children treated early for PKU with a Phe-restricted diet achieved normal IQs. Dobson et al. reported that those children for whom dietary treatment was initiated during the first month of life scored a mean IQ of 95 at age four.[17] Williamson et al. reported on a cohort of 132 children followed on treatment from the neonatal period to six years of age. "The mean IQ of the total sample at age 6 years was 98 on the Stanford-Binet Intelligence Scale... the most important predictors of IQ for 6-year-old children were: (1) mothers' intellectual ability (as measured on the Wechsler Adult Intelligence Scale); (2) age at which the subjects were first treated; and (3) how well the subjects adhered to the phe-restricted diet."[18]

Variant Phenotypes

After NBS for hyperphenylalaninemia was initiated, it became apparent that a very broad spectrum of patients exists and that this spectrum represents a continuum of elevated Phe levels. Attempts at classifying the continuum of patients culminated in the recognition that the majority of patients are compound heterozygotes with a different mutation in each of their PAH alleles and that the combination of different mutations can usually explain the biochemical phenotype.[10] Over 500 PAH gene mutations have been characterized worldwide (*PAHdb*; BIOPKU database). The majority are missense mutations with a number of them resulting in less than 1% residual enzyme activity in vivo. Active PAH is a tetramer of identical subunits, and for those mutant forms of the enzyme that show residual enzyme activity the interaction between subunits with different mutations is considered to be complex, explaining variant phenotypes where the biochemical phenotype cannot be predicted based on the patient's individual mutations.[19]

How Successful Is the Treatment?

While the treatment is successful in preventing intellectual disability, the long-term neuropsychological outcome may encompass complications such as attention deficit disorder (ADD) and executive function (EF) deficits in early treated PKU patients.

The "brain phenotype" is significantly influenced by the high Phe levels as severe intellectual disability is prevented by lowering the plasma Phe level. However, Phe levels and *PAH* mutations cannot solely explain the intellectual outcome. Especially now that an effective dietary treatment has been available for several decades, shortcomings of the treatment and its outcome are an important research focus along with the development of new treatment options to ease the difficulty of dietary compliance.

Alternative or Adjunct Treatment Options Currently Used or in Clinical Trials

Chaperone Therapy for Phenylketonuria

The use of a synthetic form (sapropterin) of the natural cofactor (BH4) as a chaperone for a defective enzyme is now an established therapy and was already described under "Treatment." It is effective in up to 50% of patients with hyperphenylalaninemeia. It is typically used in patients with a milder form of the disease. Other possible chaperones that could be explored have been proposed.[20]

Adjunct Large Neutral Amino Acid Substitution Therapy

Currently one of the main hypotheses regarding the cause of the brain damage in PKU is that competitive inhibition of large neutral amino acid (LNAA) transport across the blood–brain barrier (BBB) by high blood Phe levels leads to deficiency of Tyr and tryptophan and consequently reduced neurotransmitter and protein synthesis in the central nervous system. This hypothesis and the measurement of seemingly reduced intracerebral Phe levels under Tyr substitution initially led to additional Tyr supplementation and now LNAA supplementation during dietary therapy as a treatment concept, especially in adolescent and adult patients off diet or on a relaxed diet. Tyr supplementation by itself however—without dietary restriction of Phe intake—was early on shown to be unable to prevent severe brain damage.[21] (Also see "Decreased Neurotransmitter Synthesis" section for a discussion of this issue.)

It was also thought that Phe transport could be blocked at the intestinal mucosa by LNAA substitution, that is, that LNAAs could block Phe uptake in the gut. Berger et al., however, reported that only one of the transport mechanisms of Phe at the intestinal mucosa is sensitive to LNAA inhibition.[22]

The effectiveness of LNAA substitution for the treatment of PKU is a key question regarding PKU treatment today. The "Comparative Effectiveness Review of Adjuvant Treatment for Phenylketonuria (PKU)"[13] assessed that of the three studies that investigated the effect of LNAA substitution in PKU, one reported an improvement in executive functioning. "Overall, participants who were using a Phe-free medical food for their nutritional needs did not experience a decrease in Phe, although those not adhering to diet or not using their formula did. In all three studies, blood Phe decreased after 1 week of treatment but remained above clinically acceptable levels." The review concluded that there was insufficient evidence to suggest that LNAAs could be a viable treatment option for reducing Phe levels or increasing Phe tolerance.

Phenylalanine Ammonia Lyase Treatment:

Another adjunct therapy is the administration of phenylalanine ammonia lyase (PAL), an enzyme that converts Phe to transcinnamic acid. The initial intent was to develop an oral medication that would metabolize Phe ingested with the diet in the gut before it was absorbed. However, PAL is destroyed by low gastric pH and intestinal proteolysis when given orally. The drug that has been developed for patient use and is currently in clinical trials is a pegylated PAL that must be administered by subcutaneous injection.

The use of a genetically modified probiotic expressing PAL in the gut is also proposed as an alternative to subcutaneous injection and is currently under investigation.[23]

Induction of Mutant Phenylalanine Hydroxylase by High Phenylalanine Levels

Langenbeck et al. saw evidence that certain PAH mutants might respond to higher Phe levels with induction of the mutant enzyme.[24] It is thus important to determine the Phe tolerance of every patient empirically unless the respective molecular data are available.

Enzyme Replacement Therapy by Organ Transplant or Hepatocyte Transfer

Lichter-Konecki et al. demonstrated that besides the liver, considerable amounts of PAH activity also exists in the human kidney and that the PAH transcript is also present in the pancreas, adrenal, testes, and brain,[6] Since 10% of PAH enzyme activity is sufficient to maintain normal Phe levels in heterozygotes[5] not only liver transplant but also kidney transplant could potentially be curative in PKU. This could be assessed if a PKU patient could be investigated who needed a kidney transplant due to kidney failure. However, since PKU is amenable to dietary management and does not cause life-threatening metabolic crises, theoretically curative but potentially life-threatening organ transplant does not appear easily justified in PKU patients.

Short of whole organ replacement, liver cell transplantation has been performed in PKU[25]; however, at this point a long-lasting effect has not been demonstrated. The use of a patient's own induced pluripotent stem cells that would undergo correction of the gene defect by gene editing and then be transferred back into the patient is also being proposed as autologous cell-based therapy.[26]

Gene Therapy

PAH is a very labile, cytosolic enzyme that is hard to purify and needs a complex intracellular cofactor synthesis and regeneration system to function. For a long time, PAH was said to be expressed in the liver and kidney in rodents and only in the liver in humans.[5] As an alternative to a very rigorous, Phe-restricted diet, gene therapy approaches to PKU treatment have been explored since the mid-1980s. Retroviral and adenoviral gene transfer into primary hepatocytes (and hepatocyte transplantation[27,28]), as well as into muscle cells[29] were performed in animal models. Current experimental approaches are using adeno-associated virus gene therapy in the liver[30] or are considering vector-mediated gene therapy in hepatocytes that would then re-populate the liver of PAH-deficient recipients.[31]

Current Paradigm on Pathogenesis and Interaction With Other Metabolic Pathways

Besides clinical outcome studies, other areas of PKU research in the past two and a half decades have focused on exploring genotype/phenotype correlation,[10,11,32] gene therapy,[27,28,31] population genetics,[33] the cause of the severe brain damage,[34] and cognitive outcome.[35] The pathophysiology of the severe brain damage in PKU has not been elucidated, and it is clear that it must be related to a high Phe level since lowering the Phe level prevents severe brain damage but the mechanism by which high Phe levels harm the brain has not been satisfactory elucidated.

Phe is an essential amino acid, and in the PAH enzyme deficiency state Tyr becomes an essential amino acid. This illustrates that Phe hydroxylation is not only a breakdown pathway in the metabolism of Phe but also a synthesis pathway for the very important neurotransmitter precursor Tyr. Phe thus is important to protein synthesis as an essential amino acid and to neurotransmitter synthesis as a precursor. PAH shares the same cofactor, BH4, with the other two aromatic amino acid hydroxylases, TH and TPH, which are essential for neurotransmitter synthesis. BH4 is also the cofactor for DβH, nitric oxide synthase, and glyceryl-ether monooxygenase.

Impact of Phenylketones

As mentioned above, classic PKU and its variants are caused by a deficiency of the apo-enzyme PAH, which catalyzes the hydroxylation of Phe to Tyr and is mainly expressed in the human liver and kidney. PAH deficiency leads to elevated plasma Phe levels and low Tyr levels and increased formation of alternative Phe metabolites such as phenylpyruvate and phenyllactate through transamination and phenylacetate through decarboxylation of Phe.

In the 1970s and early 1980s there was active research investigating these alternative Phe metabolites as the main cause of the brain damage in PKU but there was poor correlation between the amount of alternative Phe metabolites excreted in the urine and clinical phenotypes. In addition, Phe metabolites were not found in sufficiently high concentrations in PKU patients to be toxic to the brain,[36] which led to less interest in this area of research.

Additional evidence that the alternative metabolites are not causing the brain damage in PKU stems from a pair of siblings with "chemical phenylketonuria".[37] Two sisters who excreted a large amount of phenylketones, had normal Phe levels, and did not develop brain damage (Trefz et al., unpublished results).

Large Neutral Amino Acid Transport at the Blood–Brain Barrier, Hypomyelination, and Protein Synthesis

The currently most favored hypothesis regarding the cause of the severe brain damage in PKU postulates that brain damage in PKU is caused by competitive inhibition of the transport of LNAA (namely, branched-chain amino acids and Tyr and tryptophan) by high plasma Phe levels at the BBB, resulting in decreased neurotransmitter synthesis and decreased cerebral protein synthesis and consequently dopamine and norepinephrine deficiency and hypomyelination.[34,38]

Reduced Cerebral Protein Synthesis and Hypomyelination

Of all the pathological changes described in the brains of untreated PKU patients, hypomyelination and gliosis are the prevailing findings[39]; hypomyelination was also observed in the PKU mouse $Pah^{enu2/2}$.[40]

Nuclear magnetic resonance spectroscopy demonstrated that brain Phe levels are considerably lower than plasma Phe levels and that there is a poor correlation between the two.[41,42] The authors of these reports explained their results again with Phe transport kinetics at the BBB. Significant interindividual variations in LNAA transport kinetics at the BBB were suggested to cause the different degrees of brain damage observed in patients. These transport variations were proposed to be due to different alleles of the L-type amino acid transporters (LAT) for LNAA; however, an association between LAT1 alleles and brain Phe concentrations could not be substantiated.[43]

The hypomyelination hypothesis seemed to be of immediate clinical relevance when areas of increased signal intensity on T2-weighted images in the periventricular white matter of previously treated adult PKU patients off-diet were discovered by magnetic resonance imaging. The images were reminiscent of demyelinating diseases, but the phenomenon was reversible by reinstitution of a rigorous diet and appeared related to the water content of the myelin sheath.[44] Manara et al. investigated this phenomenon in 20 early-treated PKU patients still on diet using diffusion-weighted imaging (DWI) and found that no patient with mean Phe levels below 460 μmol/L showed white matter abnormalities.[45] In patients with higher Phe levels there were significantly more white matter abnormalities detected on DWI than on T2- images. DWI showed a progressive involvement of frontotemporal, occipital, and parietal white matter. Changes seen on T2 and DWI showed strong correlation with the mean Phe level the year prior to the exam but no correlation with the Tyr level. Peng et al. reported significantly restricted mean diffusivity, normal fractional anisotropy, and restricted axial and radial diffusivity in several white matter tracts in early treated young adults.[46] White matter changes were more evident in older patients with higher Phe than younger patients with lower Phe levels. White et al. reported significant improvement of microstructural white matter integrity measured by mean diffusivity in patients that responded to BH4 supplementation with a 37% decrease in Phe levels.[47] This seemed to be consistent with the initial findings of Bick et al. (193).[44]

Smith and Kang investigated cerebral protein synthesis in the PKU mouse and found reduced neutral amino acid (NAA) contribution from plasma to the tRNA-bound pool in brain, but no reduction in the brain concentration of tRNA-bound NAA.[48] They concluded that in the PKU mouse brain a greater fraction of NAA in the precursor pool for protein synthesis is derived from protein degradation and that a reduction in cerebral protein synthesis may not be the cause of the brain damage in PKU.

Inhibition of Cholesterol Synthesis

A different cause of hypomyelination in PKU was discussed by Shefer et al. who investigated whether high Phe levels inhibit cholesterol synthesis in the genetic mouse model for PKU.[49] They found select tracts to be hypomyelinated in the forebrain of adult PKU mice. Furthermore they showed that 3-hydroxy-3 methylglutaryl coenzyme A reductase (HMGR) activity was decreased by 30% in forebrain while it was normal in hindbrain. They proceeded to demonstrate that Phe is a noncompetitive inhibitor of HMGR and concluded that Phe leads to moderate HMGR inhibition in PKU mouse forebrain where a subset of oligodendrocytes is unable to overcome the inhibition.

Phenylalanine Fibrils

Adler-Abramovich et al. reported that at abnormally high concentrations phenylalanine forms fibrils that resemble amyloid and are toxic to the cell.[50] They detected such fibrils in the hippocampus of the mouse model and in parietal cortex of PKU patients and discussed whether amyloidosis explains the brain damage in PKU.

Attention Deficit Disorder in Phenylketonuria Patients and Offspring of Phenylketonuria Mothers

Many patients with inborn errors of metabolism have ADD/attention deficit hyperactivity disorder (ADHD), in particular, patients with PKU and high Phe levels, patients with maple syrup urine disease and high leucine levels, and patients with urea cycle disorders. ADD/ADHD is considered to be a dopamine deficiency disorder.[51] Given the studies described below there appears to be evidence for dopamine deficiency in PKU, and ADD/ADHD might then be a logical consequence in this condition.

Antshel and Waisbren studied 7- to 16-year-old PKU patients and offspring of mothers with PKU, comparing them to unaffected siblings of PKU patients, and found that early-treated PKU patients had ADHD-inattentive type while offspring of PKU mothers treated during pregnancy had ADHD-combined type.[52] The authors formulated the hypothesis that ADHD in both groups of patients was due to the toxic effect Phe had on the same neurological systems at different time points during central nervous system development. Antshel and Waisbren noted that early-treated PKU patients had a normal IQ and showed normal development but had subtle neuropsychological deficiencies in visuospatial skills, sustained attention, processing speed, and EF, while offspring of PKU mothers treated during pregnancy scored lower on parameters of general cognition and had behavioral problems.[52] In addition, PKU patients may show white matter abnormalities in the frontal and parieto-occipital region while MPKU offspring did not. Antshel and Waisbren tested these patients with measures of selective attention and cognitive flexibility, auditory learning and memory, visuospatial skills, visual memory, visual motor integration, and executive functioning as well as an ADHD rating scale for inattentive and hyperactive-impulsive symptoms.[52] The EF difficulties seen in PKU patients were consistent with ADHD-inattentive subtype while the ones seen in MPKU offspring were consistent with ADHD-combined subtype. In both groups there was a robust relationship between EF, processing speed, and degree of Phe exposure.

Channon et al. tested adult PKU patients on a life-long diet and described cognitive slowing but did not find EF deficits, including with regard to working memory load and inhibitory conflict.[53] They did not employ the same test battery in these adult patients as had been used by Antshel and Waisbren.[52]

The "Comparative Effectiveness Review of Adjuvant Treatment for Phenylketonuria (PKU)"[13] assessed that overall, while Phe levels correlate with various assessments of EF in some papers, the degree to which they are correlated and the correlation on individual measures are inconsistent.

Decreased Neurotransmitter Synthesis

Very early on there was a hypothesis that Tyr deficiency was the cause of the brain damage in PKU by compromising protein synthesis and that Tyr supplementation would be the appropriate therapy.[54] One patient was treated according to this hypothesis with Tyr supplementation only and developed severe brain damage.[55]

Decreased neurotransmitter synthesis due to Tyr deficiency, however, has been a continued concern in PKU and the subject of many investigations. Lykkelund et al. showed decreased amounts of dopamine metabolites in cerebrospinal fluid of PKU patients.[56] Based on the hypothesis of competitive inhibition of LNAA transport at the BBB by high Phe, this observation led to the recommendation of LNAA supplementation to increase neurotransmitter synthesis in PKU patients.[57]

Lou reviewed that there is evidence for reduced Tyr concentration in the central nervous system in PKU, which implies that there will not be enough substrate for catecholamine synthesis.[58] He attributed the low Tyr level to, for example, inhibition of BBB transport. Lou reported that taking high doses of Tyr leads to shortening of reaction time and improvement of psychological test scores.

Paans et al. reported that in patients with plasma Phe levels above the maximum therapeutic concentration (> 700 μmol/l) the protein synthesis rate for Tyr was decreased when compared to controls and patients with plasma Phe concentrations within the therapeutic range, indicating a decreased availability of Tyr for neurotransmitter synthesis and explaining reduced cerebral catecholamine concentrations.[59,60]

Pietz et al.[61] and Smith et al.[62] reported that high-dose Tyr supplementation had no effect on neuropsychological performance of PKU patients. Subsequently, Pietz et al.[63] reported that giving adult PKU patients supplemental LNAA, including tryptophan and Tyr, during an oral Phe challenge blocked Phe influx into the brain and prevented the mild acute slowing of the EEG background activity (seen by EEG spectral analysis) associated with the Phe load when no LNAA supplementation was given. However, this effect of LNAA supplementation was demonstrated only in their short-term specific trial.

Positron Emission Tomography Studies of Tyrosine and Dopamine Synthesis in Adult Phenylketonuria Brain

Paans et al. used labeled Tyr (L-[1-^{11}C]-Tyr) and FESP (^{18}F-fluoro-ethyl-spiperone), a D_2-receptor ligand, to study Tyr availability in the brains of patients on low-Phe diet.[59] As already mentioned above, in two patients with Phe levels over 700 μmol/l the protein synthesis rate for Tyr was decreased, indicating decreased availability of Tyr. D_2-receptor availability seemed unchanged.

Landvogt et al. used PET to measure [^{18}F]fluoro-L-dopamine (FDOPA) usage in the brain of adult PKU patients with elevated Phe levels but normal neurological function and normal performance on the neuropsychological tests administered.[64] They found that the flux of FDOPA to brain was impaired in adult PKU patients versus controls and that this was not correlated with individual serum Phe levels. They presumed that this impairment reflected the inhibition of the LNAA carrier by elevated Phe levels as the carrier has a higher affinity for Phe than for FDOPA. They also found evidence for decreased dopa-decarboxylase activity converting L-DOPA into dopamine and speculated that this may also be due to competitive inhibition by Phe. Finally, they saw an inhibition of L-DOPA efflux from brain and suspected elevated brain Phe to impede the efflux. Since PKU patients do not have symptoms of Parkinson disease, the authors speculated whether the different effects of high Phe on dopamine metabolism and transport may in the end balance each other out. They also considered that postsynaptic dopamine receptors may be upregulated in PKU as seen in Parkinson disease patients compensating for the decreased dopamine levels.

The Prefrontal Cortex Dysfunction Hypothesis

First Welsh et al.[65] and then Diamond et al.[66] showed in systematic studies that early treated children with PKU have EF deficits, with EF being a cognitive ability that has been linked to the prefrontal cortex. Prefrontal dysfunction in PKU had been proposed before[67,68] and attributed to decreased dopamine levels in PKU patients, presumably caused by high Phe levels inhibiting Tyr transport into brain. Diamond et al.[69] explained that the prefrontal cortex is particularly vulnerable to decreased dopamine levels because its dopaminergic neurons have higher firing rates and higher dopamine turnover rates than other dopaminergic neurons.[70] They also appear to lack an autoregulatory mechanism (synthesis-modulating autoreceptors) present in other dopaminergic neurons.[71]

Diamond at al. also showed reduced levels of dopamine and the dopamine metabolite, homovanillic acid in prefrontal cortex of an animal model in which PAH was chemically inhibited.[69] The animals showed impaired performance on a task attributed to prefrontal cortex function. Noradrenaline levels were not affected, but serotonin levels and dopamine levels outside the prefrontal cortex were somewhat reduced.

Visual Evoked Potential Abnormalities in PKU

PKU patients may show prolonged latencies of visual evoked potentials, and the same symptom in patients with Parkinson disease resolves with L-dopa administration.[72]

Neuropsychological testing demonstrated that choice reaction time as assessed in visual attention task tests was influenced by the concurrent Phe level in PKU patients. Selection and inhibition of different stimuli assessed by the Colour Word Interference Task can be impaired in patients with Parkinson disease depending on their L-dopa therapy and in adolescent PKU patients dependent on their Phe level. The performance on the Colour Word Interference Task test is associated with activation of frontal cortex,[72] also felt to be particularly sensitive to decreases in dopamine levels.[69] According to a later study by Diamond,[73] a possible connection between visual performance and frontal and prefrontal cortex performance is indicated by the fact that retinal dopaminergic neurons have similar characteristics as prefrontal cortex neurons and therefore can be expected to be similarly sensitive to even mild dopamine deficiency. However, Ullrich et al. saw no effect of two weeks of L-dopa therapy on choice reaction time tasks, sustained attention, frontal lobe function, or latencies of visual evoked potentials in untreated adult PKU patients.[72]

Pascucci et al. conducted a very careful study specifically targeting the medial prefrontal cortex (mpFC) of the PAH^{enu2} PKU mouse model (ENU2).[74] They found reduced plasma and brain levels of Tyr in these mice and reduced TH protein levels as well as activity in the mpFC of these mice and hypothesized that this was due to inhibition of TH by elevated Phe, although down-regulation of the enzyme due to less dopamine synthesis could not be ruled out. The Tyr BBB ratio was not significantly different between ENU2 and wild type mice. They took this as evidence that the transport of Tyr into brain is not inhibited by high Phe.

Because of the reduced TH activity, they did not think that Tyr supplementation would be successful in normalizing dopamine levels and used low dose L-DOPA instead. L-DOPA administration caused a significant increase of extracellular dopamine levels. The authors then tested the stress response of the mice on low-dose L-DOPA. They had previously shown that the mice had deficits in serotonergic and dopaminergic neurotransmission and an abnormal noradrenergic response under stress. On the other hand, dopamine turnover was also reduced in ENU2 mice, which may help maintain normal basal dopamine levels. L-DOPA restored dopamine transmission in the mpFC to normal levels despite of high Phe levels. Extracellular norepinephrine levels were not normalized in the mpFC by L-DOPA administration. It is thus not clear which neurons decarboxylated L-DOPA to dopamine in this setting as serotonergic neurons could also have been involved. Based on this work, reduced dopamine levels in ENU2 mouse brain are due to decreased Tyr availability, less TH protein, and less TH activity in brain.

Previously Pascucci et al. also showed that less serotonin synthesis in the ENU2 mouse brain is due to inhibition of tryptophan hydroxylase activity by high Phe.[75]

Relation Between Myelin Production and Dopamine Synthesis in Phenylketonuria
Joseph and Dyer performed a comprehensive study in ENU2 mice to address hypomyelination and dopamine deficiency in PKU.[76] They measured Phe, Tyr, and dopamine in the blood, frontal cortex, and striatum of affected animals versus heterozygous littermates off diet and during a four-week course on diet. At the same time, they also measured myelin basic protein (MBP), TH, and phosphorylated neurofilament levels in the frontal cortex to analyze the relationship between myelination, axonal maturation, Tyr levels, and dopamine synthesis. Consistent with previous findings in humans, they found lower Phe levels in the frontal cortex and striatum than in the blood. Tyr levels in these brain regions in untreated PKU mice were about half of control levels but higher than the blood Tyr levels in these animals. On the other hand, Tyr levels increased to only 65% to 68% of controls during dietary intervention when Phe levels decreased substantially and blood Tyr levels normalized. Most interestingly, dopamine levels were about 60% of controls in the frontal cortex and 34% of

controls in the striatum prior to treatment and normalized despite of the fact that Tyr levels did not. Moreover, dopamine levels normalized rapidly in the striatum and gradually (over the course of four weeks) in the frontal cortex. MBP, TH, and phosphorylated neurofilament levels were approximately 75% of control values in the frontal cortex. MBP (105%) and phosphorylated neurofilament levels (115%) rose to above control levels in the frontal cortex within one week of treatment while there was no change in the amount of TH protein until the second week. MBP levels in the frontal cortex continued to increase throughout the four-week treatment period.

In the striatum, MBP and TH levels were about 74%, and 78% of control and phosphorylated neurofilament levels were normal in untreated PKU mice. All three increased to above control or close to control (TH) levels within one week on diet, and only phosphorylated neurofilament levels increased further in the second week. Based on these data, Joseph and Dyer concluded that (i) Tyr levels are not key regulators of dopamine synthesis and (ii) there appears to be a relationship between myelination and dopamine production. They interpreted their results as supporting their "myelin/dopamine theory" (as compared to a "tyrosine/dopamine theory"), which postulates that myelination influences dopamine synthesis.[76] They added that an influence of myelin on axon maturation is established although the molecular mechanism was not known. The authors suggested that myelin/axon contact triggers signaling pathways that up-regulate neurotransmitter synthesis (e.g., via phosphorylation of TH leading to increased TH activity and dopamine production without a change in the amount of TH protein present).

Joseph and Dyer also discussed the possibility that TH hydroxylates Phe in the brain of PKU mice, that dopamine synthesis is reduced because of decreased protein synthesis, and that the BBB neutral amino acid transport system may have adapted during the lifetime of the mice to elevated Phe levels such that amino acid levels in the brain, especially Tyr levels, are adapted to the brain's needs, explaining the higher brain than blood Tyr levels in the untreated animals.[76]

A large advantage of this study over studies in previous decades was that it was performed in an animal model that mimicked most closely the untreated human disease, namely, in mouse brains that had been exposed to elevated Phe levels since birth rather than only to a short-term Phe load.

Hypopigmentation

In addition to the severe intellectual disability, another unexplained classical symptom of PKU is hypopigmentation. Untreated or poorly treated PKU patients of Western European descent have fair skin and are blond and blue-eyed; patients of other ethnic groups also show signs of hypopigmentation (such as lighter skin and hair color). Initiation of dietary therapy reverses the hypopigmentation and leads to darker hair and skin color in humans and darker coat color in the PKU mouse model. This indicates that melanin biosynthesis is inhibited by high Phe levels in a reversible fashion. Fitzpatrick and Miyamoto showed that high Phe concentrations inhibit tyrosinase activity by 15% to 30% in vitro and concluded that excess Phe competitively inhibits the Tyr-tyrosinase reaction leading to the hypopigmentation.[77] However, a 15% to 30% reduction in tyrosinase activity is not sufficient to cause visible depigmentation (V. Hearing, personal communication). Schallreuther et al. reported PAH expression in melanocytes and undifferentiated keratinocytes.[78] They also reported that Phe is actively transported into melanocytes, while Tyr transport into melanocytes occurs by facilitated diffusion.[79] Gahl et al., on the other hand, demonstrated that a Tyr transport system exists in the melanosomal membrane.[80]

Maternal Phenylketonuria

Besides PKU, another significant disease entity caused by high Phe levels is MPKU or maternal yperphenylalaninemia, where high Phe levels in the mother have a severe teratogenic effect causing an embryopathy and a fetopathy that bears some resemblance to fetal alcohol syndrome.[16] As with the severe brain damage of untreated PKU patients, how high Phe levels cause this embryo-fetopathy has not been established but the observed symptoms point to a possible interference with neural crest cell migration by high Phe levels at crucial times of development. Interference with neural crest cell migration has also been discussed in other embryo-fetopathies such as fetal alcohol syndrome, with which it shares some phenotypic similarities.

The Neuropathology of Phenylketonuria

Bauman and Kemper systematically studied the brains of three untreated, profoundly intellectually disabled adult males against age-matched controls with special focus on the developmental stage of the brains in morphological and histoanatomical terms.[39] Their criteria included myelination, the width of the cortical plate, cell packing density, neuronal cell size, dendritic arborization, and synaptic spine populations. They noted that previously reported morphological findings in the brains of PKU patients were inconsistent except for brain weight, which was consistently reduced. Some but not all previous reports described changes in myelin such as myelin pallor, breakdown or necrosis, gliosis, and status spongiosus. On the other hand, neuronal changes like paucity of cortical neurons, faintly stained neurons, and immature appearing neurons were frequently observed. In one report, even depigmentation of the substantia nigra was noted.[81]

Their own findings indicated a severe inhibition of maturation in the structural development of the postnatal brain in PKU. In their study, pallor of myelin staining was limited to fiber systems with prolonged postnatal myelination and was interpreted as decreased myelination. There were also signs of delay or arrest in the development of the cytoarchitecture of the cortical plate in all cortical areas studied. Neurons with a long postnatal developmental time course such as the Betz cells showed decreased or halted maturation while neurons that are fully developed at birth were unchanged compared to controls. Cortical neurons showed paucity of dendritic arborization and reduced number of synaptic spines. Bauman and Kemper concluded that the neuron was the primary target in PKU.[39]

Animal Models for Phenylketonuria

Early on animal models for PKU were generated by feeding or injecting rodents with p-chlorophenylalanine or α-methylphenylalanine, both PAH inhibitors with p-chlorophenylalanine having toxic side effects.[5]

Genetic mouse models generated by chemical mutagenesis became available in 1988. The genetic mouse model that has been made available to the scientific community and can be obtained from Jackson Laboratories is the *Pah^{enu2}* mouse, which has a point mutation in exon 7 of the gene and shows a number of the features of the human disease, including some cognitive impairment.[82]

Unanswered Questions, Future Directions of Research, Impact on Common or Complex Disease

From a clinical perspective, the currently immediately pressing issues introduced at the beginning of this chapter are

- Establishing new pretreatment Phe level ranges that allow for the classification of patients with hyperphenylalaninemia based on their pretreatment Phe level obtained by early NBS.
- Collecting genotype/phenotype correlation data of homozygous and compound heterozygous patients with every possible mutation combination (as is done in the BioPKU database) nationally and internationally so that these data are available to the genetic community for classification of newborns with hyperphenylalaninemia.
- Answering the question whether there is efficacy in LNAA supplementation and whether it is safe through carefully designed clinical studies and animal experiments.
- Establishing the long-term efficacy of cofactor chaperone therapy.
- Developing a home monitor for Phe level measurements to empower patients to achieve better Phe level control on a day-to-day basis.

From a broader perspective of understanding the pathophysiology of PKU as a prerequisite to designing new therapies and improving outcome, the following studies are needed:

PKU has served as the paradigm and proof of concept for treating inborn errors of metabolism with a diet devoid of the offending molecule (i.e., the amino acid phenylalanine). It subsequently became a paradigm for NBS and an example for the fact that successful treatment of a deleterious genetic condition will lead to new challenges during the lifetime of the patient, such as the challenge of MPKU in female adult PKU patients. Determining the cause of the intellectual disability in PKU and of the embryofetopathy in MPKU could lead to PKU also becoming a paradigm for the pathophysiology of intellectual disability, attention deficit hyperactivity disorder (ADHD), EF, and birth defects.

To date, all patients with PKU are treated if the country they live in has the resources to provide them with NBS and dietary and or cofactor therapy. All pregnant mothers with PKU are also treated if they seek treatment and resources are available. Nevertheless, the outcome of dietary management is not perfect. Although adult PKU patients live independent lives and have successful careers, some patients are significantly compromised by learning disabilities, EF deficits, and ADHD, as are offspring of mothers with PKU. Whether these latter symptoms are a result of deficiencies of the treatment or rather due to residual disease and could be improved with more rigorous therapy, as was suggested by Diamond has not been determined with certainty.[83] As described in the previous paragraphs, symptoms generally improve with improved Phe level control, supporting the hypothesis that the symptoms are due to insufficient dietary control. This observation justified life-long strict dietary control that has consequently been recommended since the 1990s.

In summary, considering the findings described previously, it is not clear how Phe and Tyr levels in the brain of PKU patients and PKU mice are regulated. Lower brain Phe than plasma Phe levels at high plasma Phe levels could be due to a saturation of the carrier system.[84,85] Joseph and Dyer, on the other hand, reported higher brain Tyr than plasma Tyr in untreated PKU mice.[76] However, Tyr levels were overall reduced in the brain, which would either be due to adaptive transport kinetics for Tyr in affected animals or to brain synthesis of Tyr—possibly only in specific brain areas and possibly by TH. In addition, reduced TH activity was observed in the brain. Pascucci et al. also reported overall low Tyr levels but an unaltered blood/brain ratio for Tyr in the mpFC supporting normal transport of Tyr at the BBB.[74] They also observed reduced TH activity and reduced TH protein in the brain, making Tyr supplementation to raise brain dopamine levels less likely to be successful. However, they were able to show that L-DOPA supplementation increases extracellular dopamine levels but not norepinephrine levels in the ENU2 cortex. Bauman and Kemper saw decreased myelination, arrest of development of the cytoarchitecture of the cortical plate, disturbed neuronal maturation, paucity of dendritic arborization, and less synaptic spines.[39] Several direct and indirect lines of evidence, including direct measurements in specific brain regions of the ENU2 mouse, thus confirm decreased dopamine levels (whatever the cause), decreased norepinephrine levels, decreased myelin levels, and problems with neuronal development and synapse formation in PKU.

Phenylketonuria: A White Matter Disease?

PKU is still widely regarded as a white matter disease. As outlined previously, there is evidence for hypomyelination in PKU; however, it is not clear whether this is the primary or a secondary defect in PKU. Several lines of reasoning make it plausible that hypomyelination may be secondary and neuronal damage primary.

The hypothesis that the cause of the intellectual disability in PKU is hypomyelination due to decreased protein synthesis caused by the inhibition of the BBB transport of large neutral amino acids by high plasma Phe levels is put into question by the following considerations:

1. If high levels of one LNAA can inhibit the transport of the others, thus hampering protein biosynthesis, why is the phenomenon of disturbed protein biosynthesis and hypomyelination not a major factor in tyrosinemia type II and histidinemia, where plasma concentrations of Tyr and histidine comparable to Phe levels in PKU are reached?[86]

One might explain this with Phe having a higher affinity for LAT1 than Tyr or histidine but,

2. If the mechanism is transport inhibition, followed by decreased protein biosynthesis causing hypomyelination, why is the spinal cord, which is part of the central nervous system and beyond the BBB, not affected like the brain?

3. The work of Smith and Kang showed no reduction in the brain concentration of tRNA-bound NAA.[48] They concluded that a reduction in cerebral protein synthesis may not be the cause of the brain damage in PKU.

However, as hypomyelination is observed, the question is whether it is the primary defect or a secondary problem. Joseph and Dyer suggested that myelin/axon interaction triggers signals that lead to neurotransmitter synthesis—assuming that myelination influences dopamine synthesis—and axon maturation and that PKU is primarily a myelin disorder.[76] Pascucci et al. showed decreased dopamine synthesis due to TH inhibition and reduced norepinephrine synthesis both presumably due to elevated Phe levels, raising the question whether neurons or myelin are the primary site of injury in PKU.[74]

Just as myelin affects axon maturation, axons and neurons also affect myelination.[87] Neurotrophins on the one hand initiate signaling pathways in axons that control their myelination and on the other hand act on myelinating glia directly.[88] The findings of Joseph and Dyer may thus also be explained by lack of axonal activity generating signals that lead to myelination.[76] When taken together with the findings of Bauman and Kemper about developmental arrest in the PKU brain, a new view of the hypomyelination in PKU as a phenomenon that occurs secondary to neuronal damage or secondary to arrest of neuronal development could be considered.[39]

Phenylketonuria: A Disturbance in the Development of Neuronal Networks?
As described in previously, children with PKU and offspring of MPKU have ADHD and EF deficits. White matter lesions and disturbed white matter integrity in white matter tracts are viewed as the underlying cause of EF deficits.[89] While some aspects of EF are attributed to white matter damage and while hypomyelination of white matter tracts is observed in ADHD, ADHD itself is mainly regarded as a neurotransmitter disease caused by primarily dopamine and also norepinephrine deficiency.[90] Modern neuroimaging techniques have shown structural changes in patients with ADHD that indicate abnormal development in key brain regions such as the prefrontal cortex (especially left hemisphere), striatum, and parietal cortex (especially right hemisphere).[91,92] Functional imaging studies have shown functional abnormalities in the prefrontal cortex, striatum, and parietal cortex in ADHD patients,[92] and a new understanding of ADHD has evolved viewing it as a dysfunction of larger functional networks that serve attention, cognition, and self-regulation,[92] networks that did not develop properly.[92,93]

Silk et al. performed a diffusion tensor imaging study in patients with ADHD and controls and described white matter anomalies in fronto-temporal and right parietal-occipital regions and in tracts connecting prefrontal and parieto-occipital areas with the striatum and the cerebellum.[92] They interpreted the results of especially their fractional anisotropy analyses as indicating that the observed white matter anomalies might be due to less neural branching within affected white matter pathways, and they concluded that their data support the notion of abnormal development within fronto-parietal cortical networks important for attention and cognition. Because of differences observed between treated and untreated patients with ADHD, they suggested that medication may have long-term effects on brain development in patients with ADHD and that fractional anisotropy could be used to measure response to medication.

When extrapolating from this understanding of ADHD in general to PKU in particular and taking the current knowledge about PKU into account, it appears that several disciplines—neuroanatomy, neuroradiology, and neuropsychology—suggest a disturbance in brain development, neural transmission, neuronal connectivity, and neuronal networks. A new view of PKU could thus be developed that includes disturbed development of neuronal networks as a primary problem in PKU rather than a white matter disease caused by reduced protein synthesis due to an essential amino acid deficiency.

One could hypothesize that developing neurons secrete neurotrophins that stimulate myelin formation and that changes in neuronal development, synapse formation, and neurotransmitter signaling could lead to abnormal development of white matter tracts—for example, those connecting prefrontal and parieto-occipital areas with the striatum and the cerebellum.

The Role of Neurotransmitters in Brain Development

Summarizing the findings about neurotransmitters described previously, there is evidence for reduced dopamine and norepinephrine synthesis that may be the cause and the effect of a disturbed development of neuronal networks in PKU.

If the prefrontal cortex dysfunction hypothesis about dopamine deficiency causing the cognitive deficits in treated PKU patients is correct and if these region-specific cognitive deficits are residual symptoms of the classic disease in treated patients that mirror the much more severe and more generalized pathophysiology in untreated patients, then one would have to be able to explain the brain phenotype of classical untreated PKU patients with dopamine deficiency. Considering the findings by Bauman and Kemper,[39] Joseph and Dyer,[76] and Pascucci et al.,[74] dopamine deficiency may explain the developmental arrest and neuronal pathology and the hypomyelination of specific brain areas observed in untreated PKU patients and in PKU mice. Welsh et al. explained that dopaminergic projections of the neocortex primarily go to the frontal lobes.[65]

With regard to dopamine and brain development, dopamine receptors are expressed very early in embryonic development, and the interplay of their different functions is important for normal brain development. Dopamine receptor activity has been shown to affect neurogenesis, neuronal differentiation, and neural cell migration in the developing cerebral cortex.[94] Dopamine is one of the first neurotransmitters that occurs in the developing brain. The dopamine receptor 1 ko mouse has morphologic changes only in dopamine-rich cortical areas such as the prefrontal cortex and anterior cingulate. During embryonic development, dopamine receptor 1 ko mice have fewer gamma-aminobutyric acid interneurons prefrontally, and D2 ko mice have more cortical gamma-aminobutyric acid interneurons.[94] These different functions of dopamine and its receptors indicate an important and complex role for dopamine in brain development.

In treated patients, only specific vulnerable areas (e.g., the prefrontal cortex) and the networks associated with them may be affected by decreased dopamine synthesis and the function of the area, and the network may be restored when the neuronal environment is devoid of high Phe levels. Thus in treated patients an alteration in a neuronal network may only be temporal unless there is prolonged exposure to high Phe.

Lichter-Konecki et al. demonstrated a low but significant amount of the PAH transcript in the human brain.[6] If PAH is indeed expressed in the brain, this may occur only in certain brain areas where Tyr synthesis (phenylalanine hydroxylation) is vital to specific cell types for maintaining normal dopamine and norepinephrine levels. Lichter-Konecki et al. also isolated large antisense transcripts of the PAH locus (Lichter-Konecki et al. unpublished data). Such transcripts could regulate the expression of genes involved in Phe metabolism and neurotransmitter synthesis in a complex fashion and could possibly be involved in the down-regulation of the expression of genes involved in these pathways. Furthermore, the expression of antisense transcripts of the PAH locus may not be affected by missense mutations in the coding region of the PAH gene.

Hypopigmentation

With regard to the fact that melanin biosynthesis is inhibited by high Phe levels in a reversible fashion and the conclusion by Fitzpatrick and Miyamoto[77] that high Phe levels competitively inhibit the Tyr-tyrosinase reaction leading to hypopigmentation, the reported 15% to 30% reduction in tyrosinase activity was not deemed sufficient to cause visible depigmentation (V. Hearing, personal communication). Gahl et al. demonstrated that a Tyr transport system exists at the melanosomal membrane.[80] As is postulated for Tyr transport at the BBB in the context of neurotransmitter synthesis, melanosomal Tyr transport could be inhibited by high Phe levels, causing decreased melanin synthesis.

However, there could also be a disturbance in the signaling pathways crucial for melanin formation. Alterations in pigmentation are often effected at the transcriptional level.[95] An effect of high Phe on, for example, the expression of signaling molecules such as the microphthalmia-associated transcription factor, the key transcription factor of melanogenesis, would affect the expression of a number of genes regulating melanin synthesis.

If the assumptions stated by Fitzpatrick and Miyamoto were correct,[77] however, that high Phe levels interfere with tyrosinase activity, then high Phe levels would interfere with dopamine, norepinephrine, and melanin synthesis by affecting the key enzymes of their pathways, TH, and tyrosinase. Since norepinephrine synthesis was not restored when dopamine synthesis was restored by L-DOPA in a high Phe environment, one can only speculate that DβH activity may also be reduced in a high Phe environment.

Future Directions

As described earlier, there have been somewhat conflicting results in neuroimaging studies and neuropsychological studies with regard to signs of dopamine deficiency, ADHD, and EF deficits.

A number of the studies were performed in adults that either had remained on treatment or had been off treatment for years. Although acute Phe levels and sometimes the mean of the Phe level in the previous year were taken into account, the studies described did not usually say much about the type of PKU of the patients; at most they stated that classic PKU patients were studied. As described previously, the biochemical phenotypes of patients with hyperphenylalaninemia form a continuum between very mild and severe phenotypes, depending in large part on the PAH genotype of the patient.

Patients with some residual activity are at an advantage over patients with no activity.[96] It thus is important that clinical investigations are designed in the future that employ functional imaging studies in patients with PKU similar to those performed by Silk at al. in patients with ADHD,[92] which assessed the prefrontal cortex, the parietal cortex, and the striatum as well as the tracts that connect them. Such studies should be combined with highly differentiating neuropsychological tests such as the ones used by Antshel and Waisbren[52] and with careful biochemical and genetic characterization of the patients such as the long-term Phe level control and PAH genotype. Although PAH mutations cannot predict the brain phenotype, they by and large allow the prediction of the biochemical phenotype.[10,11] The biochemical phenotype, however, determines how difficult it is to maintain dietary control,[96] and a correlation between the Phe level and the brain phenotype is demonstrated in most clinical studies. As done by Antshel and Waisbren,[52] these studies should be performed in children and teenagers whose brains are still developing and not in adults. In addition, these studies should be complemented by imaging studies that are able to determine neurotransmitter levels, especially dopamine levels, in different brain areas. The results of such investigations should form a solid basis for designing new therapeutic approaches and for making recommendations regarding the degree of needed dietary control, supplemental LNAA/Tyr therapy, or ADHD treatment for PKU patients. These data would also form a basis for testing the hypothesis of abnormal brain circuitry in PKU and support the development of new drugs to treat the effects of abnormal brain circuitry and in an even more advanced state of research the development of new ways to prevent the formation of abnormal brain circuitry.

Future experiments in mice should employ only genetic mouse models such as the *PAH^{enu2}* mouse and should be designed such that the experiments investigate abnormal brain development and the contribution of dopamine and norepinephrine as well as of signaling molecules such as neurotrophic factors and transcription factors to brain development in these mice. Experiments need to be designed that will determine with certainty if high Phe reduces TH synthesis and activity as well as tyrosinase and DβH activity, that is, if there is a direct Phe effect on these enzymes or if the regulation of these enzymes is disturbed at the level of gene expression.

A future experiment in the genetic mouse model for PKU on a high Phe diet should analyze expression of the dopamine and norepinephrine synthesis pathways and of dopamine receptors as well as signaling molecules affecting these pathways and receptors in different brain areas during postnatal development of these animals. In addition, it should also include a detailed assessment of the morphology of their brains, especially of specific myelinated tracts to be able to link the morphology to known dopamine, dopamine receptor, and norepinephrine functions during brain development as well as to neuronal circuitries.

HMGR activity and expression could also be assessed at the same time in the same tissues to determine whether inhibition of HMGR activity by Phe in select oligodendrocytes contributes to the PKU brain phenotype.

A broader assessment of signaling pathways by microarray expression analysis of PKU mouse brain would allow the simultaneous assessment of the expression of signaling molecules that may be effectors of the myelin/axonal interaction and important to the development of brain circuits.

Preliminary gene expression analysis using cDNA arrays and PAH^{enu2} mouse brain mRNA revealed the expression of some but not all dopamine receptors to be altered (Lichter-Konecki et al., unpublished results).

In addition, special attention should be paid to signaling molecules that are present in the brain and in melanocytes and keratinocytes and that are involved in neuronal differentiation as well as melanin synthesis. Of these signaling molecules particular attention should be paid to those whose expression is affected by high Phe conditions. Signaling molecules that are involved in neuronal differentiation and melanin synthesis are, for instance, those of the microphthalmia-associated transcription factor signaling pathway, which is crucial to neural crest development and melanogenesis. An alteration in this pathway could for instance apply to the MPKU syndrome.

Maternal Phenylketonuria

Studies suggested above during postnatal PKU mouse brain development can be expanded to prenatal PKU mouse brain development to test whether high Phe disturbs the same systems in pre- and postnatal mouse brain development resulting in somewhat different outcomes as proposed by Antshel and Waisbren[52] or whether different systems are affected.

Modifier Genes That May Contribute to Variable Phenotypes

It would not be surprising if even carefully designed, comprehensive studies would show variability between patients, making interpretation of results difficult. Given the many pathways that appear to be affected in a high Phe level environment, one would expect variability to occur due to modifier genes. Diamond discussed modifier genes that would have an effect on dopamine levels and could explain some phenotypic variations.[73] Diamond stated that the prefrontal cortex depends more than other brain regions on the catechol-*O*-methyltransferase (COMT) enzyme for dopamine inactivation because it has fewer dopamine transporters than other brain regions. She explained that the COMT enzyme accounts for more than 60% of the dopamine degradation in prefrontal cortex but for less than 15% of the dopamine degradation in the striatum. COMT gene variants may thus have an effect on the phenotype of patients by causing differences in extracellular dopamine levels in the prefrontal cortex. Diamond et al. showed that children with a less active COMT enzyme performed better on tasks requiring the prefrontal cortex functions working memory and inhibition.[97]

Prefrontal Cortex and ADHD-Inattentive Type

Based on the fact that prefrontal cortex has less dopamine transporters than the striatum, Diamond also discussed that one would postulate that variants of the dopamine transporter gene have a greater effect on striatum function than on prefrontal cortex function while variants of the dopamine receptor D4, which is prevalent in the prefrontal cortex, should affect the prefrontal cortex.[73] This hypothesis would imply that ADHD with hyperactivity should be influenced by the dopamine transporter gene variants while symptoms consistent with ADHD-inattentive type should be influenced by D4 variants. Diamond described scientific evidence for the correctness of these assumptions. ADHD that includes hyperactivity should then best be treated with methylphenidate as it affects the dopamine transporter and ADHD-inattentive type with amphetamines. While methylphenidate and amphetamines both inhibit reuptake of dopamine and norepinephrine, only amphetamines also induce their release. When taking the results of Antshel and Waisbren into account,[52] amphetamines should be more successful in the treatment of ADHD in PKU patients.

References

1. Wolosker H, Dumin E, Balan L, Foltyn VN. D-amino acids in the brain: D-serine in neurotransmission and neurodegeneration. *FEBS J*. 2008; 275(14): 3514–3526. doi: 10.1111/j.1742-4658.2008.06515.x
2. Scolari MJ, Acosta GB. D-serine: a new word in the glutamatergic neuro-glial language. *Amino Acids*. 2007; 33(4): 563–574.
3. Halassa MM, Fellin T, Haydon PG.The tripartite synapse: roles for gliotransmission in health and disease. *Trends Mol Med*. 2007; 13(2): 54–63.
4. Hamosh A, Johnston MV: Nonketotic hyperglycinemia. In: Scriver CR, Beaudet AL, Sly WS, Valle D, eds. *The Metabolic & Molecular Bases of Inherited Disease*, Vol. II, 8th ed. New York: McGraw-Hill; 2001:2065–2078.
5. Kaufman S. Phenylketonuria: biochemical mechanisms. In: Agranoff BW, Aprison MH, eds. *Advanced Neurochemistry*, Vol. 2. New York: Plenum Press; 1976: 1–132.
6. Lichter-Konecki U, Hipke CM, Konecki DS. Human phenylalanine hydroxylase gene expression in kidney and other non-hepatic tissues. *Mol Genet Metab*. 1999; 67: 308–316.
7. Bickel H, Gerrard J, Hickmans EM. The influence of phenylalanine intake on the chemistry and behaviour of a phenyl-ketonuric child. *Acta Paediatr*. 1954; 43(1): 64–77.
8. Guthrie R, Susi A. A simple phenylalanine method for detecting phenylketonuria in large populations of newborn infants. *Pediatrics*. 1963; 32: 338–343.
9. Blau N, Hennermann JB, Langenbeck U, Lichter-Konecki U. Diagnosis, classification, and genetics of phenylketonuria and tetrahydrobiopterin (BH4) deficiencies. *Mol Genet Metab*. 2011;104(Suppl.): S2–S9.
10. Okano Y, Eisensmith R, Guettler F, et al. Molecular basis of phenotypic heterogeneity in phenylketonuria. *N Engl J Med*. 1991; 324: 1232–1238.
11. Guldberg P, Rey F, Zschocke J, et al. A European multicenter study of phenylalanine hydroxylase deficiency: classification of 105 mutations and a general system for genotype-based prediction of metabolic phenotype. *Am J Hum Genet*. 1998; 63(1): 71–79. Erratum in *Am J Hum Genet* 1998; 63(4): 1252–1253.
12. U. Lichter-Konecki 2011. unpublished results.
13. Lindegren ML, Krishnaswami S, Fonnesbeck C, et al. Adjuvant treatment for phenylketonuria (PKU): Comparative Effectiveness Review No. 56. (Prepared by the Vanderbilt Evidence-based Practice Center under Contract No. HHSA 290-2007-10065-I.) AHRQ Publication No. 12- EHC035-EF. Rockville, MD: Agency for Healthcare Research and Quality; February 2012. www.effectivehealthcare. ahrq.gov/reports/final.cfm
14. Mabry CC, Denniston JC, Nelson TL, Son CD. Maternal phenylketonuria: a cause of mental retardation in children without the metabolic defect. *N Engl J Med*. 1963; 269: 1404–1408.
15. Lenke RR, Levy HL. Maternal phenylketonuria and hyperphenylalaninemia: an international survey of the outcome of untreated and treated pregnancies. *N Engl J Med*. 1980; 303(21): 1202–1208.
16. Rouse B, Azen C, Koch R, et al. Maternal Phenylketonuria Collaborative Study (MPKUCS) offspring: facial anomalies, malformations, and early neurological sequelae. *Am J Med Genet*. 19973; 69(1): 89–95.
17. Dobson JC, Williamson ML, Azen C, Koch R. Intellectual assessment of 111 four-year-old children with phenylketonuria. *Pediatrics*. 1977; 60(6): 822–827.

18. Williamson ML, Koch R, Azen C, Chang C. Correlates of intelligence test results in treated phenylketonuric children. *Pediatrics*. 1981; 68(2): 161–167.
19. Waters PJ, Scriver CR, Parniak MA. Homomeric and heteromeric interactions between wild-type and mutant phenylalanine hydroxylase subunits: evaluation of two-hybrid approaches for functional analysis of mutations causing hyperphenylalaninemia. *Mol Genet Metab*. 2001; 73(3): 230–238.
20. Jaffe EK, Stith L, Lawrence SH, Andrake M, Dunbrack RL Jr. A new model for allosteric regulation of phenylalanine hydroxylase: implications for disease and therapeutics. *Arch Biochem Biophys*. 2013; 530(2): 73–82. doi: 10.1016/j.abb.2012.12.017
21. Batshaw ML, Valle D, Bessman SP. Unsuccessful treatment of phenylketonuria with tyrosine. *J Pediatr*. 1981; 99(1): 159–160.
22. Berger V, Larondelle Y, Trouet A, Schneider YJ. Transport mechanisms of the large neutral amino acid L-phenylalanine in the human intestinal epithelial caco-2 cell line. *J Nutr*. 2000; 130(11): 2780–2788.
23. Al Hafid N, Tong XZ, Carpenter K, et al. Towards an alternative therapy for PKU: in vitro and in vivo assessment of a genetically modified probiotic (lactococcus lactis nz9000) expressing Phenylalanine Ammonia Lyase (PAL). *J Inherit Metab Dis*. 2013; 36(Suppl. 2): S92–S93.
24. Langenbeck U, Burgard P, Wendel U, Lindner M, Zschocke J. German collaborative study on phenylketonuria (PKU) / hyperphenylalaninemia (HPA): metabolic phenotypes of phenylketonuria. Kinetic and molecular evaluation of the Blaskovics protein loading test. *J Inherit Metab Dis*. 2009; 32(4): 506–513. doi: 10.1007/s10545-009-1152-6
25. Stéphenne X, Debray FG, Smets F, et al. Hepatocyte transplantation using the domino concept in a child with tetrabiopterin nonresponsive phenylketonuria. *Cell Transplant*. 2012; 21(12): 2765–2770. doi: 10.3727/096368912X653255
26. Yusa K, Rashid ST, Strick-Marchand H, et al. Targeted gene correction of α1-antitrypsin deficiency in induced pluripotent stem cells. *Nature*. 2011; 478(7369): 391–394. doi: 10.1038/nature10424
27. Liu TJ, Kay MA, Darlington GJ, Woo SL. Reconstitution of enzymatic activity in hepatocytes of phenylalanine hydroxylase-deficient mice. *Somat Cell Mol Genet*. 1992; 18(1): 89–96.
28. Cristiano RJ, Smith LC, Woo SL. Hepatic gene therapy: adenovirus enhancement of receptor-mediated gene delivery and expression in primary hepatocytes. *Proc Natl Acad Sci USA*. 1993; 90(6): 2122–2126.
29. Rebuffat A, Harding CO, Ding Z, Thöny B. Comparison of adeno-associated virus pseudotype 1, 2, and 8 vectors administered by intramuscular injection in the treatment of murine phenylketonuria. *Hum Gene Ther*. 2010; 21(4): 463–477. doi: 10.1089/hum.2009.127
30. Harding CO, Gillingham MB, Hamman K, et al. Complete correction of hyperphenylalaninemia following liver-directed, recombinant AAV2/8 vector-mediated gene therapy in murine phenylketonuria. *Gene Ther*. 2006; 13(5): 457–462.
31. Hamman KJ, Winn SR, Harding CO. Hepatocytes from wild-type or heterozygous donors are equally effective in achieving successful therapeutic liver repopulation in murine phenylketonuria (PKU). *Mol Genet Metab*. 2011; 104(3): 235–240. doi: 10.1016/j.ymgme.2011.07.027
32. Guldberg P, Levy HL, Hanley WB, et al. Phenylalanine hydroxylase gene mutations in the United States: report from the Maternal PKU Collaborative Study. *Am J Hum Genet*. 1996; 59(1): 84–94.
33. Konecki DS, Lichter-Konecki U. The phenylketonuria locus: current knowledge about alleles and mutations of the phenylalanine hydroxylase gene in various populations (review). *Hum Genet*. 1991; 87: 377–388.
34. Scriver CR, Kaufman S. Hyperphenylalaninemia: phenylalanine hydroxylase deficiency. In: Scriver CR, Beaudet AL, Sly WS, Valle D, eds. *The Metabolic & Molecular Bases of Inherited Disease*, Vol. II, 8th ed. New York: McGraw-Hill; 2001: 1667–1724.
35. van Spronsen FJ, Huijbregts SC, Bosch AM, Leuzzi V. Cognitive, neurophysiological, neurological and psychosocial outcomes in early-treated PKU-patients: a start toward standardized outcome measurement across development. *Mol Genet Metab*. 2011; 104(Suppl.): S45–S51. doi: 10.1016/j.ymgme.2011.09.036
36. Kaufman S. An evaluation of the possible neurotoxicity of metabolites of phenylalanine. *J Pediatr*. 1989; 114: 895–900.
37. Wadman SK, Ketting D, deBree PK, van der Heiden C, Grimberg MT, Kruijswijk H. Permanent chemical phenylketonuria and a normal phenylalanine tolerance in two sisters with a normal mental development. *Clin Chim Acta*. 1975; 65: 197–204.
38. Pardridge W. M. (1998) Blood–brain barrier carrier-mediated transport and brain metabolism of amino acids. *Neurochem. Res*. 23, 635–644.

39. Bauman ML, Kemper T. Morphologic and histoanatomic observations of the brain in untreated human phenylketonuria. *Acta Neuropathol*. 1982; 58: 55–63.
40. Dyer CA, Kendler A, Philibotte T, Gardiner P, Cruz J, Levy HL. Evidence for central nervous system glial cell plasticity in phenylketonuria. *J Neuropathol Exp Neurol*. 1996; 55: 795–814.
41. Avison MJ, Herschkowitz N, Novotny EJ, et al. Proton NMR observation of phenylalanine and an aromatic metabolite in the rabbit brain in vivo. *Pediatr Res*. 1990; 27: 566–570.
42. Novotny EJ, Avison MJ, Herschkowitz N, et al. *In vivo* measurement of phenylalanine in human brain by proton nuclear magnetic resonance spectroscopy. *Pediatr Res*. 1995; 37: 244–249.
43. Møller LB, Paulsen M, Koch R, Moats R, Guldberg P, Güttler F. Inter-individual variation in brain phenylalanine concentration in patients with PKU is not caused by genetic variation in the 4F2hc/LAT1 complex. *Mol Genet Metab*. 2005; 86(Suppl. 1):S119–S123.
44. Bick U, Ullrich K, Stoeber U, et al. White matter abnormalities in patients with treated hyperphenylalaninaemia: magnetic resonance relaxometry and proton spectroscopy findings. *Eur J Pediatr*. 1993; 152: 1012–1020.
45. Manara R, Burlina AP, Citton V, et al. Brain MRI diffusion-weighted imaging in patients with classical phenylketonuria. *Neuroradiology*. 2009; 51(12): 803–812. doi: 10.1007/s00234-009-0574-z.
46. Peng H, Peck D, White DA, Christ SE. Tract-based evaluation of white matter damage in individuals with early-treated phenylketonuria. *J Inherit Metab Dis*. 2014; 37(2): 237–243.
47. White DA, Antenor-Dorsey JA, Grange DK, et al. White matter integrity and executive abilities following treatment with tetrahydrobiopterin (BH4) in individuals with phenylketonuria. *Mol Genet Metab*. 2013; 110(3): 213–217. doi: 10.1016/j.ymgme.2013.07.010
48. Smith CB, Kang J. Cerebral protein synthesis in a genetic mouse model of phenylketonuria. *Proc Natl Acad Sci USA*. 2000; 97(20): 11014–11019.
49. Shefer S, Tint GS, Jean-Guillaume D, et al. Is there a relationship between 3-hydroxy-3-methylglutaryl coenzyme a reductase activity and forebrain pathology in the PKU mouse? *J Neurosci Res*. 2000; 61(5): 549–563.
50. Adler-Abramovich L, Vaks L, Carny O, et al. Phenylalanine assembly into toxic fibrils suggests amyloid etiology in phenylketonuria. *Nat Chem Biol*. 2012; 8(8): 701–706. doi: 10.1038/nchembio.1002
51. Pennington BF, Groisser D, Welsh MC. Contrasting neuropsychological deficits in attention deficit disorder versus reading disability. *Dev Psychobiol*. 1993; 29: 511–523.
52. Antshel KM, Waisbren SE. Timing is everything: executive functions in children exposed to elevated levels of phenylalanine. *Neuropsychology*. 2003; 17(3): 458–468.
53. Channon S, Mockler C, Lee P. Executive functioning and speed of processing in phenylketonuria. *Neuropsychology*. 2005; 19(5): 679–86.
54. Bessman SP. The justification theory: the essential nature of the non-essential amino acids. *Nutr Rev*. 1979; 37(7): 209–220.
55. Batshaw ML, Valle D, Bessman SP. Unsuccessful treatment of phenylketonuria with tyrosine. *J Pediatr*. 1981; 99(1): 159–160.
56. Lykkelund C, Nielsen JB, Lou HC, et al. Increased neurotransmitter biosynthesis in phenylketonuria induced by phenylalanine restriction or by supplementation of unrestricted diet with large amounts of tyrosine. *Eur J Pediatr*. 1988; 148(3): 238–245.
57. Lou H. Large doses of tryptophan and tyrosine as potential therapeutic alternative to dietary phenylalanine restriction in phenylketonuria. *Lancet*. 1985; 2(8447): 150–151.
58. Lou HC. Dopamine precursors and brain function in phenylalanine hydroxylase deficiency. *Acta Paediatr Suppl*. 1994; 407: 86–88.
59. Paans AM, Pruim J, Smit GP, Visser G, Willemsen AT, Ullrich K. Neurotransmitter positron emission tomographic-studies in adults with phenylketonuria, a pilot study. *Eur J Pediatr*. 1996; 155(Suppl. 1): S78–S81.
60. Scriver CR, Hurtubise M, Konecki D, et al. PAHdb 2003: what a locus-specific knowledgebase can do. *Hum Mutat*. 2003 21(4): 333–344.
61. Pietz J, Landwehr R, Kutscha A, Schmidt H, de Sonneville L, Trefz FK. Effect of high-dose tyrosine supplementation on brain function in adults with 1phenylketonuria. *J Pediatr*. 1995; 127(6): 936–943.
62. Smith ML, Hanley WB, Clarke JT, et al. Randomised controlled trial of tyrosine supplementation on neuropsychological performance in phenylketonuria. *Arch Dis Child*. 1998; 78(2): 116–121.

63. Pietz J, Kreis R, Rupp A, et al. Large neutral amino acids block phenylalanine transport into brain tissue in patients with phenylketonuria. *J Clin Invest*. 1999; 103(8): 1169–78.
64. Landvogt C, Mengel E, Bartenstein P, et al. Reduced cerebral fluoro-L-dopamine uptake in adult patients suffering from phenylketonuria. *J Cereb Blood Flow Metab*. 2008; 28(4): 824–831.
65. Welsh MC, Pennington BF, Ozonoff S, Rouse B, McCabe ER. Neuropsychology of early-treated phenylketonuria: specific executive function deficits. *Child Dev*. 1990; 61(6): 1697–1713.
66. Diamond A, Prevor MB, Callender G, Druin DP. Prefrontal cortex cognitive deficits in children treated early and continuously for PKU. *Monogr Soc Res Child Dev*. 1997; 62(4): i–v, 1–208.
67. Chamove AS, Molinaro TJ. Monkey retardate learning analysis. *J Ment Defic Res*. 1978; 22(1): 37–48.
68. Pennington BF, van Doorninck WJ, McCabe LL, McCabe ER. Neuropsychological deficits in early treated phenylketonuric children. *Am J Ment Defic*. 1985; 89(5): 467–474.
69. Diamond A, Ciaramitaro V, Donner E, Djali S, Robinson MB. An animal model of early-treated PKU. *J Neurosci*. 1994; 14(5 Pt 2): 3072–3082.
70. Tam SY, Elsworth JD, Bradberry CW, Roth RH. Mesocortical dopamine neurons: high basal firing frequency predicts tyrosine dependence of dopamine synthesis. *J Neural Transm Gen Sect*. 1990; 81(2): 97–110.
71. Chiodo LA, Bannon MJ, Grace AA, Roth RH, Bunney BS. Evidence for the absence of impulse-regulating somatodendritic and synthesis-modulating nerve terminal autoreceptors on subpopulations of mesocortical dopamine neurons. *Neuroscience*. 1984; 12(1): 1–16.
72. Ullrich K, Weglage J, Oberwittler C, Pietsch M, Fünders B, von Eckardstein H, Colombo JP. Effect of L-dopa on visual evoked potentials and neuropsychological tests in adult phenylketonuria patients. *Eur J Pediatr*. 1996; 155(Suppl. 1): S74–S77.
73. Diamond A. Genetic background that may selectively be affecting dopamine dependent prefrontal cortex functions:consequences of variations in genes that affect dopamine in prefrontal cortex. *Cereb Cortex*. 2007; 17(Suppl 1): 161–170.
74. Pascucci T, Giacovazzo G, Andolina D, et al. In vivo catecholaminergic metabolism in the medial prefrontal cortex of ENU2 mice: an investigation of the cortical dopamine deficit in phenylketonuria. *J Inherit Metab Dis*. 2012; 35(6): 1001–1009. doi: 10.1007/s10545-012-9473-2
75. Pascucci T, Andolina D, Mela IL, et al. 5-Hydroxytryptophan rescues serotonin response to stress in prefrontal cortex of hyperphenylalaninaemic mice. *Int J Neuropsychoph*. 2009; 12(8): 1067–1079.
76. Joseph B, Dyer CA. Relationship between myelin production and dopamine synthesis in the PKU mouse brain. *J Neurochem*. 2003; 86(3): 615–626.
77. Fitzpatrick TB, Miyamoto M. Competitive inhibition of mammalian tyrosinase by phenylalanine and its relationship to hair pigmentation in phenylketonuria. *Nature*. 1957; 179(4552): 199–200.
78. Schallreuter KU, Wood JM, Pittelkow MR, et al. Regulation of melanin biosynthesis in the human epidermis by tetrahydrobiopterin. *Science*. 1994; 263(5152): 1444–1446.
79. Schallreuter KU, Wood JM. The importance of L-phenylalanine transport and its autocrine turnover to L-tyrosine for melanogenesis in human epidermal melanocytes. *Biochem Biophys Res Commun*. 1999; 262(2): 423–428.
80. Gahl WA, Potterf B, Durham-Pierre D, Brilliant MH, Hearing VJ. Melanosomal tyrosine transport in normal and pink-eyed dilution murine melanocytes. *Pigment Cell Res*. 1995; 8(5): 229–233.
81. Fellman JH. Epinephrine metabolites and pigmentation in the central nervous system in a case of phenylpyruvic oligophrenia. *J Neurol Neurosurg Psychiat*. 1958; 21: 58–62.
82. Zagreda L, Goodman J, Druin DP, McDonald D, Diamond A. Cognitive deficits in a genetic mouse model of the most common biochemical cause of human mental retardation. *J Neurosci*. 1999; 19(14): 6175-82.
83. Diamond A. Phenylalanine levels of 6-10 mg/dl may not be as benign as once thought. *Acta Paediatr Suppl*. 1994; 407: 89–91.
84. Moeller HE, Vermathen P, Ullrich K, Weglage J, Koch HG, Peters PE. In-vivo NMR spectroscopy in patients with phenylketonuria: changes of cerebral phenylalanine levels under dietary treatment. *Neuropediatrics*. 1995; 26: 199–202.
85. Moeller HE, Weglage J, Wiedermann D, Vermathen P, Bick U, Ullrich K. Kinetics of phenylalanine transport at the human blood–brain barrier investigated *in vivo*. *Brain Res*. 1997; 778: 329–337.
86. Hommes FA. On the mechanism of permanent brain dysfunction in hyperphenylalaninemia. *Biochem Med Metab Biol*. 1991; 46: 277–287.

87. Coelho RP, Yuelling LM, Fuss B, Sato-Bigbee C. Neurotrophin-3 targets the translational initiation machinery in oligodendrocytes. *Glia*. 2009; 57(16): 1754–1764. doi: 10.1002/glia.20888
88. Rosenberg SS, Ng BK, Chan JR. The quest for remyelination: a new role for neurotrophins and their receptors. *Brain Pathol*. 2006; 16: 288–294.
89. Clark DB, Chung T, Thatcher DL, Pajtek S, Long EC. Psychological dysregulation, white matter disorganization and substance use disorders in adolescence. *Addiction*. 2012; 107(1): 206–214. doi: 10.1111/j.1360-0443.2011.03566.x
90. Del Campo N, Fryer TD, Hong YT, et al. A positron emission tomography study of nigro-striatal dopaminergic mechanisms underlying attention: implications for ADHD and its treatment. *Brain*. 2013; 136(Pt 11): 3252–3270. doi: 10.1093/brain/awt263
91. Makris N, Buka SL, Biederman J, et al. Attention and executive systems abnormalities in adults with childhood ADHD: a DT-MRI study of connections. *Cereb Cortex*. 2008; 18(5): 1210–1220.
92. Silk TJ, Vance A, Rinehart N, Bradshaw JL, Cunnington R. White-matter abnormalities in attention deficit hyperactivity disorder: a diffusion tensor imaging study. *Hum Brain Mapp*. 2009; 30(9): 2757–2765. doi: 10.1002/hbm.20703
93. Stanley JA, Kipp H, Greisenegger E, et al. Evidence of developmental alterations in cortical and subcortical regions of children with attention-deficit/hyperactivity disorder: a multivoxel in vivo phosphorus 31 spectroscopy study. *Arch Gen Psychiatry*. 2008; 65(12): 1419–1428.
94. Bhide PG. Dopamine, cocaine and the development of cerebral cortical cytoarchitecture: a review of current concepts. *Semin Cell Dev Biol*. 2009; 20(4): 395–402. doi: 10.1016/j.semcdb.2009.01.006
95. Lei TC, Virador V, Yasumoto K, Vieira WD, Toyofuku K, Hearing VJ. Stimulation of melanoblast pigmentation by 8-methoxypsoralen: the involvement of microphthalmia-associated transcription factor, the protein kinase a signal pathway, and proteasome-mediated degradation. *J Invest Dermatol*. 2002; 119(6): 1341–1349.
96. Lichter-Konecki U, Rupp A, Konecki DS, Trefz FK, Schmidt H, Burgard P. Relation between phenylalanine hydroxylase genotypes and phenotypic parameters of diagnosis and treatment of hyperphenylalaninemic disorders. *J Inherit Metab Dis*. 1994; 17: 362–365.
97. Davidson MC, Amso D, Anderson LC, Diamond A. Development of cognitive control and executive functions from 4 to 13 years: evidence from manipulations of memory, inhibition, and task switching. *Neuropsychologia*. 2006; 44(11): 2037–2078.

SECTION 3

Therapeutic Approaches

12

Cell and Organ Transplantation for Inborn Errors of Metabolism

Alberto Burlina, Andrea Bordugo, Georg F. Hoffmann, and Jochen Meyburg

Introduction

Many primary genetic diseases have been "cured" by replacement of the entire organ in which expression of the mutant gene causes disease. This is a rather indiscriminant form of gene transfer therapy, for not only is the disease-producing mutant gene replaced but also every other gene in the transplanted tissue. At present, organ transplantation is the principal mode of gene therapy.

Treatment of enzyme deficiency diseases by organ transplantation may involve one or both of two principles. If the deficient enzyme is normally produced mainly by only one organ, as in ornithine transcarbamylase deficiency, replacement of the defective organ by a healthy organ can be expected to cure the disease. The second principle is demonstrated in patients with glycogenosis type 1. Following kidney transplantation, because of end-stage renal disease, the transplanted kidney functions not only as an excretory organ but also as the sole producer of the formerly deficient enzyme. This concept of an implanted functional source of enzyme activity is of widespread application.

Until now, inborn errors of metabolism have been treated by transplanting different organs such as bone marrow, liver, kidney (or a combination), and recently by cell transplantations.

Bone Marrow and Hematopoietic Stem Cell Transplantation

Some of the earliest organ transplantations in man were bone marrow transplantation. This method of gene transfer therapy has been successfully used in the management of inherited metabolic disorders of hematopoietic tissues, such as severe combined immunodeficiency caused by adenosine deaminase deficiency. In disorders in which hematopoietic tissues are not primarily compromised, bone marrow transplantation is used as a vehicle for delivering gene products to other tissues in the body.

Since the first transplantation done in mucopolysaccaridosis type I (Hurler syndrome), many attempts have been made to treat almost all of the lysosomal disorders by this method.[1]

After transplantation of hematopoietic stem cells (HSCTs), it is suggested that the donor cells are able to form enough enzymes to correct the enzyme deficiency partly, or even completely, and to stop or reverse the course of disease. In preparation for cell transplantation, stem cells of the patient are reduced with chemotherapy and/or radiation, allowing donor cells to grow. This process is called conditioning. Subsequently, patients receive infusions of HSCT of the donor. Depending on the kind of stem cells, production of blood cells will reconstitute after 10 to 28 days. HSCTs can come from different sources. Traditionally, bone marrow is used for the production of these cells. Recently, HSCTs are isolated from peripheral or cord blood.

With regard to the indication of bone marrow transplantation in inborn errors of metabolism, several issues have to be considered. Stem cell transplantation is still connected with considerable morbidity and mortality rates. Especially during the first days after transplantation, until the production of neutrophils (white blood cells) starts again, there is a high danger of infection for the patients. The renewed production of blood cells also has its risks, particularly the development of so-called graft-versus-host-reactions. In this process, immunocyte from the transplanted graft attack several tissues of the patient, which is often accompanied by severe symptoms like dermatorrhagia, severe diarrhea, liver insufficiency, respiratory failure, and shock.

Based on the present clinical experience with bone marrow transplantation in lysosomal storage diseases, HSCT should be considered in the following diseases: MPS type I (Hurler syndrome), MPS type VI (Marateaux-Lamy syndrome), MPS type VII (Sly syndrome), Krabbe disease, metachromatic leukodystrophy, alpha-fucosidosis, alpha-mannosidosis, Gaucher disease (although enzyme replacement therapy is available and is the first-line treatment for type 1), and Niemann-Pick disease type B.[2,3] Bone marrow transplantation has been recently reported as a suitable treatment option in glycogen storage disease type Ib with severe neutrophil dysfunction, inflammatory bowel disease, and recurrent infections.[4] For most other lysosomal defects, there is only limited or discouraging data in favor of HSCT. Because of the progressive nature and variability of each disease, a comprehensive, multidisciplinary approach should be used in each case to determine whether a patient is a suitable candidate.

Hematopoietic Stem Cells

The largest clinical experience exists for the mucopolysaccaridoses.[5] Transplantation seems to produce a variety of beneficial effects on specific symptoms of mucopolysaccharidoses. Improvement has been confirmed for MPS I regarding hepatosplenomegaly, clouding of cornea, and joint contractures, whereas skeletal changes, as in dysostosis multiplex, could not be influenced sufficiently. This is one of the reasons why this kind of therapy will not be beneficial for patients with Morquio syndrome. In patients with Sanfilippo syndrome, it was not possible to influence the mental regression. On the other hand, the intellectual development ratio of very young patients with Hurler syndrome seems to remain on the level they had reached prior to the procedure and not to decline further.[6]

Although significant successful clinical results have been reported in patients with lysosomal defects after HSCT—provided the transplantation was performed early in life—the success of stem cell therapy has been limited by donor availability, high rates of graft failure, mixed chimerism, and treatment-related morbidity and mortality. Recent studies, using cord blood as a stem cell source for cell therapy in inherited metabolic disorders showed high rates of full donor chimerism associated with normal enzyme levels following cell engraftment.[7] Because full donor chimerism and normal enzyme levels are suggested to be associated with a superior neurocognitive outcome after stem cell therapy, cord blood has been proposed as an alternative option or even preferential stem cell source for lysosomal patients. A concern, however, might be the relatively higher rate of (mainly moderate) graft versus host disease found in this study. Better matching and selection possibilities in the future might further improve these outcomes by increasing the number of cord blood units banked.

For disease types with significant central nervous system deterioration, HSCT is know only to be effective in the neonatal or presymptomatic stage of the disease. Taken together, HSCT remains a viable option for some individuals with lysosomal storage disorders (LSDs) and should be ideally performed in a centre with experience in LSDs.[8]

Liver Transplantation

During recent years, liver transplantation (LT), orthotopic or auxiliary, has become a realistic alternative for the treatment of hepatic-based inborn errors of metabolism.[9]

The long-term patient survival rates for children with inborn errors or metabolism after LT are excellent (more than 90% after five years), especially when structural liver damage is absent.[10] These are very good results that, in combination with the increasingly widespread use of split techniques that have augmented the pediatric donor pool, have extended the transplant indications in metabolic disorders during the last few years.

The indication and timing for LT in metabolic disorders depend on the underlying defect.[11] Some metabolic disorders cause progressive liver injury, eventually leading to cirrhosis and liver failure, making LT a life-saving procedure. Wilson disease, alpha-1-antitrypsin deficiency, tyrosinemia type I, glycogen storage diseases (type I a/b, IV), and disorders of bile acid synthesis and transport are classic metabolic indications.[12] The management of these disorders does not significantly differ from other structural liver diseases.

Other metabolic disorders do not cause structural liver damage, but their toxic metabolites exert severe extra hepatic effects. Diseases such as organic acidurias (e.g., propionic aciduria, methylmalonic acidurias [MMA]), maple syrup urine disease (MSUD), urea cycle defects (UCDs), primary hyperoxaluria type 1, Crigler-Najjar syndrome type 1, and others are suitable for LT. In these patients, LT is aimed to correct the enzyme deficiency, when alternative therapeutic options are not adequate or fail to prevent metabolic decompensation. In each case, the donor liver essentially represents a "factory" provided for the metabolism of circulating metabolites responsible for the symptoms of disease. Patients with liver-based metabolic defects but otherwise a normally functioning liver could benefit from auxiliary partial orthotopic liver transplantation (APOLT), leaving the option open for future gene therapy. APOLT has been successfully performed in UCD, Crigler-Najjar syndrome type 1, and glycogen storage disease type I patients.[13] Because about one-third of the donor liver is replaced in APOLT, it makes the recipient comparable to a healthy heterozygous carrier.

In glycogen storage disease type I, patients can have severe problems in following a strict diet and are always at risk for episodes of hypoglycemia, seizures, and possible brain damage. Moreover, long-term complications such as gout, growth failure, and hepatic adenomas with the risk of malignant transformations are related to the quality of metabolic control through therapy.

LT is frequently performed in order to optimize metabolic control and when malignant transformation of adenomas is suspected. Long-term outcome following transplantation is good, but immunosuppressive therapy can worsen the progression of associated kidney disease.

In MMA and propionic acidurias, given the poor long-term prognosis, LT has been more recently attempted as an alternative therapy to conventional medical treatment to cure the underlying metabolic defect.[14,15,16,17] However, the persistent excretion of urinary metabolites in transplanted patients demonstrated that replacement of the liver would only partly correct the enzymatic defect because of the persistence of the enzymatic block in other organs and tissues.[18] LT in MMA may not prevent the progressive renal and/or neurological deterioration even when intervention occurs very early in life. The overall experience reported concluded that children with organic acidurias appear to be at a higher risk of complications from transplantation than other metabolic disorders. While quality of life may be improved, transplantation does not cure patients who remain at risk of complications.

To date, the criteria for solid organ transplantation in organic acidurias have not been well established. The decision to undertake transplantation is a complicated one that involves a comprehensive understanding of the disease and then balancing the risks and benefits of transplantation, as there is still a high morbidity and even mortality after orthotopic liver transplantation (OLT). Furthermore, neurological damage can still occur years after transplantation.[19,20] In conclusion, consideration of the natural history of the disease, current therapeutic alternatives, potential future developments, and quality of life must be carefully evaluated before making such a decision. It is to be hoped that further experience and optimisation of transplant strategies in these disorders will provide more solid information and result in more predictable and better outcomes.

In UCDs, a considerable number of patients with carbamoyl phosphate synthetase deficiency (CPSD), ornithine transcarbamylase deficiency (OTCD), argininosuccinic aciduria, and citrullinemia types 1 and 2 have undergone LT in the past few decades.[21,22,23,24]

The first case reports from the end of the 1980s could demonstrate that LT could permanently normalize elevated ammonia levels in patients with UCDs.

Due to the nearly exclusive hepatic expression especially of the proximal urea cycle, the success of LT for UCDs is not surprising. Only small amounts of defective enzymes localized in the kidney and gut are not replenished by LT, and LT for UCDs may thus be regarded as a gene respectively enzyme replacement therapy. An open question is, however, the physiological importance of substantial systemic, and especially cerebral, expression of the distal urea cycle enzymes, including argininosuccinate synthetase, argininosuccinate lyase, and arginase. Therefore, reduced (OTCD and CPSD) or still elevated (citrullinemia) concentrations of citrulline may still be observed after LT in the systemic circulation. However, there is convincing evidence that further neurological impairment can be prevented by LT and that even neurological improvement could be observed in individual cases.

In the neonatal forms of proximal disorders (OTCD, CPSD, and citrullinemia), with a dramatic initial presentation and very poor long-term prognosis, only early LT can prevent severe brain damage and gives the chance for a reasonable to good outcome. In the rare case that a UCD presents as acute liver failure, an emergency LT can rescue the patient.

Special considerations must be made for female OTCD patients because the disease is inherited in X-linked fashion. All affected girls can pass on the defected gene as conductors, but some may themselves develop severe progressive symptoms often starting in early adulthood. For these patients, APOLT appears conceptually an attractive therapeutic option. APOLT has also been successfully performed in adult patients with citrullinemia type II. Although small patient cohorts indicate that OLT might be superior to APOLT, recent results in children with noncirrhotic metabolic diseases indicate good long-term results similar to OLT.

In mitochondrial disorders, the question of whether LT is an appropriate treatment option is even more difficult.[25,26,27] The unique genetic feature of mitochrondrial heteroplasmy accounts for a wide range of clinical courses, from acute liver failure to mild chronic disease. Progressive extrahepatic manifestations, especially progressive brain damage, develop in the majority of patients. The key question is whether neuromuscular involvement is present at the time when LT is considered. This decision is most difficult in patients with a combination of epilepsy and liver failure and the possible diagnosis of Alpers disease. The latter must be excluded by mutation analysis before LT.

In tyrosinemia type I, an autosomal recessively inherited metabolic disease caused by the deficiency of fumarylacetoacetase, liver involvement may cause acute liver failure, progressive deterioration leading to cirrhosis, recurrent decompensation during intercurrent illness, and hepatocellular carcinoma. LT was the only potentially curative treatment before 1991 and was associated with good outcomes. The introduction of 2-(2-nitro-4-trifluoromethylbenzyol)-1,3 cyclohexanedione (NTBC) has restricted LT to nonresponsiveness to this drug and suspicion of hepatocellular carcinoma.[28,29]

OLT has also been investigated as a treatment for MSUD.[30,31] Patients receiving OLT no longer require a diet restricted in branched-chain amino acids, and the activity of the branched-chain α–keto acid dehydrogenase complex is restored to at least the level of very mild MSUD patients. Thus OLT represents a viable cure for some patients. However, in addition to OLT being a highly invasive and very costly procedure, there remains a high risk for the development of serious complications, and most patients are required to take immunosuppressant drugs for the rest of their lives. Clearly, there is a need for alternative therapies to combat this disorder, but OLT has revealed an important fact. Although the branched-chain α–keto acid dehydrogenase complex does function in other tissues, restoration of activity of the branched-chain α–keto acid dehydrogenase complex in the liver alone is sufficient to correct metabolic abnormalities in MSUD, thus providing significant rationale for focusing on liver-directed therapies, such as cell transplantation (i.e., hepatocytes, embryonic stem cells, cord-blood cells) or gene therapy.

Liver Cell Transplantation

Although less invasive than orthotopic LT, liver cell transplantation (LCT) is still an experimental method, and the expected benefit for the patient must outweigh the known and unknown risks of the new therapy. Since only small amounts of liver cells can be transferred by LCT, not every condition that can be treated with LT is also suitable for LCT.[32]

The safety of LCT is related to the number of cells transfused. If a certain threshold is reached, shunting of the transplanted cells into extrahepatic organs may occur and the risk of portal vein thrombosis is increased. However, relevant side effects in clinical applications have so far been observed only in adults with coexisting diseases, especially structural pathology of the liver. Two precautions are essential in order to keep the number of side effects low: serial applications and thorough monitoring of cell infusion. Keeping this in mind, LCT is a safe and only slightly invasive technique. It does not carry the risk associated with permanent removal of the liver by LT. Furthermore, it has the potential of repeated applications over long time intervals. It has been shown before that cryopreserved liver cells may provide metabolic stability in inborn errors of metabolism. If cryopreserved cells could be developed into a biological drug distributable to metabolic centres within hours, this would be an important prerequisite for the necessary clinical trials and future therapies.

Hepatocyte transplantation is a promising therapy for patients with inherited metabolic diseases, which offers a less invasive and fully reversible approach.[33] Crigler-Najjar syndrome can be regarded as a model disease for LCT in metabolic disorders. In metabolic patients, LCT aims at addition of cells rather than at replacement of diseased cells as in acute liver failure. In Crigler-Najjar patients, the effect of transplanted cells can easily be monitored by the amount of reduction of plasma bilirubin. This has been shown very convincingly in the first patient (Crigler-Najjar syndrome type 1), a 10-year-old girl, whose case is frequently regarded as the breakthrough in human LCT and which prompted the initiation of several clinical programs. The initial success could be confirmed in four other children who all experienced substantial reduction of plasma bilirubin and duration of daily phototherapy. Data on the long-term clinical courses in these children are, however, incomplete. Two patients are known to have received a whole-organ transplantation after 30 and five months, respectively. Reported duration of beneficial effects was from three to 11 months.

Monitoring the success of LCT in UCD patients is much more difficult.[34,35,36] Unlike in Crigler-Najjar syndrome, multiple factors may contribute to the development of hyperammonemic crises. Affected children may experience periods of complete clinical well-being with normal laboratory values, the duration of which is almost impossible to predict. Moreover, the patient cohort hitherto treated with LCT is heterogenous in terms of patient age (one day, five years) and type of UCD (CPSD, OTCD, argininosuccinate lyase deficiency, and citrullinemia). Nevertheless, most patients experienced considerable metabolic improvement following LCT. The majority of treated children could be safely bridged to OLT without further metabolic decompensation and subsequent neurological damage. Recently, a first prospective study on LCT for the treatment of severe neonatal UCD has been started with encouraging preliminary results.

Hepatocyte transplantations have been proposed in a very restricted group of metabolic diseases. In a severe peroxisomal disorder (Infantile Refsum disease) where OLT was not regarded as appropriate because of her marked psychomotor retardation, LCT was surprisingly encouraging.[37] Not only did key laboratory parameters improve, but she also made considerable development progress. Finally, LCT has been performed in patients with glycogen storage diseases.[38] Because of the nature of the disease, monitoring of transplantation success is difficult, but some medium-term metabolic improvement has been reported in both patients.

Kidney Transplantation

An increasing number of children with inborn errors of metabolism survive the acute metabolic crises or are even found presymptomatically through extended newborn screening programs. In the long term, renal and neurologic complications often develop and become problematic. Renal failure is a particular complication of MMA and is not seen in other organic acidurias.[39] The exact pathogenesis of the renal injury is still unclear; the pathology is that of chronic tubulointerstitial nephritis progressing to end stage renal disease or disabling polyuria in adolescence. Kidney transplantation has been reported in MMA patients with renal failure, but the amount of enzyme activity provided by the kidney tissue is relatively small compared to the liver. Hence, kidney transplantation alone is not sufficient to prevent acute metabolic episodes, and disease recurrence will compromise the kidney allograft.[40]

Combined liver–kidney transplantation could represent a better strategy than liver or kidney transplantation alone in some patients. Combined liver–kidney transplantation has been reported in patients with MMA and renal dysfunction with good results.[41,42] Of five reported cases, all were alive three to 60 months after transplantation. One child required retransplantation of the liver for hepatic artery thrombosis. A further child underwent liver and kidney retransplantation and native nephrectomy for persistent polyuria, and, despite a postoperative intracranial haemorrhage, she recovered. A 95% to 97% reduction in serum and urine methylmalonic acid posttransplant was reported, allowing for significant liberalization of dietary restrictions with a consequent increase in body mass index, muscle strength, and energy. In addition, renal function normalized and neurologic status stabilized in these children. A small number of combined liver–kidney transplantations have also been successfully performed in patients with glycogen storage disease type Ia.

Conclusion

This review has summarized the theoretical considerations and some of the positive and negative aspects of transplantations for inborn errors of metabolism. There is reason to to be optimistic but at the same time cautious. Treatment of metabolic diseases with transplantation has proved efficacious. The decision process has become more complex. Questions arise as to which disease and which patients are amenable to transplantation, the appropriate age, the limitations imposed by donor availability, and the long-term results. We have learned what we may and may not anticipate from the transplantation process in several of these disorders. The time has come for prospective and comparative analyses, so that we can provide more specific recommendations and optimize outcomes in the future.

References

1. Valayannopoulos V and Wijburg FA. Therapy for the mucopolysaccharidoses. *Rheumatology.* 2011; 50: 49–59.
2. Parenti G1, Pignata C, Vajro P, Salerno M. New strategies for the treatment of lysosomal storage diseases. *Int J Mol Med.* 2013; 31: 11–20.
3. Orchard PJ and Tolar J. Transplant outcomes in leukodystrophies. *Semin Hematol.* 2010; 47: 70–78.
4. Pierre G, Chakupurakal G, McKiernan P, Hendriksz C, Lawson S, Chakrapani A. Bone marrow transplantation in glycogen storage disease type 1b. *J Pediatr.* 2008; 152: 286–288.
5. de Ru MH, Boelens JJ, Das AM, et al. Enzyme replacement therapy and/or hematopoietic stem cell transplantation at diagnosis in patients with mucopolysaccharidosis type I: results of a European consensus procedure. *Orphanet J Rare Dis.* 2011; 6: 55.
6. Prased UK, Kurtzberg J. Transplant outcomes in mucopolysaccharidosis. *Semin Hematol.* 2010;47:59–69.
7. Orchard PJ, Blazar BR, Wagner J, et al. Hematopoietic cell therapy for metabolic disease. *J Pediatr.* 2007; 151: 340–346.
8. Wynn RF, Wraith JE, Mercer J, et al. Improved metabolic correction in patients with lysosomal storage disease treated with hematopoietic stem cell transplant compared with enzyme replacement therapy. *J Pediatr.* 2009; 154: 609–611.
9. Mazariegos G, Shneider B, Burton B, Fox IJ, Hadzic N, Kishnani P, Morton DH, McIntire S, Sokol RJ, Summar M, White D, Chavanon V, Vockley J. Liver transplantation for pediatric metabolic disease. *Mol Genet Metab.* 2014; 111:418–27
10. Kayler LK, Merion RM, Lee S, et al. Long-term survival after liver transplantation in children with metabolic disorders. *Pediatr Transplant.* 2002; 6: 295–300.
11. Meyburg J, Hoffmann GF. Liver transplantation for inborn errors of metabolism. *Transplantation.* 2005; 80: S135.
12. Sze YK, Dhawan A, Taylor RM, et al. Pediatric liver transplantation for metabolic liver disease: experience at King's College Hospital. *Transplantation.* 2009; 87: 87–93.
13. Reddy SK, Austin SL, Spencer-Manzon M, et al. Liver transplantation for glycogen storage disease type Ia. *J Hepatol.* 2009; 51(3): 483–490.
14. Barshes NR, Vanatta JM, Patel AJ, et al. Evaluation and management of patients with propionic acidemia undergoing liver transplantation: A comprehensive review. *Pediatr Transplant.* 2006; 10: 773–781.
15. Yorijuji T, Kawai M, Mamada M, et al. Living-donor liver transplantation for propionic acidaemia. *J Inherit Metab Dis.* 2004; 27: 205–210.
16. Kaplan P, Ficicioglu C, Mazur AT, Palmieri M, Berry GT. Liver transplantation is not curative for methylmalonic acidopathy caused by methylmalonyl-CoA mutase deficiency. *Mol Genet Metab.* 2006; 88: 322–326.
17. Kasahara M, Horikawa R, Tagawa M, et al. Current role for transplantation for methylmalonic acidemia: A review of the literature. *Pediatr Transplant.* 2006; 10: 943–947.
18. Morioka D, Kasahara M, Horikawa R et al. Efficacy of living donor transplantation for patients with methylmalonic aciduria. *Am J Transplant.* 2007; 7: 2782–2787.

19. Nyhan WL, Gargus JJ, Boyle K, Selby R, Koch R. Progressive neurologic disability in methylmalonic acidemia despite transplantation of the liver. *Eur J Pediatr.* 2002; 161: 377–379.
20. Chakrapani A, Sivakumar P, McKiernan P, Leonard JV. Metabolic stroke in methylmalonic acidemia five years after liver transplantation. *J Pediatr.* 2002; 140: 261–263.
21. McBride KL, Miller G, Carter S, Karpen S, Goss J, Lee B. Developmental outcomes with early orthotopic liver transplantation for infants with neonatal-onset urea cycle defects and a female patient with late-onset ornithine transcarbamylase deficiency. *Pediatrics.* 2004; 114: e523–e526.
22. Morioka D, Kasahara M, Takada Y, et al. Current role of liver transplantation for the treatment of urea cycle disorders: a review of the worldwide English literature and 13 cases at Kyoto University. *Liver Transplant.* 2005; 11: 1332.
23. Teufel U, Weitz J, Flechtenmacher C, et al. High urgency liver transplantation in ornithine transcarbamylase deficiency presenting with acute liver failure. *Pediatr Transplantation.* 2009; 15(6): 49–53.
24. Whitington PF, Alonso EM, Boyle JT, et al. Liver transplantation for the treatment of urea cycle disorders. *J Inherit Metab Dis.* 1998; 21(Suppl. 1): 112–118.
25. Grabhorn El, Tsiakas K, Herden U, et al. Long-term outcomes after liver transplantation for deoxyguanosine kinase deficiency: a single-center experience and a review of the literature. *Liver Transpl.* 2014; 20: 464–472.
26. De Greef El, Christodoulou J, Alexander IE, et al. Mitochondrial respiratory chain hepatopathies: role of liver transplantation. A case series of five patients. *J Inherit Metab Dis.* 2012; 4: 5–11.
27. El-Hattab AW1, Scaglia F. Mitochondrial DNA depletion syndromes: review and updates of genetic basis, manifestations, and therapeutic options. *Neurotherapeutics.* 2013; 10: 186–198.
28. de Laet C1, Dionisi-Vici C, Leonard JV, et al. Recommendations for the management of tyrosinaemia type 1. *Orphanet J Rare Dis.* 2013; 11: 8–8.
29. Bartlett DC1, Preece MA, Holme E, et al. Plasma succinylacetone is persistently raised after liver transplantation in tyrosinaemia type 1. *J Inherit Metab Dis.* 2013; 36: 15–20.
30. Badell IR, Hanish SI, Hughes CB, Hewitt WR, Chung RT, Spivey JR, Knechtle SJ. Domino liver transplantation in maple syrup urine disease: a case report and review of the literature. *Transplant Proc.* 2013 Mar;45:806–809.
31. Mazariegos GV, Morton DH, Sindhi R, et al. Liver transplantation for classical maple syrup urine disease: long-term follow-up in 37 patients and comparative United Network for Organ Sharing experience. *J Pediatr.* 2012 160:116–121.
32. Jorns C, Ellis EC, Nowak G, et al. Hepatocyte transplantation for inherited metabolic diseases of he liver. *J Int Med.* 2012; 272: 201–223.
33. Vogel KR, Kennedy AA, Whitehouse LA, Gibson KM. Therapeutic hepatocyte transplant for inherited metabolic disorders: functional considerations, recent outcomes and future prospects. *J Inherit Metab Dis.* 2014; 37(2): 165–176.
34. Fox IJ, Chowdhury JR, Kaufman SS, et al. Treatment of the Crigler-Najjar syndrome type I with hepatocyte transplantation. *N Engl J Med.* 1998; 338: 1422–1446.
35. Horslen SP, McCowan TC, Goertzen TC, et al. Isolated hepatocyte transplantation in an infant with a severe urea cycle disorder. *Pediatrics.* 2003; 111: 1262–1267.
36. Meyburg J, Das AM, Hoerster F, et al. One liver for four children: first clinical series of liver cell transplantation for severe neonatal urea cycle defects. *Transplantation.* 2009; 87: 636–641.
37. Sokal EM, Smets F, Bourgois A, et al. Hepatocyte transplantation in a 4-year-old girl with peroxisomal biogenesis disease: technique, safety and metabolic follow-up. *Transplantation.* 2003; 76: 735–738.
38. Muraca M, Gerunda G, Neri D, et al. Hepatocyte transplantation as a treatment for glycogen storage disease type 1a. *Lancet.* 2002; 359: 317–318.
39. Morath MA1, Hörster F, Sauer SW. Renal dysfunction in methylmalonic acidurias: review for the pediatric nephrologist. *Pediatr Nephrol.* 2013; 28: 227–235.
40. Brassier A1, Boyer O, Valayannopoulos V, et al. Renal transplantation in 4 patients with methylmalonic aciduria: a cell therapy for metabolic disease. *Mol Genet Metab.* 2013; 110: 106–110.
41. Van't Hoff W, Dixon M, Taylor J, et al. Successful liver-kidney transplantation in a child with methylmalonic aciduria. *J Pediatr.* 1998; 132: 1043–1044.
42. McGuire P, Lim-Melia E, Diaz G, et al. Combined liver-kidney transplantation for the management of methylmalonic aciduria: a case report and review of the literature. *Mol Genet Metab.* 2008; 93: 22–29.

13

Gene Replacement Therapy for Inborn Errors of Metabolism

Nicola Brunetti-Pierri

Introduction

Inborn errors of metabolism have historically played an important role in the development of gene therapy. One of the first attempts to treat a human disease by gene transfer can be dated to the prerecombinant DNA era when argininemia patients were injected with the papilloma Shope virus on the incorrect assumption that the virus genome encoded for the arginase gene that is mutated in argininemia.[1] Although the infection of human fibroblasts resulted in increased arginase activity, intravenous injections of the virus in patients had no effect on arginine levels.[1] Several years later, Lesch-Nyhan disease became one of the first disease targets for viral vector mediated gene therapy. In this earliest attempt, a genetically modified retrovirus carrying the human hypoxanthine phosphoribosyltransferase was used to infect mouse bone marrow cells ex vivo, and tranduced cells were subsequently transplanted into mice.[2]

Inborn errors of metabolism continue to be logical targets for gene therapy. The prognosis of several metabolic disorders is uncertain, especially given the elevated risks of repeated crises during intercurrent illnesses. Therefore, liver and/or hematopoietic stem cell transplantation has been considered in several of these disorders. The invasive nature of the transplant procedure and the limitations of donor organ availability could make gene therapy an attractive alternative or adjunctive treatment. Moreover, expanded newborn screening is allowing early detection of several disorders, and the availability of clinical gene therapy to be initiated at the time of newborn screening, prior to the onset of symptoms and before development of tissue damage, has the potential to dramatically change the natural history of these diseases.

The recent successes of gene therapy by multiple groups in severe combined immune deficiency (SCID) due to adenosine deaminase deficiency or to mutations in the X-linked interleukin receptor common γ chain[3-5], and in Leber's congenital amaurosis[6-8] clearly support the development of gene replacement therapies.

Gene Therapy: Definitions and General Principles

The basic concept of gene therapy is simple: introduce genes into the target cells to either cure the disease or to slow down its progression. To accomplish this goal, gene therapy requires technologies capable of transferring genetic material into a variety of cells, tissues, and organs. The genetic material to transfer includes the expression cassette with the therapeutic gene, a flanking promoter, and other signal sequences such as the polyA addition site. The whole process of gene delivery and expression, defined as *transduction*, can be achieved by two main tools: viral and nonviral vectors. In general, viral vectors have shown greater transduction efficiency because they exploit the virus's highly evolved biological machinery to gain access into cells and to transfer their DNA content into the nucleus. Virus-based vectors for gene therapy have been generated by deleting most or all the coding regions from the viral genome and leaving intact those sequences needed for functions such as packaging of the vector genome into the viral capsid or integration of DNA into the host chromatin. The expression cassette of choice is inserted into the viral backbone in place of the deleted sequences (Figure 13.1). The viral vectors are produced in cell factory systems in which essential components are provided *in trans* to enable vectors to be packaged and to maintain their ability to deliver genes to the target cells. Viral vectors lacking the essential components for viral propagation can only produce dead-end infections, which result in transfer of their genetic content only to the infected cells without subsequent spread of infection.

Genes can be potentially transferred to germline or somatic cells. Germline gene transfer involves the insertion of a normal gene into germ cells such that it will be transmitted in a Mendelian fashion to the offspring. For ethical reasons, germline gene therapy is not acceptable. Somatic gene therapy is the insertion of therapeutic genes in somatic cells. By this approach the therapeutic gene is transferred only to a portion of the somatic cells without the occurrence of germline transmission.

Most of the gene therapy approaches for inborn errors of metabolism are based on delivering a corrected copy of the defective gene without removal of the endogenous mutated gene. This approach is defined as *gene addition* or *gene replacement*. Gene addition is best suited for

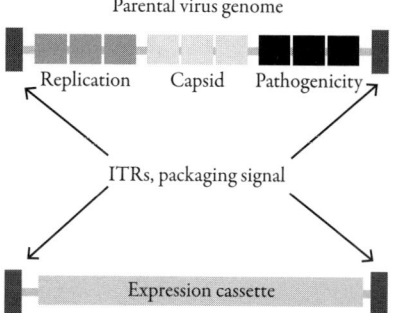

FIGURE 13.1 Schematic of a viral genome containing genes involved in replication, virion structure (capsid), and pathogenicity. Minimally, gene therapy vectors contain the essential *cis*-acting elements and the expression cassette (e.g., promoter and therapeutic gene) with the transcriptional regulatory elements replacing the viral coding sequences. *Abbreviations: ITRs = inverted terminal repeats.*

disorders due to loss-of-function mutations, and advantages of this approach include its simplicity, whereas disadvantages often include the lack of controlled gene expression. However, for the majority of the inborn errors of metabolism, a strict regulation of the expression of the therapeutic gene is not required. Other gene therapy approaches include *gene reprogramming* and *gene repair*. Gene reprogramming is based on modification of the mRNA to avoid the consequences of a mutation by inhibiting the expression of the mutated gene. This strategy, using for example small interfering RNA, is useful to prevent the expression of a mutated protein with deleterious function or to inhibit a cryptic splice site, thus preventing expression of an abnormally spliced product. Gene repair seeks to correct mutant sequences in the genomic DNA. This strategy can be achieved by chimeric proteins composed of a DNA-sequence-specific binding domain and an endonuclease capable of inducing site-specific DNA double-strand breaks. The main limitations of this approach are the low efficiency and the off-target effects. For most inborn errors of metabolism, neither gene reprogramming nor gene repair are needed and gene addition is sufficient to achieve therapeutic effects.

Gene transfer can be obtained in vivo by direct administration of the gene therapy vector to a specific tissue or organ, that is, systemic intravascular administration, intramuscular injection, and intracerebral stereotactic, intraventricular, or intrathecal injections. Alternatively, cells can be isolated from the patient, cultured and genetically modified ex vivo, and returned back into the patient.

Gene Delivery Systems

Several vectors have been investigated for gene therapy, and so far no single vector system has yet emerged as clearly superior to the others for all applications. The choice of the vector delivery system is generally dictated by the nature of the disease and by the target tissue. Because inborn errors of metabolism are chronic conditions, a major requirement for gene transfer vectors is the ability to drive long-term expression of the therapeutic gene. Ideally, the gene correction should be achieved with one or a few administrations. However, in the case of viral vectors, readministration is complicated by the development of neutralizing antibodies that prevent further vector-mediated transduction. In the following sections, we discuss the main classes of vectors that have been investigated for gene therapy of inborn errors of metabolism.

Viral Vectors

Modified, defective viruses have been extensively used to deliver foreign DNA sequences to target cells. Viral vectors can be broadly classified into vectors derived from RNA viruses (γ-retrovirus and lentivirus) used to mediate integrative gene transfer and nonintegrative vectors derived from DNA viruses (adenovirus, adeno-associated virus) (Table 13.1). The main drawback of RNA viruses is their uncontrolled integration that can cause insertional carcinogenesis while the major disadvantage of DNA viruses is their immunogenicity. The genetic material of DNA viruses does not usually integrate into cells and is not replicated at cell division. Therefore, in contrast to RNA viral vectors, applications of DNA virus-derived vector are restricted to postmitotic cells.

TABLE 13.1 Overview of Gene Therapy Vectors for Inborn Errors of Metabolism

	Genetic Material	Cloning Capacity	Vector Genome Forms in Nuclei of Transduced Cells	Advantages	Disadvantages
Retroviral vectors	RNA	8 kb	Integrated	- High efficiency integration - No viral immune response - Long-term expression	- Transduction only in dividing cells - Insertional carcinogenesis
Lentiviral vectors	RNA	8–10 kb	Integrated	- Transduction of nondividing cells - Long-term expression	- Integration into active genes - Risk of replication competent HIV
Adenoviral vectors	dsDNA	Up to 35 kb (HDAd)	Episomal	- Transduction of nondividing cells - Large cloning capacity - High transduction levels - Long-term expression (HDAd)	- Acute toxicity
AAV vectors	ssDNA	5–9 kb	Episomal (>90%) Integrated (<10%)	- Transduction of nondividing cells - Long-term expression	- Limited cloning capacity - CTL-mediated immune reaction in human livers
Naked plasmid DNA	dsDNA	Unlimited	Episomal	- Transduction of nondividing cells - No inflammatory response - Large cloning capacity - Ease preparation	- Low efficiency of transduction - Clinically relevant delivery method still to be developed

Note. dsDNA = double-stranded DNA; ssDNA = single-stranded DNA; AAV = adeno associated virus; HDAd = helper-dependent adenoviral vector; CTL = cytotoxic T lymphocyte; HIV = human immunodeficiency virus.

Retroviral vectors: γ-Retroviruses are lipid-enveloped particles containing two identical copies of a linear single-stranded RNA genome of 7 to 11 kb (Table 13.1). Retroviral vectors are traditionally derived from oncoretroviruses, such as the Moloney murine leukemia retrovirus, which was the first vector developed for gene therapy.[9] Retroviral vectors can only transduce dividing cells and require natural breakdown of the nuclear membrane, which occurs during cell division, to enter the nucleus. Therefore, actively dividing cells, such as hematopoietic stem cells, are excellent targets for retroviral vector-mediated gene therapy while nondividing cells of tissues such as brain, eye, lung, adult liver, and pancreas are less efficiently targeted by in vivo gene delivery with retroviral vectors. Following infection of target cells, the RNA genome is reverse transcribed and integrates into the host genomic DNA. Retroviruses insert into the host genome in a nonrandom manner, and up to 25% of integration events occur within 10 kb of promoter elements, particularly of transcriptionally active genes, including proto-oncogenes.[10,11] Integration provides the potential for long-term gene expression because the integrated genome is maintained in the progeny of the transduced cells. However, it also increases the risk of cancer formation through insertional mutagenesis and/or insertional activation of proximal genes, as was observed in the clinical gene therapy trial for X-linked SCID.[12] The most important and effective applications of retroviral vectors have been ex vivo hematopoietic stem cell gene

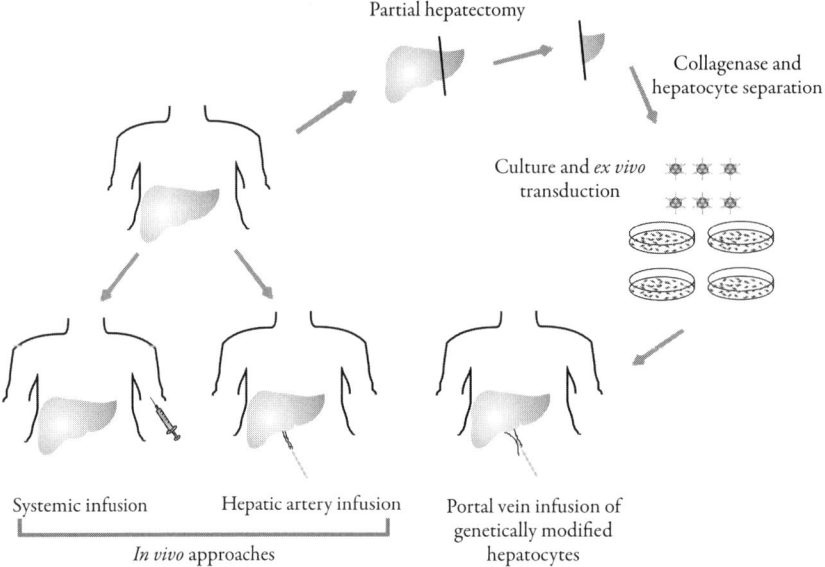

FIGURE 13.2 Strategies of ex vivo and in vivo liver-directed gene therapy.

transfer to correct congenital immune deficiencies. Nevertheless, in one of the earliest gene therapy trials, they were also used for liver-directed gene therapy. In this trial, performed in a patient with familial hypercholesterolemia due to homozygous mutations in the low-density lipoprotein receptor, autologous hepatocytes obtained from surgical removal of approximately 15% of the liver were cultured and genetically corrected ex vivo with recombinant retroviruses carrying the gene for the low-density lipoprotein receptor and then reinfused in the patient (Figure 13.2).[13] Although some modest degree of reduction in low-density lipoprotein cholesterol was observed, this was transitory. Likely, the insufficient number of corrected hepatocytes returned to the patient and/or the lack of selective advantage of corrected cells contributed to the insufficient clinical benefit, as explained in more details in the section 'Ex vivo approaches to gene therapy'.

In vivo gene therapy with retroviral vectors has been complicated because of technical issues related to generation of high titer vector preparations and because hepatocytes are nonproliferating cells under most circumstances. Effective strategies for in vivo liver-directed gene therapy using retroviral vectors require induction of hepatocyte cell division through manipulations such as partial hepatectomy or hepatocyte growth factor treatment.[14,15] Alternatively, retroviral vectors can transduce hepatocytes from newborn animals (mice and dogs) without a stimulus for replication.[16–19]

Lentiviral vectors: Lentivirus-based vectors are derived from the human immunodeficiency virus type 1 (HIV-1), which is part of the retrovirus family but has acquired the ability to also transduce nondividing cells. Compared to retroviruses, lentiviral vectors are less genotoxic and so far no insertional carcinogenesis has been reported in the experimental setting, though their integration pattern appears nonrandom. Specifically, lentiviruses integrate mostly into transcriptionally active gene units but do not target the region near the transcription start sites.[20–22] Given the limited prevalence in the general population of preexisting immunity against HIV-1 and, therefore, against lentiviral vector components,[23] the patient population potentially eligible for lentiviral-mediated gene therapy is wide (Table 13.1). Besides applications in hematological disorders, owing to their ability to transduce nondividing cells, lentiviral vectors can also be used to deliver transgenes in vivo to tissues that would not be effectively transduced by retroviral vectors, such as cells of the central nervous system, airway epithelium, and liver.

Adenoviral vectors: Adenovirus-derived vectors are the most commonly used in human gene therapy clinical trials. However, the majority of these applications are for cancer treatment. Very few trials were directed at the treatment of genetic disorders, the initial disease application for which adenoviral vectors were developed, and currently there are no clinical trials ongoing for monogenic disorders using these vectors (http://www.abedia.com/wiley/). Adenoviral vectors are excellent gene transfer vectors due to their ability to efficiently infect a variety of cell types from various species to direct high-level transgene expression. Following host cell infection, the adenoviral vector genome remains episomal in the nucleus. While early generation E1-deleted adenoviral vectors remain very useful for several applications, the transient transgene expression in vivo is a clear limitation for the therapy of inborn errors of metabolism. In contrast, helper-dependent adenoviral vectors (also referred to as gutless, gutted, mini, fully deleted, high-capacity, Δ, pseudo, or gene-deleted), which are deleted of all viral coding sequences, are clearly superior in terms of safety and efficacy for the treatment of monogenic disorders. Helper-dependent adenoviral vectors also have a large cloning capacity of up to ~37 kb, which allows delivery of whole genomic loci and large *cis*-acting elements to enhance and prolong transgene expression (Table 13.1).

In several preclinical studies for liver-directed gene therapy, helper-dependent adenoviral vectors have shown long-term and in some cases even life-long phenotypic correction without chronic toxicity.[24,25] Long-term expression by helper-dependent adenoviral vectors has also been demonstrated in clinically relevant large animal models, including nonhuman primates and dogs.[26–31] Unfortunately, relatively high vector doses are required to achieve efficient hepatic transduction following systemic intravenous injection, and these high doses are responsible for an acute toxic response.[32–34] Various strategies have been investigated to overcome this obstacle.[26,29,35–37]

Adeno-associated viral vectors: Vectors derived from adeno-associated viruses (AAV) are small, nonenveloped viruses that package a linear single-stranded DNA genome. They are attractive for in vivo gene therapy because of a favorable safety profile and the ability to drive long-term transgene expression following a single vector administration. A major limitation of AAV vectors is their packaging capacity, considered to be limited to 4.7 kb (Table 13.1). However, some groups have reported efficient packaging of up to 8.9 kb of DNA in AAV,[38–40] or transfer of large genes in vivo by splitting large gene expression cassettes into halves, each contained in one of two separate (dual) AAV vectors.[41,42] The excellent safety profile makes AAV a promising tool for clinical gene transfer. Moreover, newly isolated serotypes, such as serotype 8 AAV (AAV8), have shown improved efficiency in transducing hepatocytes.[43,44] In liver-directed gene therapy approaches, serotype 2 AAV (AAV2) have been successfully used to correct small and large animal models and have been introduced in clinical trial for hemophilia B.[45] However, in contrast to the results obtained in preclinical studies, systemic

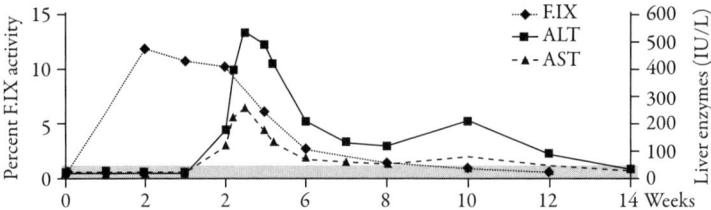

FIGURE 13.3 Circulating F.IX activity and serum transaminase (AST and ALT) levels following hepatic artery administration of 2×10^{12} vector genomes/Kg of AAV2 vector encoding F.IX in one hemophilia B subject. Taken from Manno et al.[45] with permission. The shaded gray area denotes normal range of AST and ALT.

administration of AAV2 resulted in therapeutic factor IX (F.IX) levels that were only short-term and associated with a transient subclinical increase of liver enzymes.[45] This adverse response is attributed to a cytoxic T lymphocyte response against the AAV capsid proteins that resulted in the elimination of the transduced hepatocytes and short-term F.IX expression (Figure 13.3).[46] Although occurring at higher doses, an immune reaction has been observed also in human patients receiving AAV8 vectors.[47] Immunosuppression regimens appear to overcome this obstacle and patients have benefited from AAV8 mediated F.IX expression.[47]

Nonviral Vectors

Nonviral vectors based on DNA have been developed with the goal of overcoming the obstacles of viral vectors. Compared to viral-based strategies, nonviral vectors are less toxic, do not elicit a humoral response and therefore can be readminister multiple times,[48] can drive long-term transgene expression,[49] and are simpler and cheaper to produce as clinical-grade vectors. The main problem of these vectors is the lack of an efficient in vivo delivery method, their rapid clearance in the bloodstream, the lack of organ-specific distribution, and low efficiency of cellular uptake following systemic delivery (Table 13.1). Simple injections of naked plasmid DNA into the liver,[50] muscle,[51] skin,[52] or airway[53] result in some degree of gene transfer, but this is largely insufficient for correction of human disorders. Chemical or physical methods have been used to enhance the efficiency of gene transfer. Chemical methods use synthetic or natural compounds such as cationic lipids or cationic polymers, protecting the DNA from nuclease-mediated DNA degradation. These DNA complexes are taken up by cells in the form of intracellular vesicles from which a small fraction of the DNA escapes into the cytoplasm and migrates into the nucleus, where transgene expression takes place. Some promising strategies for in vivo delivery of naked plasmid DNA have been developed.[54,55] Nevertheless, the limitation to date of nonviral gene transfer remains the low level of gene expression compared to viral vectors.

Genetic Regulation of Transgene Expression

The design of the expression cassette is important for long-term transgene expression that is required for inborn errors of metabolism. However, in the context of specific gene therapy applications, our knowledge of optimal promoters and expression cassettes is often limited. The use of strong, tissue-specific expression cassette is important for secreted proteins because high levels of expression of the therapeutic gene may allow the use of smaller doses of vector particles. However, the use of potent promoters may be unnecessary or may cause unwanted toxicity. Moreover, enzymes responsible for metabolic disorders are often part of multisubunit complexes, and overexpression of one component does not necessarily result in higher activity of the whole complex.

While promoter strength is a significant issue, ability to drive long-term expression and tissue specificity are also important. The cytomegalovirus promoter, for example, is susceptible to down-modulation[56] and therefore, it is not ideal in the context of diseases requiring long-term expression of therapeutic genes. Tissue specificity is another important factor to consider in the choice of the promoter, as ubiquitous expression may result in an immune response due to transgene expression into immune cells.

Transgene expression following vector delivery can indeed trigger an immune response against the therapeutic protein, which will prevent long-term phenotypic correction. Besides the choice of promoter, several other factors can influence this immune response, including the underlying genetic defects (single amino acid substitution resulting in expression of a mutated protein are less likely to result in formation of antibodies against the vector-encoded therapeutic protein compared to mutations causing complete lack of the protein), route of vector administration, dose of vector, status and nature of the target tissue (underlying disease or immune-privileged sites), and patient-related factors (age, immune status, comorbid diseases).

Gene Therapy for Inborn Errors of Metabolism

The treatment for inborn errors of metabolism, including gene therapy, is first based on our understanding of biochemistry and pathophysiology of the disease target. In general terms, the pathogenesis of inborn errors of metabolism can be explained by few models: (i) deficiency of essential product/enzyme, (ii) deleterious systemic effects of circulating toxic metabolites, and (iii) cell autonomous disease process. In the first two groups of disorders, overexpression of the defective protein by gene transfer in a limited number of cells may be sufficient for phenotypic correction. In cell autonomous disorders, correction of one cell does not improve adjacent cells, and, therefore, phenotypic correction requires gene transfer in a large number of cells.

Hemophilia A and B, due to deficiency of factor VIII (F.VIII) and F.IX respectively, are disorders due to the deficiency of enzymes. Hemophilias have been the focus of a large number of studies aimed at developing gene therapy because the pathophysiology of the disease is well known, small and large animal models are available, and expression of a small amount of clotting factor can result in significant amelioration of the disease. It is well established that 2% to 3% of wild-type levels of F.VIII or F.IX result in substantial reduction of the clinical manifestations of the disease while expression greater than 30% of wild-type levels would result in a phenotypically normal patient under most circumstances.[57] Therefore, hemophilia A and B could be significantly improved if 2% to

3% of the hepatocytes are transduced with a vector expressing the clotting factor in the transduced cells at the same levels of the hepatic endogenous promoter. This percentage could be even lower if transduced cells express the clotting factor at levels that are higher than the hepatic endogenous promoter.

With respect to the pulmonary disease, α-1-antitrypsin deficiency is similar to hemophilias because it results from the reduced plasma levels of α-1-antitrypsin, a plasma antiprotease synthesized by hepatocytes. For treatment of the lung disease of α-1-antitrypsin deficiency, the goal is to achieve plasma α-1-antitrypsin of at least 11 μM because concentration below this level is associated with an increased risk of chronic lung disease.[58] In contrast to the pulmonary disease, the liver phenotype is due to a cell-autonomous process and severe hepatic disease can currently be treated only by liver transplantation.

In lysosomal storage disorders, cells are affected by lysosomal accumulation of undegraded products, but the defective enzyme can be transferred from one cell to another through the mannose-6-phosphate receptor pathway. As a consequence, the enzyme can be produced in a single target tissue, secreted into the circulation, and taken up by other diseased tissues.

For defects in proteins that are not secreted, as in the case of diseases due to accumulation of toxic metabolites or cell autonomous disorders, establishing the levels of therapeutic gene needed for correction is more complicated. This information is important because it will dictate the therapeutic dose of the gene transfer vector and ultimately the safety and feasibility of the clinical trial. Data from preclinical studies in animal models and from clinical transplantation trials have been used to estimate these levels. Hepatocyte transplantation trials are helpful to estimate the percentage of correction. In these trials, the number of transplanted cells is usually between 5% and 10% of the theoretical liver mass, and some degree of correction has been observed in Crigler-Najjar syndrome type 1,[59] glycogen storage disease type Ia,[60] ornithine transcarbamylase (OTC) deficiency,[61] Refsum disease,[62] and factor VII deficiency,[63] thus suggesting that this percentage of hepatocyte correction by gene transfer is sufficient to obtain clinical benefit.

For inborn errors of liver metabolism producing excessive or abnormal metabolites, such as primary hyperoxaluria type 1, a large portion of the liver, although structurally normal, has to be replaced/corrected. Orthotopic liver transplantation is able to correct the metabolic defect (i.e., elevated oxalate synthesis and excretion) to prevent the pathological consequences of chronic oxalate deposition in tissues throughout the body. In a gene therapy context, it is expected that a large proportion of hepatocytes has to be transduced by gene therapy to minimize the deleterious effect of uncorrected hepatocytes which will continue to synthesize oxalate. Although hepatocytes suffer no damage from the enzymatic defect, primary hyperoxaluria type 1 appears to behave like cell-autonomous defects in which one corrected hepatocyte cannot compensate for overproduction of toxic metabolites in its neighbor cells.[64]

In disorders due to organ dysfunction secondary to cell autonomous disease processes, the metabolic defect results in toxicity within each affected cell, and for the gene therapy to be effective, the functional gene needs to be delivered to a large percentage of cells. For example, while a high level of correction is not needed to protect from the development of the pulmonary disease, high levels of hepatocyte transduction are needed to treat the cell-autonomous liver disease of α-1-antitrypsin deficiency. In this disorder, unlike the lung disease, the liver damage occurs through a gain-of-function mechanism caused by retention of hepatotoxic mutant α1-antitrypsin in the endoplasmic reticulum of liver cells. Several studies have focused on the delivery of the normal α-1-antitrypsin gene into hepatocytes or airway cells to restore normal α-1-antitrypsin production and to protect lung tissue.[65-68] However, while effective for the lung phenotype these approaches do not affect the liver disease. Gene therapy strategies for the liver disease must be designed to down-regulate expression of the endogenous α1-antitrypsin in a large percentage of hepatocytes[69,70] or promote clearance of toxic α1-antitrypsin polymers.[71]

The defect of fumarylacetoacetate hydrolase responsible for tyrosinemia type 1 also results in a cell autonomous disease, damaging hepatocytes and cells of renal proximal tubules.[72,73] Fumarylacetoacetate is strongly mutagenic and causes small insertions and deletions and large genomic rearrangements,[74] resulting in an increased risk of hepatocellular carcinoma. The achievement of 100% of hepatocyte correction would be required to reduce the risk of cancer. This scenario is likely similar in glycogen storage disease type 1, which is also associated with an increased risk of hepatic adenomas leading to life-threatening complications such as bleeding or malignant transformation.[75,76] The pathogenesis of adenomas is unclear, but the risk of developing adenomas does not appear to be related to dietary treatment, compliance to treatment, or metabolic control.[77] Although a level of expression as low as 8% to 10%[78,79] is sufficient for the control of hypoglycemia, levels of correction to reduce the risk of hepatocellular adenomas are likely higher.

Ex Vivo Approaches to Gene Therapy

Cell transplantation can be used in an autologous setting in which the patient's own cells are genetically manipulated ex vivo and then transplanted back in the patient. Ex vivo gene transfer was proven to be effective in a number of immunological disorders in which expression of the therapeutic gene provides a selective growth advantage over untransduced cells. For example, in the case of adenosine deaminase deficiency, corrected cells have a strong selective-amplification effect, allowing even a small amount of engrafted cells to completely restore the immune system.[3] Similar approaches would be desirable as an alternative to liver transplantation in inborn errors of metabolism because they would be less invasive and not require life-long immunosuppression. However, for liver-directed approaches, ex vivo gene therapy has been less encouraging mostly because of limited engrafment of genetically modified hepatocytes. In contrast to adenosine deaminase-SCID, hepatocytes corrected for an enzymatic defect usually lack of a selective advantage over defective cells. Liver repopulation by corrected hepatocytes only occurs if recipient hepatocytes are affected by a cytotoxic cell-autonomous disease process. Therefore, to achieve successful liver repopulation with corrected cells, transplanted cells must have a selective growth advantage over uncorrected cells or endogenous hepatocytes must be removed from the liver to *make space* for transplanted cells to proliferate and expand. In tyrosinemia type 1, hepatocytes corrected for fumarylacetoacetate hydrolase deficiency have a strong selective growth advantage and *space* is made by the genetic defect affecting hepatocyte viability.[80] Interestingly, it has been rarely observed that liver samples from patients with tyrosinemia type 1 contained fumarylacetoacetate hydrolase enzyme activity because of somatic reversion of the disease-causing inherited mutation followed by clonal selection of reverted hepatocytes. Besides providing the first example of spontaneous gene correction in the liver, this observation demonstrated the strong selective growth advantage of spontaneously reverted fumarylacetoacetate hydrolase-positive hepatocytes.[81] This observation illustrates the principle that in tyrosinemia type 1 genetically repaired hepatocytes have a selective growth advantage and proliferate to efficiently repopulate mutant livers thus, curing the underlying metabolic disease. Nevertheless, for the majority of inborn errors of liver metabolism repopulation by corrected hepatocytes cannot occur because of lack of a selective growth advantage of normal cells over the defective cells.

Ex vivo approaches for liver gene therapy are also complicated by the need of multiple surgeries for removal of the hepatic tissue to obtain hepatocytes and for reinfusion of genetically modified cells via portal vein infusion into the patient's liver (Figure 13.2). The limited viability of cultured primary hepatocytes, which undergo a few rounds of cell division but not enough to substantially expand the population, is another important issue.

Ex vivo gene therapy directed at hematopoietic stem cells has also found applications for treatment of multi-systemic diseases, including brain disorders, lysosomal storage and peroxisomal diseases. As in the case of liver transplantation, bone marrow transplantation has been important to predict the results of ex vivo gene therapy for these disorders. Following bone marrow transplantation, donor cells with normal function populate the bone marrow, and bone marrow-derived stem cells differentiating into monocytes can migrate into the brain and further differentiate into microglial cells.[82–85] Interestingly, it has also been shown that transduction of genetically modified bone marrow-derived cells overexpressing lysosomal enzymes can migrate into the central nervous system and mediate cross-correction of neighboring brain cells. This approach resulted in very encouraging outcomes in patients with metachromatic leukodytrophy.[86] Patients with X-linked adrenoleukodystrophy have also been treated by ex vivo gene therapy with lentiviral vector, which resulted in stable expression of the therapeutic gene and evidence of clinical benefits.[87] For X-linked adrenoleukodystrophy, the data generated so far show that gene therapy provides a benefit similar to allogenic hematopoietic stem cells transplantation, despite a relatively low level of gene correction. In addition, as in the case of SCID, ex vivo gene therapy overcomes the problems related to allogenic bone marrow transplantation, including the development of graft-versus-host disease, graft rejection, early death from infections, and regimen associated toxicity.

In Vivo Approaches to Gene Therapy

For in vivo approaches, the therapeutic gene is introduced directly into the host. Therefore, in vivo gene therapy circumvents the need for invasive procedures of cellular harvesting and reimplantation. In vivo gene therapy for inborn errors of metabolism has been mostly focused on the liver, muscle, and brain. The liver has been a major target because several inborn errors of metabolism are due to enzymes that are expressed primarily in the liver. Therefore, liver-directed gene transfer can result in correction of other affected districts as previously shown by organ transplantation studies. Organ transplantation is in fact not different from gene therapy, and every disease that is treated with such therapy is amenable to correction with gene therapy as well.[88] Some urea cycle disorders, for example, are almost completely corrected by liver transplantation.[88] For several other disorders, such as organic acidemias, glycogen storage disease type 1, and fatty acid oxidation defects, it is still unclear whether liver-directed gene therapy will correct all manifestations of the diseases.[89] In glycogen storage disease type 1, it is unknown whether correction of the liver will prevent development of slowly progressing renal disease.[90–92] Preclinical studies in the mouse model of very long-chain acyl-CoA dehydrogenase deficiency with liver-directed gene therapy resulted in correction of the acylcarnitine profile and prevention of stress-induced hypoglycemia. However, it is not clear whether transduction of cardiac and muscle is also required to prevent the other manifestations of the disease.[93] A better understanding of the pathophysiology of these disorders will help clarifying these issues.

Liver-directed gene therapy: The goal of liver-directed gene therapy is to deliver genes to the hepatocytes. Hepatocytes are accessible to intravenously injected vectors. However, vector-hepatocyte interactions are limited by two major obstacles: Kupffer cells and liver sinusoidal endothelial cells. Liver sinusoidal endothelial cells form a structural barrier between the hepatic blood and the extracellular fluid in the space of Disse, a vascular space that prevents the access of large molecules to the hepatocytes. The endothelial cells of the liver have fenestrations of about 100 nm in diameter that allow viral particles from the bloodstream to cross the endothelium and to reach the hepatocytes (Figure 13.4). Uptake of viral particles, such as adenoviral vectors, may be dependent on the size of these fenestrations.[94–96] Within the sinusoids, Kupffer cells, which are attached to endothelial and parenchymal cells, remove from the circulation foreign and damaged materials, including viral vector particles, and therefore they limit the efficiency of hepatocyte gene transfer (Figure 13.4).

The main problems of in vivo approaches are essentially related to the immune reactions that viral vectors elicit once they are infused in the blood. The outcomes of the clinical trials for OTC and hemophilia B have clearly shown these problems. Systemic injection of adenoviral vectors is associated to toxicity caused by the capsid proteins. This capsid-mediated toxic response is dose-dependent, occurs shortly after vector administration, and is characterized by high levels of serum proinflammatory cytokines and chemokines due to activation of an innate inflammatory immune response.[32,97] Furthermore, systemic administration of adenoviral vectors likely results in widespread transduction of a large number of extrahepatic cell types (e.g., blood cells, endothelium, spleen, lung, etc.), which contributes to inefficient hepatocyte transduction and likely to toxicity. The toxic reaction against the adenoviral vector has indeed been involved in the death of one patient included in the clinical trial aimed at correction of OTC deficiency using a second generation (E1- and E4-deleted) adenoviral vector. The trial, which enrolled 18 subjects, was interrupted when one of the two subjects injected at the highest dose suffered fatal complications. In all remaining subjects, the clinical outcome was characterized by mild and transient toxicity.[98,99]

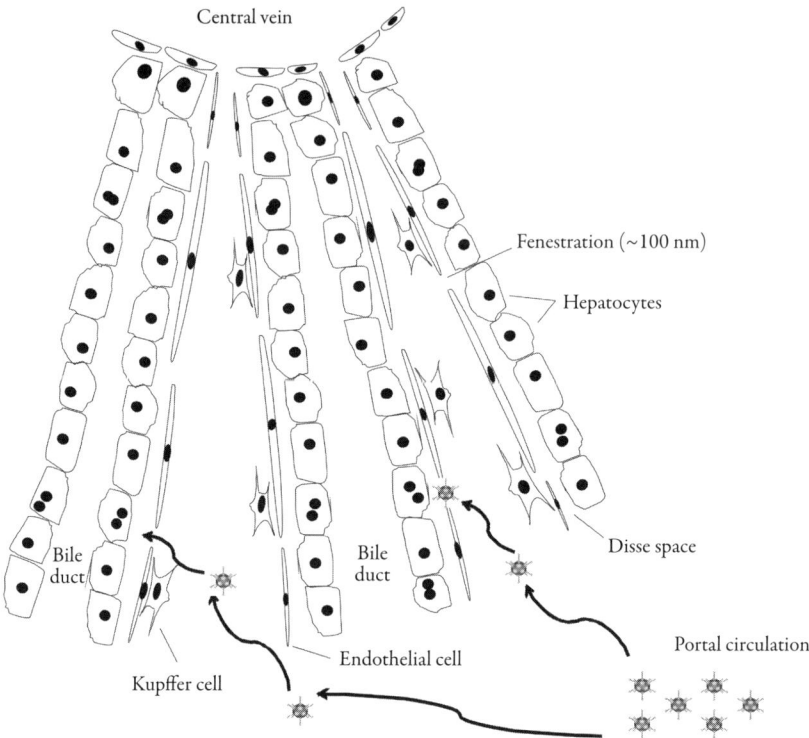

FIGURE 13.4 Liver microarchitecture and in vivo gene therapy. Kupffer cells and liver sinusoidal endothelial cells are two major cell types affecting both the efficiency and the toxicity of gene transfer vectors. Liver sinusoidal endothelial cells with their fenestrated structure form a structural barrier between the hepatic blood and the extracellular fluid in the space of Disse, a vascular space which prevent the access of large molecules to the hepatocytes. The liver fenestrations are approximately 100 nm in diameter and allow viral particles from the bloodstream to cross the endothelium and to reach the hepatocytes. Kupffer cells, avidly remove bloodborne viral vector particles.

The clinical course of the patient who died was completely different, as within 24 hours he developed liver injury, coagulopathy, and hyperammonemia followed by the development of respiratory distress syndrome and multiple organ failure leading to death. It is important to note that the same dose of vector, on a viral particles/kg basis, was well tolerated in another patient enrolled in the same trial.[98] The main difference between these two subjects was that the patient who survived was a female, had essentially normal ^{15}N incorporation into urea, and had no documented hyperammonemic episodes. In contrast, the patient who died was a male with symptomatic partial OTC deficiency with a 20-fold reduction in ^{15}N incorporation into urea. It is unclear whether the underlying more severe OTC deficiency in the patient who died may have contributed to the fatal outcome. Improvements in the safety of the vector (helper-dependent adenoviral vectors) and strategies to achieve high-efficiency hepatic transduction using low vector doses that are less toxic may allow further clinical application of these vectors for metabolic disorders.[35]

Although no severe adverse events were observed, the results of in vivo AAV-mediated liver-directed clinical gene therapy have been initially disappointing. Upon AAV2 systemic administration in hemophilia B patients, therapeutic F.IX levels were achieved only transiently, and their decrease was associated with a subclinical increase in serum transaminases (Figure 13.3).[45] This reaction was due to a cytoxic T lymphocyte response to the AAV capsid resulting in the elimination of the transduced hepatocytes, which prevented long-term F.IX expression, as previously discussed. Based on the discovery that other serotypes of AAV displayed higher liver tropism compared to AAV2, another clinical trial for liver-directed gene therapy was more recently started in hemophilia B patients using AAV8. In this trial, no immune reaction was observed at the lower doses, while two participants who received the higher dose of vector developed a transient, asymptomatic elevation of serum transaminase levels, which was associated with the detection of AAV8-capsid-specific T cells in the peripheral blood. Both of these subjects received a short course of glucocorticoid therapy, which rapidly normalized transaminase levels and maintained F.IX in the therapeutic range. In all patients, AAV8 administration resulted in therapeutic F.IX levels at 2% to 11% of normal levels; four of the six discontinued F.IX prophylaxis and remained free of spontaneous hemorrhage, and in the other two the interval between prophylactic clotting factor infusions was increased.[47]

Muscle-directed gene therapy: Although correction of the deficient enzymatic activity in the affected organ would be most straightforward, expression within an ectopic tissue (different from the natural production site) can either result in secretion of a deficient protein into the boodstream or in clearance of toxic metabolites from the circulation. For this strategy to be effective, the enzyme produced in the ectopic site must be functional. The muscle has been the preferred tissue for these goals because of its simple access through intramuscular injections and for safety. Muscle-directed gene therapy with AAV vectors has generated encouraging preclinical results in hemophilia B mice and dogs. These studies have led to a human clinical trial that has shown excellent safety data and evidence of gene transfer. However, no clinical benefit was observed.[100] In a trial investigating intramuscular administrations of serotype 1 AAV (AAV1) in patients with lipoprotein lipase deficiency,[101] loss of correction was associated with a transient increase in serum creatinine phosphokinase in the higher vector dose cohort as a consequence of a T-cell response against AAV capsid proteins, similar to what was observed in liver-directed hemophilia B gene therapy clinical trials.[47,102] Patients receiving higher doses were also treated with immunosuppressants from the time of vector administration and up to 12 weeks post-injection. Overall, vector administration was well tolerated and was associated with sustained transgene expression, transient reduction of fasting plasma tryglicerides, long-term changes in trygliceride-rich lipoprotein characteristics, and fewer pancreatitis attacks.[103,104] The encouraging results of this trial led to official approval by the European Medicine Agency of Glybera (alipogene tiparvovec) as the first gene-therapy medicine recommended for authorization in the European Union.[105,106]

Like F.IX, α-1-antitrypsin functions as a circulating plasma protein and the mechanism underlying the lung disease in α-1-antitrypsin deficiency is the lack of α-1-antitrypsin. The therapy for the lung phenotype is dependent on replacement of plasma levels regardless of the site of production of α-1-antitrypsin. Therefore, as in the case of hemophilia, gene augmentation for α-1-antitrypsin deficiency can be accomplished by delivery of the gene to a variety of different tissues as long as these are able to secrete α-1-antitrypsin.[107] The muscle-directed approach for α-1-antitrypsin deficiency has entered in clinical trials.[108] This clinical trial using AAV expressing α-1-antitrypsin delivered by intramuscular injections showed a favorable safety profile and sustained levels of α-1-antitrypsin for at least one year after vector administration. However, α-1-antitrypsin levels were below the therapeutic levels.[58,65,109]

Skeletal muscle expression of the normal enzyme involved in bile glucuronidation has also been found to be effective in decreasing the serum bilirubin levels in the animal model of Crigler-Najjar syndrome.[110,111] However, enzymes often require subunits or cofactor that may not be available in the ectopic tissue. For example, phenylalanine hydroxylase expression in skeletal muscle only if supplied with the necessary cofactors can effectively clear phenyl alanine from the circulation in phenylketonuria animal models. By expressing the complete phenylalanine hydroxylase system (phenylalanine hydroxylase and BH_4-biosynthetic enzymes guanosine triphosphate cyclohydrolase I and 6-pyruvoyltetrahydrobiopterin synthase) in skeletal muscle of phenylketonuria mice, long-term phenylalanine reduction can be achieved.[112]

The major limitation of muscle-directed gene therapy is the limited number of muscle fibers that are transduced following an intramusclar injection. Future directions for clinical muscle-directed gene therapy will require the distribution of the vector to a larger muscle mass through limb perfusion as well as some form of immune modulation to allow AAV-mediated long-term expression.

Lung-directed gene therapy: Gene delivery by airway administration has been investigated to convert the lung into a metabolic factory for production and systemic delivery of therapeutic proteins into the blood such as F.IX[113] and α-galactosidase.[114] However, cells of the airway epithelium have a considerable high turnover, and likely the expression of the transgene from a nonintegrative vector will be progressively lost, thus requiring readministration of the vector to have sustained transgene expression. Readministration of viral vectors is a challenge because of the humoral response provoked against the viral capsid following the first administration. Potential strategies to overcome this obstacle include serotype switching and immunosuppression at the time of the administration.

Brain-directed gene therapy: Several inborn errors of metabolism have major involvement of the central nervous system. Intravascular delivery of viral vectors is in general ineffective at treating the brain disease because the blood–brain barrier prevents access of most gene therapy vectors to the central nervous system. In contrast, serotype 9 AAV (AAV9) administered intravascularly at high doses results in efficient widespread brain gene transfer in both neonatal or adult mice, and thus it overcomes the obstacle of the blood–brain barrier.[115] This unique capacity of AAV9 vectors could pave the way to a multitude of therapeutic applications. In contrast, most viral vectors do not cross the blood–brain barrier, and have been investigated for direct intracranial injections. AAV and lentiviral vectors have been the most commonly used viral vectors for gene transfer to the brain.

Successful proof-of-concept studies of gene replacement via direct intracranial administration of viral vectors in animal models of inborn errors of metabolism include, among others: MPS I,[116,117] MPS IIIA,[118,119] MPS IIIB,[120–123] MPS VII,[124–126] Krabbe disease,[127,128] metachromatic leukodystrophy,[129-131] Niemann-Pick disease type A,[132-135] infantile and late-infantile forms of neuronal ceroid lipofuscinosis,[136-141] and Canavan disease.[142-144]

Human trials testing safety and efficacy of intracranial administrations of AAV have been performed in patients with Canavan disease, late-infantile neuronal ceroid lipofuscinosis and mucopolysaccharidosis type IIIA. Patients with Canavan disease have received intraparenchymal injections of AAV2 encoding the human aspartoacylase via six cranial burr holes.[145] The vector injections were well tolerated with no evidence of toxicity or immune response to the vector or transgene over a five-year follow-up period.[146,147] Patients treated with gene therapy showed reduction in cerebral N-acetyl-aspartate, slowed progression of brain atrophy, slight improvement in seizure frequency, and stabilization of overall clinical status.[146]

AAV2 expressing the human CLN2 was also administered to 12 sites in the brain of children with late-infantile neuronal ceroid lipofuscinosis. Compared with control subjects, the measured rates of decline of all brain MRI parameters were slower in vector-injected patients, albeit the numbers were not sufficient to reach statistical significance. Moreover, the clinical assessment of the neurologic status showed a significantly reduced rate of decline compared with control subjects.[148]

Patients with mucopolysaccharidosis IIIA received serotype rh.10 AAV vector by intracerebral injections and an immunosuppressive treatment to prevent theoretical risk of immunomediated elimination of transduced cells. Brain atrophy evaluated by magnetic resonance imaging appeared stable in two out of four treated subjects but worsened in the remaining two subjects. A possible although moderate improvement in behavior was noted in three subjects.[149]

Given the invasiveness of intracranial administration, alternative strategies aiming at correction of central nervous system disease are highly desirable. Interestingly, lysosomal enzymes can be delivered across the blood–brain barrier if administered at higher doses than those used in conventional therapy.[150] Such high levels of enzymes have also been achieved through liver-directed gene therapy in animal models of MPSVII[126] and MPSII.[151,152]

Conclusions

The concept of treating inborn errors of metabolism by gene therapy has long appealed to researchers because it promises to treat the primary cause of these disorders. In the past few years gene therapy has become widely accepted and has emerged as a novel form of medicine with potential impact on several human disorders. However, these studies have also revealed several problems, such as unexpected toxicity and insertional oncogenesis. Despite these problems, the abundant progress made on the preclinical front and the encouraging results of recent clinical trials for SCID, retinal diseases, hemophilia B, and leukodystrophies clearly support further development of gene therapies. The experience in clinical gene therapy gained so far clearly indicates that a careful risk/benefit assessment must be made for each condition, incorporating the underlying pathophysiology, long-term prognosis, and inherent and potential unforeseen risks of the different gene transfer approaches.

References

1. Terheggen HG, Lowenthal A, Lavinha F, Colombo JP, Rogers S. Unsuccessful trial of gene replacement in arginase deficiency. *Z Kinderheilkd*. 1975; 119: 1–3.
2. Miller AD, Eckner RJ, Jolly DJ, Friedmann T, Verma IM. Expression of a retrovirus encoding human HPRT in mice. *Science*. 1984; 225: 630–632.
3. Aiuti A, Cattaneo F, Galimberti S, et al. Gene therapy for immunodeficiency due to adenosine deaminase deficiency. *N Engl J Med*. 2009; 360: 447–458.
4. Hacein-Bey-Abina S, Hauer J, Lim A, et al. Efficacy of gene therapy for X-linked severe combined immunodeficiency. *N Engl J Med*. 2010; 363: 355–364.
5. Gaspar HB, Cooray S, Gilmour KC, et al. Hematopoietic stem cell gene therapy for adenosine deaminase-deficient severe combined immunodeficiency leads to long-term immunological recovery and metabolic correction. *Sci Transl Med*. 2011; 3:97ra80.
6. Bainbridge JW, Smith AJ, Barker SS, et al. Effect of gene therapy on visual function in Leber's congenital amaurosis. *N Engl J Med*. 2008; 358: 2231–2239.
7. Cideciyan AV, Aleman TS, Boye SL, et al. Human gene therapy for RPE65 isomerase deficiency activates the retinoid cycle of vision but with slow rod kinetics. *Proc Natl Acad Sci USA*. 2008; 105: 15112–15117.
8. Maguire AM, Simonelli F, Pierce EA, et al. Safety and efficacy of gene transfer for Leber's congenital amaurosis. *N Engl J Med*. 2008; 358: 2240–2248.
9. Rosenberg SA, Aebersold P, Cornetta K, et al. Gene transfer into humans-immunotherapy of patients with advanced melanoma, using tumor-infiltrating lymphocytes modified by retroviral gene transduction. *N Engl J Med*. 1990; 323:570–578.
10. Cattoglio C, Facchini G, Sartori D, et al. Hot spots of retroviral integration in human CD34+ hematopoietic cells. *Blood*. 2007; 110: 1770–1778.
11. Wu X, Li Y, Crise B, Burgess SM. Transcription start regions in the human genome are favored targets for MLV integration. *Science*. 2003; 300: 1749–1751.
12. Hacein-Bey-Abina S, Von Kalle C, Schmidt M, et al. LMO2-associated clonal T cell proliferation in two patients after gene therapy for SCID-X1. *Science*. 2003; 302: 415–419.
13. Grossman M, Raper SE, Kozarsky K, et al. Successful ex vivo gene therapy directed to liver in a patient with familial hypercholesterolaemia. *Nat Genet*. 1994; 6: 335–341.
14. Ferry N, Duplessis O, Houssin D, Danos O, Heard JM Retroviral-mediated gene transfer into hepatocytes in vivo. *Proc Natl Acad Sci USA*. 1991; 88: 8377–8381.
15. Kay MA, Rothenberg S, Landen CN, et al. In vivo gene therapy of hemophilia B: sustained partial correction in factor IX-deficient dogs. *Science*. 1993; 262: 117–119.
16. Ponder KP, Melniczek JR, Xu L, et al. Therapeutic neonatal hepatic gene therapy in mucopolysaccharidosis VII dogs. *Proc Natl Acad Sci USA*. 2002; 99: 13102–13107.
17. VandenDriessche T, Vanslembrouck V, Goovaerts I, et al. Long-term expression of human coagulation factor VIII and correction of hemophilia A after in vivo retroviral gene transfer in factor VIII-deficient mice. *Proc Natl Acad Sci USA*. 1999; 96: 10379–10384.
18. Xu L, Gao C, Sands MS, et al. Neonatal or hepatocyte growth factor-potentiated adult gene therapy with a retroviral vector results in therapeutic levels of canine factor IX for hemophilia B. *Blood*. 2003; 101: 3924–3932.
19. Xu L, Mango RL, Sands MS, Haskins ME, Ellinwood NM, Ponder KP. Evaluation of pathological manifestations of disease in mucopolysaccharidosis VII mice after neonatal hepatic gene therapy. *Mol Ther*. 2002; 6: 745–758.
20. Montini E, Cesana D, Schmidt M, et al. The genotoxic potential of retroviral vectors is strongly modulated by vector design and integration site selection in a mouse model of HSC gene therapy. *J Clin Invest*. 2009; 119: 964–975.
21. Mitchell RS, Beitzel BF, Schroder AR, et al. Retroviral DNA integration: ASLV, HIV, and MLV show distinct target site preferences. *PLoS Biol*. 2004; 2: E234.
22. Schroder AR, Shinn P, Chen H, Berry C, Ecker JR, Bushman F. HIV-1 integration in the human genome favors active genes and local hotspots. *Cell*. 2002; 110: 521–529.
23. Vu MQ, Steketee RW, Valleroy L, Weinstock H, Karon J, Janssen R. HIV incidence in the United States, 1978–1999. *J Acquir Immune Defic Syndr*. 2002; 31: 188–201.

24. Kim IH, Jozkowicz A, Piedra PA, Oka K, Chan L. Lifetime correction of genetic deficiency in mice with a single injection of helper-dependent adenoviral vector. *Proc Natl Acad Sci USA*. 2001; 98: 13282–13287.
25. Toietta G, Mane VP, Norona WS, et al. Lifelong elimination of hyperbilirubinemia in the Gunn rat with a single injection of helper-dependent adenoviral vector. *Proc Natl Acad Sci USA*. 2005; 102: 3930–3935.
26. Brunetti-Pierri N, Ng T, Iannitti DA, et al. Improved hepatic transduction, reduced systemic vector dissemination, and long-term transgene expression by delivering helper-dependent adenoviral vectors into the surgically isolated liver of nonhuman primates. *Hum Gene Ther*. 2006; 17: 391–404.
27. Brunetti-Pierri N, Nichols TC, McCorquodale S, et al. Sustained phenotypic correction of canine hemophilia B after systemic administration of helper-dependent adenoviral vector. *Hum Gene Ther*. 2005; 16: 811–820.
28. Brunetti-Pierri N, Stapleton GE, Law M, et al. Efficient, long-term hepatic gene transfer using clinically relevant HDAd doses by balloon occlusion catheter delivery in nonhuman primates. *Mol Ther*. 2009; 17: 327–333.
29. Brunetti-Pierri N, Stapleton GE, Palmer DJ, et al. Pseudo-hydrodynamic delivery of helper-dependent adenoviral vectors into non-human primates for liver-directed gene therapy. *Mol Ther*. 2007; 15: 732–740.
30. Morral N, O'Neal W, Rice K, et al. Administration of helper-dependent adenoviral vectors and sequential delivery of different vector serotype for long-term liver-directed gene transfer in baboons. *Proc Natl Acad Sci USA*. 1999; 96: 12816–12821.
31. Brunetti-Pierri N, Ng T, Iannitti D, et al. Transgene expression up to 7 years in nonhuman primates following hepatic transduction with helper-dependent adenoviral vectors. *Hum Gene Ther*. 2013; 24: 761–765.
32. Brunetti-Pierri N, Palmer DJ, Beaudet AL, Carey KD, Finegold M, Ng P. Acute toxicity after high-dose systemic injection of helper-dependent adenoviral vectors into nonhuman primates. *Hum Gene Ther*. 2004; 15: 35–46.
33. Morral N, O'Neal WK, Rice K, et al. Lethal toxicity, severe endothelial injury, and a threshold effect with high doses of an adenoviral vector in baboons. *Hum Gene Ther*. 2002; 13: 143–154.
34. Nunes FA, Furth EE, Wilson JM, Raper SE. Gene transfer into the liver of nonhuman primates with E1-deleted recombinant adenoviral vectors: safety of readministration. *Hum Gene Ther*. 1999; 10: 2515–2526.
35. Brunetti-Pierri N, Liou A, Patel P, et al. Balloon catheter delivery of helper-dependent adenoviral vector results in sustained, therapeutic hFIX expression in rhesus macaques. *Mol Ther*. 2012; 20: 1863–1870.
36. Croyle MA, Le HT, Linse KD, et al. PEGylated helper-dependent adenoviral vectors: highly efficient vectors with an enhanced safety profile. *Gene Ther*. 2005; 12: 579–587.
37. Mok H, Palmer DJ, Ng P, Barry MA. Evaluation of polyethylene glycol modification of first-generation and helper-dependent adenoviral vectors to reduce innate immune responses. *Mol Ther*. 2005; 11: 66–79.
38. Allocca M, Doria M, Petrillo M, et al. Serotype-dependent packaging of large genes in adeno-associated viral vectors results in effective gene delivery in mice. *J Clin Invest*. 2008; 118: 1955–1964.
39. Grieger JC, Samulski RJ. Packaging capacity of adeno-associated virus serotypes: impact of larger genomes on infectivity and postentry steps. *J Virol*. 2005; 79: 9933–9944.
40. Lu H, Chen L, Wang J, et al. Complete correction of hemophilia A with adeno-associated viral vectors containing a full-size expression cassette. *Hum Gene Ther*. 2008; 19: 648–654.
41. Yan Z, Zhang Y, Duan D, Engelhardt JF. Trans-splicing vectors expand the utility of adeno-associated virus for gene therapy. *Proc Natl Acad Sci USA*. 2000; 97: 6716–6721.
42. Ghosh A, Yue Y, Lai Y, Duan D. A hybrid vector system expands adeno-associated viral vector packaging capacity in a transgene-independent manner. *Mol Ther*. 2008; 16: 124–130.
43. Gao G, Alvira MR, Somanathan S. Adeno-associated viruses undergo substantial evolution in primates during natural infections. *Proc Natl Acad Sci USA*. 2003; 100: 6081–6086.
44. Davidoff AM, Gray JT, Ng CY, et al. Comparison of the ability of adeno-associated viral vectors pseudo-typed with serotype 2, 5, and 8 capsid proteins to mediate efficient transduction of the liver in murine and nonhuman primate models. *Mol Ther*. 2005; 11: 875–888.
45. Manno CS, Pierce GF, Arruda VR, et al. Successful transduction of liver in hemophilia by AAV-Factor IX and limitations imposed by the host immune response. *Nat Med*. 2006; 12: 342–347.
46. Mingozzi F, Maus MV, Hui DJ, et al. CD8(+) T-cell responses to adeno-associated virus capsid in humans. *Nat Med*. 2007; 13: 419–422.
47. Nathwani AC, Tuddenham EG, Rangarajan S, et al. Adenovirus-associated virus vector-mediated gene transfer in hemophilia B. *N Engl J Med*. 2011; 365: 2357–2365.

48. Niidome T, Huang L. Gene therapy progress and prospects: nonviral vectors. *Gene Ther.* 2002; 9: 1647–1652.
49. Miao CH, Thompson AR, Loeb K, Ye X. Long-term and therapeutic-level hepatic gene expression of human factor IX after naked plasmid transfer in vivo. *Mol Ther.* 2001; 3: 947–957.
50. Hickman MA, Malone RW, Lehmann-Bruinsma K, et al. Gene expression following direct injection of DNA into liver. *Hum Gene Ther.* 1994; 5: 1477–1483.
51. Wolff JA, Malone RW, Williams P, et al. Direct gene transfer into mouse muscle in vivo. *Science.* 1990; 247: 1465–1468.
52. Choate KA, Khavari PA. Direct cutaneous gene delivery in a human genetic skin disease. *Hum Gene Ther.* 1997; 8: 1659–1665.
53. Meyer KB, Thompson MM, Levy MY, Barron LG, Szoka FC Jr. Intratracheal gene delivery to the mouse airway: characterization of plasmid DNA expression and pharmacokinetics. *Gene Ther.* 1995; 2: 450–460.
54. Alino SF, Herrero MJ, Noguera I, Dasi F, Sanchez M. Pig liver gene therapy by noninvasive interventionist catheterism. *Gene Ther.* 2007; 14: 334–343.
55. Eastman SJ, Baskin KM, Hodges BL, et al. Development of catheter-based procedures for transducing the isolated rabbit liver with plasmid DNA. *Hum Gene Ther.* 2002; 13: 2065–2077.
56. Zabner J, Wadsworth SC, Smith AE, Welsh MJ. Adenovirus-mediated generation of cAMP-stimulated Cl- transport in cystic fibrosis airway epithelia in vitro: effect of promoter and administration method. *Gene Ther.* 1996; 3: 458–465.
57. Pollak ES, High KA. *Hemophilia B: factor IX deficiency*, New York: McGraw-Hill; 2001.
58. American Thoracic Society/European Respiratory Society. Statement: standards for the diagnosis and management of individuals with α-1 antitrypsin deficiency. *Am J Respir Crit Care Med.* 2003; 168: 818–900.
59. Fox IJ, Chowdhury JR, Kaufman SS, et al. Treatment of the Crigler-Najjar syndrome type I with hepatocyte transplantation. *N Engl J Med.* 1998; 338: 1422–1426.
60. Muraca M, Gerunda G, Neri D, et al. Hepatocyte transplantation as a treatment for glycogen storage disease type 1a. *Lancet.* 2002; 359: 317–318.
61. Horslen SP, McCowan TC, Goertzen TC, et al. Isolated hepatocyte transplantation in an infant with a severe urea cycle disorder. *Pediatrics.* 2003; 111: 1262–1267.
62. Sokal EM, Smets F, Bourgois A, et al. Hepatocyte transplantation in a 4-year-old girl with peroxisomal biogenesis disease: technique, safety, and metabolic follow-up. *Transplantation.* 2003; 76: 735–738.
63. Dhawan A, Mitry RR, Hughes RD, et al. Hepatocyte transplantation for inherited factor VII deficiency *Transplantation.* 2004; 78: 1812–1814.
64. Danpure CJ. Molecular etiology of primary hyperoxaluria type 1: new directions for treatment. *Am J Nephrol.* 2005; 25: 303–310.
65. Flotte TR, Trapnell BC, Humphries M, et al. Phase 2 clinical trial of a recombinant adeno-associated viral vector expressing alpha1-antitrypsin: interim results. *Hum Gene Ther.* 2011; 22: 1239–1247.
66. Jaffe HA, Danel C, Longenecker G, et al. Adenovirus-mediated in vivo gene transfer and expression in normal rat liver. *Nat Genet.* 1992; 1: 372–378.
67. Kay MA, Baley P, Rothenberg S, et al. Expression of human alpha 1-antitrypsin in dogs after autologous transplantation of retroviral transduced hepatocytes. *Proc Natl Acad Sci USA.* 1992; 89: 89–93.
68. Song S, Morgan M, Ellis T, et al. Sustained secretion of human alpha-1-antitrypsin from murine muscle transduced with adeno-associated virus vectors. *Proc Natl Acad Sci USA.* 1998; 95: 14384–14388.
69. Duan YY, Wu J, Zhu JL, et al. Gene therapy for human alpha1-antitrypsin deficiency in an animal model using SV40-derived vectors. *Gastroenterology.* 2004; 127: 1222–1232.
70. Mueller C, Tang Q, Gruntman A, et al. Sustained miRNA-mediated knockdown of mutant AAT with simultaneous augmentation of wild-type AAT has minimal effect on global liver miRNA profiles. *Mol Ther.* 2012; 20: 590–600.
71. Pastore N, Blomenkamp K, Annunziata F, et al. Gene transfer of master autophagy regulator TFEB results in clearance of toxic protein and correction of hepatic disease in alpha-1-anti-trypsin deficiency. *EMBO Mol Med.* 2013; 5: 397–412.
72. Kubo S, Sun M, Miyahara M, et al. Hepatocyte injury in tyrosinemia type 1 is induced by fumarylacetoacetate and is inhibited by caspase inhibitors. *Proc Natl Acad Sci USA.* 1998; 95: 9552–9557.
73. Sun MS, Hattori S, Kubo S, Awata H, Matsuda I, Endo F. A mouse model of renal tubular injury of tyrosinemia type 1: development of de Toni Fanconi syndrome and apoptosis of renal tubular cells in Fah/Hpd double mutant mice. *J Am Soc Nephrol.* 2000; 11: 291–300.

74. Manning K, Al-Dhalimy M, Finegold M, Grompe M. In vivo suppressor mutations correct a murine model of hereditary tyrosinemia type I. *Proc Natl Acad Sci USA*. 1999; 96: 11928–11933.
75. Lee PJ. Glycogen storage disease type I: pathophysiology of liver adenomas. *Eur J Pediatr*. 2002; 161(Suppl. 1): S46–S49.
76. Rake JP, Visser G, Labrune P, Leonard JV, Ullrich K, Smit GP. Glycogen storage disease type I: diagnosis, management, clinical course and outcome: results of the European Study on Glycogen Storage Disease Type I (ESGSD I). *Eur J Pediatr*. 2002; 161(Suppl. 1): S20–S34.
77. Di Rocco M, Calevo MG, Taro M, Melis D, Allegri AE, Parenti G. Hepatocellular adenoma and metabolic balance in patients with type Ia glycogen storage disease. *Mol Genet Metab*. 2008; 93: 398–402.
78. Beaty RM, Jackson M, Peterson D, et al. Delivery of glucose-6-phosphatase in a canine model for glycogen storage disease, type Ia, with adeno-associated virus (AAV) vectors. *Gene Ther*. 2002; 9: 1015–1022.
79. Keller KM, Schutz M, Podskarbi T, Bindl L, Lentze MJ, Shin YS. A new mutation of the glucose-6-phosphatase gene in a 4-year-old girl with oligosymptomatic glycogen storage disease type 1a. *J Pediatr*. 1998; 132: 360–361.
80. Ruppert S, Kelsey G, Schedl A, Schmid E, Thies E, Schutz G. Deficiency of an enzyme of tyrosine metabolism underlies altered gene expression in newborn liver of lethal albino mice. *Genes Dev*. 1992; 6: 1430–1443.
81. Kvittingen EA, Rootwelt H, Berger R, Brandtzaeg P. Self-induced correction of the genetic defect in tyrosinemia type I. *J Clin Invest*. 1994; 94: 1657–1661.
82. Asheuer M, Pflumio F, Benhamida S, et al. Human CD34+ cells differentiate into microglia and express recombinant therapeutic protein. *Proc Natl Acad Sci USA*. 2004; 101: 3557–3562.
83. Aubourg P, Blanche S, Jambaque I, et al. Reversal of early neurologic and neuroradiologic manifestations of X-linked adrenoleukodystrophy by bone marrow transplantation. *N Engl J Med*. 1990; 322: 1860–1866.
84. Walkley SU, Thrall MA, Dobrenis K, et al. Bone marrow transplantation corrects the enzyme defect in neurons of the central nervous system in a lysosomal storage disease. *Proc Natl Acad Sci USA*. 1994; 91: 2970–2974.
85. Biffi A, Capotondo A, Fasano S, et al. Gene therapy of metachromatic leukodystrophy reverses neurological damage and deficits in mice. *J Clin Invest*. 2006; 116: 3070–3082.
86. Biffi A, Montini E, Lorioli L, et al. Lentiviral hematopoietic stem cell gene therapy benefits metachromatic leukodystrophy. *Science*. 2013; 341: 1233158.
87. Cartier N, Hacein-Bey-Abina S, Bartholomae CC, et al. Hematopoietic stem cell gene therapy with a lentiviral vector in X-linked adrenoleukodystrophy. *Science*. 2009; 326: 818–823.
88. Meyburg J, Hoffmann GF. Liver transplantation for inborn errors of metabolism. *Transplantation*. 2005; 80: S135–S137.
89. Leonard JV, Walter JH, McKiernan PJ. The management of organic acidaemias: the role of transplantation. *J Inherit Metab Dis*. 2001; 24: 309–311.
90. Ghosh A, Allamarvdasht M, Pan CJ, et al. Long-term correction of murine glycogen storage disease type Ia by recombinant adeno-associated virus-1-mediated gene transfer. *Gene Ther*. 2006; 13: 321–329.
91. Labrune P. Glycogen storage disease type I: indications for liver and/or kidney transplantation. *Eur J Pediatr*. 2002; 161(Suppl. 1): S53–S55.
92. Matern D, Starzl TE, Arnaout W, et al. Liver transplantation for glycogen storage disease types I, III, and IV. *Eur J Pediatr*. 1999; 158(Suppl. 2): S43–S48.
93. Merritt JL II, Nguyen T, Daniels J, Matern D, Schowalter DB. Biochemical correction of very long-chain acyl-CoA dehydrogenase deficiency following adeno-associated virus gene therapy. *Mol Ther*. 2009; 17: 425–429.
94. Brunetti-Pierri N, Palmer DJ, Mane V, Finegold M, Beaudet AL, Ng P. Increased hepatic transduction with reduced systemic dissemination and proinflammatory cytokines following hydrodynamic injection of helper-dependent adenoviral vectors. *Mol Ther*. 2005; 12: 99–106.
95. Lievens J, Snoeys J, Vekemans K, et al. The size of sinusoidal fenestrae is a critical determinant of hepatocyte transduction after adenoviral gene transfer. *Gene Ther*. 2004; 11: 1523–1531.
96. Snoeys J, Lievens J, Wisse E, et al. Species differences in transgene DNA uptake in hepatocytes after adenoviral transfer correlate with the size of endothelial fenestrae. *Gene Ther*. 2007; 14: 604–612.
97. Muruve DA, Barnes MJ, Stillman IE, Libermann TA. Adenoviral gene therapy leads to rapid induction of multiple chemokines and acute neutrophil-dependent hepatic injury in vivo. *Hum Gene Ther*. 1999; 10: 965–976.

98. Raper SE, Yudkoff M, Chirmule N, et al. A pilot study of in vivo liver-directed gene transfer with an adenoviral vector in partial ornithine transcarbamylase deficiency. *Hum Gene Ther*. 2002; 13: 163–175.
99. Raper SE, Chirmule N, Lee FS, et al. Fatal systemic inflammatory response syndrome in an ornithine transcarbamylase deficient patient following adenoviral gene transfer. *Mol Genet Metab*. 2003; 80: 148–158.
100. Kay MA, Manno CS, Ragni MV, et al. Evidence for gene transfer and expression of factor IX in haemophilia B patients treated with an AAV vector. *Nat Genet*. 2000; 24: 257–261.
101. Stroes ES, Nierman MC, Meulenberg JJ, et al. Intramuscular administration of AAV1-lipoprotein lipase S447X lowers triglycerides in lipoprotein lipase-deficient patients. *Arterioscler Thromb Vasc Biol*. 2008; 28: 2303–2304.
102. Mingozzi F, Meulenberg JJ, Hui DJ, et al. AAV-1-mediated gene transfer to skeletal muscle in humans results in dose-dependent activation of capsid-specific T cells. *Blood*. 2009; 114: 2077–2086.
103. Carpentier AC, Frisch F, Labbe SM, Gagnon R, de Wal J, Greentree S, Petry H, Twisk J, Brisson D, Gaudet D 2012; Effect of alipogene tiparvovec (AAV1-LPL(S447X)) on postprandial chylomicron metabolism in lipoprotein lipase-deficient patients. *J Clin Endocrinol Metab*. 2012; 97: 1635–1644.
104. Gaudet D, Methot J, Dery S, et al. Efficacy and long-term safety of alipogene tiparvovec (AAV1-LPL(S447X)) gene therapy for lipoprotein lipase deficiency: an open-label trial. *Gene Ther*. 2012; 20: 361–369.
105. European Medicines Agency. European Medicines Agency recommends first gene therapy for approval. Press release; 2012 (July 20).
106. Yla-Herttuala S. Endgame: glybera finally recommended for approval as the first gene therapy drug in the European union. *Mol Ther*. 2012; 20: 1831–1832.
107. Mueller C, Flotte TR Clinical gene therapy using recombinant adeno-associated virus vectors. *Gene Ther*. 2008; 15: 858–863.
108. Flotte TR, Brantly ML, Spencer LT, et al. Phase I trial of intramuscular injection of a recombinant adeno-associated virus alpha 1-antitrypsin (rAAV2-CB-hAAT) gene vector to AAT-deficient adults. *Hum Gene Ther*. 2004; 15: 93–128.
109. Brantly ML, Spencer LT, Humphries M, et al. Phase I trial of intramuscular injection of a recombinant adeno-associated virus serotype 2 alphal-antitrypsin (AAT) vector in AAT-deficient adults. *Hum Gene Ther*. 2006; 17: 1177–1186.
110. Jia Z, Danko I. Long-term correction of hyperbilirubinemia in the Gunn rat by repeated intravenous delivery of naked plasmid DNA into muscle. *Mol Ther*. 2005; 12: 860–866.
111. Pastore N, Nusco E, Vanikova J, et al. Sustained reduction of hyperbilirubinemia in Gunn rats after adeno-associated virus-mediated gene transfer of bilirubin UDP-glucuronosyltransferase isozyme 1A1 to skeletal muscle. *Hum Gene Ther*. 2012; 23: 1082–1089.
112. Ding Z, Harding CO, Rebuffat A, Elzaouk L, Wolff JA, Thony B. Correction of murine PKU following AAV-mediated intramuscular expression of a complete phenylalanine hydroxylating system. *Mol Ther*. 2008; 16: 673–681.
113. Auricchio A, O'Connor E, Weiner D, et al. Noninvasive gene transfer to the lung for systemic delivery of therapeutic proteins. *J Clin Invest*. 2002; 110: 499–504.
114. Li C, Ziegler RJ, Cherry M, et al. Adenovirus-transduced lung as a portal for delivering alpha-galactosidase A into systemic circulation for Fabry disease. *Mol Ther*. 2002; 5: 745–754.
115. Foust KD, Nurre E, Montgomery CL, Hernandez A, Chan CM, Kaspar BK. Intravascular AAV9 preferentially targets neonatal neurons and adult astrocytes. *Nat Biotechnol*. 2009; 27: 59–65.
116. Ciron C, Desmaris N, Colle MA, et al. Gene therapy of the brain in the dog model of Hurler's syndrome. *Ann Neurol*. 2006; 60: 204–213.
117. Watson G, Bastacky J, Belichenko P, et al. Intrathecal administration of AAV vectors for the treatment of lysosomal storage in the brains of MPS I mice. *Gene Ther*. 2006; 13: 917–925.
118. Fraldi A, Hemsley K, Crawley A, et al. Functional correction of CNS lesions in an MPS-IIIA mouse model by intracerebral AAV-mediated delivery of sulfamidase and SUMF1 genes. *Hum Mol Genet*. 2007; 16: 2693–2702.
119. McIntyre C, Derrick Roberts AL, Ranieri E, Clements PR, Byers S, Anson DS. Lentiviral-mediated gene therapy for murine mucopolysaccharidosis type IIIA. *Mol Genet Metab*. 2008; 93: 411–418.
120. Cressant A, Desmaris N, Verot L, et al. Improved behavior and neuropathology in the mouse model of Sanfilippo type IIIB disease after adeno-associated virus-mediated gene transfer in the striatum. *J Neurosci*. 2004; 24: 10229–10239.

121. Di Domenico C, Villani GR, Di Napoli D, et al. Intracranial gene delivery of LV-NAGLU vector corrects neuropathology in murine MPS IIIB. *Am J Med Genet A*. 2009; 149A: 1209–1218.
122. Fu H, Kang L, Jennings JS, et al. Significantly increased lifespan and improved behavioral performances by rAAV gene delivery in adult mucopolysaccharidosis IIIB mice. *Gene Ther*. 2007; 14: 1065–1077.
123. McCarty DM, Dirosario J, Gulaid K, Muenzer J, Fu H. Mannitol-facilitated CNS entry of rAAV2 vector significantly delayed the neurological disease progression in MPS IIIB mice. *Gene Ther*. 2009; 16: 1340–1352.
124. Liu G, Chen YH, He X, et al. Adeno-associated virus type 5 reduces learning deficits and restores glutamate receptor subunit levels in MPS VII mice CNS. *Mol Ther*. 2007; 15: 242–247.
125. Liu G, Martins I, Wemmie JA, Chiorini JA, Davidson BL. Functional correction of CNS phenotypes in a lysosomal storage disease model using adeno-associated virus type 4 vectors. *J Neurosci*. 2005; 25: 9321–9327.
126. Sferra TJ, Backstrom K, Wang C, Rennard R, Miller M, Hu Y. Widespread correction of lysosomal storage following intrahepatic injection of a recombinant adeno-associated virus in the adult MPS VII mouse. *Mol Ther*. 2004; 10: 478–491.
127. Rafi MA, Zhi Rao H, Passini MA, et al. AAV-mediated expression of galactocerebrosidase in brain results in attenuated symptoms and extended life span in murine models of globoid cell leukodystrophy. *Mol Ther*. 2005; 11: 734–744.
128. Shen JS, Watabe K, Ohashi T, Eto Y. Intraventricular administration of recombinant adenovirus to neonatal twitcher mouse leads to clinicopathological improvements. *Gene Ther*. 2001; 8: 1081–1087.
129. Consiglio A, Quattrini A, Martino S, et al. In vivo gene therapy of metachromatic leukodystrophy by lentiviral vectors: correction of neuropathology and protection against learning impairments in affected mice. *Nat Med*. 2001; 7: 310–316.
130. Iwamoto N, Watanabe A, Yamamoto M, et al. Global diffuse distribution in the brain and efficient gene delivery to the dorsal root ganglia by intrathecal injection of adeno-associated viral vector serotype 1. *J Gene Med*. 2009; 11: 498–505.
131. Sevin C, Benraiss A, Van Dam D, et al. Intracerebral adeno-associated virus-mediated gene transfer in rapidly progressive forms of metachromatic leukodystrophy. *Hum Mol Genet*. 2006; 15: 53–64.
132. Dodge JC, Clarke J, Song A, et al. Gene transfer of human acid sphingomyelinase corrects neuropathology and motor deficits in a mouse model of Niemann-Pick type A disease. *Proc Natl Acad Sci USA*. 2005; 102: 17822–17827.
133. Dodge JC, Clarke J, Treleaven CM, et al. Intracerebroventricular infusion of acid sphingomyelinase corrects CNS manifestations in a mouse model of Niemann-Pick A disease. *Exp Neurol*. 2009; 215: 349–357.
134. Passini MA, Bu J, Fidler JA, et al. Combination brain and systemic injections of AAV provide maximal functional and survival benefits in the Niemann-Pick mouse. *Proc Natl Acad Sci USA*. 2007; 104: 9505–9510.
135. Passini MA, Macauley SL, Huff MR, et al. AAV vector-mediated correction of brain pathology in a mouse model of Niemann-Pick A disease. *Mol Ther*. 2005; 11: 754–762.
136. Cabrera-Salazar MA, Roskelley EM, Bu J, et al. Timing of therapeutic intervention determines functional and survival outcomes in a mouse model of late infantile Batten disease. *Mol Ther*. 2007; 15: 1782–1788.
137. Griffey M, Bible E, Vogler C, Levy B, Gupta P, Cooper J, Sands MS. Adeno-associated virus 2-mediated gene therapy decreases autofluorescent storage material and increases brain mass in a murine model of infantile neuronal ceroid lipofuscinosis. *Neurobiol Dis*. 2004; 16: 360–369.
138. Griffey MA, Wozniak D, Wong M, et al. CNS-directed AAV2-mediated gene therapy ameliorates functional deficits in a murine model of infantile neuronal ceroid lipofuscinosis. *Mol Ther*. 2006; 13: 538–547.
139. Haskell RE, Hughes SM, Chiorini JA, Alisky JM, Davidson BL. Viral-mediated delivery of the late-infantile neuronal ceroid lipofuscinosis gene, TPP-I to the mouse central nervous system. *Gene Ther*. 2003; 10: 34–42.
140. Passini MA, Dodge JC, Bu J, et al. Intracranial delivery of CLN2 reduces brain pathology in a mouse model of classical late infantile neuronal ceroid lipofuscinosis. *J Neurosci*. 2006; 26: 1334–1342.
141. Sondhi D, Peterson DA, Giannaris EL, et al. AAV2-mediated CLN2 gene transfer to rodent and non-human primate brain results in long-term TPP-I expression compatible with therapy for LINCL. *Gene Ther*. 2005; 12: 1618–1632.

142. Leone P, Janson CG, Bilaniuk L, et al. Aspartoacylase gene transfer to the mammalian central nervous system with therapeutic implications for Canavan disease. *Ann Neurol*. 2000; 48: 27–38.
143. Matalon R, Surendran S, Rady PL, et al. Adeno-associated virus-mediated aspartoacylase gene transfer to the brain of knockout mouse for Canavan disease. *Mol Ther*. 2003; 7: 580–587.
144. McPhee SW, Francis J, Janson CG, et al. Effects of AAV-2-mediated aspartoacylase gene transfer in the tremor rat model of Canavan disease. *Brain Res Mol Brain Res*. 2005; 135: 112–121.
145. Janson C, McPhee S, Bilaniuk L, et al. Clinical protocol. Gene therapy of Canavan disease: AAV-2 vector for neurosurgical delivery of aspartoacylase gene (ASPA; to the human brain. *Hum Gene Ther*. 2002; 13: 1391–1412.
146. Leone P, Shera D, McPhee SW, et al. Long-term follow-up after gene therapy for Canavan disease. *Sci Transl Med*. 2012; 4: 165ra163.
147. McPhee SW, Janson CG, Li CA, et al. Immune responses to AAV in a phase I study for Canavan disease. *J Gene Med*. 2006; 8: 577–588.
148. Worgall S, Sondhi D, Hackett NR, et al. Treatment of late infantile neuronal ceroid lipofuscinosis by CNS administration of a serotype 2 adeno-associated virus expressing CLN2 cDNA. *Hum Gene Ther*. 2008; 19: 463–474.
149. Tardieu M, Zérah M, Husson B, et al. Intracerebral Administration of Adeno-Associated Viral Vector Serotype rh.10 Carrying Human SGSH and SUMF1 cDNAs in Children with Mucopolysaccharidosis Type IIIA Disease: Results of a Phase I/II Trial. *Hum Gene Ther*. 2014; 25: 506–516.
150. Vogler C, Levy B, Grubb JH, et al. Overcoming the blood-brain barrier with high-dose enzyme replacement therapy in murine mucopolysaccharidosis VII. *Proc Natl Acad Sci USA*. 2005; 102: 14777–14782.
151. Cardone M, Polito VA, Pepe S, et al. Correction of Hunter syndrome in the MPSII mouse model by AAV2/8-mediated gene delivery. *Hum Mol Genet*. 2006; 15: 1225–1236.
152. Polito VA, Cosma MP. IDS crossing of the blood-brain barrier corrects CNS defects in MPSII mice. *Am J Hum Genet*. 2009; 85: 296–301.

14

Enzyme Replacement and Other Therapies for the Lysosomal Storage Disorders

GREGORY M. PASTORES AND CHRISTINE M. ENG

Introduction

Enzyme replacement therapy (ERT) as an option for the treatment of inborn errors of metabolism due to single enzyme defects was first proposed and studied in the 1970s using enzyme purified from human blood or tissue products. Using the lysosomal storage disorders (LSDs) Gaucher disease (GD) and Fabry disease (FD) as models for these early proof-of-concept experiments, the infusion of small quantities of purified enzyme was shown to transiently decrease substrate levels in blood and urine.[1,2] These early studies utilized human enzyme isolated from sources such as human placental tissue and involved limited numbers of doses in individual patients due to the difficulty of isolating sufficient quantities of enzyme. Subsequently, a collaborative effort between academia and industry was established to isolate sufficient quantities of enzyme to allow the development and evaluation of ERT in clinical trials involving patients with non-neuropathic GD (type 1). The first product to gain US Food and Drug Administration (FDA) approval was a human placenta-derived preparation called alglucerase (Ceredase; Genzyme Corporation, Cambridge, MA.) indicated for the treatment of GD type 1. Clinical response to this agent was rapid and measurable, and patients on alglucerase showed a decrease in hepatosplenomegaly and normalized hematologic profiles.[3] FDA approval was granted in 1991 on the basis of a single center, open label study that demonstrated an increase in platelet count as a primary outcome measure.[4] In 1994, a recombinant product, imiglucerase, produced by transfection of the human acid beta glucosidase gene in Chinese hamster ovary cells was developed and evaluated in clinical trials (imiglucerase, Cerezyme; Genzyme Corporation, Cambridge, MA).[5] The approval of imiglucerase was followed by major investments in research and development for the treatment of other LSDs. This interest from industry was stimulated by the financial success of the treatments for GD as well as orphan drug legislation adopted by the United States and the European Union offering exclusivity and protection from competition for several years as an incentive to develop treatments for rare diseases. Subsequently, several recombinant enzymes were developed for other LSDs and studied in clinical trials. These agents have gained US and worldwide marketing approval, enabling ERT for Mucopolysaccharidosis type I (MPS-I; 2003), FD (2003), MPS-VI, MPS-II, and Pompe disease. As a further testament to the activity in this area, two additional recombinant enzyme replacement products for GD have been developed by other biotechnology companies and are or will be alternatives to imiglucerase. The two new acid beta glucosidase (*GBA1*) formulations include (i) velaglucerase alfa (Shire HGT, Lexington, MA), which is produced by gene activation of human fibrosarcoma cell line,[6] and (ii) taliglucerase alfa, generated from carrot cell lines that have been transduced with the human *GBA1*.[7]

With approximately one to two decades of clinical experience with these various ERTs, a picture is emerging for the spectrum of clinical response and predictors of individual patient response or nonresponse. For each disease we have learned that different organs and tissues respond differently, when patients should be offered treatment, and that, for some diseases, monitoring the efficacy of treatment can be challenging. While the ERTs have been shown to have beneficial effects in multiple organ systems for each of the relevant disorders, the long-term outcome as measured by improved life expectancy and quality of life still awaits analysis of the next generation of patients who are diagnosed early in their disease course and have the benefit of early intervention with ERT. The increased awareness and attention that these disorders have received as a result of treatments becoming available has also led to improvements in concomitant therapies for specific organ dysfunction. For example, as a result of analysis of phase 4 FD clinical trial data for agalsidase beta, a relationship was demonstrated between baseline proteinuria and outcome on ERT. As a consequence, the use of angiotensin converting enzyme (ACE) inhibitors or sartans has been recommended as an adjunct therapy.

In this review, we focus on lessons learned through clinical trials and clinical (post-marketing) experience with ERT for GD, FD, and MPS-VI (as a model for the MPS disorders). GD provides the opportunity to evaluate the effects of ERT over the longest period of time since the availability of therapy. In addition, the disease characteristics of GD provide relatively straightforward parameters for the evaluation of treatment efficacy. The broadest experience with individualizing treatment to address different populations of patients exists for GD and has served as a model for the other disorders. Discussion of the experience with ERT for FD provides a contrasting picture of a disease that is slowly progressive and provides a challenge to measure incremental improvements in outcome. Finally, discussion of the experience of treatment for the mucopolysaccharidoses is demonstrated by MPS-VI, which shares many of the somatic features of the other MPS disorders but generally does not have cognitive involvement. We also review the risks and potential limitations of ERT, particularly adverse events and immunogenicity and other factors that may limit efficacy of ERT. Finally, new therapeutic approaches for the lysosomal disorders are discussed.

Gaucher Disease

GD, an autosomal recessively inherited disorder of glycosphingolipid metabolism, results from dysfunction of the lysosomal membrane-associated glycoprotein acid beta-glucosidase. As a consequence, there is intracellular accumulation of glucosylceramide and other glycolipids in cells of monocyte lineage. Although the gene defect and relevant biochemical pathways have been defined, the mechanisms by which substrate accumulation causes disease manifestations are not completely understood. The direct effects of a build-up of substrate laden cells may account for some aspects of disease, but the overall pathology is likely to be more complex with deleterious effects on a variety of intra- and extra-cellular functions. ERT has been available since 1991; although proof of concept was initially shown using a placental-derived extract, there are several recombinant enzymes currently available (e.g., imiglucerase, velaglucerase and taliglucerase).[4,5,8] Essentially, the provision of exogenous enzyme compensates for the patient's intrinsic deficiency. In this case, a key to delivering the recombinant enzyme to various sites of pathology was recognition of the need to modify the native enzyme, to expose the mannose residues of its carbohydrate side-chain.[5] Uptake by cells of the reticuloendothelial system in GD is mediated by mannose receptors; this is distinct from the other recombinant enzymes that are available for other LSDs that rely on the mannose-6-phosphate receptor system. Interestingly, unlike most other lysosomal enzymes that transit through mannose-6-phosphate receptors, endogenous acid beta-glucosidase has been shown to be delivered to the lysosome via lysosomal integral membrane protein-2.[9]

Several studies have demonstrated the safety and efficacy of ERT with imiglucerase, in a range of doses from 15 to 60 units/kg, administered at two-week intervals. The effectiveness of ERT after two to five years of treatment was documented in 1,028 patients (48% <18 years old) in a report from the Gaucher Registry.[10] The following results were noted: hemoglobin concentrations typically increased to normal or near normal levels within six to 12 months, with a sustained response throughout five years. Patients with intact spleens had the greatest response of improved platelet counts within two years and had slower improvement thereafter. There was a smaller response if baseline thrombocytopenia was severe, presumably on account of persistent hypersplenism due to fibrosis of the spleen in long-term disease. In splenectomized patients, platelet counts returned to normal in six to 12 months. Hepatomegaly and splenomegaly decreased by up to 60%, but spleen volume may remain more than five times normal in some patients. In patients who had bone pain or bone crises before treatment, symptoms resolved in 52% and 94%, respectively.

Guidelines for the use of ERT in patients with neuronopathic GD are less well established. The recombinant enzyme does not cross the blood-brain barrier (BBB) and thus would be expected to have limited ability to impact the neurologic disease. However, other somatic effects of GD should respond to ERT, which would be considered palliative in these cases.[11,12] In some studies, ERT was found to reverse almost all of the systemic manifestations and appeared to stabilize the neurologic disease in some patients with the subacute variant, that is, GD type 3.[13-15] This was illustrated in a series of 21 patients, ages eight months to 35 years, who were treated with individually adjusted doses of enzyme and followed for two to eight years.[14] Improvement occurred in hemoglobin levels, platelet count, and acid phosphatase values. ERT decreased spleen and liver volume and improved bone structure. Neurologic responses were variable. Supranuclear gaze palsy in 19 patients was unchanged; one improved, and one worsened. ABR improved or was unchanged in 19 patients and deteriorated in two. In another report, all eight children receiving high-dose ERT had deterioration in ABR.[16] Cognitive function was unchanged or improved in 13 patients and worsened in eight. Asymptomatic interstitial lung disease, present in 19 patients, did not respond to treatment.

ERT can and should be considered as palliative therapy for patients with type 3 disease and severe visceral symptoms.[17] In particular, it should be offered in patients known to be at risk for neuronopathic GD due to genotype or family history who are identified early in the disease course before the onset of neurologic signs or symptoms. It may also have beneficial palliative effects in type 2 disease but does not alter the ultimate outcome and is not generally used.[18] Unfortunately, there is no evidence that hematopoietic stem cell transplantation (HSCT) is efficacious in patients with GD type 2.

The timeline of response to treatment varies, but analysis of data from the Gaucher Registry demonstrates the following trends. Improvements usually occur within six months after initiation of therapy and include reduction of spleen and liver volume, resolution of thrombocytopenia and anemia, reduction in fatigue, and improvement in bone complaints.[10] Skeletal improvement may not be evident until two to three years of therapy, bone mineralization may stabilize and slowly improve, and the risk of pathologic fracture may be reduced.[10]

Treatment of children with ERT may mitigate or prevent the complications that occur later in life, particularly skeletal abnormalities.[16,19] If started during the first decade, ERT can normalize growth and possibly the onset of pubertal development.[20]

Modification of the Treatment Algorithm to Individualize Care

Dose adjustments must be made on an individual basis. An increased dose may be indicated if visceromegaly, anemia, thrombocytopenia, and biomarkers fail to improve after six months.[19] If bone crises continue, the dose should be increased by 50%.[21] Dose increases also may be necessary to achieve therapeutic goals or for relapse following dose reduction.[22] However, an increased dose is unlikely to be effective with certain types of irreversible pathology (i.e., femoral head osteonecrosis and fibrosis of the liver, spleen, or lung). Additional evaluation may be necessary for patients who are unable to achieve their therapeutic goals after three to six months. Dose reductions should be considered only after all relevant therapeutic goals have been met.[23] Decisions regarding dose reduction should be made with caution. Dose reductions should occur no more frequently than every six months and must be accompanied by reassessment of disease severity to ensure the maintenance of therapeutic goals. Although certain patients may do well on lower doses, in general maintenance regimen involves a dose ≥30 mg/kg every two weeks.[19]

Recent studies suggest a dose–response relationship, with patients on a higher dose showing better outcomes.[24] Imiglucerase infusions given once a month also appear to be effective in stabilizing key disease parameters, when compared to those on an every-two-weeks interval on the same cumulative dose over a four-week period;[25] These observations have been confirmed in a significant number of patients treated with imiglucerase for four years,[10] although varying proportions of patients failed to achieve all therapeutic goals, as previously defined.[22]

Although effective in controlling systemic disease, ERT has not been shown to alter ultimate prognosis in patients with neurologic disease, likely because the BBB prevents the build-up of sufficient amounts of the infused enzyme within the central nervous system (CNS).[26] Investigations are actively pursuing various strategies for directly delivering the enzyme into the cerebrospinal fluid or brain parenchyma, or modifying the recombinant protein so that it can be readily taken across the BBB. For instance, the gene fusion of acid beta glucosidase with apolipoprotein B delivered intravascularly with a lentiviral vector resulted in uptake of the secreted protein via apolipoprotein B receptors on the BBB.[27]

An alternative approach to reduce substrate accumulation involves the use of substrate synthesis inhibitors (see chapter 16 in this volume). This approach has been shown to be beneficial in GD with an iminosugar called miglustat (Zavesca, Actelion, Pharmaceuticals) and also with a more potent investigational P-4 analogue, eliglustat. There is active screening of other small molecules that may be potentially useful.

Various therapeutic options are being examined as a means for addressing the different problems that develop in GD patients, although ERT currently represents the standard of care. Given the spectrum of disease expression and the likely multifactorial basis of disease, additional therapeutic strategies may be required to optimize treatment outcome.

Fabry Disease

FD is one of three LSDs caused by a defective gene on the X-chromosome. Interestingly, the disorder does not follow the usual pattern of X-linked recessive clinical expression; rather, the disorder manifests in males but also in females, although to a more variable degree. Deficiency of the hydrolase, alpha-galactosidase A leads to the typical signs and symptoms—such as acroparesthesias, angiokeratoma, corneal opacities, and hypohidrosis, which begin in childhood and adolescence. Progressive accumulation of the substrate globotriaosylceramide (GL-3) leads to microvascular ischemia and eventual compromise of the function of vital organs, particularly the kidney, heart, and brain. The progressive nature of FD reflects different cascades of disease processes that may precede clinical symptoms by a significant time period. Lysosomal accumulation can lead to cellular dysfunction, which triggers various tissue responses, such as inflammation. Ultimately, there is irreversible damage and renal, cardiac, and CNS complications. Additionally, vascular endothelial cell storage may lead to luminal encroachment and occlusion, as well as to altered vascular reactivity and a prothrombotic state[28,29] leading to ischemic events affecting various sites. Pathophysiologic observations in tissue specimens of FD patients were recently summarized in Eng, Germain, et al.[30] As there is no fixed combination or order of organ involvement and disease progression, all relevant organ systems need to be assessed, treated, and monitored individually.

ERT for FD received approval from the European Medicines Agency in 2001 and the FDA in 2003. Two similar and competing intravenous therapies, agalsidase alfa (Replagal, Shire HGT, Lexington, MA) and agalsidase beta (Fabrazyme, Genzyme Corporation, Cambridge, MA), were approved for use by the European Medicines Agency, while Orphan Drug legislation limited the FDA to approval of one drug for a 10-year period of exclusivity. Agalsidase beta has been the only ERT available for FD in the United States except for a small number of patients treated through investigator-initiated investigational new drug applications (INDs) or sponsored clinical trials for agalsidase alfa. The recommended dosage and administration for agalsidase alfa is 0.2 mg/kg body weight given intravenously over 40 minutes to 1 hr once every two weeks, whereas agalsidase beta is given at 1 mg/kg every two weeks over 2 to 4 hr.

Findings from a double-blind, randomized controlled trial with agalsidase beta, derived from transfected Chinese hamster ovary cells, at a dose of 1 mg/kg every two weeks indicate that this enzyme therapy exerts a positive impact on major clinical outcomes emphasizing the benefit of early therapeutic intervention in patients with FD.[31] Both the reduction of symptoms and prevention of late complications of FD are key therapeutic goals for ERT.[32]

Agalsidase alfa is a recombinant protein manufactured using a human fibroblast cell line, subjected to "activation" of the encoding gene for AGAL. Prior to marketing approval, agalsidase alfa was studied in two clinical trials. The first trial involved treatment of 10 male FD patients with single infusions of five escalating doses of agalsidase alfa, each dose given to two patients prior to advancing to the next dosing level (Schiffmann, Murray et al. 2000).[33] Liver biopsies showed a decrease in substrate accumulation in the liver as well as presence of the enzyme in every cell type, suggesting diffuse uptake via the mannose-6-phosphate receptor. The tissue half-life in the liver was greater than 24 hours. The pivotal trial was a single site randomized double-blind placebo controlled study conducted in 26 male FD patients.[34] Patients randomized to study drug received 12 doses of 0.2 mg/kg body weight over six months. The primary efficacy endpoint was the effect of treatment on pain without concomitant pain medication as measured by the "pain at its worst" question 3 on the Brief Pain Inventory. Pain scores showed a progressive decrease in the treatment group compared to no change in the placebo group with some measures reaching statistical significance. Long term results of 25 patients from the pivotal study were reported as part of an extension study.[35] During the four to four and a half years of ERT, eight of 25 patients developed persistent IgG antibodies to agalsidase alfa, but none demonstrated IgE antibodies. Estimated glomerular filtration rate (GFR) remained stable in patients with Stage I (GFR >90 ml/min) or Stage II (GFR 60–89 ml/min) chronic kidney disease as measured at baseline. However, in the subgroup of patients with Stage III chronic kidney disease (GFR 30–59 ml/min), the eGFR declined, but the slope of the decline in GFR was reduced compared with historical controls. This trend toward preservation and stabilization of renal function particularly in patients with mild to moderate kidney dysfunction at baseline and proteinuria less than 1 g/day was further demonstrated through combined retrospective analysis of the renal function data from the pivotal and extension study, together with data from two other clinical trials of agalsidase alfa.[36,37]

Similarly, agalsidase beta was studied in a phase 1/2 clinical trial, a placebo controlled pivotal (phase 3) trial, and a placebo controlled phase 4 study that was fully enrolled prior to FDA approval, but continued post-approval. The phase 1/2 trial was conducted in 15 male FD patients who were randomized to one of five treatment groups: 0.3, 1.0, or 3.0 mg/kg body weight administered every other week for five doses, or 1.0 or 3.0 mg/kg given every other day for five doses.[38] This study demonstrated that all dose levels achieved a reduction in plasma GL-3 to normal levels following five doses, however the 1.0 and 3.0 mg/kg groups achieved the reduction at a faster rate than the lowest dose group. Since the 1.0 mg/kg dose was associated with fewer infusion reactions than the highest dose, 1.0 mg/kg was chosen as the dose for the pivotal trial. This study was a randomized double-blind, placebo controlled multicenter study of 56 males and females with FD who received 11 doses given once every two weeks.[39] The primary endpoint of clearance of GL-3 from the renal capillary endothelium as a surrogate of improved kidney function was achieved ($p < 0.0005$) and a composite endpoint of clearance of GL-3 from capillary endothelium in kidney, heart, and skin biopsies was also highly statistically significant ($p < 0.0005$). Patients in this study were subsequently enrolled in long-term, open-label extension studies. These patients achieved or maintained normal or near-normal renal capillary endothelial histology on repeat biopsy after six months of open-label treatment.[39] A detailed histological assessment of the agalsidase beta phase III extension trial biopsies found that after 11 months of agalsidase beta treatment, there was complete clearance of GL-3 from the vascular endothelium, glomerular mesangial cells, and cortical interstitial cells.[31,40] Moderate clearance was noted from the smooth muscle cells of arterioles and small arteries. GL-3 clearance from podocytes and distal tubular epithelium was not as complete as that observed in other cell types.

In a double-blind, placebo-controlled, phase 4 clinical trial (2:1 randomization), 51 male and female FD patients received biweekly infusions of 1 mg/kg of agalsidase beta, while 31 patients received a placebo.[31] The median treatment duration of the study population, who all had mild to moderate renal disease at baseline, was 18.5 months. The results of this study showed that beneficial effects of agalsidase beta on estimated GFR and serum creatinine levels were more pronounced in patients who began ERT at less advanced stages of renal dysfunction. In addition, renal function, as measured by estimated GFR slope, was better preserved ($p = 0.03$) in agalsidase beta-treated group compared to the placebo group (1.5 vs. 5.1 mL/min/1.73m^2/year). Importantly, agalsidase beta significantly reduced the risk of reaching the composite endpoint of major renal, cardiac, cerebrovascular events, or death by 61% ($p = 0.034$) in the per protocol population, after adjusting for the baseline imbalance in proteinuria between the treatment groups.

Complete prevention of renal or other major events was not seen in the phase 4 study and probably cannot be expected in patients with advanced disease. As with other forms of chronic kidney disease, it may not be realistic to expect improvement in kidney function in patients with advanced kidney disease, but the reduction in the rate at which the chronic kidney disease progresses is a salutary outcome. The need for close monitoring and additional therapies, such as the use of ACE inhibitors or statins and other agents, may be necessary to achieve an optimal outcome.[30]

To date, there has been over 10 years of experience with the use of agalsidase alfa and beta in the clinical environment, and there have been multiple small prospective and retrospective studies, as well as reports of large cohorts of patients enrolled in registries for both drugs. Review of these studies and reports can begin to shape the outlook for long-term safety and efficacy of these agents when used in routine clinical settings and in heterogeneous groups of patients.

Renal function is of paramount concern to FD patients as it is the organ most typically involved in affected males and also causes signficant morbidity in affected females. As reviewed above, long-term follow-up studies conducted for both agents describe patients treated for nearly five years; this experience is meant to establish subgroups of patients who respond well and others who may be poor responders to therapy.[37,41] At this point in our understanding, the factors that influence preservation of renal function are baseline GFR, renal pathology (e.g., interstitial fibrosis, tubular atrophy, glomerulosclerosis), and degree of proteinuria at the initiation of treatment. For example, a stable eGFR was reported with 54 months of ERT; however, proteinuria greater than 1 gm/day or GFR < 90 predicted continued loss of GFR during ERT.[41,42] The degree of proteinuria appears to be a strong predictor: the same study showed that in patients with baseline proteinuria of less than 1 gm/day, the slope of GFR decline was −1.005 over 54 months. However in patients with proteinuria of > 1 gm/day, the slope of decline was −7.399. Although there may be continued loss of GRF over time, the slope of decline may be improved with ERT as opposed to no therapy, as estimated from studies of historical controls.[43] There are many advocates for aggressive treatment of proteinuria in FD patients through the use of ACE inhibitors and sartans. Smaller case reports also describe stabilization of kidney function in patients with moderately impaired renal function who are treated with ERT in combination with ACE inhibitor and sartans aiming to reduce proteinuria.[44] Another study in moderately to severely impaired patients (mean baseline eGFR <60 mL/min/1.73m2) showed some improvement in renal response but continued progression of disease.[45] The use of these agents to achieve maximal reduction of proteinuria can be problematic in FD patients as they are generally normotensive until advanced stages of renal insufficiency, and they may experience hypotension and other adverse effects of ACE and sartans. Thus treated patients will require close monitoring.

Cardiac involvement that can be attributed to FD includes LV hypertrophy, valvular disease, conduction abnormalities, and congestive heart failure as an end event. With the exception of conduction abnormalities, which may commence at an early age, the age of occurrence of cardiac events generally follows renal events in both males and females.[46] The mean ages at occurrence of cardiovascular events (myocardial infarction, arrhythmia, angina, congestive heart failure, significant cardiac procedure) and cerebrovascular events (stroke) were lower in males compared to females. Cardiovascular events were reported for 19% of the males and 14% of females at mean (standard deviation) ages of 39.0 (12) years and 47.6 (13) years, respectively. ERT has been shown to reduce myocardial storage of glycosphingolipids. During the open-label portion of the agalsidase beta phase 3 extension study, a significant reduction in LV mass and improvement in intracardiac conduction (QRS complex) were achieved.[44] Another study has shown that agalsidase beta treatment resulted in a significant improvement in cardiac morphological parameters with improvement of myocardial regional function and reduction of LV mass.[47] The latter observation was also made in a separate study of agalsidase alfa in females.[48] In a placebo-controlled study of 15 males with FD treated with agalsidase alfa, a significant reduction in LV mass occurred in the treatment group in the first six months of the study.[36] In two years of open-label follow-up, decreases in LV posterior wall and septal wall thickness were observed, which may be consistent with cardiac remodeling.[36]

Agalsidase beta was studied in 32 male and female patients with FD who were naïve to treatment.[49] Baseline MRI studies were performed and the degree of myocardial fibrosis at baseline was determined, leading to grouping of patients into no fibrosis, low, or medium fibrosis groups. The change in LV longitudinal function as measured by the longitudinal peak systolic strain rate of the septum increased on ERT ($p = 0.045$) in patients with no fibrosis. In addition, a mild but significant improvement in exercise capacity was demonstrated for patients with no fibrosis ($p = 0.014$). The authors concluded that the effect of ERT depended on stage at initiation of treatment in that patients with no fibrosis and mild hypertrophy at baseline showed normalization of LV wall thickness and mass, improved LV radial and longitudinal septal function, and exercise tolerance with ERT. Death from cardiac-related complications have remained a major source of mortality in FD, likely because of advanced disease despite control of renal pathology.[50]

The long-term effectiveness of ERT on decreasing stroke risk and other CNS-related disease manifestations remains to be delineated. Strokes have been reported to occur in patients while on agalsidase alfa and beta, and the number of white matter lesions have also been observed to increase while on therapy.[34,42,48,51] The use of aspirin may reduce the risk of embolic stroke, but this requires further investigation. Statins have also been recommend, as a measure of risk reduction.

Regarding early symptoms, ERT has been reported to have a beneficial effect on the frequency and severity of pain episodes and early treatment in young males and symptomatic females, and children.[48,52,53] It should be noted however, that statistically significant reduction of pain in a placebo-controlled trial of agalsidase beta has not been demonstrated, although trends in reduction have been observed.[34,39] However, there has been significant improvement in small nerve fiber function and intradermal vibration receptors with agalsidase beta.[54] Improvement in sweating has also been shown in a three-year study.[55]

The frequency of gastrointestinal (GI) symptoms in individuals with FD is high and can be debilitating and lead to decreased quality of life.[32,46] It has been frequently observed that GI symptoms, particularly diarrhea, markedly improve with ERT; however, published reports are few. In one study, GI symptoms, such as abdominal cramps and frequent bowel movements, had markedly improved after six to seven months of treatment.[56] Although the results of this small case series need to be confirmed in a larger population of patients, the findings are striking. After six months of agalsidase beta treatment, all four patients reported "no" or "only occasional" abdominal pain or diarrhea, had discontinued their GI medications, and had gained 3 to 8 kg in weight.

The evidence is building with regard to improved outcomes seen with early initiation of ERT prior to the development of irreversible changes such as myocardial fibrosis, renal pathology, or proteinuria.[49,57] Results from recent clinical trials of ERT in pediatric patients provides further evidence of tolerability of ERT in this age group as well as improvement in the early signs and symptoms of the disease.[58] Wraith et al. reported the results of a multicenter open-label trial with participants between seven and 15 years, Tanner III or below, documented FD plus one of following: history of FD pain crises, uncontrolled chronic pain, urine albumin >30 mg/dl, eGFR < 80 ml/min, history of GI disturbance, autonomic neuropathy, low BMI, or abbreviated EKG. The treatment phase was preceded by a 12-week observation and baseline data collection period in order to document frequency and severity of symptoms such as pain and GI disturbance. After a 48-week treatment period (agalsidase beta at 1 mg/kg every two weeks), it was determined that ERT was well tolerated, there was superficial dermal capillary GL-3 clearance, and GI symptoms showed statistically significant improvement by week 24. While renal and cardiac manifestations were not present in this cohort, three adolescent males with hyperfiltration did not show progression, and a trend toward quality of life improvements was seen. Thus these studies suggest that pediatric-age patients tolerate the infusions well and may benefit from improvement of early signs and symptoms. Similar observations have been made in pediatric patients treated with agalsidase alfa.[53]

While the clinical trial experience and subsequent clinical experience with the enzyme replacement therapies for FD has shown positive effects in several measured parameters and clinical endpoints, the long-term effect on morbidity, mortality, and life expectancy is still unknown. It appears clear that to achieve an optimal patient outcome, ERT must be started early in the disease course, before irreversible damage occurs. For males with predicted classic FD, this implies that treatment be initiated in late childhood to adolescence. However, the challenge continues to be the failure to recognize and diagnose the majority of patients without a known family history prior to the third decade of life. Other challenges that remain in the optimization of treatment of individuals with FD include development of noninvasive markers of disease progression as a method to monitor patient response to therapy, as well as the development of models to help predict which females are at risk for severe disease. Finally, the current optimal treatment of FD includes initiation of ERT early in the disease course and continued monitoring and institution of concomitant therapies such as ACE inhibitors and antiplatelet agents as indicated.

Mucopolysaccharidoses

The disorders collectively called the mucopolysaccharidoses (MPS) are inborn errors of the metabolic pathways responsible for the sequential degradation of glycosaminoglycan (GAG). With the exception of MPS-IVA and -VI, the MPS are characterized by both somatic and neurologic (cognitive) pathology; there is also heterogeneity of severity within some disorders, notably MPS-I and -II, resulting in some patients with a severe neurologic phenotype and other groups that are cognitively normal. Of the nine different MPS disorders, enzyme replacement therapy is available for three—MPS-I, -II, and -VI. ERT is under development for MPS-IVA; preliminary reports suggest benefit in some patients, with regulatory approval anticipated. Intrathecal ERT in a subset of patients with MPS-II (Hunter syndrome) and cognitive impairment is currently underway and being planned for patients with MPS-III-A.

MPS-VI or Maroteaux-Lamy syndrome is an autosomal recessive LSD caused by the deficiency of arylsulfatase B also known as N-acetylgalactosamine-4-sulfatase.[59] Deficiency of arylsulfatase B leads to accumulation of dermatan sulfate in various tissues of the body leading to classic signs and symptoms common to several of the MPS disorders. These include short stature, dysostosis multiplex, joint contractures, characteristic facial features, corneal clouding, hepatosplenomegaly, and cardiac, pulmonary, and airway compromise. The population of individuals affected with MPS-VI demonstrates a continuum of disease severity, mainly related to age of onset and rate of progression of disease, and may be loosely predicted by pretreatment urinary GAG levels.[60] Urinary GAG levels greater than 100 μg/mg creatinine are generally considered to be a poor prognostic indicator. The highest urinary GAG levels are associated with individuals with onset of disease symptoms before two to three years of age and a lifespan extending into the second or third decade. Growth velocity slows after the first year of life and typically ceases at three to four years of age. These patients usually manifest the full spectrum of severe organ system involvement and associated complications. There is a slowly progressive form of MPS-VI characterized by lower levels of dermatan sulfate and appearance of signs and symptoms after five years of age or later in the second or third decades. While these patients have an attenuated form of the disease, most will develop serious complications including joint contractures, cardiac valve disease, airway compromise, or sleep apnea.

Following recognition and diagnosis, individuals with MPS-VI have two therapeutic options: bone marrow/HSCT or enzyme replacement therapy. Results of bone marrow/HSCT have been reviewed.[61,62] ERT for MPS-VI (galsulfase, Naglazyme; Biomarin, Novato, CA) received FDA approval in May 2005 and EU approval in January 2006, based on the results of Phase 1/2, phase 2, and phase 3 clinical trials in affected patients.[63-66] The Phase 1/2 and Phase 2 studies demonstrated that galsulfase was well tolerated in patients and caused a reduction in urinary GAG levels. The 24-week, randomized double-blind, placebo-controlled phase 3 clinical trial showed significant improvement among treated patients in a 12-min walk test, with a reduction in urinary GAG levels and nearly significant improvement in a 3-min stair-climb test. All three clinical trials of galsulfase were followed by open-label extension studies, allowing for analysis of data for 56 participants treated for up to five years. Reduction in urinary GAG levels was sustained, and, in general, improvements gained in walk distance were maintained in follow up. There were several patients for whom the improvement in walk capacity was transient, and this has been attributed to advanced skeletal compromise at baseline. Further analysis of growth patterns in this cohort of 56 patients found that mean height increased by 2.9 cm after 48 weeks and 4.3 cm after 96 weeks on galsulfase, with the greatest height increases seen in patients less than 16 years of age. Taking into account age and pubertal status, there may also be improvement in growth velocity on treatment. Finally, evidence of catch-up pubertal development was suggested by progression or completion of pubertal development in 10 patients who had delayed puberty at baseline.

Evidence supporting early intervention for improved outcomes with ERT is given by a case report of two siblings with MPS-VI who initiated ERT at different stages of disease progression.[67] The older sibling began ERT at 3.6 years of age and demonstrated scoliosis, limitation of joint range of motion, cardiac valve involvement, and coarsening of the facial features. The younger sibling, who was diagnosed shortly after birth due to a known family history began ERT at eight weeks of age. At 3.6 years of age, he had none of the disease features that the older sibling demonstrated at the same age without treatment.

Experiments in animal models of MPS-I, -II, and –III-A have shown that ERT delivered via the intrathecal route distributes throughout the CNS and penetrates brain tissue, where it promotes clearance of lysosomal storage material. Studies are underway to investigate the safety and efficacy of intrathecal ERT in patients with MPS-I and signs of spinal cord compression.[68,69]

Other studies are examining alternative formulations of the enzyme. In experiments involving the mouse model of MPS-VII (β-glucuronidase deficiency), inactivation of the exposed carbohydrate recognition markers by sodium metaperiodate/sodium borohydride led to effective deglycosylation of β-glucuronidase and greater brain uptake, with marked reduction of neuronal storage when compared with unmodified enzyme.[70]

Safety of the Enzyme Replacement Therapies

ERT involves the regular infusion of a protein that may be foreign to the patient, particularly those with null alleles. This form of treatment is associated with the risk of developing antibodies that may lead to allergic reactions or that may neutralize activity of the administered protein.[71] All available ERTs result in the formation of the IgG class of antibodies in some or the majority of treated patients, depending on the disorder. Typically, antibodies develop after the first three to five infusions, the titers rise over several additional infusions, followed by a reduction in titers for the long term, suggesting the development of immune tolerance to the infused protein. Although the development of antibodies and the occurrence of infusion reactions are often temporally related, there does not appear to be a strict correlation between the two occurrences. Infusion reactions to ERTs are generally defined as an adverse reaction occurring during the infusion or until the end of the day of infusion. The most commonly experienced infusion reaction consists of rigors, chills, and increase in body temperature that is self-limited over 20 min to 1 hr. This type of reaction is generally managed by stopping the infusion during the reaction and administration of an antipyretic and antihistamine. When the rigors and chills subside, the infusion can be restarted at a slower rate, generally without recurrence of the infusion reaction. Once a patient experiences this type of infusion reaction, he or she is at increased risk of having similar reactions during subsequent infusions and will typically react for several infusions followed by cessation of the reaction. Antipyretics and antihistamines can be administered as premedications for prophylaxis in subsequent infusions. Steroids may also be used in more severe or refractory cases with usual success. The most effective management of these reactions and allergic reactions in general is to slow the infusion of the protein to rates as low as 0.1 mg/min, dilution of the protein in a larger volume of the diluent (typically normal saline), with an increase in infusion rate undertaken every 15 to 30 min, as tolerated. It is generally thought that this type of reaction is mediated by the complement cascade and probably not by IgG, as evidenced by the reports of rigors and chills in both IgG-positive and IgG-negative patients.

Infusion reactions of a more serious nature have also been described for all of the available ERTs. These may consist of urticaria, wheezing, angioedema, hypotension, and anaphylactic reactions. These may occur at any time during the course of treatment and may be associated with IgG or IgE antibody formation. In a study of six male patients treated with agalsidase beta who experienced adverse events associated with detection of IgE antibodies and/or skin-test reactivity to agalsidase beta, four patients were successfully rechallenged.[72] The rechallenge protocol consisted of half the standard dose (0.5 mg/kg) given once per week instead of once every two weeks and an infusion rate ramp that started at 0.01 mg/min with doubling every 30 min to a maximum rate of 0.25 mg/min. If patients tolerated the protocol without adverse reactions, the dose and rate were liberalized. One of the six patients had positive IgE antibodies while the remaining five were IgE negative but skin-test positive. The IgE positive patient was a 66-year-old patient who experienced hypotension, rhonchi, chills, pyrexia, nausea, and vomiting but no urticaria at the fifth infusion. After more than 400 days off therapy, this patient was successfully rechallenged and received agalsidase beta at the standard dose of 1 mg/kg every two week. One of the five patients who was IgE negative but skin-test positive withdrew from the study after one dose due to recurrence of adverse events, but the study reports that the patient was able to tolerate infusions off protocol. Thus in patients who experience the most severe infusion reactions and/or have demonstrated IgE antibody formation, successful readministration and long-term maintenance of therapy has been achieved using a modified, stepwise protocol of reintroduction.

While formation of IgG antibodies is common to most of the enzyme replacement therapies, the effect of antibodies on clinical efficacy is less clear. Treatment of patients with GD using imiglucerase or velaglucerase may have the lowest incidence of IgG antibody formation; approximately 13% of GD patients receiving imiglucerase develop IgG antibodies usually within the first year after initiation of therapy, but these patients appear to reach and maintain therapeutic goals. However, several reports exist of patients developing inhibitory antibodies to imiglucerase.[73-75] One such patient with GD type 1 responded during the first year of alglucerase treatment (placental glucocerebrosidase) with reduction in liver and spleen volumes, decreased fatigue, and decreased frequency and severity of bone pain.[74] Within 12 months of initiation of therapy, the patient experienced mild infusion reactions, but from months 13 to 21 of treatment had a recurrence of fatigue and bone pain, as well as a 25% increase in spleen volume. High inhibitory antibody titers were detected, and the patient started an immune tolerance protocol consisting of cyclophosphamide with consistent enzyme therapy and conservative management of infusion reactions. Clinical manifestations improved, and the patient has been able to remain stable with decreased doses of the enzyme. A second patient was also reported who had initial improvement of GD-related signs and symptoms, followed by plateau and then worsening in the second year of treatment, accompanied by an increase in liver and spleen volume. Persistent high inhibitory antibody titers were detected from at least months 29 to 41 of enzyme therapy. The patient showed clinical improvement to increased dose of imiglucerase. Inhibitory antibodies have also been reported in MPS-II patients receiving idursulfase (Elaprase, Shire HGT, Lexington, MA) with a report of four of 32 IgG-positive patients having inhibitory antibodies. The effect of these inhibitory antibodies on efficacy of recombinant idursulfase is not yet known.

Antibody production appears to have a more profound impact on efficacy of ERT in Pompe disease, particularly in the infantile phenotype, which is characterized by rapidly progressive muscle weakness, hypertrophic cardiomyopathy, feeding problems, failure to thrive, and respiratory insufficiency. The usual time frame of presentation and diagnosis in these patients is three to five months of age, and without treatment death occurs at a mean age of 6.0 to 8.7 months of age. In a retrospective comparison of 21 cross-reactive immunologic material (CRIM)-positive and 11 CRIM-negative participants in clinical trials of recombinant acid α-glucosidase (Myozyme, Genzyme Corporation, Cambridge, MA), a difference in outcome was observed between the groups.[76] At baseline, all patients were six months of age or less and ventilator-independent. After 52 weeks of treatment with recombinant α-glucosidase, six of 11 CRIM-negative patients were deceased or ventilator-dependent as contrasted with one of 21 CRIM-positive patients. By 27 months of age on treatment, all CRIM-negative patients were deceased or ventilator dependent, as opposed to four of 21 CRIM-positive patients. All CRIM-negative patients and 90% of CRIM-positive patients developed IgG antibodies; however, the titers of antibody were significantly higher in the CRIM-negative patients. The mean peak titer level of CRIM-negative patients was 1:204,000 and showed continued increase in titers through week 52. In contrast, the median peak titer level for CRIM-positive patients was 1:1800, and these patients showed decline in titers over time, similar to the immune tolerance pattern seen in other LSDs treated with ERT. Since approximately 20% of infantile Pompe disease patients are CRIM-negative, strategies for immune modulation via tolerance-inducing protocols are being investigated in infantile Pompe disease; however, from early accounts it appears that reversing an established immune response has limited success. Currently, efforts are being directed to identify CRIM-negative patients early in the course of diagnosis and begin immune modulation concomitantly with the initiation of ERT or soon after.[77] If this approach is successful, it may close the gap between outcomes for CRIM-positive and CRIM-negative patients. An algorithm for the management of these complex patients has recently been proposed.[78]

Alternatives to Enzyme Replacement Therapy: Small Molecule-Based Therapies

Several small molecules have been identified that exhibit properties that make them suitable as prospective treatment options for LSDs; putative advantages include oral administration, wide volume of distribution, and access to potentially sequestered sites (e.g., across the BBB); the absence of antibody formation (which in some cases reduce the benefit derived from ERT); and the need for immunomodulation (as required for HSCT and for CRIM-negative infantile Pompe disease patients). For the long term, the safety and efficacy of these drugs will need to be closely monitored in light of the chronic exposure that will be necessary to maintain disease control.[78] In particular, drugs that are internally processed may compete with the metabolism of other medications the patient may be on, or exhibit interactions with other agents that can be potentially deleterious. Moreover, nonspecificity of drug action may involve off-target effects and raise additional concerns about its safety. With certain approaches, patients may be screened for particular mutations that may be corrected by a specific strategy, such a premature stop codon read-through option or the rescue of a misfolded protein by pharmacologic chaperones. This molecular-based personalized therapy may allow patients to be guided to the safest, most convenient, and most effective form of therapy for their particular disease. Ultimately, in vitro screening strategies must be correlated with in vivo effects that are predictive of positive clinical outcomes.

Substrate Reduction Therapy

Substrate reduction therapy (also see chapter 15 in this volume) is designed to partially reduce the synthesis of the substrate or its precursor and to approximate the residual capacity of the mutant enzyme and thereby strike a metabolic balance within the cell.[79] This approach was initially demonstrated clinically in patients with GD type 1 given miglustat, an alkylated iminosugar that inhibits the activity of glucosylceramide synthase.[80] Miglustat's mechanism of action is nonspecific to a particular disease; by limiting precursor synthesis it reduces not only glucocerebroside accumulation but also the buildup of G_{M2}-ganglioside (i.e., the offending lipid in Tay-Sachs disease, Sandhoff disease and Niemann-Pick, type C (NPC). In patients with NPC, improved supranuclear gaze palsy and swallowing has been observed following miglustat treatment.[81] However, miglustat does not appear to alter ultimate neurologic prognosis in NPC patients with progressive disease. NPC2, caused by a deficiency of a soluble (noncatalytic) protein, is a potential candidate for HSCT.[82]

Miglustat has been used as a maintenance therapy in selected patients, and a significant number of patients with GD type 1 were switched to this drug following the shortage of imiglucerase.[83] Patients have been shown to experience a reduction in liver/spleen volume and normalization of hematologic parameters on long-term treatment and maintenance of ERT-derived therapeutic benefits. Unfortunately, a trial of miglustat in patients with GD type 3 on ERT did not conclusively show combination therapy to provide additional benefits.[26]

Side effects reported with the use of miglustat include GI problems (mainly diarrhea in 80% of patients, particularly during the initial exposure to treatment), tremor, and peripheral neuropathy.[84] The diarrhea probably results from miglustat's inhibition of other glucosidases in the GI tract; these problems tend to diminish with ongoing therapy and respond well to low-carbohydrate diet, although compliance with miglustat is often negatively affected by this side effect. The peripheral neuropathy noted in smaller cohorts exposed to miglustat has not been as frequently reported with subsequent clinical experience.

A second SRT formulation, eliglustat, has been shown to achieve therapeutic outcomes in treated GD type 1 patients that are comparable to ERT.[85]

For the MPS disorders, genistein, a component of soy extract, has been shown to reduce the accumulation of GAGs in human MPS-I, -II, -III–A, and –III-B fibroblasts.[86] Interestingly, these findings are achieved not by directly inhibiting GAG synthesis but through the inhibition of epidermal growth factor receptor, which is involved with modulating expression of enzymes involved in GAG synthesis. Mouse models of MPS-II with defects of iduronate-2-sulphatase were given two doses of genistein, 5 or 25 mg/kg/day, added to the diet for 10 or 20 weeks. Urinary GAG levels were reduced after 10 weeks' treatment with genistein in both dose groups. In tissue samples from the liver, spleen, kidney, and heart, a reduction in GAG content was observed after 10 weeks' treatment. Decreased GAG deposits in brain were observed after genistein treatment in some animals. This approach is probably best described as substrate modulation therapy; a term also appropriate for approaches to modify GAGs into a form that allows its degradation by intact pathways to which it is diverted, as proposed by Zacharon Pharmaceuticals.[87]

In an open-label study of 10 MPS patients given genistein for 12 months, there was significant reduction in heparan sulphate levels in urine and improvements of hair morphology and cognitive function. No adverse reactions were observed. Additional studies are underway to ascertain its safety and efficacy in patients with MPS-III.

Substrate Depletion Therapy

Cystinosis is an autosomal recessive LSD caused by defective transport of the amino acid cystine out of lysosomes. The stored cystine is poorly soluble and crystallizes within the lysosomes of many cell types, leading to widespread tissue and organ damage, particularly of the kidney, eye, liver, and brain. The disorder is due to mutations in the gene encoding the transmembrane transport protein cystinosin. In 1994, the FDA approved the use of an oral aminothiol cystine-depleting agent cysteamine (Cystagon, CVS Procare) that promotes the lowering of cystine content in lysosomes of patients with cystinosis. The drug is a weak base that enters the lysosome and reacts with cystine, forming a mixed disulfide of half-cystine and cysteamine. This mixed disulfide exits the lysosome via the transport system for cationic amino acids, which is unaffected in cystinosis. Treated patients show maintenance of renal function and improved growth.[88] Cysteamine eye drops help to dissolve the corneal crystals that can develop in these individuals, including postkidney transplant cases.

Chemical-Chaperone Enzyme Enhancement Therapy

The use of pharmacological chaperones has been proposed as a therapeutic approach for certain LSDs, based on demonstration that particular agents acting as active-site inhibitors can serve as a template to promote the refolding and correct trafficking of mutant proteins (see chapter 16 in this voume for further details).[89] As protein rescue may only occur in certain cases (e.g., missense mutations that do not lead to a major loss or destruction of the enzyme or inactivate the catalytic site), disease-specific treatments would be limited to a subset of patients and not the entire spectrum of enzyme-deficient patients (such as those with null alleles or mutations leading to premature protein truncation).

Pharmacologic chaperones appear to work best in the presence of residual enzyme activity. As these are patients who may follow an atypical course of disease, it will be necessary to identify the subgroup of patients most likely to show disease progression and the appropriate time to introduce the treatment in these cases. This is a practical issue, not currently fully addressed by information regarding patient genotype or the monitoring of biomarkers. Furthermore, certain pharmacologic chaperones have inhibitory properties, which potentially complicate determination of the right combination of dose and frequency of drug administration to maximize enhancement of enzymes activity. There may also be differences in enzyme enhancement across cell types in individual patients that could result in variable clinical outcomes.

Two formulations, isofagomine and migalastat, are the subject of clinical trials for GD and FD, respectively.[90] For both drugs, the rationale for advancing to human subjects was established through proof of principle studies in vitro using cells obtained from affected individuals and in animal models of disease. Interestingly, studies in affected cells from patients with Pompe disease suggest the use of pharmacologic chaperones may also improve uptake and stability of exogenous enzyme, thereby providing potential justification for combination therapy.[91]

Recently, it has been suggested that mutant proteins may be rescued from premature degradation through enhancement of other factors involved with promoting proper folding within the endoplasmic reticulum. For instance, celastrol and MG 132 have been demonstrated to partially restore enzyme activity in cell lines obtained from patients with GD and Tay-Sachs disease.[92] Also, verapamil and diltiazem, which act as calcium antagonists, partially restored lysosomal enzyme activity in cell lines from patients with GD, MPS-III-A (Sanfilippo syndrome), and mannosidosis.[93] Presumably, blocking calcium channels enhances the proper folding of mutant enzyme by up-regulating a subset of molecular chaperones within the endoplasmic reticulum. The latter process has been referred to as proteostasis regulation; wherein protein rescue is mediated indirectly, by up-regulating endogenous chaperones rather than acting as a folding template for the mutant enzyme.[92] Thus in contrast to the pharmacologic chaperones that are specific to the mutant enzyme in any given disease, proteostasis regulators may serve a broad spectrum of disease.

Recently, the use of histone deacetylase inhibitors was shown to increase the quantity and activity of acid beta-glucosidase activity in firbroblast obtained from GD patients. The changes were attributed to limitation of the deacetylation of heat shock protein 90, resulting in less recognition of the mutant peptide and acid beta-glucosidase degradation.[94]

Premature Stop-Codon Read-Through

In several LSDs, the underlying defect is a premature stop-codon mutation. Several drugs, such as gentamicin, have been shown to selectively target premature stop codons and modify the tRNA recognition process to insert preferentially specific amino acids, essentially enabling the potential for read-through and translation of the encoded protein.[95,96] Obviously, agents will have to be carefully selected to ensure that processes involved with native stop codons of other genes are not dysregulated.

In severe MPS-I (Hurler syndrome) the premature stop codons Q70X and W402X are two of the most common α-L-iduronidase gene mutations. In Chinese hamster ovary cells-K1 cells expressing these mutations, gentamicin-enhanced stop-codon read-through restored a low level of α-L-iduronidase activity and reduced lysosomal GAG accumulation.[95,97] A recent report noted 4,5-disubstituted aminoglycosides (lividomycin and NB54) induced more read-through for the W402X mutation, while 4,6-disubstituted aminoglycosides promoted more read-through for the Q70X mutation. These observations were attributed to differences in predicted mRNA secondary structure, a potential consideration in the design of trials and selection of patients.[98]

Gene Therapy

Gene therapy remains a promising treatment approach for the LSDs. Although several animal studies suggest therapeutic benefits, application in human patients remains investigational. Several studies have been performed primarily in mouse models of disease and in most cases with a viral-vector mediated approach, including systemic and direct injection into CSF or brain parenchyma. Improvements have been observed in animal models of MPS-III-A, -III–B, and -VII, infantile neuronal ceroid lipofuscinosis, Niemann–Pick disease, metachromatic leukodystrophy (MLD), and Krabbe disease injected with an adeno-associated viral vector and the relevant cognate gene.[99] Meanwhile, there is growing interest in demonstrating proof of principle in larger animal models, such as sheep, cats, and dogs.[100]

Modification of donor cells used in transplant may also enable overexpression of the cognate enzyme and enhance the benefit derived from HSCT alone. In studies involving the mouse model of MLD, ex vivo gene transfer into hematopoietic cells led to improved outcomes when compared with transplant of unmodified cells.[101] Recently, this approach was undertaken in three asymptomatic patients diagnosed with late-infantile MLD (ages seven to 21 months) and reported to lead to a high enzyme expression throughout hematopoietic lineages and in cerebrospinal fluid. The disease in these patients did not manifest or progress beyond the predicted age of symptom onset.[102]

A trial to examine the safety of gene therapy in patients with late-infantile neuronal ceroid lipofuscinosis has also been conducted, using direct injection of AAV2 containing the CLN2 gene (encoding tripeptidyl-peptidase I).[103] A brain MRI showed a trend toward a lesser deterioration in atrophy and cortical apparent diffusion coefficient, compared with the relentless progression of the condition in the 18 months prior to the trial. In addition, the decline in the condition of the eight treated subjects for whom data were available for more than six months was significantly slower than that in a number of historical control groups. Enzyme infusion relied on preoperative stereotactic planning to optimize a parenchymal target and diffuse administration, which have recently been described.[104]

Antisense Splicing Modulation Therapy

Certain mutations create novel splice sites, resulting in an altered transcript and dysfunctional protein product that can be prematurely degraded, leading to absent or reduced enzyme activity within the lysosome. Antisense oligonucleotides force the use of the natural splice sites by modulating the splicing pattern through steric hindrance of the recognition and binding of the splicing apparatus to selected sequences.[105] As a consequence, there is greater recovery of normally spliced transcripts encoding the functional protein. Currently identified agents with antisense oligonucleotides properties include aminoglycosides (e.g., gentamicin and G418) and nonaminoglycosides (e.g., PTC124 and RTC13), but screening for additional drug is ongoing.[106]

In studies using cells from NPC patients, antisense oligonucleotides treatment has been shown to reverse aberrant splicing due to an intronic mutation (c.1554-1009G>A located in intron 9), which causes an inclusion of a pseudo-exon. The mutation in this case generates a premature termination codon and a transcript that is degraded by the nonsense-mediated mRNA decay mechanism. Normal splicing was restored in fibroblasts from the treated patient using a specific antisense morpholino oligonucleotide targeted to the cryptic splice site.[107]

Organ Transplantation

In LSDs associated with failure of the kidneys (e.g., FD, cystinosis), liver (GD), or heart (FD), organ transplantation has been undertaken as a life-saving measure.[108–110] Although donor organs from living relatives or cadavers express normal enzyme activity and are spared from reaccumulation of the substrate, it is unlikely that sufficient amounts of the enzyme are secreted or adequate microchimerism develops to effect clearance of the systemic disease burden. Thus ERT may still be necessary to achieve overall disease stability or control. As with HSCT, it is important to exclude the possibility the organ donor may be a carrier, in particular, the transfer of a presumed healthy kidney from a female relative in a family segregating for FD (an X-linked trait).

Adjunctive Therapies

Increased understanding of downstream disease mechanisms implicated in LSD pathology may lead to identification of potential targets for therapeutic intervention.[111]

Animal studies suggest cellular changes develop prior to onset of disease manifestations, and thus there is a critical need for early diagnosis and intervention to optimize clinical outcome.[112,113] However, pathology may be initiated prenatally, in which case even newborn screening to identify affected individuals may not be adequate. Obviously, in the latter instance identification of families at risk may enable preimplantation genetic or prenatal diagnosis to reduce recurrence risk.

Aberrant inflammation has been described in several LSDs, including G_{M1}-gangliosidosis, G_{M2}-gangliosidosis (Sandhoff disease), and NPC.[114] Nonsteroidal anti-inflammatory agents reduced brain inflammation, improved motor function, and increased survival rates when given alone or in combination with miglustat in mouse models of Sandhoff disease and NPC.[115] In the mouse model for NPC, the use of the c-Abl-specific inhibitor imatinib also improved neurological symptoms.[116]

Osteopenia has been described in GD, FD, and Pompe disease.[117–119] Anti-bone-resorbing agents, such as alendronate, have been shown to improve bone density in GD patients receiving ERT.[120] Additional studies are necessary before this approach is implemented, as the incidence of pathologic fractures in relation to decreased bone density in patients with LSD is not known.

As noted above, in FD the use of ACE inhibitors has been advocated in patients with proteinuria.[121] In addition, anti-platelet-aggregating agents have been recommended to reduce risk of developing stroke.

Thus adjunctive therapies may be useful in combination with available targeted treatments for improved results; although it would be ideal for controlled studies to be undertaken prior to general implementation. In practice, prospective studies or longitudinal follow with data collected through registry programs and outcomes compared to a historical data set may be acceptable, given the understandable difficulty of conducting trials in rare diseases.

Disease Prevention

Not to be overlooked are strategies aimed at disease prevention through carrier detection and appropriate genetic counseling. For the more common of the LSDs, such as GD and Tay-Sachs disease, carrier screening programs based on biochemical or DNA-based detection of carriers have been offered to at-risk populations (mainly based on ethnicity) for several decades. The effectiveness of these programs has been demonstrated for Tay–Sachs disease in the Ashkenazi Jewish community wherein the incidence of the disorder in this population has significantly declined and is now less than in the general population.[122] With cost-effective improvements in high-throughput genotyping or next-generation sequencing approaches, the possibility of carrier detection for the ultra-rare LSDs in the general population may soon be a reality. Information about reproductive risks can offer families the option of preimplantation or prenatal genetic diagnosis.[123] In addition to preconception or prenatal genetic screening, newborn screening for the LSDs may offer the benefit of early detection and treatment for affected individuals. In these instances, the true potential for enhancement of quality of life and reduction of morbidity and mortality for the available treatment modalities may be fully realized.

Summary

The field of LSDs is being rapidly transformed by advances in our understanding of disease mechanisms and the introduction of various therapeutic options. None of these approaches are necessarily exclusive but hold the promise of introducing combination therapies to improve clinical outcome. However, it will be critical to initially demonstrate that singular strategies do alter disease course. Obviously, given the rarity of these diseases, clinical trials will have to demonstrate that there is indeed a benefit to be gained with a combination approach. The latter is not a trivial issue, as current and projected costs of care for patients with LSDs are huge. Meanwhile, significant inroads have not been made in the management of primary CNS disease, although supportive care can improve the lives of affected individuals and their families.

References

1. Brady RO, Pentchev PG, et al. Replacement therapy for inherited enzyme deficiency. Use of purified glucocerebrosidase in Gaucher's disease. *N Engl J Med*. 1974; 291(19): 989–993.
2. Desnick RJ, Dean KJ, et al. Enzyme therapy in Fabry disease: differential in vivo plasma clearance and metabolic effectiveness of plasma and splenic alpha-galactosidase A isozymes. *Proc Natl Acad Sci USA* 1979; 76(10): 5326–5330.
3. Barton NW, Brady RO, et al. Dose-dependent responses to macrophage-targeted glucocerebrosidase in a child with Gaucher disease. *J Pediatr*. 1992; 120(2 Pt 1): 277–280.
4. Barton NW, Brady RO, et al. Replacement therapy for inherited enzyme deficiency—macrophage-targeted glucocerebrosidase for Gaucher's disease. *N Engl J Med*. 1991; 324(21): 1464–1470.

5. Grabowski GA, Barton NW, et al. Enzyme therapy in type 1 Gaucher disease: comparative efficacy of mannose-terminated glucocerebrosidase from natural and recombinant sources. *Ann Intern Med.* 1995; 122(1): 33–39.
6. Gonzalez DE, Turkia HB, Lukina EA, et al. Enzyme replacement therapy with velaglucerase alfa in Gaucher disease: results from a randomized, double-blind, multinational, Phase 3 study. *Am J Hematol.* 2013; 88(3): 166–171.
7. Zimran A, Brill-Almon E, Chertkoff R, et al. Pivotal trial with plant cell-expressed recombinant glucocerebrosidase, taliglucerase alfa, a novel enzyme replacement therapy for Gaucher disease. *Blood.* 2011; 118(22): 5767–5773.
8. Zimran A, Altarescu G, et al. Phase 1/2 and extension study of velaglucerase alfa replacement therapy in adults with type 1 Gaucher disease: 48-month experience. *Blood.* 2010; 115(23): 4651–4656.
9. Reczek D, Schwake M, Schröder J, et al. LIMP-2 is a receptor for lysosomal mannose-6-phosphate-independent targeting of beta-glucocerebrosidase. *Cell.* 2007; 131(4): 770–783.
10. Weinreb NJ, Charrow J, et al. Effectiveness of enzyme replacement therapy in 1028 patients with type 1 Gaucher disease after 2 to 5 years of treatment: a report from the Gaucher Registry. *Am J Med.* 2002; 113(2): 112–119.
11. Prows CA, Sanchez N, et al. Gaucher disease: enzyme therapy in the acute neuronopathic variant. *Am J Med Genet.* 1997; 71(1): 16–21.
12. Grabowski GA. Recent clinical progress in Gaucher disease. *Curr Opin Pediatr.* 2005; 17(4): 519–524.
13. Schiffmann R, Heyes MP, et al. Prospective study of neurological responses to treatment with macrophage-targeted glucocerebrosidase in patients with type 3 Gaucher's disease. *Ann Neurol.* 1997; 42(4): 613–621.
14. Altarescu G, Hill S, et al. The efficacy of enzyme replacement therapy in patients with chronic neuronopathic Gaucher's disease. *J Pediatr.* 2001; 138(4): 539–547.
15. Beutler E. Gaucher disease: muldZtiple lessons from a single gene disorder. *Acta Paediatr Suppl.* 2006; 95(451): 103–109.
16. Grabowski GA, Andria G, et al. Pediatric non-neuronopathic Gaucher disease: presentation, diagnosis and assessment: consensus statements. *Eur J Pediatr.* 2004; 163(2): 58–66.
17. Jmoudiak M, Futerman AH. Gaucher disease: pathological mechanisms and modern management. *Br J Haematol.* 2005; 129(2): 178–188.
18. Bove KE, Daugherty C, et al. Pathological findings in Gaucher disease type 2 patients following enzyme therapy. *Hum Pathol.* 1995; 26(9): 1040–1045.
19. Baldellou A, Andria G, et al. Paediatric non-neuronopathic Gaucher disease: recommendations for treatment and monitoring. *Eur J Pediatr.* 2004; 163(2): 67–75.
20. Charrow J. Enzyme replacement therapy for Gaucher disease. *Expert Opin Biol Ther.* 2009; 9(1): 121–131.
21. Cohen IJ, Katz K, et al. Low-dose high-frequency enzyme replacement therapy prevents fractures without complete suppression of painful bone crises in patients with severe juvenile onset type I Gaucher disease. *Blood Cell Mol Dis.* 1998; 24(3): 296–302.
22. Pastores GM, Weinreb NJ, et al. Therapeutic goals in the treatment of Gaucher disease. *Semin Hematol.* 2004; 41(4 Suppl. 5): 4–14.
23. Andersson HC, Charrow J, et al. Individualization of long-term enzyme replacement therapy for Gaucher disease. *Genet Med.* 2005; 7(2): 105–110.
24. de Fost M, Hollak CE, et al. Superior effects of high-dose enzyme replacement therapy in type 1 Gaucher disease on bone marrow involvement and chitotriosidase levels: a 2-center retrospective analysis. *Blood.* 2006; 108(3): 830–835.
25. Kishnani PS, DiRocco M, et al. A randomized trial comparing the efficacy and safety of imiglucerase (Cerezyme) infusions every 4 weeks versus every 2 weeks in the maintenance therapy of adult patients with Gaucher disease type 1. *Mol Genet Metab.* 2009; 96(4): 164–170.
26. Schiffmann R, Fitzgibbon EJ, et al. Randomized, controlled trial of miglustat in Gaucher's disease type 3. *Ann Neurol.* 2008; 64(5): 514–522.
27. Spencer BJ, Verma, IM. Targeted delivery of proteins across the blood-brain barrier. *Proc Natl Acad Sci USA.* 2007; 104(18): 7594–7599.
28. DeGraba T, Azhar S, et al. Profile of endothelial and leukocyte activation in Fabry patients. *Ann Neurol.* 2000; 47(2): 229–233.

29. Kampmann C, Wiethoff CM, et al. The heart in Anderson Fabry disease. *Z Kardiol*. 2002; 91(10): 786–795.
30. Eng CM, Germain DP, et al. Fabry disease: guidelines for the evaluation and management of multi-organ system involvement. *Genet Med*. 2006; 8(9): 539–548.
31. Banikazemi M, Bultas J, et al. Agalsidase-beta therapy for advanced Fabry disease: a randomized trial. *Ann Intern Med*. 2007; 146(2): 77–86.
32. Mehta A, Ricci R, et al. Fabry disease defined: baseline clinical manifestations of 366 patients in the Fabry Outcome Survey. *Eur J Clin Invest*. 2004; 34(3): 236–242.
33. Schiffmann R, Murray GJ, et al. Infusion of alpha-galactosidase A reduces tissue globotriaosylceramide storage in patients with Fabry disease. *Proc Natl Acad Sci USA*. 2000; 97(1): 365–370.
34. Schiffmann R., Kopp JB, et al. Enzyme replacement therapy in Fabry disease: a randomized controlled trial. *JAMA*. 2001; 285(21): 2743–2749.
35. Schiffmann R, Ries M, et al. Long-term therapy with agalsidase alfa for Fabry disease: safety and effects on renal function in a home infusion setting. *Nephrol Dial Transplant*. 2006; 21(2): 345–354.
36. Hughes DA, Elliott PM, et al. Effects of enzyme replacement therapy on the cardiomyopathy of Anderson-Fabry disease: a randomised, double-blind, placebo-controlled clinical trial of agalsidase alfa. *Heart*. 2008; 94(2): 153–158.
37. West M, Nicholls K, et al. Agalsidase alfa and kidney dysfunction in Fabry disease. *J Am Soc Nephrol*. 2009; 20(5): 1132–1139.
38. Eng CM, Banikazemi M, et al. A phase 1/2 clinical trial of enzyme replacement in fabry disease: pharmacokinetic, substrate clearance, and safety studies. *Am J Hum Genet*. 2001; 68(3): 711–722.
39. Eng CM, Guffon N, et al. Safety and efficacy of recombinant human alpha-galactosidase A—replacement therapy in Fabry's disease. *N Engl J Med*. 2001; 345(1): 9–16.
40. Thurberg BL, Rennke H, et al. Globotriaosylceramide accumulation in the Fabry kidney is cleared from multiple cell types after enzyme replacement therapy. *Kidney Int*. 2002; 62(6): 1933–1946.
41. Germain DP, Waldek S, et al. Sustained, long-term renal stabilization after 54 months of agalsidase beta therapy in patients with Fabry disease. *J Am Soc Nephrol*. 2007; 18(5): 1547–1557.
42. Wilcox WR, Banikazemi M, et al. Long-term safety and efficacy of enzyme replacement therapy for Fabry disease. *Am J Hum Genet*. 2004; 75(1): 65–74.
43. Schiffmann R, Warnock DG, et al. Fabry disease: progression of nephropathy, and prevalence of cardiac and cerebrovascular events before enzyme replacement therapy. *Nephrol Dial Transplant*. 2009; 24(7): 2102–2111.
44. Feriozzi S, Schwarting A, et al. Agalsidase alfa slows the decline in renal function in patients with Fabry disease. *Am J Nephrol*. 2009; 29(5): 353–361.
45. Tahir H, Jackson LL, et al. Antiproteinuric therapy and fabry nephropathy: sustained reduction of proteinuria in patients receiving enzyme replacement therapy with agalsidase-beta. *J Am Soc Nephrol*. 2007; 18(9): 2609–2617.
46. Eng CM, Fletcher J, et al. Fabry disease: baseline medical characteristics of a cohort of 1765 males and females in the Fabry Registry. *J Inherit Metab Dis*. 2007; 30(2): 184–192.
47. Breunig F, Knoll A, et al. Enzyme replacement therapy in Fabry disease: clinical implications. *Curr Opin Nephrol Hypertens*. 2003; 12(5): 491–495.
48. Whybra C, Miebach E, et al. A 4-year study of the efficacy and tolerability of enzyme replacement therapy with agalsidase alfa in 36 women with Fabry disease. *Genet Med*. 2009; 11(6): 441–449.
49. Weidemann F, Niemann M, et al. Long-term effects of enzyme replacement therapy on fabry cardiomyopathy: evidence for a better outcome with early treatment. *Circulation*. 2009; 119(4): 524–529.
50. Mehta A, Clarke JT, Giugliani R, et al. Natural course of Fabry disease: changing pattern of causes of death in FOS—Fabry Outcome Survey. *J Med Genet*. 2009; 46(8): 548–552.
51. Vedder AC, Linthorst GE, et al. Treatment of Fabry disease: outcome of a comparative trial with agalsidase alfa or beta at a dose of 0.2 mg/kg. *PLoS One*. 2007; 2(7): e598.
52. Ries M, Clarke JT, et al. Enzyme-replacement therapy with agalsidase alfa in children with Fabry disease. *Pediatrics*. 2006; 118(3): 924–932.
53. Ramaswami U, Wendt S, et al. Enzyme replacement therapy with agalsidase alfa in children with Fabry disease. *Acta Paediatr*. 2007; 96(1): 122–127.
54. Hilz MJ, Brys M, et al. Enzyme replacement therapy improves function of C-, Adelta-, and Abeta-nerve fibers in Fabry neuropathy. *Neurology*. 2004; 62(7): 1066–1072.

55. Schiffmann R, Floeter MK, et al. Enzyme replacement therapy improves peripheral nerve and sweat function in Fabry disease. *Muscle Nerve.* 2003; 28(6): 703–710.
56. Dehout F, Roland D, et al. Relief of gastrointestinal symptoms under enzyme replacement therapy [corrected] in patients with Fabry disease. *J Inherit Metab Dis.* 2004; 27(4): 499–505.
57. Warnock DG, Daina E, et al. Enzyme replacement therapy and Fabry nephropathy. *Clin J Am Soc Nephrol.* 2010; 5(2): 371–378.
58. Wraith JE, Tylki-Szymanska A, et al. Safety and efficacy of enzyme replacement therapy with agalsidase beta: an international, open-label study in pediatric patients with Fabry disease. *J Pediatr.* 2008; 152(4): 563–570, 570 e561.
59. Valayannopoulos V, Nicely H, et al. Mucopolysaccharidosis VI. *Orphanet J Rare Dis.* 2010; 5: 5.
60. Swiedler SJ, Beck M, et al. Threshold effect of urinary glycosaminoglycans and the walk test as indicators of disease progression in a survey of subjects with Mucopolysaccharidosis VI (Maroteaux-Lamy syndrome). *Am J Med Genet A.* 2005; 134A(2): 144–150.
61. Herskhovitz E, Young E, et al. Bone marrow transplantation for Maroteaux-Lamy syndrome (MPS VI): long-term follow-up. *J Inherit Metab Dis.* 1999; 22(1): 50–62.
62. Rovelli AM. The controversial and changing role of haematopoietic cell transplantation for lysosomal storage disorders: an update. *Bone Marrow Transplant.* 2008; 41(Suppl. 2): S87–S89.
63. Harmatz P, Ketteridge D, et al. Direct comparison of measures of endurance, mobility, and joint function during enzyme-replacement therapy of mucopolysaccharidosis VI (Maroteaux-Lamy syndrome): results after 48 weeks in a phase 2 open-label clinical study of recombinant human N-acetylgalactosamine 4-sulfatase. *Pediatrics.* 2005; 115(6): e681–e689.
64. Harmatz P, Kramer, WG, et al. Pharmacokinetic profile of recombinant human N-acetylgalactosamine 4-sulphatase enzyme replacement therapy in patients with mucopolysaccharidosis VI (Maroteaux-Lamy syndrome): a phase I/II study. *Acta Paediatr Suppl.* 2005; 94(447): 61–68; discussion 57.
65. Harmatz P, Giugliani R, et al. 2006; Enzyme replacement therapy for mucopolysaccharidosis VI: a phase 3, randomized, double-blind, placebo-controlled, multinational study of recombinant human N-acetylgalactosamine 4-sulfatase (recombinant human arylsulfatase B or rhASB) and follow-on, open-label extension study. *J Pediatr.* 2006; 148(4): 533–539.
66. Harmatz P, Giugliani R, et al. Long-term follow-up of endurance and safety outcomes during enzyme replacement therapy for mucopolysaccharidosis VI: Final results of three clinical studies of recombinant human N-acetylgalactosamine 4-sulfatase. *Mol Genet Metab.* 2008; 94(4): 469–475.
67. McGill JJ, Inwood AC, et al. Enzyme replacement therapy for mucopolysaccharidosis VI from 8 weeks of age—a sibling control study. *Clin Genet.* 2010; 77(5): 492–498.
68. Dickson PI, Chen AH. Intrathecal enzyme replacement therapy for mucopolysaccharidosis I: translating success in animal models to patients. *Curr Pharm Biotech.* 2011; 12(6): 946–955.
69. Vera M, Le S, Kan SH, et al. Immune response to intrathecal enzyme replacement therapy in mucopolysaccharidosis I patients. *Pediatr Res.* 2013; 74(6): 712–720
70. Sands MS, Vogler CA, et al. Biodistribution, kinetics, and efficacy of highly phosphorylated and non-phosphorylated beta-glucuronidase in the murine model of mucopolysaccharidosis VII. *J Biol Chem.* 2001; 276(46): 43160–43165.
71. Brooks DA, Kakavanos R, et al. Significance of immune response to enzyme-replacement therapy for patients with a lysosomal storage disorder. *Trends Mol Med.* 2003; 9(10): 450–453.
72. Bodensteiner D, Scott CR, et al. Successful reinstitution of agalsidase beta therapy in Fabry disease patients with previous IgE-antibody or skin-test reactivity to the recombinant enzyme. *Genet Med.* 2008; 10(5): 353–358.
73. Brady RO, Murray GJ, et al. Management of neutralizing antibody to Ceredase in a patient with type 3 Gaucher disease. *Pediatrics.* 1997; 100(6): E11.
74. Germain DP, Kaneski CR, et al. Mutation analysis of the acid beta-glucosidase gene in a patient with type 3 Gaucher disease and neutralizing antibody to alglucerase. *Mutat Res.* 2001; 483(1–2): 89–94.
75. Zhao H, Bailey LA, et al. Enzyme therapy of gaucher disease: clinical and biochemical changes during production of and tolerization for neutralizing antibodies. *Blood Cells Mol Dis.* 2003; 30(1): 90–96.
76. Banugaria SG, Prater SN, et al. The impact of antibodies on clinical outcomes in diseases treated with therapeutic protein: lessons learned from infantile Pompe disease. *Genet Med.* 2011; 13(8): 729–736.
77. Koeberl DD, Kishnani PS. Immunomodulatory gene therapy in lysosomal storage disorders. *Curr Gene Ther.* 2009; 9(6): 503–510.

78. Banugaria SG, Prater SN, Patel TT, et al. Algorithm for the early diagnosis and treatment of patients with cross reactive immunologic material-negative classic infantile pompe disease: a step towards improving the efficacy of ERT. *PLoS One.* 2013; 8(6): e67052.
79. Platt FM, Jeyakumar M. Substrate reduction therapy. *Acta Paediatr Suppl.* 2008; 97(457): 88–93.
80. Cox T, Lachmann R, et al. Novel oral treatment of Gaucher's disease with N-butyldeoxynojirimycin (OGT 918) to decrease substrate biosynthesis. *Lancet.* 2000; 355(9214): 1481–1485.
81. Patterson MC, Vecchio D, et al. Miglustat for treatment of Niemann-Pick C disease: a randomised controlled study. *Lancet Neurol.* 2007; 6(9): 765–772.
82. Breen C, Wynn RF, O'Meara A, et al. Developmental outcome post allogenic bone marrow transplant for Niemann Pick Type C2. *Mol Genet Metab.* 2013; 108(1): 82–84.
83. Giraldo P, Alfonso P, et al. Real-world clinical experience with long-term miglustat maintenance therapy in type 1 Gaucher disease: the ZAGAL project. *Haematologica.* 2009; 94(12): 1771–1775.
84. Hollak CE, Hughes D, et al. Miglustat (Zavesca) in type 1 Gaucher disease: 5-year results of a post-authorisation safety surveillance programme. *Pharmacoepidemiol Drug Saf.* 2009; 18(9): 770–777.
85. Lukina E, Watman N, Arreguin EA, et al. Improvement in hematological, visceral, and skeletal manifestations of Gaucher disease type 1 with oral eliglustat tartrate (Genz-112638) treatment: 2-year results of a phase 2 study. *Blood.* 2010; 116(20): 4095–4098.
86. Piotrowska E, Jakobkiewicz-Banecka J, et al. Genistein-mediated inhibition of glycosaminoglycan synthesis as a basis for gene expression-targeted isoflavone therapy for mucopolysaccharidoses. *Eur J Hum Genet.* 2006; 14(7): 846–852.
87. Brown JR., Crawford BE, et al. Glycan antagonists and inhibitors: a fount for drug discovery. *Crit Rev Biochem Mol Biol.* 2007; 42(6): 481–515.
88. Kleta R, Gahl WA. Pharmacological treatment of nephropathic cystinosis with cysteamine. *Expert Opin Pharmacother.* 2004; 5(11): 2255–2262.
89. Fan JQ. Pharmacological chaperone therapy for lysosomal storage disorders—leveraging aspects of the folding pathway to maximize activity of misfolded mutant proteins. *Febs J.* 2007; 274(19): 4943.
90. Lieberman RL, D'Aquino AJ, et al. Effects of pH and iminosugar pharmacological chaperones on lysosomal glycosidase structure and stability. *Biochemistry.* 2009; 48(22): 4816–4827.
91. Porto C, Cardone M, Fontana F, et al. The pharmacological chaperone N-butyldeoxynojirimycin enhances enzyme replacement therapy in Pompe disease fibroblasts. *Mol Ther.* 2009; Jun; 17(6): 964–971.
92. Mu TW, Ong DS, et al. Chemical and biological approaches synergize to ameliorate protein-folding diseases. *Cell.* 2008; 134(5): 769–781.
93. Ong DS, Mu TW, et al. Endoplasmic reticulum Ca2+ increases enhance mutant glucocerebrosidase proteostasis. *Nat Chem Biol.* 2010; 6(6): 424–432.
94. Yang C, Rahimpour S, Lu J, et al. Histone deacetylase inhibitors increase glucocerebrosidase activity in Gaucher disease by modulation of molecular chaperones. *Proc Natl Acad Sci USA.* 2013; 110(3): 966–971.
95. Hein LK, Bawden M, et al. Alpha-L-iduronidase premature stop codons and potential read-through in mucopolysaccharidosis type I patients. *J Mol Biol.* 2004; 338(3): 453–462.
96. Brooks DA, Muller VJ, et al. Stop-codon read-through for patients affected by a lysosomal storage disorder. *Trends Mol Med.* 2006; 12(8): 367–373.
97. Keeling KM, Brooks DA, et al. Gentamicin-mediated suppression of Hurler syndrome stop mutations restores a low level of alpha-L-iduronidase activity and reduces lysosomal glycosaminoglycan accumulation. *Hum Mol Genet.* 2001; 10(3): 291–299.
98. Kamei M, Kasperski K, Fuller M, et al. Aminoglycoside-induced premature stop codon read-through of mucopolysaccharidosis type i patient Q70X and W402X mutations in cultured cells. *JIMD Rep.* 2013 Nov 6.
99. Cearley CN, Wolfe JH. A single injection of an adeno-associated virus vector into nuclei with divergent connections results in widespread vector distribution in the brain and global correction of a neurogenetic disease. *J Neurosci.* 2007; 27(37): 9928–9940.
100. Haskins M. Gene therapy for lysosomal storage diseases (LSDs) in large animal models. *ILAR J.* 2009; 50(2): 112–121.
101. Biffi A, De Palma M, et al. Correction of metachromatic leukodystrophy in the mouse model by transplantation of genetically modified hematopoietic stem cells. *J Clin Invest.* 2004; 113(8): 1118–1129.

102. Biffi A, Montini E, Lorioli L, et al. Lentiviral hematopoietic stem cell gene therapy benefits metachromatic leukodystrophy. *Science*. 2013; 341(6148): 1233158.
103. Worgall S Sondhi D, et al. Treatment of late infantile neuronal ceroid lipofuscinosis by CNS administration of a serotype 2 adeno-associated virus expressing CLN2 cDNA. *Hum Gene Ther*. 2008; 19(5): 463–474.
104. Souweidane M, Fraser JF, Arkin LM, et al. Gene therapy for late infantile neuronal ceroid lipofuscinosis: neurosurgical considerations. *J Neurosurg Pediatr*. 2010; 6(2): 115–122.
105. Du L, Gatti RA. Progress toward therapy with antisense-mediated splicing modulation. *Curr Opin Mol Ther*. 2009; 11(2): 116–123.
106. Du L, Jung ME, Damoiseaux R, et al. A new series of small molecular weight compounds induce read through of all three types of nonsense mutations in the ATM gene. *Mol Ther*. 2013; 21(9): 1653–1660.
107. Rodriguez-Pascau L, Coll MJ, et al. Antisense oligonucleotide treatment for a pseudoexon-generating mutation in the NPC1 gene causing Niemann-Pick type C disease. *Hum Mutat*. 2009; 30(11): E993–E1001.
108. Karras A, De Lentdecker P, et al. Combined heart and kidney transplantation in a patient with Fabry disease in the enzyme replacement therapy era. *Am J Transplant*. 2008; 8(6): 1345–1348.
109. Nesterova G, Gahl W. Nephropathic cystinosis: late complications of a multisystemic disease. *Pediatr Nephrol*. 2008; 23(6): 863–878.
110. Ayto RM, Hughes DA, et al. Long-term outcomes of liver transplantation in type 1 Gaucher disease. *Am J Transplant*. 2010; 10(8): 1934–1939.
111. Platt FM, Boland B, van der Spoel AC. The cell biology of disease: lysosomal storage disorders: the cellular impact of lysosomal dysfunction. *J Cell Biol*. 2012; 199(5): 723–734.
112. Hemsley KM, Hopwood JJ. Delivery of recombinant proteins via the cerebrospinal fluid as a therapy option for neurodegenerative lysosomal storage diseases. *Int J Clin Pharmacol Ther*. 2009; 47(Suppl. 1): S118–S123.
113. Hemsley KM, Luck AJ, et al. Examination of intravenous and intra-CSF protein delivery for treatment of neurological disease. *Eur J Neurosci*. 2009; 29(6): 1197–1214.
114. Jeyakumar M, Thomas R, et al. Central nervous system inflammation is a hallmark of pathogenesis in mouse models of GM1 and GM2 gangliosidosis. *Brain*. 2003; 126(Pt 4): 974–987.
115. Jeyakumar M, Smith DA, Williams IM, et al. NSAIDs increase survival in the Sandhoff disease mouse: synergy with N-butyldeoxynojirimycin. *Ann Neurol*. 2004; 56(5): 642–649.
116. Alvarez AR, Klein A, et al. Imatinib therapy blocks cerebellar apoptosis and improves neurological symptoms in a mouse model of Niemann-Pick type C disease. *Faseb J*. 2008; 22(10): 3617–3627.
117. Pastores GM, Wallenstein S, et al. Bone density in Type 1 Gaucher disease. *J Bone Miner Res*. 1996; 11(11): 1801–1807.
118. Germain DP, Benistan K, et al. Osteopenia and osteoporosis: previously unrecognized manifestations of Fabry disease. *Clin Genet*. 2005; 68(1): 93–95.
119. van den Berg LE, Zandbergen AA, et al. Low bone mass in Pompe disease: muscular strength as a predictor of bone mineral density. *Bone*. 2010; 47(3): 643–649.
120. Wenstrup RJ, Bailey L, et al. Gaucher disease: alendronate disodium improves bone mineral density in adults receiving enzyme therapy. *Blood*. 2004; 104(5): 1253–1257.
121. Ortiz A, Oliveira JP, et al. Recommendations and guidelines for the diagnosis and treatment of Fabry nephropathy in adults. *Nature Clin Pract Nephr*. 2008; 4(6): 327–336.
122. Kaback MM. Screening and prevention in Tay-Sachs disease: origins, update, and impact. *Adv Genet*. 2001; 44: 253–265.
123. Hwu WL, Chien YH, et al. Newborn screening for neuropathic lysosomal storage disorders. *J Inherit Metab Dis*. 2010; 33(4): 381–386.

15

Chaperone Therapy for the Lysosomal Storage Disorders

ALEXANDER J. CHOI, ROBERT BURNETT, EHUD GOLDIN,
WEI ZHENG, AND ELLEN SIDRANSKY

Introduction—Principles of Chaperone Therapy

Lysosomal storage disorders (LSDs) are a group of more than 50 rare, inborn errors of metabolism that result from defects in lysosomal function.[1] In these disorders, genetic mutations lead to the deficiency of a specific lysosomal enzyme or a transporter, resulting in the build-up of its corresponding substrate. The deficiency of lysosomal enzymes can occur as a result of (i) reduced synthesis of the mutant enzyme; (ii) misfolding of the mutant enzyme, which decreases biological activity; or (iii) instability of the mutant protein that leads to degradation, though the mutant protein may have normal activity.[2] The consequent accumulation of the substrate in lysosomes results in the associated symptoms. In most LSDs, the amount of the mutated protein in lysosomes is greatly reduced, although they usually retain some residual function. Therefore, increasing the amount of mutant protein in the lysosome is a potential therapeutic approach for the treatment of LSDs. Therapies currently available for several of the LSDs include enzyme replacement therapy (ERT) and substrate reduction therapy (SRT); however, the majority of the LSDs still lack any effective treatment.

In recent years, scientific insights into the cell biology of lysosomal pathways have led to a new therapeutic approach involving pharmacological chaperones. These drugs can be administered orally and have the potential to penetrate the blood–brain barrier (BBB) to exert functional activity in neuronal tissues. Pharmacological chaperones are small molecule drugs designed to selectively bind specific proteins. They increase enzyme integrity by stabilizing the misfolded protein, thereby assisting the trafficking of the mutant enzyme to the target site, e.g., the lysosome.[3] Most lysosomal enzymes are glycosylated and folded at a neutral pH in the endoplasmic reticulum (ER) before being transported to the lysosome. During protein synthesis and post-translational modification, cellular chaperones, such

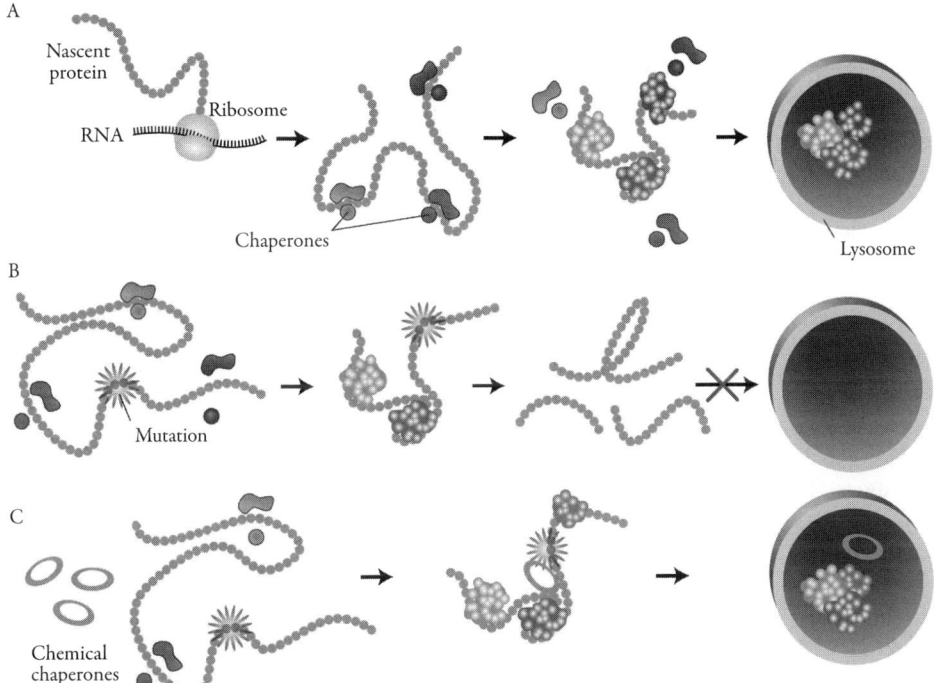

FIGURE 15.1 (A) Wild-type enzyme: The normal protein folding process is shown. The enzyme is synthesized and folded with the assistance of cellular chaperones. After post-translational modification, the folded enzyme is transported into the lysosome. (B) Mutant enzyme: The mutant enzyme is synthesized but cannot fold properly due to the mutation. The protein is subsequently degraded or aggregates into an aberrant protein; the enzyme is not transported to the lysosome. (C) Mutant enzyme corrected with a pharmacologic chaperone: As in (B), the mutant enzyme is synthesized but cannot fold properly. However, the pharmacological chaperone binds to the active site of the misfolded enzyme, preventing its premature degradation and facilitating its trafficking into the lysosome.

as Hsp90 and Hsp70, commonly assist in the protein folding processes (Figure 15.1A). However, genetic mutations or sequence errors can occur during protein synthesis, causing misfolding of the newly synthesized protein. This leads to early degradation or aggregation of the aberrant protein (Figure 15.1B). Chaperone therapy targets this pathophysiologic process, aiming to prevent or correct misfolding and mistrafficking of mutant proteins. Many pharmacologic chaperones are competitive inhibitors of the target enzyme that bind to the active site of the misfolded enzyme. They assist in proper folding of the enzyme, prevent premature degradation, and facilitate trafficking of the mutant protein from the ER to the lysosome, where the drug is outcompeted and displaced by the abundant substrates accumulated in the lysosome (Figure 15.1C). In the lysosome, the properly folded mutant enzyme is able to hydrolyze and remove the accumulated substrates, resulting in an improvement in the associated clinical symptoms. Because most of these small molecules bind at the active site of the wild-type enzyme, this approach best targets mutations that do not affect the topology of the enzyme's active site. Although many enzyme inhibitors have been explored as pharmacological chaperones in several LSDs, a small molecule chaperone with the property to bind and activate the enzyme is a better choice for chaperone therapy.

Current Therapy for the Lysosomal Storage Disorders
Enzyme Replacement Therapy

Currently, the preferred therapy for the LSDs is ERT, which has been developed for several specific disorders. By supplying patients with the exogenous enzyme, ERT aims to restore the functional enzyme quantity, to reduce the amount of accumulated substrate in the lysosome. The introduction of ERT has led to the successful management of diseases that were once considered untreatable. Currently approved ERTs target Fabry disease,[4, 5] Gaucher disease (GD),[6] several mucopolysaccharidoses (MPS I,[7] MPS II,[8] and MPS VI[9]), and Pompe disease.[10] Although ERT was once considered a panacea for the LSDs, it does have several important limitations.

The first successful ERT was developed for type 1 GD. The infusion of recombinant glucocerebrosidase (GCase) to patients with GD successfully reversed most of the visceral manifestations presented with the disease.[11] However, the therapy has not been successful in treating the neurologic manifestations found in the neuronopathic forms of GD (types 2 and 3). Currently, three different ERT products—imiglucerase (Genzyme), velaglucerase alfa (Shire), and taliglucerase alfa (Protalix BioTherapeutics)—have been approved for the treatment of GD. The intravenously administered enzyme does not cross the BBB, and fails to ameliorate the central nervous system (CNS) pathology associated with this disorder.[12, 13] Different strategies have been considered to circumvent this problem with CNS delivery in patients with neuronopathic involvement.[14] One strategy to facilitate the enzyme entry into the brain involves Trojan horse technology in which a monoclonal antibody is attached to both the human insulin receptor and the enzyme. Another potential method for transporting the recombinant enzyme across the BBB is to add the protein transduction domain of HIV-1 Tat protein to the enzyme. To date, none of these strategies have been used in clinical settings to reduce neurologic complications of the LSDs, but they may play a role in the development of future treatment options for the LSDs.

Despite the success in treating non-neuronopathic GD with the recombinant enzyme, other LSDs did not have the same dramatic therapeutic effect with ERT treatments. For example, in Fabry disease, ERT seems most effective when given to mildly affected patients. Treatment in patients with Fabry disease with near normal renal function at baseline often can preserve renal function and prevent progression of cardiac hypertrophy. However, patients with significant renal dysfunction are less likely to see improvements in disease manifestations, e.g., cardiac hypertrophy and/or renal function. Moreover, unlike in GD, male patients with Fabry disease frequently have no residual enzymatic activity, and thus are more likely to develop antibodies to the infused enzyme.[15, 16]

In Pompe disease, the effectiveness of ERT is also limited. While infants with this disease have shown astounding improvements in cardiac function, growth, and development, the overall clinical response is still restricted by insufficient uptake of the enzyme by skeletal muscles.[17] In addition, the development of antibodies in response to ERT in infants without residual enzymatic activity has devastating effects, ultimately resulting in death.[18] In some adults, the overall efficacy of ERT can also be decreased due to the above phemomena.[19]

Similar to neuronopathic forms of GD, ERT for MPS I did not result in an improvement of neurological symptoms in patients with neuronopathic manifestations, although improvements were seen in upper respiratory and visceral symptoms. ERT may have limited efficacy in the attenuated forms of MPS I, where patients primarily exhibit skeletal features.[20]

While ERT has extended and saved many lives, it has significant limitations. It is not a cure but a palliative treatment that is inconvenient because the exogenous enzyme must be infused intravenously every two weeks, requiring frequent visit to a physician for the duration of one's life. Also, the average cost of ERT ranges from $40,000 to $500,000 per patient per year, which is burdensome to both patients and society as a whole.[21] This high cost also limits the distribution of the therapy in developing countries.

Substrate Reduction Therapy

A second available therapy for several of the LSDs is SRT, which reduces substrate accumulation by inhibiting the synthesis of the substrate or the precursor of the mutant enzyme. The goal of SRT is not to completely inhibit the formation of these substrates, but to balance and stabilize the rate of their metabolism. Since many of the glycosphingolipids implicated in the LSDs are required by the body and have important roles in cellular lipid homeostasis, the concept of SRT was initially viewed with some concern.[22] Another challenge of SRT is finding a proper target enzyme that can be inhibited, without risking the development of another type of LSD. For example, unesterified cholesterol accumulates in lysosomes of patients with Niemann Pick disease type C due to mutations in the NPC1 or NPC2 protein. The unesterified cholesterol is the product of acid lipase that hydrolyzes cholesteryl ester to unesterified cholesterol in lysosomes. Reduction of free cholesterol formation by inhibiting acid lipase in the lysosome could theoretically result in Wolman disease, a different LSD caused by the deficiency of acid lipase. Despite these theoretical concerns, successful preclinical and mouse studies with SRT have led to progress toward clinical trials for Sandhoff disease.[23, 24]

Currently, only one SRT, miglustat (N-butyldeoxynojirimycin, "Zavesca"), has been approved by the the US Food and Drug Administration for patients with type 1 GD. Miglustat reversibly inhibits glucosylceramide synthase, the enzyme that catalyzes the biosynthesis of glucosylceramide. Clinical trials of miglustat demonstrated visceral and hematopoietic improvements in patients with a mild form of type 1 GD. However, the results can be variable, and side effects and a high withdrawal rate have led to disinterest among some patients.[25, 26] Some studies evaluating whether it would be feasible for patients currently on ERT to switch to SRT[27-29] indicate that SRT may be an effective treatment for long-term maintenance. In addition, miglustat has also been approved in Europe for the treatment of Niemann-Pick disease type C, although its mechanism of action is still unclear.[30]

SRT is a relatively new approach for drug development, and several other drugs are under development and in clinical trials. One promising substrate reduction therapy for type 1 GD is eliglustat tartrate.[31] The drug can be administered orally and has been shown to specifically inhibit glucosylceramide synthase, the enzyme that produces glucosylceramide. Preliminary studies show improvements in anemia, thrombocytopenia, hepatosplenomegaly, and skeletal manifestations over a 52-week period.[31] These results show that SRT presents a safe, effective, and convenient means of treatment for certain types of LSDs.

A study of miglustat in neuronopathic GD indicated that the drug failed to impact the neurologic parameters being evaluated.[32] While no human studies have yet to demonstrate clear improvements in neurological symptoms, scientists and physicians are hard at work continuing to improve the SRT for neuronopathic GD. A recently developed glucosylceramide synthase inhibitor, GZ 161, has been shown to decrease neurological complications in type 2 GD mouse models.[33] The compound, when systemically administered to these mice, was found to reduce brain neuropathology and extend lifespan. Future discoveries and manipulations of drugs like GZ 161 may have the potential as a therapy for patients afflicted with neuronopathic LSDs.

The Concept of Pharmacologic Chaperones

Compared to ERT and SRT, pharmacological chaperones may offer a less expensive, easily administered, and more convenient regimen for the treatment of the LSDs. Because they are small molecule drugs, pharmacological chaperones can usually be administered orally and can reach the tissues efficiently. An added benefit is that they can be optimized for penetration into the brain by crossing the BBB, rendering them to be attractive therapeutics for alleviating neurological symptoms of LSDs. Moreover, their size and specificity to the enzyme can thwart the development of antibodies and limit side effects once the specificity of the drug is optimized. The convenience of administration and reduced production costs allow for a more regular and continuous treatment for the patients, when compared to ERT.

While not all mutations would be amenable to the actions of chaperones, many of the mutations identified in patients with LSDs are missense mutations, leading to a misfolded enzyme that could be degraded prematurely. Protein misfolding and subsequent dysfunction of the mutant enzymes lead to lysosomal storage of related lipids. The degradation of misfolded and dysfunctional enzymes is constantly monitored by the cells via the process of endoplasmic reticulum associated degradation (ERAD).[34] This quality-control system monitors the integrity and conformation of the proteins in the ER by weeding out the misfolded proteins for degradation before they are delivered to the target cellular organelles. Proteins that are incorrectly folded in the ER are subsequently translocated to the cytosol where they are degraded by proteasomes before they reach their target site in cells.[34]

Pharmacological chaperones ameliorate the enzymatic deficiency in the cells by binding to the newly synthesized mutant protein, stabilizing its conformation, and preventing its premature degradation. The pharmacological chaperone often binds to the active sites of the enzymes, rendering them as competitive enzyme inhibitors by nature. The pharmacological chaperone-stabilized mutant enzyme escapes ERAD after protein synthesis and then translocates to lysosomes. It is assumed that in the low pH environment, the high substrate concentration in the lysosome releases the noncovalently bound chaperone molecule from the enzyme. The active site on the mutant enzyme is then replaced with the endogenous substrates that have accumulated in the lysosomes due to the enzyme deficiency.[35] However, for such chaperone therapy to work effectively, the active site of the mutant enzyme must remain intact and should have residual activity. Pharmacological chaperones are not useful when the protein is not produced, as in the case of null alleles, and they may not be potent when the mutation affects the active site.

In cases where the active site topology has been changed such that the natural substrate is unable to bind, or the protein is not produced at all due to a null allele, pharmacological chaperones could potentially increase the efficacy of ERT.[36] A compound that stabilizes the exogenous protein in the lysosome may increase the half-life of the recombinant enzyme, thus reducing the inconvenience of frequent intravenous infusion of the recombinant proteins and the financial burden of ERT.

Animal Studies and Clinical Trials of Pharmacologic Chaperones for Lysosomal Storage Disorders

Recently, three small molecule chaperones have been advanced to clinical trials for the LSDs: isofagomine (IFG) for type 1 GD, 1-deoxygalactonojirimycin (DGJ) for Fabry disease, and 1-deoxynojirimycin (DNJ) for Pompe disease.[2]

IFG (AT2101, "Plicera") is an active site inhibitor of GCase. Treatment of skin fibroblasts from patients with GD homozygous for the p.Asn409Ser ("N370S") mutation of GCase with IFG resulted in an increased amount of mutant enzyme and enhanced activity in the lysosome,[37] although the response was much less robust in p.Leu483Pro ("L444P") mutated fibroblasts.[38] Administration of IFG to mice with human WT GCase, as well as endogenous V394L GCase, resulted in increased GCase activity in both forms of the enzyme over an eight-week period. Another study showed that IFG delayed the onset of neurological symptoms and extended the life of V394L homozygous mice, suggesting that pharmacological chaperones have the ability to cross the BBB and to alleviate central nervous system symptoms.[39] IFG increased the activity of GCase in cell lysates by two- to five-fold and enhanced lysosomal translocation in disease-relevant tissues, including the brain.[3,38] Unfortunately, initial results of IFG in a phase 2 clinical trial of patients with GD type 1 who had not been treated with ERT or SRT were disappointing, although IFG treatment was continued for six months. While it was found that GCase enzymatic activity increased in white blood cells, there was no significant improvement in disease manifestations. The study is currently on hold and a phase 3 clinical trial of IFG has been cancelled.[40] Another compound, ambroxol, identified through a screen of approved drugs, is being explored as a potential therapy for GD.[41] A pilot study indicated that ambroxol increased platelet counts and decreased spleen volumes in patients with type 1 GD over a 52-week period.[41,42] Moreover, ambroxol, administered to patients with neuronopathic GD with mutation p.N188S, was reported to improve neurological symptoms, specifically oculomotor dysfunction and myoclonus.[2] However, there have not been adequate controlled studies conducted with this drug.

DGJ (AT1001, "Amigal") is a competitive inhibitor of alpha-galactosidase A (α-gal). DGJ was reported to enhance the activity of α-gal in transgenic R301Q mutant mice and in human fibroblast cell lines from patients with Fabry disease.[43,44] One study showed that introducing DGJ to fibroblasts of a transgenic mouse expressing mutated human α-gal prevented the mutated enzyme from forming a complex with BiP, one of the cellular chaperones involved in ERAD.[45] Immunofluorescence data showed that in mutant mice treated with DGJ, the rescued α-gal was translocated to the lysosome. Moreover, in fibroblasts from patients with Fabry disease, administration of DGJ significantly reduced the amount of the accumulated substrate globotriaosylceramide in the lysosome. Positive results from the phase 2 safety and tolerability clinical study were reported, and the development of DGJ as an oral therapy for Fabry disease looks promising. The effectiveness of DGJ in phase 3 clinical trials is currently being evaluated.[40]

DNJ (AT2220) is a competitive inhibitor of alpha-glucosidase (α-glu). Based on *in vitro* studies, DNJ was shown to significantly increase enzyme levels and activity in patient-derived fibroblasts from patients with Pompe disease and in transiently transfected COS-7 cells.[46] As with DGJ, the data from immunofluorescence studies in patient fibroblasts demonstrated an increased amount of α-glu in the lysosome after the administration of DNJ, indicating stabilization of the mutant enzyme and subsequent translocation to lysosomes.[46] DNJ is currently being tested in a phase 1 clinical study to evaluate the pharmacokinetics of binding in muscle from healthy adult subjects.[40]

It has been proposed that a combination therapy using both pharmacological chaperone therapy and ERT could result in a better therapeutic regimen for patients. Some *in vitro* studies have shown that pharmacological chaperones can be used as an enhancement and a sustenance agent for the exogenous enzymes to prolong and augment the effect of functional enzyme (endogenous or exogenous) and thereby reduce the frequency of intravenous administration of the exogenous enzymes. One such study showed that when DGJ was administered with recombinant α-gal A in a mouse model of Fabry disease, the half-life of the recombinant enzyme increased, improving enzymatic activity and reducing substrate levels in tissues compared to mice treated with recombinant enzyme alone.[47] Such studies suggest that incubation of the recombinant enzyme with its respective pharmacological chaperone can result in increased activity and stability of the exogenous enzyme, as well as improvement of its lysosomal trafficking.[48,49] However, the *in vivo* data is still preliminary and must be validated in further experiments.

Enzyme Activators as Pharmacological Chaperones

Most of the pharmacological chaperones that are currently in the literature or under development for LSDs are enzyme inhibitors. This is due to the presence of readily available enzyme inhibitors, and because enzyme inhibitors are easier to identify. However, the use of enzyme inhibitors for chaperone therapy may have inherent disadvantages, as there is a need to balance a compound's chaperone activity with its direct inhibition of enzyme activity. Most of the pharmacological chaperones discussed above are potent enzyme inhibitors. The use of an inhibitor to enhance the activity of a mutant enzyme is a somewhat uncertain prospect *in vivo*. With inhibitors, drug dosing and the interval length between drug administrations must be specifically designed to offset the enzyme inhibitory effect of the drugs. It has been reported that once mutant enzymes are translocated to lysosomes by pharmacological chaperones, they can remain functional for several days.[50] Thus, it is postulated that inhibitors might need to be given at intervals as every one to two weeks.[51] Based on these shortcomings, enzyme activators appear to be a naturally better choice as pharmacological chaperones.

An enzyme activator will similarly bind to the mutant protein and help correct its folding and trafficking to the lysosome. Moreover, the activator can directly enhance the residual activity of the mutant enzymes that are newly translocated or already present in the lysosome. In theory, both the chaperoning and enzyme stimulatory ability of the activator chaperone would synergistically restore the function of a mutant enzyme in the lysosome. However, enzyme activators bind to nonenzymatic pockets on the enzyme's surface, making them difficult to identify compared to inhibitors. Nevertheless, the discovery and development of small molecule activators may provide a new approach for chaperone therapy for the treatment of LSDs. Indeed, we have recently found a series of chaperone compounds with enzyme activator capability for mutant α-glu via a high throughput screening (HTS).[52] Several promising lead compounds have been identified that can chaperone mutant glucosidase to the lysosome in patient fibroblasts[53] but at the same time do not inhibit the enzyme, as shown through immunostaining studies.

Small molecule chaperones are usually identified by screening compound libraries using the wild-type enzyme in the screening assay. During the assay development and optimization process, the enzymatic activity is usually optimized to near maximal activity by changing buffer components, the amount of enzyme and substrate, and incubation times in order to increase the window and sensitivity of a screen assay. The wild-type enzyme is usually used for the development of the screening assay due to its availability and because it has the inherent enzymatic activity needed for appropriate assay window and sensitivity. Since the enzymatic activity in most screening assays has already reached the highest detectable level, these assays can easily identify inhibitors from the compound libraries, but not the enzyme activators. In the LSDs, the mutant forms of the enzymes have reduced activity. Thus it is logical to use the mutant, rather than the wild-type enzyme for the screening assay to identify the enzyme activators as pharmacological chaperones. For example, in the case of GD, specific activators were identified by using the p.Asn409Ser ("N370S") mutant form of the enzyme for compound screening.[54]

The other type of pharmacological chaperone is neither an enzyme activator nor inhibitor but binds to the mutant enzyme and stabilizes its structure. The screening assay with high throughput capability for such compounds is difficult to develop because of the nature of small molecule-protein binding assays. It will be necessary to develop new technologies and methods for HTS in order to identify this new type of chaperone compound from compound library screens.

Ultimately, pharmacological chaperones function to correct the enzyme deficiency by rebalancing cellular proteostasis. The function of protein degradation by way of the proteasome is tightly regulated with regard to protein concentration, conformation, binding interactions, and trafficking into subcellular locations by transcriptional and translational mechanisms.[55] Protein folding, as well as an intricate network of interactive proteins, can

TABLE 15.1 **Types of Different Chaperones**

Name	Molecular Nature	Description
Cellular or Protein Chaperone	Proteins, naturally occurring	A protein factor that aids in the correct folding of a newly synthesized protein. It also protects the nascent polypeptide chain from undesirable associations until it can fold properly. Examples are calnexin, calreticulin, and BiP.
Chemical Chaperone	Small molecule	These are small molecules that can stabilize mutant proteins. In contrast to pharmacological chaperones, they are nonspecific, and high compound concentrations are required. Chemical chaperones nonspecifically bind to and stabilize many proteins without a specific binding site. Examples of chemical chaperones include glycerol, DMSO, and trehalose.
Pharmacological Chaperone	Small molecule	These small molecules are designed specifically to bind to a target protein.
Proteostasis Regulator	Small molecule	These molecules enhance protein formation after synthesis at the level of the ER by lifting the overly strict checkpoint controls. They may be broadly applicable for a series of enzymes. Examples include proteasomal inhibitors and agents that modulate calcium influx such as verapamil, diltiazem, and celastrol.

Note. DMSO = dimethyl sulfoxide; ER = endoplasmic reticulum.

affect the balance and regulation in proteostasis.[56] Thus, another approach in chaperone therapy is the identification of small molecules that can enhance protein maturation after synthesis by lifting overly strict checkpoint controls. "Proteostasis regulators" are small molecules that can have an effect on the production of many different proteins. Some of the proteostasis regulators being considered for the LSDs include proteasomal inhibitors and calcium channel blockers such as verapamil, diltiazem, and celastrol (Table 15.1). However, this therapeutic strategy still requires validation in disease models, and better proteostasis compounds are needed for future studies.

The Process of Pharmacological Chaperone Discovery

The promising preclinical and clinical results, along with the logical hypothesis of pharmacological chaperone therapy, have stimulated further investigation and development of these small molecules as a new therapy for rare genetic diseases. Still, the process of drug discovery and development of pharmacological chaperones involves multiple steps and can take many years (Figure 15.2).

Target Identification

Target identification is the first step of small molecule drug discovery, where a biological target protein for drug therapy is identified and validated. For example, the most direct target in GD is the enzyme GCase, since its enzymatic activity is reduced in lysosomes due to genetic mutations. Correction of the deficiency in lysosomal GCase activity by a pharmacological chaperone is a clear goal of drug development. In addition, enhancement of the residual mutant GCase activity in the lysosome may be considered as well. Other targets, such as the ERAD pathway for post-translational protein processing, might also be considered as a means to decrease premature degradation of mutant enzymes, enhancing translocation to the lysosomes. Histone deacetylase inhibitors (HDACis) were shown to be effective

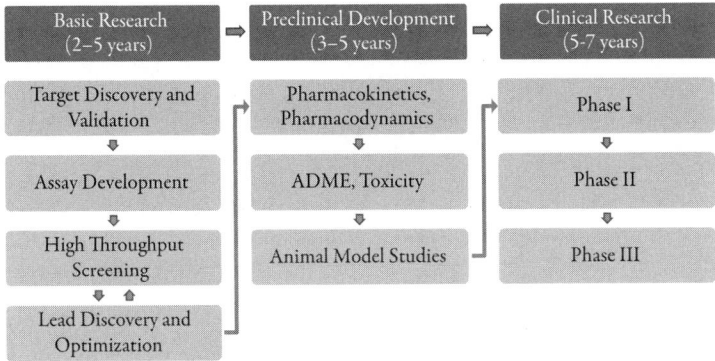

FIGURE 15.2 Timeline of drug discovery and development.

proteostasis regulators in the GD pathway.[57] HDACis remove acetyl groups from cellular chaperones, including Hsp90β, the protein responsible for directing the mutant GCase through a valosin-containing protein degradation process.[58] HDACis decrease binding of mutant GCase with Hsp90 and increase its binding to Hsp70 and the TCP1 ring complex, both of which stabilize GCase, allowing the mutant GCase to escape premature degradation and be delivered to the lysosome to perform its biological function. Treatment of patient-derived GD fibroblasts with mutations N370S or L444P with two broad-spectrum HDACis, SAHA (vorinistat) and LB-205, showed increased GCase activity and protein levels. These results indicate that pharmacological manipulation of the cellular chaperone system could provide another potential treatment option for LSDs. However, focusing on targets other than enzymes may have negative consequences, as other misfolded enzymes that are normally degraded by the ERAD pathway would also be affected. Thus, drugs targeting the gating pathway of protein synthesis and processing must be carefully tested to ensure their specificity for the disease-related proteins in order to avoid adverse effects.

Assay Development

Once a drug target is determined, the next step is to develop a homogeneous, reproducible, and sensitive assay to screen for potential lead compounds. It is important to establish a screening assay with the capability for HTS of compound libraries. HTS requires that the assays be miniaturized into a small well format, such as 1536-well plates, to increase screening throughput and to reduce the use of reagents. A fluorogenic enzyme assay is usually the first choice, since many of the enzymes implicated in the LSDs are hydrolases.[59] Moreover, fluorogenic enzyme assays are homogeneous, facile to perform, and are suitable for HTS. In the case of GD, purified recombinant GCase serves as an excellent source of wild-type enzyme for HTS, because the enzyme is available in large quantities. Red fluorescence labels, such as resorufin and BODIPY, are usually recommended for fluorogenic substrates because they are less prone to the interference by the fluorescent compounds in the compound library, even though a small percentage of the total compound library can be in the blue and green fluorescence wavelength spectrum. Alternatively, the use of a native substrate may be considered if the enzyme assay meets the requirements for HTS, as described above.

In addition, several other factors can greatly facilitate drug screening. The best primary screening assays should have short incubation times, use inexpensive reagents, and involve as few assay steps as possible. An ideal assay for HTS would have no more than six steps and an incubation time of less than a few hours, excluding plate wash steps. In addition, whenever possible, the screen assay should have clear physiological relevance. A novel approach for improving physiological relevance is to use lysosomal hydrolases in a tissue-homogenate preparation, which more closely resembles the natural cellular environment. A successful example of this approach is a HTS using enzyme extracts prepared from a splenectomy sample from a patient with GD (genotype N370S/N370S). The mutant GCase from this preparation was in its native physiological environment and yielded more reliable numbers of high quality noninhibitory chaperones.[54]

During assay development and prior to screening, various conditions such as the buffer components, pH, incubation time and temperature, enzyme and substrate concentrations, and compound solvent tolerability (i.e. compound stability in an organic solvent such as dimethyl sulfoxide [DMSO]) must be evaluated and optimized. For assays of lysosomal enzymes, an acidic buffer and the least amount of enzyme possible (usually at nanomolar concentration) should be used. The incubation time should be in the linear portion of the time course curve with sufficient fluorescence signal. Substrate concentration should be around or below the K_m value in order to maintain the high sensitivity for compound screens. A screen assay optimized for these conditions will have increased sensitivity, thus enabling the identification of valuable lead compounds.

Known inhibitors or activators are commonly used to validate the sensitivity and reproducibility of a screen assay. Potencies (IC_{50} or EC_{50} values) of the control compounds should usually be within two-fold of the reported value. A DMSO solvent plate without compounds is usually used to determine the assay parameters, including the signal-to-basal ratio and the Z' factor. A signal-to-basal ratio greater than two-fold and a Z' factor greater than 0.5 are considered acceptable for HTS. The stability of both the enzyme and substrate should also be evaluated over a 24-hr time period to ensure that the signal-to-basal ratio remains constant throughout the time it takes for continuous robotic screening. A test screen using a small compound library, such as the Ligands of Pharmacologically Active Compounds library from Sigma-Aldrich containing 1,280 compounds, is usually used to evaluate the performance of the optimized assay for HTS.[60]

Performing the High Throughput Screen

Screening of the compound library is initiated after development of an optimized assay. In an academic screening center, the size of the optimized chemical compound library is usually between 100,000 to 400,000 compounds, while the numbers in the pharmaceutical industry can be between 2 and 3 million compounds. The compounds in the library should be specifically selected and checked to meet the criteria of high quality (greater than 90% purity) "drug-like" properties, and chemical diversity. All of the compounds in the library are dissolved in DMSO solution at 1 to 10 mM concentrations, and are stored in 96-, 384-, or 1536-well plates. The compound solution is usually diluted 100- to 200-fold in the assay plates during the screens in order to keep the DMSO concentration less than 1% in most biochemical assays and less than 0.5% in cell-based assays. Since hundreds to thousands of plates need to be screened in the primary screen, a robotic system is commonly applied in this process. The screen robot mainly consists of four parts: the liquid handling system for reagent/compound dispensing, incubators and storage system for assay and compound plates, plate readers for assay plate detection, robotic arms and controlling software. In addition, a large quantity of reagents needs to be prepared that will be stable in buffer solution for at least 12 to 24 hrs. Using a robotic screening system, the primary screen can usually be completed within one week.

Data Analysis to Identify the Primary Hits

The next step after the primary screen is to perform data analysis, using specially designed software. In most screening centers, a single compound concentration is used in the primary screen, and 50% inhibition or activation is usually used as the cutoff point for hit (active compound) selection. The commonly accepted hit rate from primary screens usually ranges

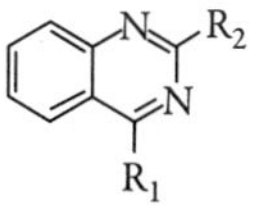

Compound number	R1	R2	AC_{50} (μM)
1	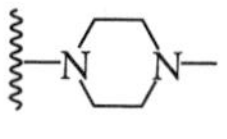 -N(piperazine)N-	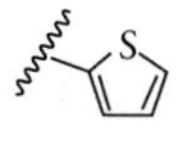 thiophene-CH₂	Inactive
2	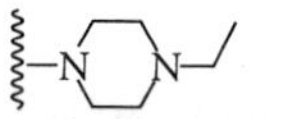 -N(piperazine)N-CH₃	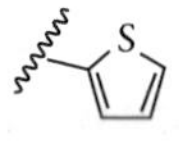 thiophene-CH₂	Inactive
3	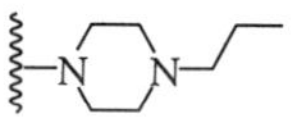 -N(piperazine)N-C₂H₅	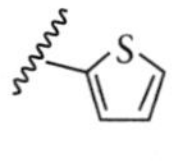 thiophene-CH₂	Inactive
4	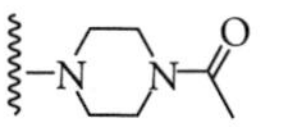 -N(piperazine)N-C(=O)-	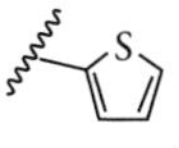 thiophene-CH₂	79.97
5	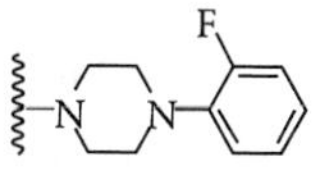 -N(piperazine)N-(2-F-phenyl)	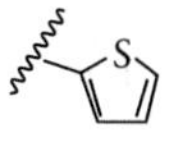 thiophene-CH₂	63.52
6	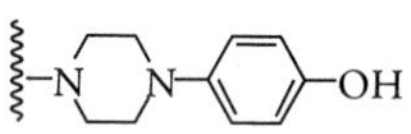 -N(piperazine)N-(4-OH-phenyl)	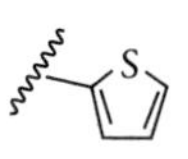 thiophene-CH₂	63.52
7	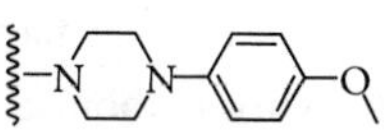 -N(piperazine)N-(4-Cl-phenyl)	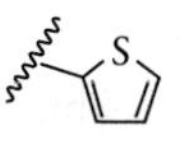 thiophene-CH₂	79.97

FIGURE 15.3 An example of structure-activity relationship (SAR) of a pharmacological chaperone. The different R1 and R2 groups result in chemicals with differing AC50 values.

between 0.1% and 1% of the total compound collection. On the other hand, the selection of primary hits in a quantitative HTS in which several compound concentrations are tested is based on compound potency (EC_{50}/IC_{50}) and its maximal response (usually greater than 70% control activity or inhibition). The information–rich data from a quantitative HTS enables early structure–activity relationships analysis and immediate structure clustering for the active compounds (Figure 15.3). The wealth of information resulting from the primary screen allows for more efficient selection of appropriate leads, as well as fewer required compounds for the next step of hit confirmation.

Hit Cherry-Picking and Confirmation

The initial primary hits, usually hundreds to a few thousand compounds, are then specifically selected ("cherry-picked") for confirmation and secondary screens. Each of the cherry-picked compounds is titrated, and their potencies are determined again in the same assay used in the primary screen to confirm their activities. The false positive and nonspecific compounds are eliminated from the list of primary hits by the counter-screens. The specificity of active compounds for the target protein is also assessed. In the case of LSDs, since the screening assays are often fluorogenic enzyme assays, other lysosomal enzyme assays using similar fluorogenic substrates can be used in counter-screens. For example, α-gal and α-glu enzyme assays have been used as counter-screens for GCase in order to eliminate the fluorescent compounds, as well as nonspecific compounds. After elimination of fluorescent and nonspecific compounds, powder samples of the confirmed and specific compounds are purchased for tertiary screens to further validate pharmacological activities and drug-like properties.

Tertiary Screens for Further Confirmation of Active Compounds

The selected active compounds, usually fewer than 30, are tested for enzyme kinetic properties. The K_i values for each compound are determined using software programs such as Prism® (Graphpad, San Diego, CA) or Sigma plot (Systat Software, Inc. San Jose, CA). A rapid K_i assessment method has been developed permitting measurement of the K_i values of six compounds in one 384-well plate using a fluorogenic enzyme assay.[36] The mechanism of action of identified compounds, such as competitive, noncompetitive, or uncompetitive inhibition, is commonly evaluated using a Lineweaver-Burk (double reciprocal) plot.

In addition, cell-based assays are needed for compound testing to evaluate whether the enzymes inhibitors or activators possess chaperone activity in cells. One approach is to utilize patient-derived skin fibroblasts, which are primary cells that can be maintained for 15 to 20 passages in culture. The whole-cell enzymatic activity is measured with a fluorogenic substrate in both the absence and presence of the test compound. An acidic assay buffer with pH of 4 to 4.2, consisting of 0.2 M sodium acetate-PBS buffer (1:1 ratio), is used to permeabilize the cell membrane to allow substrates to enter the cells.[61] The compounds that enhance enzymatic activity in enzyme-deficient patient cell lines are considered potential pharmacological chaperones. Although this cell-based assay generates valuable information about the chaperone's activity in a whole-cell system, investigators must also show that enzymatic activity is enhanced in specific cellular compartments, such as in the lysosome. A complementary

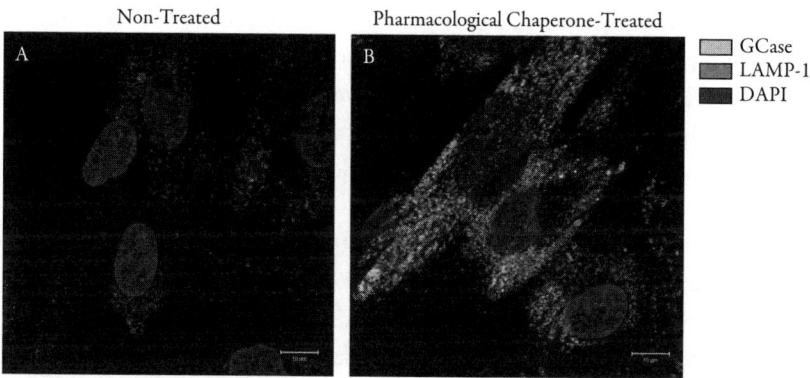

FIGURE 15.4 Confocal immunofluorescence imaging of fibroblasts from a patient. The non-treated (wild-type) cells exhibit baseline expression of GCase and LAMP-1 (lysosomal associated membrane protein) while the pharmacological chaperone-treated cells exhibit increased overall expression of GCase.

approach to the whole-cell enzyme assay is an immunofluorescence experiment in which the target enzyme is stained with an enzyme-specific fluorescent antibody and colocalization of the target enzyme with an organelle-specific marker is assessed. Examples of such markers are lysosomal markers, including Lysotracker dye (Invitrogen) and LAMP1 antibody staining.[62] Figure 15.4 shows the colocalization of one specific lysosomal enzyme with LAMP1, demonstrating an increase in the amount of mutant enzyme delivered to lysosomes after compound administration in patient-derived cells.[45] The combination of both the whole-cell enzymatic activity and the immunofluorescence colocalization help to define the chaperone activity of the lead compounds. In addition, Western blotting can be used to confirm the ability of the chaperone to stabilize and translocate the mutant enzyme, based on the protein size of the different forms of the enzyme observed.

In the case of GCase, a fluorescent probe has been synthesized that binds specifically to the GCase enzyme, which is more specific than available antibodies. The probe, a structural relative of the GCase inhibitor condrytol beta epoxide, is a novel reagent with a BODIPY fluorescent tag attached for imaging.[63] The probe's high specificity for GCase makes it a powerful tool for quantification, trafficking, and cell imaging studies. The probe has proven to be a useful reagent for *in vivo* assays in mice, and has the potential to open up new avenues for HTS assays.

Additionally, a thermal shift assay or a functional temperature shift assay can be used to determine if a compound is binding to the protein. The thermal shift assay measures the denaturation temperature (T_m) of a protein in the presence or absence of the candidate small chaperone molecule. The protein is denatured slowly while the temperature is gradually increased, thus exposing hydrophobic inner domains that can bind to a dye, resulting in an increase in fluorescence intensity. In a thermal shift assay, the small chaperone molecule binds to the target protein and increases the temperature needed for protein denaturation, thus shifting the thermodenaturation curve to the right.[64] Similarly, a functional temperature shift assay measures the particular temperature at which the enzymatic activity is significantly reduced in the presence or absence of the small molecule chaperone compound as the temperature is gradually increased. The enzymatic activity is diminished once the enzyme is denatured. However, in the presence of a small molecule chaperone, the denaturation may occur at higher temperatures, as reflected by persistent enzymatic activity and its increased resistance to rising temperatures. Both assays provide information regarding the extent of binding of the small molecules to the proteins, which serves as the basis for chaperone therapy. Once a compound is verified in these tertiary assays, it is considered to be an early lead, which can proceed to the next step of drug development–lead optimization.

Lead Optimization

Lead optimization includes the synthesis of hundreds to thousands of new chemical analogs of a lead compound identified from HTS and the methods described above to improve the potency, bioavailability, pharmacokinetic properties, and solubility of the compound, as well as to reduce the compound toxicity. Experienced medicinal chemists usually direct the lead optimization effort, in collaboration with biologists and pharmacologists. After the optimization, the potency of a lead compound is usually improved to within the nanomolar range for enzyme modulators, and other drug-like properties are enhanced. The efficacy of the optimized lead compound is then tested on animal models, when available, to confirm its *in vivo* efficacy.

Preclinical Development

Once the efficacy of an improved lead compound has been established and the lead compound shows appropriate drug properties without significant toxicity, it can enter preclinical development. A further late-stage lead optimization may be necessary after the assessment of drug toxicity in animals. The pharmacokinetics and oral bioavailability of the optimized lead compound in animal species are evaluated for further pharmacodynamic and toxicology studies. Ultimately, when the lead compound demonstrates the required drug properties, and no obvious toxicity is seen in animal models, an Investigational New Drug application to the Food and Drug Administration is prepared for the long-awaited phase I clinical trial.

Conclusion

Recent advances in drug discovery have led to the development of various small molecules for the treatment of LSDs. While many require further validation to establish their therapeutic effect and toxicity, several emerging pharmacological chaperones for the treatment of specific lysosomal storage diseases are already being evaluated in Food and Drug Administration-approved clinical trials. All of the pharmacological chaperones developed to date are enzyme inhibitors whose inherent inhibitory nature may compromise therapeutic benefits because of the challenge to balance the activity of enzyme binding/inhibition with the restoration of enzyme activity in the lysosome. As an alternative, new strategies are being developed to identify novel small molecule chaperones that either have no enzyme inhibitory properties, or have the ability to activate the enzyme. Chemical modification of the lead chaperone compounds may reduce inhibitory activity, while their chaperone function remains. New screening assays, such as ones performed on native enzyme preparations, may enhance our ability to identify more ideal lead chaperone compounds, including activators from compound library screens. In addition to their application as chaperone therapy, selected small molecule compounds could also be useful in combination with existing ERT and SRT to enhance therapeutic effects. In the case of ERT, the chaperone compound may potentially stabilize the infused recombinant protein, leading to reduced frequency of drug administration. Thus, continued progress in the development of optimized pharmacological chaperones should bring about new and effective therapies for patients with LSDs in the near future.

Acknowledgments

This work was supported by the intramural research program of the National Human Genome Research Institute and the National Institutes of Health and the Molecular Libraries Initiative of the National Institutes of Health Roadmap for Medical Research. Darryl Leja assisted with the preparation of Figure 15.1 and Dr. Wendy Westbroek with Figure 15.4.

References

1. Lachmann R. Treatments for lysosomal storage disorders. *Biochem Soc Trans.* 2010; 38(6): 1465–1468.
2. Suzuki Y. Chaperone therapy update: Fabry disease, GM1-gangliosidosis and Gaucher disease. *Brain Dev.* 2013; 35(6): 515–523.
3. Lieberman RL, Wustman BA, Huertas P, et al. Structure of acid beta-glucosidase with pharmacological chaperone provides insight into Gaucher disease. *Nat Chem Biol.* 2007; 3(2): 101–107.
4. Schiffmann R, Murray GJ, Treco D, et al. Infusion of alpha-galactosidase A reduces tissue globotriaosylceramide storage in patients with Fabry disease. *Proc Natl Acad Sci USA.* 2000; 97(1): 365–370.
5. Lee K, Jin X, Zhang K, et al. A biochemical and pharmacological comparison of enzyme replacement therapies for the glycolipid storage disorder Fabry disease. *Glycobiology.* 2003; 13(4): 305–313.
6. Cox TM. Gaucher disease: clinical profile and therapeutic developments. *Biologics.* 2011; 4: 299–313.
7. Tolar J, Orchard PJ. Alpha-L-iduronidase therapy for mucopolysaccharidosis type I. *Biologics.* 2008; 2(4):743–751.
8. Muenzer J, Gucsavas-Calikoglu M, McCandless SE, Schuetz TJ, Kimura A. A phase I/II clinical trial of enzyme replacement therapy in mucopolysaccharidosis II (Hunter syndrome). *Mol Genet Metab.* 2007; 90(3): 329–337.
9. Harmatz P, Giugliani R, Schwartz I, et al. Enzyme replacement therapy for mucopolysaccharidosis VI: a phase 3, randomized, double-blind, placebo-controlled, multinational study of recombinant human N-acetylgalactosamine 4-sulfatase (recombinant human arylsulfatase B or rhASB) and follow-on, open-label extension study. *J Pediatr.* 2006; 148(4): 533–539.
10. Beck M. Alglucosidase alfa: Long term use in the treatment of patients with Pompe disease. *Ther Clin Risk Manag.* 2009; 5: 767–772.
11. Barton NW, Brady RO, Dambrosia JM, et al. Replacement therapy for inherited enzyme deficiency—macrophage-targeted glucocerebrosidase for Gaucher's disease. *N Engl J Med.* 1991; 324(21): 1464–1470.
12. Erikson A. Remaining problems in the management of patients with Gaucher disease. *J Inherit Metab Dis.* 2001; 24(Suppl 2):122–126; discussion 187–128.
13. Beck M. New therapeutic options for lysosomal storage disorders: enzyme replacement, small molecules and gene therapy. *Hum Genet.* 2007; 121(1): 1–22.
14. Brady RO, Yang C, Zhuang Z. An innovative approach to the treatment of Gaucher disease and possibly other metabolic disorders of the brain. *J Inherit Metab Dis.* 2013; 36(3): 451–454.
15. Breunig F, Weidemann F, Strotmann J, Knoll A, Wanner C. Clinical benefit of enzyme replacement therapy in Fabry disease. *Kidney Int.* 2006; 69(7): 1216–1221.
16. Hollak CE, Linthorst GE. Immune response to enzyme replacement therapy in Fabry disease: impact on clinical outcome? *Mol Genet Metab.* 2009; 96(1): 1–3.
17. Raben N, Danon M, Gilbert AL, et al. Enzyme replacement therapy in the mouse model of Pompe disease. *Mol Genet Metab.* 2003; 80(1–2): 159–169.

18. Kishnani PS, Goldenberg PC, DeArmey SL, et al. Cross-reactive immunologic material status affects treatment outcomes in Pompe disease infants. *Mol Genet Metab*. 2010; 99(1): 26–33.
19. de Vries JM, van der Beek NA, Kroos MA, et al. High antibody titer in an adult with Pompe disease affects treatment with alglucosidase alfa. *Mol Genet Metab*. 2010; 101(4): 338–345.
20. Wraith JE, Beck M, Lane R, et al. Enzyme replacement therapy in patients who have mucopolysaccharidosis I and are younger than 5 years: results of a multinational study of recombinant human alpha-L-iduronidase (laronidase). *Pediatrics*. 2007; 120(1): e37–e46.
21. Beutler E. Lysosomal storage diseases: natural history and ethical and economic aspects. *Mol Genet Metab*. 2006; 88(3): 208–215.
22. Pastores GM. Miglustat: substrate reduction therapy for lysosomal storage disorders associated with primary central nervous system involvement. *Recent Pat CNS Drug Discov*. 2006; 1(1): 77–82.
23. Platt FM, Neises GR, Dwek RA, Butters TD. N-butyldeoxynojirimycin is a novel inhibitor of glycolipid biosynthesis. *J Biol Chem*. 1994; 269(11): 8362–8365.
24. Jeyakumar M, Butters TD, Cortina-Borja M, et al. Delayed symptom onset and increased life expectancy in Sandhoff disease mice treated with N-butyldeoxynojirimycin. *Proc Natl Acad Sci USA*. 1999; 96(11): 6388–6393.
25. Cox T, Lachmann R, Hollak C, et al. Novel oral treatment of Gaucher's disease with N-butyldeoxynojirimycin (OGT 918) to decrease substrate biosynthesis. *Lancet*. 2000; 355(9214): 1481–1485.
26. Pastores GM, Barnett NL, Kolodny EH. An open-label, noncomparative study of miglustat in type I Gaucher disease: efficacy and tolerability over 24 months of treatment. *Clin Ther*. 2005; 27(8): 1215–1227.
27. Giraldo P, Latre P, Alfonso P, et al. Short-term effect of miglustat in every day clinical use in treatment-naive or previously treated patients with type 1 Gaucher's disease. *Haematologica*. 2006; 91(5): 703–706.
28. Elstein D, Dweck A, Attias D, et al. Oral maintenance clinical trial with miglustat for type I Gaucher disease: switch from or combination with intravenous enzyme replacement. *Blood*. 2007; 110(7): 2296–2301.
29. Giraldo P, Alfonso P, Atutxa K, et al. Real-world clinical experience with long-term miglustat maintenance therapy in type 1 Gaucher disease: the ZAGAL project. *Haematologica*. 2009; 94(12): 1771–1775.
30. Patterson MC, Vecchio D, Prady H, Abel L, Wraith JE. Miglustat for treatment of Niemann-Pick C disease: a randomised controlled study. *Lancet Neurol*. 2007; 6(9): 765–772.
31. Lukina E, Watman N, Arreguin EA, et al. A phase 2 study of eliglustat tartrate (Genz-112638), an oral substrate reduction therapy for Gaucher disease type 1. *Blood*. 2010; 116(6): 893–899.
32. Schiffmann R, Fitzgibbon EJ, Harris C, et al. Randomized, controlled trial of miglustat in Gaucher's disease type 3. *Ann Neurol*. 2008; 64(5): 514–522.
33. Cabrera-Salazar MA, Deriso M, Bercury SD, et al. Systemic delivery of a glucosylceramide synthase inhibitor reduces CNS substrates and increases lifespan in a mouse model of type 2 Gaucher disease. *PLoS One*. 2012; 7(8): e43310.
34. Meusser B, Hirsch C, Jarosch E, Sommer T. ERAD: the long road to destruction. *Nat Cell Biol*. 2005; 7(8): 766–772.
35. Lieberman RL, D'Aquino JA, Ringe D, Petsko GA. Effects of pH and iminosugar pharmacological chaperones on lysosomal glycosidase structure and stability. *Biochemistry*. 2009; 48(22): 4816–4827.
36. Benito JM, Garcia Fernandez JM, Ortiz Mellet C. Pharmacological chaperone therapy for Gaucher disease: a patent review. *Expert Opin Ther Pat*. 2011; 21(6): 885–903.
37. Steet RA, Chung S, Wustman B, Powe A, Do H, Kornfeld SA. The iminosugar isofagomine increases the activity of N370S mutant acid beta-glucosidase in Gaucher fibroblasts by several mechanisms. *Proc Natl Acad Sci USA*. 2006; 103(37): 13813–13818.
38. Khanna R, Benjamin ER, Pellegrino L, et al. The pharmacological chaperone isofagomine increases the activity of the Gaucher disease L444P mutant form of beta-glucosidase. *Febs J*. 2010; 277(7): 1618–1638.
39. Sun Y, Ran H, Liou B, et al. Isofagomine in vivo effects in a neuronopathic Gaucher disease mouse. *PLoS One*. 2011; 6(4): e19037.
40. Amicus Therapeutics I. Fabry disease : AT1001 clinical trials. (http://www.amicustherapeutics.com/clinicaltrials).
41. Maegawa GH, Tropak MB, Buttner JD, et al. Identification and characterization of ambroxol as an enzyme enhancement agent for Gaucher disease. *J Biol Chem*. 2009; 284(35): 23502–23516.
42. Zimran A, Altarescu G, Elstein D. Pilot study using ambroxol as a pharmacological chaperone in type 1 Gaucher disease. *Blood Cells Mol Dis*. 2013; 50(2): 134–137.

43. Fan JQ, Ishii S, Asano N, Suzuki Y. Accelerated transport and maturation of lysosomal alpha-galactosidase A in Fabry lymphoblasts by an enzyme inhibitor. *Nat Med.* 1999; 5(1): 112–115.
44. Benjamin ER, Flanagan JJ, Schilling A, et al. The pharmacological chaperone 1-deoxygalactonojirimycin increases alpha-galactosidase A levels in Fabry patient cell lines. *J Inherit Metab Dis.* 2009; 32(3): 424–440.
45. Yam GH, Zuber C, Roth J. A synthetic chaperone corrects the trafficking defect and disease phenotype in a protein misfolding disorder. *Faseb J.* 2005; 19(1): 12–18.
46. Flanagan JJ, Rossi B, Tang K, et al. The pharmacological chaperone 1-deoxynojirimycin increases the activity and lysosomal trafficking of multiple mutant forms of acid alpha-glucosidase. *Hum Mutat.* 2009; 30(12): 1683–1692.
47. Trapero A, Llebaria A. Glucocerebrosidase inhibitors for the treatment of Gaucher disease. *Future Med Chem.* 2013; 5(5): 573–590.
48. Shen JS, Edwards NJ, Hong YB, Murray GJ. Isofagomine increases lysosomal delivery of exogenous glucocerebrosidase. *Biochem Biophys Res Commun.* 2008; 369(4): 1071–1075.
49. Porto C, Cardone M, Fontana F, et al. The pharmacological chaperone N-butyldeoxynojirimycin enhances enzyme replacement therapy in Pompe disease fibroblasts. *Mol Ther.* 2009; 17(6): 964–971.
50. Ringe D, Petsko GA. What are pharmacological chaperones and why are they interesting? *J Biol.* 2009; 8(9): 80.
51. Lockhart DC (Cranbury, NJ, US), Wustman B (Princeton, NJ, US), Inventors; Amicus Therapeutics, Inc. (Cranbury, NJ, US), assignee. Dosing regimens for the treatment of lysosomal storage diseases using pharmacological chaperones; Patent application; 2010.
52. Marugan JJ, Zheng W, Motabar O, et al. Evaluation of 2-thioxo-2,3,5,6,7,8-hexahydropyrimido[4,5-d]pyrimidin-4(1H)-one analogues as GAA activators. *Eur J Med Chem.* 2010; 45(5): 1880–1897.
53. Patnaik S, Zheng W, Choi JH, et al. Discovery, structure-activity relationship, and biological evaluation of noninhibitory small molecule chaperones of glucocerebrosidase. *J Med Chem.* 2012; 55(12): 5734–5748.
54. Goldin E, Zheng W, Motabar O, et al. High throughput screening for small molecule therapy for Gaucher disease using patient tissue as the source of mutant glucocerebrosidase. *PLoS One.* 2012; 7(1): e29861.
55. Mu TW, Ong DS, Wang YJ, et al. Chemical and biological approaches synergize to ameliorate protein-folding diseases. *Cell.* 2008; 134(5): 769–781.
56. Balch WE, Morimoto RI, Dillin A, Kelly JW. Adapting proteostasis for disease intervention. *Science.* 2008; 319(5865): 916–919.
57. Lu J, Yang C, Chen M, et al. Histone deacetylase inhibitors prevent the degradation and restore the activity of glucocerebrosidase in Gaucher disease. *P Proc Natl Acad Sci USA.* 2011; 108(52): 21200–21205.
58. Yang C, Rahimpour S, Lu J, et al. Histone deacetylase inhibitors increase glucocerebrosidase activity in Gaucher disease by modulation of molecular chaperones. *Proc Natl Acad Sci USA.* 2013; 110(3): 966–971.
59. Urban DJ, Zheng W, Goker-Alpan O, et al. Optimization and validation of two miniaturized glucocerebrosidase enzyme assays for high throughput screening. *Comb Chem High T Scr.* 2008; 11(10): 817–824.
60. Inglese J, Auld DS, Jadhav A, et al. Quantitative high-throughput screening: a titration-based approach that efficiently identifies biological activities in large chemical libraries. *Proc Natl Acad Sci USA.* 2006; 103(31): 11473–11478.
61. Zheng W, Padia J, Urban DJ, et al. Three classes of glucocerebrosidase inhibitors identified by quantitative high-throughput screening are chaperone leads for Gaucher disease. *Proc Natl Acad Sci USA.* 2007; 104(32): 13192–13197.
62. Yam GH, Bosshard N, Zuber C, Steinmann B, Roth J. Pharmacological chaperone corrects lysosomal storage in Fabry disease caused by trafficking-incompetent variants. *Am J Physiol Cell Physiol.* 2006; 290(4): C1076–C1082.
63. Witte MD, Kallemeijn WW, Aten J, et al. Ultrasensitive in situ visualization of active glucocerebrosidase molecules. *Nature Chem Bio.* 2010; 6(12): 907–913.
64. Lo MC, Aulabaugh A, Jin G, et al. Evaluation of fluorescence-based thermal shift assays for hit identification in drug discovery. *Annal Biochem.* 2004; 332(1): 153–159.

16

Substrate Deprivation Therapy

Marc C. Patterson

Substrate deprivation therapy, also known as substrate reduction[1] or substrate inhibition therapy, has entered clinical trials and practice in the past decade as an alternative approach to the management of lysosomal storage diseases. Until the 1990s, there were no disease-modifying therapies available for the lysosomal storage diseases. The development of enzyme replacement therapy for Gaucher disease, which has proven highly effective for the management of its visceral manifestations, has been followed by the development of therapies for mucopolysaccharidoses (MPS) types I, II, and VI; Pompe disease; and Fabry disease.[2] In addition to these forms of enzyme replacement therapy, hematopoietic stem cell transplantation is also available for several of these diseases, although the different therapeutic approaches have not been systematically studied in head-to-head trials.[3]

Both enzyme replacement therapy and hematopoietic stem cell transplantation are effective in many patients but in general do not treat the central nervous system manifestations of these diseases, are expensive, and, in the case of hematopoietic stem cell transplantation, carry significant risks, although these have become less prominent in recent years.

Substrate deprivation therapy is based on several principles. First, there is considerable data to suggest that the accumulation of substrate in lysosomal storage diseases plays an important role in the pathogenesis of these disorders and in their clinical phenotypes. The amount of substrate that accumulates in the tissues represents a balance between the synthesis of these large macromolecules and their catabolism, which is catalyzed by enzymes most commonly deficient in these diseases or which is facilitated by other molecules such as those involved in transport as in Niemann-Pick disease, type C (NPC). It follows that if the catabolic rate is decreased by deficiency of the primary gene product, then the amount of substrate will increase. One can approach this problem by increasing the activity of the enzyme by direct replacement, enhancement of the enzyme activity by enzyme enhancement or chaperone therapy, or by transplanting a new source of enzyme as in hematopoietic stem cell transplantation. Alternatively, the balance can be favorably altered if the synthesis of substrate can be inhibited. This latter approach is the subject of this chapter.

TABLE 16.1 **Agents Studied for Substrate Deprivation Therapy**

Class	Mechanism of Action (where known)	Examples	Diseases or Models Studied
Imino sugars	Inhibition of glucosylceramide synthase; suppression of inflammation; other	Miglustat, N-BDGJ, AMP-DMN	Gaucher, Niemann-Pick disease, type C, GM2 gangliosidosis
Morpholinopropanolol analogs	Inhibition of glucosylceramide synthase	Eliglustat	Gaucher
Flavonoids	Inhibition of glycosaminoglycan synthesis in vitro; antioxidant properties	Genistein	MPS II, III, VII
Glucose/xylose analogs	Inhibition of glycosaminoglycan synthesis in vitro	4-deoxy analogues of 2-acetamido-2-deoxy-D-glucose and 2-acetamido-2-deoxy-D-xylose; 4-deoxy-4-fluoro analogues of 2-acetamido-2-deoxy-D-glucose and 2-acetamido-2-deoxy-D-galactose[65]	Glycosaminoglycan synthesis (cell culture)
Fluorone dye	Inhibition of chain elongation	Rhodamine B	MPS III, VII (mice)
RNA	Silencing of gene expression (EXTL 2 and EXTL3–encode heparan sulfate synthesizing enzymes)	Specific shRNAs	Glycosaminoglycan synthesis (cell culture)

Note. N-BDGJ = N-butyldeoxygalactonojirimycin; AMP-DMN = N-(5-adamantane-1-yl-methoxy) pentyl)-dexoynojirimycin; MPS= mucopolysaccharidoses.

In the case of the lysosomal storage diseases, several classes of molecules have been investigated in animals and, in some cases, in humans (summarized in Table 16.1). The molecules that have been most widely studied are imino sugars, including N-butyldeoxynojirimycin (miglustat) and its congeners N-butyldeoxygalactonojirimycin (N-BDJG) and N-(5-adamantane-1-yl-methoxy-pentyl)deoxynojirimycin (AMP-DMN).

There is also a series of morpholinopropanol analogues, and, of these, eliglustat[4] has been most extensively investigated. Other classes of molecules include the flavonoids, particularly the plant-derived molecule genistein, as well as the fluorone dye rhodamine B, as well as a number of glucose and xylose analogues that have been developed to inhibit the synthesis of glycosaminoglycans. Most recently, gene silencing of the EXTL 2 and 3 genes has been investigated in animal models as a potential therapy for MPS.

Imino Sugars (Deoxynojirimycin Derivatives)

The imino sugars are glucose analogues in which the oxygen in the ring is replaced by nitrogen, attached to side chains of varying lengths. The nature of the substitutions in the side chains confers specificity and potency on the molecules so derived.

N-butyldeoxynojirimycin, (OGT-918, miglustat) has been most extensively studied. This molecule was first recognized as an inhibitor of glucosylceramide synthase in the early 1990s.[5] Glucosylceramide synthase catalyzes the rate-limiting step in the synthesis of the higher-order glycosphingolipids, which accumulate in excess within lysosomes in the sphingolipid storage diseases. Miglustat was initially found to be effective in reducing storage in a chemically induced cellular module of Gaucher disease[5] and was subsequently shown to be effective in ameliorating the biochemical changes and neuropathology in a murine model of Tay-Sachs disease (infantile GM2 gangliosidosis).[6] In control mice, glycosphingolipid accumulation was reduced by 50% to 70%, and lymphoid tissues were 50% acellular in comparison to controls; no overt pathology was found in relation to these changes.[7]

Studies of miglustat in the murine and feline models of NPC also showed efficacy in delaying clinical onset, prolonging survival, and improving neuropathological changes,[8] and subsequently clinical trials were begun for both Gaucher disease and NPC. A series of clinical trials in non-neuronopathic Gaucher disease led to approval of miglustat for the management of mild Gaucher disease in adults who were not able to tolerate enzyme replacement therapy.[9,10] The clinical studies of miglustat in Gaucher disease were challenging to perform, because by the time the molecule was available for study, most patients who had access to enzyme replacement therapy were being treated effectively with this modality. Thus, only a subset of patients was available for study. Nevertheless, miglustat was shown to improve the complete blood count and platelet count, reduce organomegaly,[11] and, over a period of time, improve bony changes in Gaucher disease.[9]

Miglustat inhibits alpha-glucosidase I and II[5] as well as disaccharidases in the gut, thus accounting for its major adverse effects, which include gastrointestinal upset with bloating and diarrhea. There was some concern in early clinical trials that the drug may be associated with peripheral neuropathy in adults with Gaucher disease.[11] but subsequent investigations have suggested that there were likely other etiologies for the peripheral neuropathy that was seen in these patients. Peripheral neuropathy has not been reported as an adverse effect of this drug when studied in patients with NPC.[12]

Some studies have suggested that the combination of enzyme replacement therapy with miglustat may be particularly efficacious.[13] There is also evidence that miglustat may function as a chaperone in addition to its substrate deprivation effect in both Gaucher disease[14] and Pompe disease fibroblasts,[15] thus acting to reduce substrate accumulation both by substrate inhibition and increased catabolism.

A controlled prospective study[12] and uncontrolled retrospective studies of miglustat[16] have been performed in NPC. The first controlled clinical study[12] suggested that miglustat stabilized or improved a number of measures of disease expression, although the study was underpowered. Long-term studies in children[17,18] and adults[19] have shown no new safety concerns and support the contention that miglustat leads to some stabilization of NPC. These findings in their entirety formed the basis of approval of this drug for management of progressive neurologic manifestations of NPC in the European Union[20] and several other countries in both hemispheres. The drug is not currently approved for this indication in the United States. Subsequently, Chinese[21] and French[22] studies have found evidence of stabilization of disease manifestations in NPC in late-infantile and juvenile groups but not in the early-infantile patients. An Italian report of two patients with early-onset disease who were treated very soon after onset[23] suggested that there could be a preventive benefit in this subset of patients if treatment is instituted sufficiently early.

As is often the case in rare diseases, clinical studies in NPC and related diseases are challenging, owing to the small number of patients available, their marked clinical heterogeneity, and the absence of widely accepted markers of disease severity and progression. These issues are most pressing in those rare disorders with central nervous system manifestations.[24]

Two studies of the effect of miglustat in GM2 gangliosidosis have been published. Neither a controlled study in adults[25] nor a case series in children[26] showed evidence of clinical benefit. A case report of the use of miglustat in juvenile Sandhoff disease described slowing of neurologic progression and stabilization of body weight.[27] It is difficult to interpret these studies. While it seems clear that there was no substantial effect in the published series, it also seems likely that patients who participated in these studies already had a significant burden of disease at the time therapy was instituted. It may be, in fact, that no intervention would be helpful once a certain threshold of disease burden has been crossed. One cannot, therefore, necessarily assume that miglustat or a similar agent would not be helpful if used in patients with very early or presymptomatic disease.

A series was published investigating the use of miglustat in MPS type III (Sanfilippo disease) and showed no clear evidence of clinical benefit.[28] Likewise, a controlled study utilizing miglustat in neuronopathic Gaucher disease (type III) showed no neurologic benefits.[29] One case report presented intriguing eye movement data suggesting that at least in the mild case described, neurologic improvement had been associated with the use of this agent.[30]

Miglustat is a viable therapeutic option in the management of non-neuronopathic Gaucher disease, particularly for patients with mild to moderate disease who are unable to tolerate enzyme replacement therapy.[9] One short-term study suggested that the efficacy of miglustat over six months was comparable to enzyme replacement therapy,[31] and the same group reported acceptable efficacy and safety over periods of up to four years of therapy.[32]

Dietary modification can be helpful in ameliorating the gastrointestinal effects of miglustat,[19] and there is evidence that a modified ketogenic diet[33] can enhance the central nervous system absorption and activity of miglustat in an animal model of Sandhoff disease. Timing of food intake does not appear to be important in regulating the exposure of an individual to miglustat.[34]

Miglustat's ability to penetrate the central nervous system is a critical attribute. The concentration can be measured by fairly simple methods in the cerebrospinal fluid[35]; the enhancement of physiological tremor in patients with NPC is further evidence of its central effects.[36]

Miglustat has many actions in addition to the inhibition of glucosylceramide synthase. In vitro studies have suggested beneficial effects in models of cystic fibrosis. Through alpha-1,2 glucosidase inhibition, miglustat prevents the interaction between the common cystic fibrosis mutation delF508-CFTR and calnexin, thus permitting the mutated protein to elude the endoplasmic reticulum degradation system and to restore the cAMP-activated chloride current in epithelial cystic fibrosis cells[37]; chronic treatment produces a stable non-cystic fibrosis phenotype in cultured epithelial cells.[38] Sodium currents are also restored in this model.[39] Nasal delivery of miglustat in F508del transgenic mice corrects both sodium and chloride currents.[40]

The relative lack of specificity of miglustat is obviated in its congener, N-BDGJ. N-BDGJ's relative specificity, with diminished effects on disaccharidases and alpha-galactosidases, has been demonstrated in a number of studies.[41,42] In addition, N-BDGJ has shown increased efficacy compared to miglustat without impairing general growth or causing lymphoid hypoplasia in the murine model of Sandhoff disease.[43] N-BDGJ has also shown efficacy in reducing the amount of GM2 ganglioside accumulating in the murine model of GM2 gangliosidosis.[44] Beneficial clinical effects have been observed in the GM1 mouse model,[45] which is paralleled by diminished storage of brain GM1 ganglioside.[46]

AMP-DMN (Genz -529468) is a hydrophobic derivative of deoxynojirimycin that is a potent inhibitor of nonlysosomal glucosylceramide synthase at nanomolar concentrations; lysosomal glucocerebrosidase and α-glucosidase, the glucosylceramide synthase, and the N-linked glycan-trimming α-glucosidases of the endoplasmic reticulum are not affected at these concentrations.[47] A comparative study of this agent and miglustat in a Sandhoff murine model demonstrated diminished GM2 ganglioside levels in the liver following treatment with both drugs, delay in the loss of motor function and coordination, reduced neuroinflammation, and histopathology.[48]

Although AMP-DMN is more potent than miglustat, there was no difference in their clinical and pathological effects. Surprisingly, exposure to both drugs was associated with marked elevation of glucosylceramide in the brain, although GM2 was reduced by miglustat and increased by AMP-DMN. These findings suggest that the neuropathological benefits of imino sugars in lysosomal storage diseases are likely mediated by actions other than substrate inhibition.[48]

Morpholinopropanol Homologues

Eliglustat is the best studied of a series of homologues of a morpholinopropanol, 1-phenyl-2-decanoylamino-3-morpholino-1-propanol,[49] whose ability to specifically inhibit glucosylceramide synthase has been investigated over the past two decades.[49,50] The inhibition of glucosylceramide synthase is accompanied by induction of its expression, which also occurs with N- butyldeoxynojirimycin.[51]

The pharmacologic profile of the compound appears to be favorable, and preliminary studies in a murine model of Gaucher disease were highly promising.[52] A phase 2 study of eliglustat in 26 patients with type 1 Gaucher disease found that 77% of participants showed improvement in at least two of three endpoints: splenomegaly, platelet count, and hemoglobin. Most patients also showed a reduction in biomarkers, in addition to normalization of plasma glucosylceramide and ganglioside GM3.[53] Nine-month data from a phase 3 study also showed positive results.[54] Detailed pharmacokinetic studies of eliglustat have been published.[55] The drug is reported to cause nausea, dizziness, and vomiting with escalating doses and mild increases in PR, QRS, and QT/QTc intervals on the electrocardiogram.

Eliglustat does not to cross the blood–brain barrier and thus is not a candidate for managing the neuronopathic forms of lysosomal storage.

Flavonoids and Other Compounds Used in Mucopolysaccharidoses

A number of compounds have been studied in animal models of the MPS. Although enzyme replacement therapy is available for MPS types I, II, and VI, the most prevalent of this family of disorders, MPS type III, or Sanfilippo disease, lacks effective disease-modifying therapy.

Genistein (4',5,7-trihydroxyisoflavone) is a flavonoid with multiple actions, which include estrogenic effects, antioxidant properties, and inhibition of glycosaminoglycan synthesis in vitro. The drug's wide range of actions has been reviewed.[56] Studies have shown reduced storage of glycosaminoglycans in the MPS IIIB mouse, albeit without evidence of effects on central nervous system storage.[57] But when higher doses of the agent were employed, improvement in the neuropathology and in the behavioral phenotype of the murine model was found.[58]

Studies in patient-derived fibroblasts from patients with MPS IIIA and VII did show evidence of reduced storage, particularly when combinations of related analogues of genistein were employed.[59] Studies in the MPS2 murine model have also shown reduced accumulation of glycosaminoglycans following treatment with Genistein.[60]

One study has been performed in a series of patients with MPS type III of various enzymatic subtypes. A 5 mg/kg/day dose was employed, but no clinical effect was seen.[61] A double-blind crossover trial of 10 mg/kg/day in 30 patients with MPS type III (all types) showed no clinical effect, although both plasma concentrations and urinary excretion of glycosaminoglycans were slightly reduced while remaining in the range for untreated patients.[62] High-dose genistein aglycone (150 mg/kg/day) has been studied in an open-label trial in 19 patients with MPS type III and three with MPS type II (all of whom had neurologic manifestations).[63] The effect on urinary glycosaminoglycan excretion was erratic, and there was no decline overall. The authors felt that the drug was safe and recommended a controlled trial to assess possible benefit.

Glucose and Xylose Analogues and Rhodamine B

Two papers have described the effectiveness of a series of glucose and xylose analogues (4-deoxy analogues of 2-acetamido-2-deoxy-D-glucose and 2-acetamido-2-deoxy-D-xylose[64] and 4-deoxy-4-fluoro analogues of 2-acetamido-2-deoxy-D-glucose and 2-acetamido-2-deoxy-D-galactose[65]) in reducing glycosaminoglycan storage in cell culture by enzyme inhibition, but no clinical trials have been pursued. Likewise, studies of rhodamine B, a fluorone dye that inhibits chain elongation,[66] have been reported. Studies in the MPS IIIA and MPS VII mice showed evidence of diminished glycosaminoglycan accumulation,[67] and, in a subsequent study, the behavioral phenotype of this murine model showed improvement.[68] Transgenerational studies of the mice suggested that it is safe to use in the long term.[69] No human studies have yet been reported.

RNA Interference

A different approach to substrate deprivation therapy has recently been reported in murine models of MPS IIIA and in fibroblast culture. This approach used RNA interference as a method of targeting substrate reduction therapy to heparan sulfate synthesizing enzymes, which are encoded by the EXTL 2 and EXTL 3 genes.[70] These studies suggested that, at least in these in vitro models, lysosomal glycosaminoglycan levels can be reduced. Incorporation of shRNAs into a lentiviral expression system reduced gene expression, and one EXTL 2 specific shRNA reduced glycosaminoglycan synthesis.

Conclusion

Substrate deprivation therapy is based on the premise that substrate accumulation is a key event in the pathophysiology of lysosomal storage diseases and that reduction of this accumulation will ameliorate the course of disease. It is approved for type 1 Gaucher disease worldwide and in several countries (but not the United States) for NPC. This small molecule approach holds promise, particularly if more specific and potent drugs can be developed, which target the central nervous system without affecting other enzyme systems. Although substrate deprivation is accomplished by these agents, it may not be their most important mechanism of action, since reduction of inflammation and chaperone effects may also be contributing to the positive effects seen in animals and humans. It is noteworthy that, given the multitude of actions of many of the molecules being investigated, there may be benefits to other unrelated diseases, as demonstrated by the effectiveness of miglustat in models of cystic fibrosis in vitro and in vivo[71] and by the effects of eliglustat in ameliorating an animal model of polycystic kidney disease.[72]

References

1. Platt FM, Jeyakumar M. Substrate reduction therapy. *Acta Paediatr Suppl*. 2008; 97: 88–93.
2. Valayannopoulos V. Enzyme replacement therapy and substrate reduction therapy in lysosomal storage disorders with neurological expression. *Handb Clin Neurol*. 2013; 113: 1851–1857.
3. Somaraju UR, Tadepalli K. Hematopoietic stem cell transplantation for Gaucher disease. *Cochrane Database Syst Rev*. 2012; 7: CD006974.
4. Shayman JA. Eliglustat tartrate: glucosylceramide synthase inhibitor treatment of type 1 Gaucher disease. *Drugs Future*. 2010; 35: 613–620.
5. Platt FM, Neises GR, Dwek RA, Butters TD. N-butyldeoxynojirimycin is a novel inhibitor of glycolipid biosynthesis. *J Biol Chem*. 1994; 269: 8362–8365.
6. Platt FM, Neises GR, Reinkensmeier G, et al. Prevention of lysosomal storage in Tay-Sachs mice treated with N-butyldeoxynojirimycin. *Science*. 1997; 276: 428–431.
7. Platt FM, Reinkensmeier G, Dwek RA, Butters TD. Extensive glycosphingolipid depletion in the liver and lymphoid organs of mice treated with N-butyldeoxynojirimycin. *J Biol Chem*. 1997; 272: 19365–19372.
8. Zervas M, Somers KL, Thrall MA, Walkley SU. Critical role for glycosphingolipids in Niemann-Pick disease type C. *Curr Biol*. 2001; 11: 1283–1287.
9. Pastores GM, Giraldo P, Cherin P, Mehta A. Goal-oriented therapy with miglustat in Gaucher disease. *Curr Med Res Opin*. 2009; 25: 23–37.
10. Ficicioglu C. Review of miglustat for clinical management in Gaucher disease type 1. *Ther Clin Risk Manag*. 2008; 4: 425–431.
11. Cox T, Lachmann R, Hollak C, et al. Novel oral treatment of Gaucher's disease with N-butyldeoxynojirimycin (OGT 918) to decrease substrate biosynthesis. *Lancet*. 2000; 355: 1481–1485.
12. Patterson MC, Vecchio D, Prady H, Abel L, Wraith JE. Miglustat for treatment of Niemann-Pick C disease: a randomised controlled study. *Lancet Neurol*. 2007; 6: 765–772.

13. Cox-Brinkman J, van Breemen MJ, van Maldegem BT, et al. Potential efficacy of enzyme replacement and substrate reduction therapy in three siblings with Gaucher disease type III. *J Inherit Metab Dis.* 2008; 31: 745–752.
14. Alfonso P, Pampin S, Estrada J, et al. Miglustat (NB-DNJ) works as a chaperone for mutated acid beta-glucosidase in cells transfected with several Gaucher disease mutations. *Blood Cells Mol Dis.* 2005; 35: 268–276.
15. Porto C, Cardone M, Fontana F, et al. The pharmacological chaperone N-butyldeoxynojirimycin enhances enzyme replacement therapy in Pompe disease fibroblasts. *Mol Ther.* 2009; 17: 964–971.
16. Pineda M, Wraith JE, Mengel E, et al. Miglustat in patients with Niemann-Pick disease Type C (NP-C): a multicenter observational retrospective cohort study. *Mol Genet Metab* 2009; 98: 243–249.
17. Patterson MC, Vecchio D, Jacklin E, et al. Long-term miglustat therapy in children with Niemann-Pick disease type C. *J Child Neurol.* 2010; 25: 300–305.
18. Pineda M, Perez-Poyato MS, O'Callaghan M, et al. Clinical experience with miglustat therapy in pediatric patients with Niemann-Pick disease type C: a case series. *Mol Genet Metab.* 2010; 99: 358–366.
19. Champion H, Ramaswami U, Imrie J, et al. Dietary modifications in patients receiving miglustat. *J Inherit Metab Dis.* 2010; 33(Suppl. 3): S379–S383.
20. European Medicines Agency. Zavesca (miglustat). http://www.ema.europa.eu/ema/index.jsp?curl=pages/medicines/human/medicines/000435/human_med_001171.jsp&murl=menus/medicines/medicines.jsp&mid=WC0b01ac058001d124. Accessed July 4, 2014.
21. Chien YH, Peng SF, Yang CC, et al. Long-term efficacy of miglustat in paediatric patients with Niemann-Pick disease type C. *J Inherit Metab Dis.* 2013; 36: 129–137.
22. Heron B, Valayannopoulos V, Baruteau J, et al. Miglustat therapy in the French cohort of paediatric patients with Niemann-Pick disease type C. *Orphanet J Rare Dis.* 2012; 7: 36.
23. Di Rocco M, Dardis A, Madeo A, Barone R, Fiumara A. Early miglustat therapy in infantile Niemann-Pick disease type C. *Pediatr Neurol.* 2012; 47: 40–43.
24. Dickson PI, Pariser AR, Groft SC, et al. Research challenges in central nervous system manifestations of inborn errors of metabolism. *Mol Genet Metab.* 2011; 102: 326–338.
25. Shapiro BE, Pastores GM, Gianutsos J, Luzy C, Kolodny EH. Miglustat in late-onset Tay-Sachs disease: a 12-month, randomized, controlled clinical study with 24 months of extended treatment. *Genet Med.* 2009; 11: 425–433.
26. Maegawa GH, Banwell BL, Blaser S, et al. Substrate reduction therapy in juvenile GM2 gangliosidosis. *Mol Genet Metab.* 2009; 98: 215–224.
27. Tallaksen CM, Berg JE. Miglustat therapy in juvenile Sandhoff disease. *J Inherit Metab Dis.* 2009; 32(Suppl. 1): S289–S293.
28. Guffon N, Bin-Dorel S, Decullier E, Paillet C, Guitton J, Fouilhoux A. Evaluation of miglustat treatment in patients with type iii mucopolysaccharidosis: a randomized, double-blind, placebo-controlled study. *J Pediatr.* 2011; 159(5): 838–844.
29. Schiffmann R, Fitzgibbon EJ, Harris C, et al. Randomized, controlled trial of miglustat in Gaucher's disease type 3. *Ann Neurol.* 2008; 64: 514–522.
30. Accardo A, Pensiero S, Ciana G, Parentin F, Bembi B. Eye movement impairment recovery in a Gaucher patient treated with miglustat. *Neurol Res Int.* 2010; 4: 1–5.
31. Giraldo P, Latre P, Alfonso P, et al. Short-term effect of miglustat in every day clinical use in treatment-naive or previously treated patients with type 1 Gaucher's disease. *Haematologica.* 2006; 91: 703–706.
32. Giraldo P, Alfonso P, Atutxa K, et al. Real-world clinical experience with long-term miglustat maintenance therapy in type 1 Gaucher disease: the ZAGAL project. *Haematologica.* 2009; 94: 1771–1775.
33. Denny CA, Heinecke KA, Kim YP, et al. Restricted ketogenic diet enhances the therapeutic action of N-butyldeoxynojirimycin towards brain GM2 accumulation in adult Sandhoff disease mice. *J Neurochem.* 2010; 113: 1525–1535.
34. van Giersbergen PL, Dingemanse J. Influence of food intake on the pharmacokinetics of miglustat, an inhibitor of glucosylceramide synthase. *J Clin Pharmacol.* 2007; 47: 1277–1282.
35. Guitton J, Coste S, Guffon-Fouilhoux N, Cohen S, Manchon M, Guillaumont M. Rapid quantification of miglustat in human plasma and cerebrospinal fluid by liquid chromatography coupled with tandem mass spectrometry. *J Chromatogr B Analyt Technol Biomed Life Sci.* 2009; 877: 149–154.
36. Wraith JE, Vecchio D, Jacklin E, et al. Miglustat in adult and juvenile patients with Niemann-Pick disease type C: long-term data from a clinical trial. *Mol Genet Metab* 2010; 99: 351–357.

37. Norez C, Noel S, Wilke M, et al. Rescue of functional delF508-CFTR channels in cystic fibrosis epithelial cells by the alpha-glucosidase inhibitor miglustat. *FEBS Lett.* 2006; 580: 2081–2086.
38. Norez C, Antigny F, Noel S, Vandebrouck C, Becq F. A cystic fibrosis respiratory epithelial cell chronically treated by miglustat acquires a non-cystic fibrosis-like phenotype. *Am J Respir Cell Mol Biol.* 2009; 41: 217–225.
39. Noel S, Wilke M, Bot AG, De Jonge HR, Becq F. Parallel improvement of sodium and chloride transport defects by miglustat (n-butyldeoxynojyrimicin) in cystic fibrosis epithelial cells. *J Pharmacol Exp Ther.* 2008; 325: 1016–1023.
40. Lubamba B, Lebacq J, Lebecque P, et al. Airway delivery of low-dose miglustat normalizes nasal potential difference in F508del cystic fibrosis mice. *Am J Respir Crit Care Med.* 2009; 179: 1022–1028.
41. Platt FM, Neises GR, Karlsson GB, Dwek RA, Butters TD. N-butyldeoxygalactonojirimycin inhibits glycolipid biosynthesis but does not affect N-linked oligosaccharide processing. *J Biol Chem.* 1994; 269: 27108–27114.
42. Andersson U, Butters TD, Dwek RA, Platt FM. N-butyldeoxygalactonojirimycin: a more selective inhibitor of glycosphingolipid biosynthesis than N-butyldeoxynojirimycin, in vitro and in vivo. *Biochem Pharmacol.* 2000; 59: 821–829.
43. Andersson U, Smith D, Jeyakumar M, et al. Improved outcome of N-butyldeoxygalactonojirimycin-mediated substrate reduction therapy in a mouse model of Sandhoff disease. *Neurobiol Dis.* 2004; 16: 506–515.
44. Baek RC, Kasperzyk JL, Platt FM, Seyfried TN. N-butyldeoxygalactonojirimycin reduces brain ganglioside and GM2 content in neonatal Sandhoff disease mice. *Neurochem Int.* 2008; 52: 1125–1133.
45. Elliot-Smith E, Speak AO, Lloyd-Evans E, et al. Beneficial effects of substrate reduction therapy in a mouse model of GM1 gangliosidosis. *Mol Genet Metab.* 2008; 94: 204–211.
46. Kasperzyk JL, El-Abbadi MM, Hauser EC, D'Azzo A, Platt FM, Seyfried TN. N-butyldeoxygalactonojirimycin reduces neonatal brain ganglioside content in a mouse model of GM1 gangliosidosis. *J Neurochem.* 2004; 89: 645–653.
47. Overkleeft HS, Renkema GH, Neele J, et al. Generation of specific deoxynojirimycin-type inhibitors of the non-lysosomal glucosylceramidase. *J Biol Chem.* 1998; 273: 26522–26527.
48. Ashe KM, Bangari D, Li L, et al. Iminosugar-based inhibitors of glucosylceramide synthase increase brain glycosphingolipids and survival in a mouse model of Sandhoff disease. *PLoS One.* 2011; 6: e21758.
49. Abe A, Wild SR, Lee WL, Shayman JA. Agents for the treatment of glycosphingolipid storage disorders. *Curr Drug Metab.* 2001; 2: 331–338.
50. Abe A, Inokuchi J, Jimbo M, et al. Improved inhibitors of glucosylceramide synthase. *J Biochem.* 1992; 111: 191–196.
51. Abe A, Radin NS, Shayman JA. Induction of glucosylceramide synthase by synthase inhibitors and ceramide. *Biochim Biophys Acta.* 1996; 1299: 333–341.
52. Cox TM. Eliglustat tartrate, an orally active glucocerebroside synthase inhibitor for the potential treatment of Gaucher disease and other lysosomal storage diseases. *Curr Opin Investig Drugs.* 2010; 11: 1169–1181.
53. Lukina E, Watman N, Arreguin EA, et al. A phase 2 study of eliglustat tartrate (Genz-112638), an oral substrate reduction therapy for Gaucher disease type 1. *Blood.* 2010; 116: 893–899.
54. Mistry P, Lukina E, Dridi M-FB, et al. A phase 3, randomized, double-blind, placebo-controlled, multicenter study to investigate the efficacy and safety of eliglustat in patients with Gaucher disease type 1 (ENGAGE): Results after 9 months of treatment. *Mol Genet Metab.* 2013; 108: S66–S67.
55. Peterschmitt MJ, Burke A, Blankstein L, et al. Safety, tolerability, and pharmacokinetics of eliglustat tartrate (Genz-112638) after single doses, multiple doses, and food in healthy volunteers. *J Clin Pharmacol.* 2011; 51: 695–705.
56. Wegrzyn G, Jakobkiewicz-Banecka J, Gabig-Ciminska M, et al. Genistein: a natural isoflavone with a potential for treatment of genetic diseases. *Biochem Soc Trans.* 2010; 38: 695–701.
57. Malinowska M, Wilkinson FL, Bennett W, et al. Genistein reduces lysosomal storage in peripheral tissues of mucopolysaccharide IIIB mice. *Mol Genet Metab.* 2009; 98: 235–242.
58. Malinowska M, Wilkinson FL, Langford-Smith KJ, et al. Genistein improves neuropathology and corrects behaviour in a mouse model of neurodegenerative metabolic disease. *PLoS One.* 2010; 5: e14192.
59. Arfi A, Richard M, Gandolphe C, Scherman D. Storage correction in cells of patients suffering from mucopolysaccharidoses types IIIA and VII after treatment with genistein and other isoflavones. *J Inherit Metab Dis.* 2010; 33: 61–67.

60. Friso A, Tomanin R, Salvalaio M, Scarpa M. Genistein reduces glycosaminoglycan levels in a mouse model of mucopolysaccharidosis type II. *Br J Pharmacol*. 2010; 159: 1082–1091.
61. Delgadillo V, O'Callaghan MD, Artuch R, Montero R, Pineda M. Genistein supplementation in patients affected by Sanfilippo disease. *J Inherit Metab Dis*. 2011; 34(5): 1039–1044.
62. de Ruijter J, Valstar MJ, Narajczyk M, et al. Genistein in Sanfilippo disease: a randomized controlled crossover trial. *Ann Neuro*. 2012; 71: 110–120.
63. Kim KH, Dodsworth C, Paras A, Burton BK. High dose genistein aglycone therapy is safe in patients with mucopolysaccharidoses involving the central nervous system. *Mol Genet Metab*. 2013; 109: 382–385.
64. Berkin A, Szarek MA, Plenkiewicz J, Szarek WA, Kisilevsky R. Synthesis of 4-deoxy analogues of 2-acetamido-2-deoxy-D-glucose and 2-acetamido-2-deoxy-D-xylose and their effects on glycoconjugate biosynthesis. *Carbohydr Res*. 2000; 325: 30–45.
65. Berkin A, Szarek WA, Kisilevsky R. Synthesis of 4-deoxy-4-fluoro analogues of 2-acetamido-2-deoxy-D-glucose and 2-acetamido-2-deoxy-D-galactose and their effects on cellular glycosaminoglycan biosynthesis. *Carbohydr Res*. 2000; 326: 250–263.
66. Kaji T, Kawashima T, Sakamoto M. Rhodamine B inhibition of glycosaminoglycan production by cultured human lip fibroblasts. *Toxicol Appl Pharmacol*. 1991; 111: 82–89.
67. Roberts AL, Thomas BJ, Wilkinson AS, Fletcher JM, Byers S. Inhibition of glycosaminoglycan synthesis using rhodamine B in a mouse model of mucopolysaccharidosis type IIIA. *Pediatr Res*. 2006; 60: 309–314.
68. Roberts AL, Rees MH, Klebe S, Fletcher JM, Byers S. Improvement in behaviour after substrate deprivation therapy with rhodamine B in a mouse model of MPS IIIA. *Mol Genet Metab*. 2007; 92: 115–121.
69. Roberts AL, Fletcher JM, Moore L, Byers S. Trans-generational exposure to low levels of rhodamine B does not adversely affect litter size or liver function in murine mucopolysaccharidosis type IIIA. *Mol Genet Metab*. 2010; 101: 208–213.
70. Kaidonis X, Liaw WC, Roberts AD, Ly M, Anson D, Byers S. Gene silencing of EXTL2 and EXTL3 as a substrate deprivation therapy for heparan sulphate storing mucopolysaccharidoses. *Eur J Hum Genet*. 2010; 18: 194–199.
71. Dechecchi MC, Nicolis E, Norez C, et al. Anti-inflammatory effect of miglustat in bronchial epithelial cells. *J Cystic Fibrosis*. 2008; 7: 555–565.
72. Natoli TA, Smith LA, Rogers KA, et al. Inhibition of glucosylceramide accumulation results in effective blockade of polycystic kidney disease in mouse models. *Nat Med*. 2010; 16: 788–792.

Index

AAV (adeno-associated viral vectors) for gene delivery, 285–286
AAV-mediated liver-directed clinical gene therapy, 293
Abu-Elheiga, L. A., 152
Acidurias, organic, 105–109
Acylcarnitine profile (ACP) analysis, 13
Acyl-CoA dehydrogenases. *See also* Fatty acid metabolism
 acyl-CoA dehydrogenase 9 deficiency, 166–167
 deficiencies in, 20–24, 27
 hypoglycemia and, 85
Adams-Oliver syndrome, 55
Adeno-associated viral vectors (AAV) for gene delivery, 285–286
Adenosine deaminase deficiency, 280
Adenoviral vectors for gene delivery, 285
Agalsidase alfa and beta, 308–311
Agency for Healthcare Research and Quality, 244
Aicardi-Goutieres syndrome, 229
Aldolase isoforms, 79–80
Alglucerase, 303
Alpers-Huttenlocher syndrome, 189
Alpha-fucosidosis, 272
Alpha-mannosidosis, 272
α-Dystroglycanopathies, 51–54
α-1-antitrypsin deficiency, 273, 288–289, 293–294
American College of Medical Genetics (ACMG), 3–4, 84, 237
Amino acid disorders. *See* Branched chain amino acid disorders
Analytes, 6–11
Anemia, congenital nonspherocytic hemolytic, 126–127
Anesthesia, in mitochondrial disorder diagnosis, 198
Antioxidants, 110, 209
Antisense splicing modulation for lysosomal storage disorders, 320–321
Antley-Bixley syndrome, autosomal recessive, 211–213
Apoptosis, 129–130, 192
Arginase 1 deficiency and spastic paraplegia, 143–144
Arginine
 compartmental regulation of, 137
 for MELAS syndrome, 197
 in UCD treatment, 144–145
 in ureagenesis and non-ureagenic functions, 140–141
Argininemia (arginase deficiency), 13
Argininosuccinate lyase and nitric oxide deficiency, 143
Argininosuccinate synthetase deficiency (citrullinemia, Type I), 14
Argininosuccinic aciduria (argininosuccinate lyase deficiency), 14
Arion's Model, 76
Attention deficit and hyperactivity disorder (ADHD), phenylketonuria and
 dopamine deficiency related to, 251–252
 inattentive type, 263–264
 as neuropsychological outcome, 247
 prefrontal cortex abnormalities in, 259–260
Audiological screening. *See* Mitochondrial disorders
Autosomal recessive Antley-Bixley syndrome, 211–213
Auxiliary partial orthotopic liver transplantation (APOLT), 274–275

Bacterial inhibition assay, 3
BCAA (branched chain amino acid) disorders. *See* Branched chain amino acid (BCAA) disorders
Beta-ketothiolase deficiency (IVA), 100, 102
Beta-ketothiolase deficiency (methylacetoacetyl-CoA thiolase deficiency), 30, 100, 102
Betaine supplementation, 230
Bickel, H., 244
Bile acids, for Smith-Lemli-Opitz syndrome, 209
Biopterin metabolism disorders, 17–19
Biotinidase, enzyme assay for, 3
Blood-brain barrier
 cerebral folate deficiency and, 229–230
 gene therapy blocked by, 294
 hyperammonemia effects on, 139
 large neutral amino acid transport at, 104, 247, 249–251
 neuroactive steroids crossing, 210

Blood-brain barrier (*cont.*)
    tauroursodeoxycholic acid (TUDCA) crossing, 209
    transcription peptide-mediated enzyme replacement therapy for delivery through, 110
Blood transfusions, for pyruvate kinase deficiency, 122–123
Bone marrow transplantation, 123, 271–273
Brain development, 50–51, 53
Brain-directed gene therapy, 294
Branched chain amino acid (BCAA) disorders, 92–118
    biochemistry, metabolism, regulation, 92–96
    differential diagnosis and secondary work-up, 103
    mitochondrial disorders and, 194
    newborn screening differential diagnosis, 99–100
    pathogenesis of, 103–109
    symptomatic diagnosis, 97–98
    treatment options
        dietary management, 109–110
        gene and cell therapies, 111–112
        mitochondria-targeted, 110
        organ transplantation, 111–112
        overview, 101–103
Branched-chain ketoacid dehydrogenase deficiency. *See* Maple syrup urine disease (MSUD)
Brunetti-Pierri, N., 280
B12 vitamin. *See* One-carbon metabolism disorders
Burdugo, A., 271
Burlina, A., 271
Burnett, R., 328

Campeau, P. M., 134
Canadian Dariusleut Hutterite population, 108
Canavan disease, 295
Carbamoyl-phosphate synthase 1 and pulmonary hypertension, 142–143
Carbohydrate deficient glycoprotein syndrome. *See* Human glycosylation disorders
Carcinogenesis, 129–130, 289
Carnitine/acylcarnitine translocase deficiency, 23
Carnitine cycle, 155–160
Carnitine palmitoyl transferase (CPT type IA), 20, 23, 85
Carnitine supplementation, 197
Carnitine uptake defect (primary carnitine deficiency), 19–20
CASTOR (coenzyme A sequestration, toxicity, or redistribution), 107
CDG (congenital disorders of glycosylation). *See* Human glycosylation disorders
CDG Family Network Foundation, 62
CDG-Ia (PMM2-CDG), disorders in, 38–43
CDG United, 62
Cell and organ transplantation, 271–279
    bone marrow and hematopoietic stem cell, 271–273
    in branched chain amino acid disorders, 111–112
    kidney, 277
    liver, 273–276
    liver cell, 276–277
    for lysosomal storage disorders, 321
    in phenylketonuria, 248

Cerebellar hypoplasia, PMM2-CDG and, 50
Cerebral folate deficiency, 228–229
Cerebral protein synthesis, 249–250
Chanarin-Dorfman syndrome, 154
Chaperone therapy. *See also* Lysosomal storage disorders, chaperone therapy for
    chemical-chaperone enzyme enhancement therapy, 318–319
    molecular, 210
    for phenylketonuria, 245, 247
Chemical-chaperone enzyme enhancement therapy, 318–319
CHILD (congenital hemidysplasia with ichthyosiform erythroderma and limb defects) syndrome, 211–213
CHIME syndrome, 58
Choi, A. J., 328
Cholesterol, sterols, and isoprenoids, 203–224
    CHILD syndrome, chondrodysplasia punctata 2, desmosterolosis, lathosterolosis, sterol C4 methyl oxidase deficiency, and autosomal recessive Antley-Bixley syndrome, 211–213
    cerebrotendinous xanthomatosis, 210–211
    mevalonate kinase deficiency, 213–216
    overview, 203–205
    phenylketonuria and, 251
    Sjögren-Larsson syndrome, 216
    Smith-Lemli-Opitz syndrome, 205–210
    steroid 5a-reductase type 3 deficiency, 216
Chondrodysplasia punctata 2, 211–213
Chondroitin sulfate defects, 57
Chronic encephalopathy, 104. *See also* Maple syrup urine disease (MSUD)
Chronic progressive external ophthalmoplegia (CPEO), 189
Citrullinemia, Type I (argininosuccinate synthetase deficiency), 14
Citrullinemia, Type II (citrin deficiency), 14–15
Cobalamin metabolism disorders, 25–26. *See also* One-carbon metabolism disorders
Coenzyme A sequestration, toxicity, or redistribution (CASTOR), 107
Cofactor supplementation, 196–197
Coffee, E. M., 68
Collaborative Study of Children Treated for Phenylketonuria, 246
College of American Pathology, 12
Colour Word Interference Task, 253
Comparative Effectiveness Review of Adjuvant Treatment for Phenylketonuria (Evidence-based Practice Center, Agency for Healthcare Research and Quality), 244–245, 247, 252
Computerized tomography (CT) scans, 194
Congenital adrenal hyperplasia, 3
Congenital disorders of glycosylation (CDG). *See* Human glycosylation disorders
Congenital hemidysplasia with ichthyosiform erythroderma and limb defects (CHILD) syndrome, 211–213
Congenital nonspherocytic hemolytic anemia, 126–127

CoQ$_{10}$ deficiency, 196–197
Costeff syndrome, 107–108
CPEO (chronic progressive external ophthalmoplegia), 189
CPT type IA (carnitine palmitoyl transferase), 20, 23, 85
Craigen, W. J., 225
Creatine monohydrate supplementation, 197
Cerebrotendinous xanthomatosis (CTX), 210–211
Crigler-Najjar syndrome, 111, 274, 276, 288, 294
CT (computerized tomography) scans, 194
CTX (cerebrotendinous xanthomatosis), 210–211
Cystathionine β-synthase deficiency (homocystinuria), 16
Cysteamine therapy, 318

Deoxynojirimycin derivatives, 347–350
Dermatan sulfate defects, 57
Dermatologic symptoms, in human glycosylation disorders, 43
Desmosterolosis, 211–213
DHAP (dihydroxyacetone phosphate), 69
Diabetes. *See* Mitochondrial disorders
Dietary management
  for branched chain amino acid disorders, 109–110
  for fatty acid oxidation disorders, 164–165
  in miglustat therapy, 349
  for mitochondrial disorders, 197–198
  for phenylketonuria, 244
  for Smith-Lemli-Opitz syndrome, 208
Dihydrofolate reductase deficiency, 230
Dihydropteridine reductase deficiency, 244
Dihydropterin reductase deficiency, 17–18
Dihydroxyacetone phosphate (DHAP), 69
Dopamine synthesis
  in brain development, 260
  myelin production in PKU and, 254–255
  PET studies of, 252–253
  visual evoked potential abnormalities in PKU and, 253–254
Dowling-Degos disease, 54

ECG (electrocardiogram), 194
Echocardiogram, 194
EEG (electroencephalogram), 194
Ehlers-Danlos syndrome, 55, 57
Eklund, E. A., 37
Electrocardiogram (ECG), 194
Electroencephalogram (EEG), 194
Electron transport chain activity, in mitochondrial disorders, 195
Electrophoresis, 5
El-Gharbawy, A., 119
El-Hattab, A. W., 180
Eliglustat tartate therapy, 331–332
Eliglustat therapy, 350
Embden-Meyerhof pathway, 123
Endocrinologic symptoms, in human glycosylation disorders, 43, 51
Endurance training, as mitochondrial disorder therapy, 197

Eng, C. M., 303
Enolase, 81–82
Enzyme-linked immunosorbent assay, 5
Enzyme replacement therapy, 248. *See also* Lysosomal storage disorders; Lysosomal storage disorders, chaperone therapy for
Epilepsy. *See* Mitochondrial disorders
Episodic hyperammonemia, 138
Erez, A., 134
Eroglu, Y., 203
Erythropoietin, for pyruvate kinase deficiency, 123
Ethylmalonic encephalopathy, 20–21
European Medicines Agency, 293, 308
Evidence-based Practice Center, Agency for Healthcare Research and Quality, 244
Exercise, as mitochondrial disorder therapy, 197
Exercise intolerance, 82, 127–128

Fabry disease
  description of, 307–312
  enzyme replacement therapy for, 330
  pharmacological chaperone therapy for, 333–334
Factor VII deficiency, 288
False negative rate (FNR), in newborn screening, 11
False negatives (FN), in newborn screening, 11
False positive rate (FPR), in newborn screening, 11
False positives (FP), in newborn screening, 114
Fanconi-Bickel syndrome, 78
Fatty acid metabolism, 152–179
  carnitine cycle, 155–160
  fatty acid β-oxidation, 152–153
  fatty acid oxidation, 160–167
    acyl-CoA dehydrogenase 9 deficiency, 166–167
    medium-chain acyl-CoA dehydrogenase deficiency, 162–163
    newborn screening for disorders in, 19–24
    overview, 160–161
    short-chain acyl-CoA dehydrogenase deficiency, 161–162
    3-hydroxyacyl-CoA dehydrogenase deficiency, 166
    trifunctional protein and long-chain 3-hydroxyacyl-CoA dehydrogenase deficiency, 165–166
    very-long-chain acyl-CoA dehydrogenase deficiency, 164–165
  ketogenesis and ketolysis defects, 168–169
  ketone bodies production and utilization, 167–168
  supply and transport, 154–155
  therapeutic developments, 169–172
FCMD (Fukuyama congenital muscular dystrophy), 53
FDA (U.S. Food and Drug Administration), 303, 308, 318
5,10-methylenetetrahydrofolate hydrogenase deficiency, 230–323
Flavonoids, 351
Fluoroimmunoassay, 4–5
FN (false negatives), in newborn screening, 11
FNR (false negative rate), in newborn screening, 11

Folate metabolism disorders. *See* One-carbon metabolism disorders
Folate supplementation, for pyruvate kinase deficiency, 122–123
Folic acid-related disorders. *See* One-carbon metabolism disorders
Folinic acid supplementation, 229–230
4-hydroxy-phenylpyruvate dioxygenase deficiency (tyrosinemia, type III), 18–19
FP (false positives), in newborn screening, 114
FPR (false positive rate), in newborn screening, 11
Freeze, H. H., 37
Fructose -1,6-biphosphate 1-phosphohydrolase, 74–75
Fructose -1,6-biphosphate aldolase, 79–80
Fructose 6-phosphate (Fru 6-P), 69
Fukuyama congenital muscular dystrophy (FCMD), 53
Fumarylacetoacetate hydrolase deficiency (tyrosinemia, type I), 18, 273

Galactokinase deficiency, 31–32
Galactose-1-phosphate uridyltransferase deficiency, 31
Galactose metabolism disorders, 3, 31–32
GAPDH (glyceraldehyde 3-phosphate dehydrogenase), 82–83
Gastrointestinal symptoms, in human glycosylation disorders, 42
Gaucher disease
  bone marrow transplantation for, 272
  chemical-chaperone enzyme enhancement therapy for, 319
  description of, 305–307
  eliglustat therapy for, 350
  enzyme replacement therapy for, 330–331
  miglustat therapy for, 348
  substrate reduction therapy for, 331–332
Gene and cell therapies
  for branched chain amino acid disorders, 111–112
  for lysosomal storage disorders, 320
  for phenylketonuria, 248–249, 263
  for Smith-Lemli-Opitz syndrome, 209–210
  for urea cycle disorders, 146
Gene replacement therapy, 280–302
  definitions and principles, 281–282
  ex vivo approaches, 289–290
  models for, 287–289
  nonviral vectors for delivery of, 286
  transgene expression regulation, 286–287
  viral vectors for delivery of, 282–286
  in vivo approaches, 290–295
Genetics of mitochondrial disorders, 181, 183–184
Glc 6-P (glucose-6-phosphate), 68
Gluconeogenesis, 68–91
  defects in enzymes distinguishing glycolysis from, 70–79
    fructose -1,6-biphosphate 1-phosphohydrolase, 74–75
    glucose 6-phosphatase, 75–79
    overview, 70–71
    phosphoenolpyruvate carboxykinase, 72–74
    pyruvate carboxylase, 71–72

human enzymes in, 69
inter-dependent pathways in, 70
liver-specific isoforms of enzymes of glycolysis and, 79–80
one-isoform enzymes of glycolysis and, 80–84
other deficiencies affecting, 84–85
Glucophosphate isomerase (GPI), 83–84
Glucose 6-phosphatase, defects in, 75–79
Glucose 6-phosphate (Glc 6-P), 68
Glucose analogues, in substrate deprivation therapy, 351
Glucosylceramide synthase inhibitor therapy, 332
Glutaric aciduria, type I, 28
Glutaric aciduria, type II, 21
Glyceraldehyde 3-phosphate dehydrogenase (GAPDH), 82–83
Glycine N-methyltransferase deficiency (hypermethioninemia), 16–17
Glycogen storage diseases (GSDs), 77, 288–289
Glycolysis, 119–133
  biochemical pathway, 119–120
  congenital nonspherocytic hemolytic anemia, 126–127
  defects in enzymes distinguishing from gluconeogenesis, 70–79
    fructose -1,6-biphosphate 1-phosphohydrolase, 74–75
    glucose 6-phosphatase, 75–79
    overview, 70–71
    phosphoenolpyruvate carboxykinase, 72–74
    pyruvate carboxylase, 71–72
  early detection of disorders in, 128–130
  enzyme deficiencies of, 121
  exercise intolerance, muscle cramps, myoglobinuria, 127–128
  hemolysis and/or neurological manifestations, 126
  liver-specific isoforms of enzymes of gluconeogenesis and, 79–80
  one-isoform enzymes of gluconeogenesis and, 80–84
  phosphofructokinase deficiency, 123–125
  pyruvate kinase deficiency, 121–123
Glycosaminoglycan synthesis defects, 55–57
Glycosaminoglycan synthesis defects (O-xylose pathway defects), 55–57
Glycosphingolipid synthesis defects, 60
Glycosylation disorders. *See* Human glycosylation disorders
Goldin, E., 328
GPI (glucophosphate isomerase), 83–84
GPI anchor synthesis deficiencies, 57–59
Graham, B. H., 3
GSDs (glycogen storage diseases), 77, 288–289
Guanosine triphosphate cyclohydrolase (GTPCH) deficiency, 17–18, 244
Guthrie, R., 3, 242

Health Resources and Services Administration of U.S. Department of Health and Human Services, 11
Hearing assessment. *See* Mitochondrial disorders
Hematopoietic stem cell transplantation, 271–273, 290

Hemochromatosis, 128–129
Hemolytic anemia, congenital nonspherocytic, 126–127
Hemolytic phenotype
  congenital nonspherocytic hemolytic anemia, 126–127
  neurological manifestations with, 126
  pyruvate kinase deficiency, 121–123
Hemophilia A and B, 287–288
HEM (hydrops-ectopic calcification-moth-eaten) skeletal dysplasia, 203
Heparan sulfate defects, 57
Hepatopathy. See Mitochondrial disorders
Hereditary folate malabsorption, 228
Hereditary fructose intolerance (HFI), 75, 80
Hereditary inclusion body myopathy, 54
HFI (hereditary fructose intolerance), 75
High performance liquid chromatography (HPLC), 5
Histone deacetylase inhibitor therapy, 319
Histopathology, in mitochondrial disorders, 194–195
HIV-1 (human immunodeficiency virus type 1), 284
Hoffmann, G. F., 271
Homocystinuria, 3, 16
HPLC (high performance liquid chromatography), 5
Human glycosylation disorders, 37–67
  diagnosis, 44–46
  glycosphingolipid synthesis defects, 60
  GPI anchor synthesis deficiencies, 57–59
  metabolic pathway in N-linked glycosylation, 46
  mucin type glycosylation defects, 60
  multiple glycosylation pathway defects, 60
  myopathic glycosylation disorders, 54
  N-linked oligosaccharide function, 46–51
  N-linked oligosaccharide synthesis or multiple glycosylation pathways, other disorders in, 43–44
  O-fucose and O-GlcNAc pathway defects, 54–55
  O-mannose pathway defects, 51–54
  overview, 37–38
  O-xylose pathway defects (glycosaminoglycan synthesis defects), 55–57
  PMM2-CDG (CDG-Ia), 38–43
  therapy and model systems, 60–61
Human immunodeficiency virus type 1(HIV-1), 284
Hunter syndrome, 312, 319
Hurler syndrome, 272–273
Hydrops-ectopic calcification-moth-eaten (HEM) skeletal dysplasia, 203
Hydroxyprolinemia, 12
Hyperammonemia, 136, 138–139
Hyperlipidemia, 78
Hypermethioninemia (methionine S-adenosyltransferase, glycine N-methyltransferase, or S-adenosylhomocysteine hydrolase deficiencies), 16–17, 109
Hyperornithinemia-hyperammonemia-homocitrullinuria syndrome, 136

Hyperphenylalaninemia. See Phenylketonuria
Hyperuricemia, 78
Hypogammaglobulinemia, from folate malabsorption, 228
Hypoglycemia
  from acyl-CoA dehydrogenase deficiencies, 85
  from gluconeogenesis enzyme deficiencies, 73–74
  hypoketotic, 162, 165
  from mtDNA depletion syndrome, 193
Hypomyelination, 249–250
Hypopigmentation, 255–256, 261

Ichthyosis prematurity syndrome, 155
Imerslund-Grasbeck disease, 232
Imiglucerase, 303, 330
Imino sugars, 347–350
Incidental detection of nontargeted disorders in newborn screening, 12
Insulin, 129, 154
Intellectual disability. See Mitochondrial disorders
Iron issues. See Glycolysis
Isobutyryl-CoA dehydrogenase deficiency (isobutyric aciduria), 26–27, 102–103
Isoelectric focusing, 5
Isoleucine. See Branched chain amino acid disorders
Isoprenoids. See Cholesterol, sterols, and isoprenoids
Isovaleric acidemia (isovaleryl-CoA dehydrogenase deficiency), 27

Jackson Laboratories, 257
Jaeken, J., 38

Kearns-Sayre syndrome (KSS), 184, 188
Ketone bodies, 167–169
Kidney transplantation, 277
Koeberl, D., 119, 131
Krabbe disease, 272, 295, 320
Krasnewich, D. M., 37
KSS (Kearns-Sayre syndrome), 184

Lactic acidemia, 72, 78
Large neutral amino acid transport at blood-brain barrier, 247, 249–251
Larsen-like syndrome, 55
Lathosterolosis, 211–213
Leber hereditary optic neuropathy (LHON), 189
Leber's congenital amaurosis, 280
Lee, B. H., 134
Leigh syndrome, 188
Leja, D., 343
Lemli, L., 205
Lentiviral vectors for gene delivery, 284–285
Lesch-Nyhan disease, 280
Leucine. See Branched chain amino acid disorders
LHON (Leber hereditary optic neuropathy), 189
Lichter-Konecki, U., 241
Limb-girdle muscular dystrophy, 53
Linkage region defects, 55–56
Lipids. See Cholesterol, sterols, and isoprenoids; Fatty acid metabolism

Liver
    gene therapy and, 290–293
    human glycosylation disorder symptoms of, 42
    isoforms of enzymes of glycolysis and gluconeogenesis specific to, 79–80
    liver cell transplantation, 276–277
    transplantation of, 111, 145–146, 248, 273–276
Long-chain 3-hydroxyacyl-CoA dehydrogenase deficiency, 23–24, 165–166
Lung-directed gene therapy, 294
Lysosomal storage disorders, 303–327
    adjunctive therapies for, 321–322
    antisense splicing modulation for, 320–321
    bone marrow transplantation for, 272
    chemical-chaperone enzyme enhancement therapy, 318–319
    disease prevention, 322
    enzyme replacement safety, 314–316
    Fabry disease, 307–312
    Gaucher disease, 305–307
    gene therapy for, 288, 320
    mucopolysaccharidoses, 312–314
    organ transplantation for, 321
    overview, 303–304
    premature stop-codon read-through, 319
    small molecule-based therapies for, 316–317
    substrate depletion therapy for, 318
    substrate reduction therapy for, 317–318
Lysosomal storage disorders, chaperone therapy for, 328–345
    animal studies and clinical trials, 333–334
    current therapies for, 330–332
    enzyme activators in, 334–336
    pharmacological chaperone discovery process, 336–342
    pharmacologic chaperones, 332–333
    principles of, 328–329

Mabry syndrome, 58
Magnetic resonance imaging (MRI), 194, 250
Magnetic resonance spectroscopy (MRS), 194
Malonic aciduria (malonyl-CoA decarboxylase deficiency), 26
Mannosidosis, 319
Manoli, I., 92
Maple syrup urine disease (MSUD)
    bacterial inhibition assay for, 3
    as branched-chain ketoacid dehydrogenase deficiency, 15
    dietary management as therapy for, 109–110
    impaired metabolism of isoleucine as cause of, 95
    liver transplantation for, 111, 273, 275–276
    newborn screening for, 96–100
    pathogenesis of, 104–105
Maroteaux-Lamy syndrome, 313
March of Dimes Foundation, 4, 84
Maternal phenylketonuria, 245–246, 251–252, 256, 263
Maternal PKU Collaborative Study, 246
McArdle disease, 124
mDNA content, in mitochondrial disorders, 195

MEB (muscle-eye-brain) disease, 51, 53
Medium-chain acyl-CoA dehydrogenase deficiency, 22, 162–163
Medium/short-chain hydroxy acyl-CoA deficiency, 21–22
Megaloblastic anemia -1, 232
MELAS (mitochondrial encephalomyopathy with lactic acidosis and stroke-like episodes), 184
MERRF (myoclonic epilepsy with ragged-red fibers), 184, 188
Metachromatic leukodystrophy (MLD), 272, 295, 320
Methionine cycle disorders. See One-carbon metabolism disorders
Methionine S-adenosyltransferase deficiency (hypermethioninemia), 16–17, 109
Methylacetoacetyl-CoA thiolase deficiency (beta-ketothiolase deficiency), 30
Methylacetoacetyl-CoA thiolase deficiency (beta-ketothiolase deficiency), 30
Methylene-tetrahydrofolate reductase deficiency, 229–230
Methylmalonic acidurias (MMA)
    differential diagnosis of, 100
    gene and cell therapies for, 111–112
    kidney transplantation for, 277
    liver transplantation for, 273–274
    newborn screening for, 24
    organ transplantation for, 111–112
    pathogenesis of, 105–107
Methylmalonyl semialdehyde deficiency, 109
Mevalonate kinase deficiency, 213–216
Meyburg, J., 271
Miglustat therapy, 317, 331, 348
Mitochondrial disorders, 180–202
    categorization of, 184–189
    cerebral folate deficiency and, 229
    clinical manifestations, 184, 193
    diagnosis of, 192–193
    electron transport chain activity, 195
    energy generation, 181–182
    genetics of, 181
    histopathology, 194–195
    inheritance, heteroplasmy, segregation, and threshold effect, 183–184
    mDNA content, 195
    mechanisms of, 189–192
    molecular testing, 195–196
    multiorgan involvement extent, 194
    protein import, 182–183
    screening tests, 193–194
    treatments, 196–198
Mitochondrial encephalomyopathy with lactic acidosis and stroke-like episodes (MELAS), 184, 188
Mitochondrial neurogastrointestinal encephalopathy (MNGIE), 184
Mitochondria-targeted treatment, 110
MLD (metachromatic leukodystrophy), 272, 295, 320
MMA (methylmalonic acidurias). See Methylmalonic acidurias (MMA)

MNGIE (mitochondrial neurogastrointestinal encephalopathy), 184
Molecular chaperones, for Smith-Lemli-Opitz syndrome, 210
Molecular Libraries Initiative, Roadmap for Medical Research, National Institutes of Health (NIH), 343
"Moon-lighting," glycolytic enzymes in, 130
Morpholinopropanol homologues, 350
MRI (magnetic resonance imaging), 194, 250
MRS (magnetic resonance spectroscopy), 194
MSUD (maple syrup urine disease). *See* Maple syrup urine disease (MSUD)
mtDNA. *See* Mitochondrial disorders
Mucin type glycosylation defects, 60
Mucopolysaccharidoses, 312–314, 330, 351
Multiple acyl-CoA dehydrogenase deficiency, 21
Multiple carboxylase deficiency, 28–29
Multiple glycosylation pathway defects, 43–44, 60
Muscle cramps, from glycolysis disorders, 127–128
Muscle-directed gene therapy, 293–294
Muscle-eye-brain (MEB) disease, 51, 53
Muscular dystrophy, 53
Myoclonic epilepsy with ragged-red fibers (MERRF), 184, 188
Myoglobinuria, from glycolysis disorders, 119, 127–128
Myopathic glycosylation disorders, 54
Myopathy phenotype. *See also* Mitochondrial disorders
    exercise intolerance, muscle cramps, myoglobinuria, 127–128
    phosphofructokinase deficiency, 123–125

Nagamani, S. C. S., 134
NARP (neurogenic weakness with ataxia and retinitis pigmentosa), 184, 188
National Heart, Lung, and Blood Institute, NIH, 131
National Human Genome Research Institute, 343
National Institutes of Health (NIH), 131, 343
NCV (nerve conduction velocity) studies, 194
nDNA. *See* Mitochondrial disorders
Neonatal hypothyroidism, 3
Nerve conduction velocity (NCV) studies, 194
Nervous system symptoms, in human glycosylation disorders, 41–42
Neural network development disturbance, phenylketonuria as, 259–260
Neurogenic weakness with ataxia and retinitis pigmentosa (NARP), 184, 188
Neuronal ceroid lipofuscinosis, 295
Neurosteroids, for Smith-Lemli-Opitz syndrome, 210
Neurotransmission and neurotoxicity. *See* Phenylketonuria
Neutropenia, 78
Newborn screening, overview of, 3–34. *See also* Phenylketonuria
    amino acid catabolism and transport disorders, 13–17
    analyte cut-off determination, 11
    biochemical *versus* molecular confirmation in, 12–13
    biopterin metabolism disorders, 17–19
    electrophoresis in, 5
    enzyme-linked immunosorbent assay in, 5
    fatty acid oxidation disorders, 19–24
    fluoroimmunoassay in, 4–5
    future directions in, 32
    galactose metabolism disorders, 31–32
    history of, 3–4
    incidental detection of nontargeted disorders, 12
    isoelectric focusing in, 5
    one-carbon metabolism disorders, 237
    organic acidemias, 24–31
    primary and secondary analyte selection, 6–11
    principle of, 4
    quality control for, 12
    radioimmunoassay in, 5
    tandem mass spectroscopy in, 6
Newborn Screening Quality Assurance Program of U.S. Centers for Disease Control and Prevention, 12
Ng, B., 62
Niemann-Pick disease, 320
Niemann-Pick disease type A, 295
Niemann-Pick disease type B, 272
Niemann-Pick disease type C, 317, 331
NIH (National Institutes of Health), 131, 343
Nitric oxide deficiency, 143, 192, 197
Nitrogen scavenging agents, 144
N-linked glycosylation, metabolic pathway in, 46
N-linked oligosaccharide
    function of, 46–51
    synthesis of, 43–44
Non-ureagenic functions. *See* Ureagenesis and non-ureagenic functions
Notch family of proteins, 54
Nuclear magnetic resonance spectroscopy, 250

OAA (oxaloacetate), 71
O-fucose pathway defects, 54–55
O-GlcNAc pathway defects, 54–55
OLT (orthotopic liver transplantation), 274–275
O-mannose pathway defects, 51–54
One-carbon metabolism disorders, 225–240
    absorption and transport disorders, 232–233
    cerebral folate deficiency, 228–229
    dihydrofolate reductase deficiency, 230
    5,10-methylenetetrahydrofolate dehydrogenase deficiency, 230–232
    hereditary folate malabsorption, 228
    intracellular processing disorders, 233–236
    methylene-tetrahydrofolate reductase deficiency, 229–230
    newborn screening for, 237
    other biological processes affected by, 236
    overview, 225–226
    pathways, 226–228
One-isoform enzymes of gluconeogenesis and glycolosis, 80–84
Opitz, J., 205
Ophthalmologic symptoms, 42. *See also* Mitochondrial disorders
Organic acidemias, 24–31
Organic acidurias, 105–109, 273

Organ transplantation. *See* Cell and organ transplantation
Ornithine carbamoyltransferase (OTC) deficiency, 288
Orphan Drug legislation, 308
Orthopedic symptoms, in human glycosylation disorders, 42
Orthotopic liver transplantation (OLT), 274–275
Osteopenia, 321
OTC (ornithine carbamoyltransferase) deficiency, 288
"Out-of-wind" phenomenon, 124
Oxaloacetate (OAA), 71
O-xylose pathway defects (glycosaminoglycan synthesis defects), 55–57

PA (propionic acidemia). *See* Propionic acidemia (PA)
PAL (phenylalanine ammonia lyase) treatment, 248
Parkinson's disease, phenylketonuria and, 253
Pastores, G. M., 303
Patterson, M. C., 346
Pearson syndrome, 188
Pentose phosphate shunt, 69
Peripheral neuropathy, 194
Peters Plus syndrome, 54
PET (positron emission tomography) studies of tyrosine and dopamine synthesis, 252–253
PGAM (phosphoglycerate mutase), 82
Pharmacologic chaperones. *See* Lysosomal storage disorders, chaperone therapy for
Phenylalanine ammonia lyase (PAL) treatment, 248
Phenylalanine hydroxylase deficiency, 17
Phenylketonuria (PKU), 241–268
  alternative or adjunct treatment options, 247–249
  attention deficit disorder and, 251–252
  background, 242–243
  decreased neurotransmitter synthesis, 252–257
  differential diagnosis, 243–244
  future research on, 257–264
    direction for, 261–263
    hypopigmentation, 261
    maternal phenylketonuria, 263
    modifier genes, 263
    as neural network development disturbance, 259–260
    neurotransmitter role in brain development, 260–261
    overview, 257–258
    prefrontal cortex and ADHD-inattentive type, 263–264
    as white matter disease, 258–259
  large neutral amino acid transport at blood-brain barrier, 249–251
  phenylketone impact, 249
  screening method for, 3
  treatment, 243–246
  variant phenotypes, 246–247
Phosphoenolpyruvate carboxykinase, 72–74
Phosphofructokinase deficiency, 123–125
Phosphoglycerate mutase (PGAM), 82
Phosphoglycerates, 69
Plasma amino acid (PPA) analysis, 12

PMM2-CDG (CDG-Ia), disorders in, 38–43
Pneumocystis jiroveci infection, 228
Pompe disease, 316, 321, 330, 333–334
Positive predictive value (PPV), in newborn screening, 11
Positron emission tomography (PET) studies of tyrosine and dopamine synthesis, 252–253
PAA (plasma amino acid) analysis, 12
PPV (positive predictive value), in newborn screening, 11
Prefrontal cortex dysfunction hypothesis, in phenylketonuria, 253
Premature stop-codon read-through, 319
Prenatal treatments, for Smith-Lemli-Opitz syndrome, 210
Presumptive positive rate, in newborn screening, 11
Primary carnitine deficiency (carnitine uptake defect), 19–20
Primary hyperoxaluria type 1, 274
Propionic acidemia (PA)
  gene and cell therapies for, 111–112
  newborn screening for, 24
  organ transplantation for, 111
  pathogenesis of, 100
Propionic acidurias, liver transplantation for, 274
Protein synthesis, cerebral, 249–250
Proteostasis regulators, 336
Pterin-4α-carbinolamine dehydratase deficiency, 17–18
Pulmonary hypertension, 142–143
Pyruvate carboxylase, 12, 71–72
Pyruvate kinase deficiency, 121–123, 128–129

Radioimmunoassay, 5
Ragged-red fibers, in histology, 184, 188, 194
Rapoport-Luebering shunt, 127
Refsum disease, 288
Region 4 Genetics Collaborative, 11
Renal impairment, 42. *See also* Mitochondrial disorders
Resistance training, as mitochondrial disorder therapy, 197
Retroviral vectors for gene delivery, 283–284
Rett syndrome, 229
Rhodamine B, 351
Riboflavin supplementation, 197
RNA interference, in substrate deprivation therapy, 351–352
Roadmap for Medical Research, National Institutes of Health (NIH), 343
Roullet, J.-B., 203

S-adenosylhomocysteine hydrolase deficiency (hypermethioninemia), 16–17, 109
Sandhoff disease, 317, 321
Sanfilippo syndrome, 319
Sapropterin dihydrochloride therapy, 245, 247
SCAD (short-chain acyl-CoA dehydrogenase deficiency), 20, 102–103, 161–162
Scaglia, F., 180
Schneckenbecken dysplasia, 57
SCID (severe combined immune deficiency), 280, 290

Secondary mitochondrial dysfunction, 106–107, 110
Sensitivity, in newborn screening, 11
Sensorineural hearing loss. See Mitochondrial disorders
Severe combined immune deficiency (SCID), 280, 290
Shchelochkov, O. A., 134
Shinawi, M. S., 152
Short/branched-chain acyl-CoA dehydrogenase deficiency (2-methylbutyrylglycinuria), 27, 102
Short-chain acyl-CoA dehydrogenase deficiency (SCAD), 20, 102–103, 161–162
Sickle cell disease, 5
Sidransky, E., 328
SIDS (sudden infant death syndrome), 73
6-pyruvoyl-tetrahydropterin synthase deficiency, 17–18
Sjögren-Larsson syndrome, 216
SLOS (Smith-Lemli-Opitz syndrome), 205–210
Sly syndrome, 272
Small molecule-based therapies, 316–317
Smith, D., 205
Smith-Lemli-Opitz syndrome (SLOS), 205–210
Spastic paraplegia, 143–144
Splenectomy, for pyruvate kinase deficiency, 122–123
SRT (substrate reduction therapy), 317–318, 328, 331–332
Statins, for Smith-Lemli-Opitz syndrome, 208–209
Steiner, R. D., 203
Steroid 5-alpha-reductase type 3 deficiency, 216
Sterol C4 methyl oxidase deficiency, 211–213
Sterols. See Cholesterol, sterols, and isoprenoids
Substrate depletion therapy, 318
Substrate deprivation therapy, 346–355. See also Substrate reduction therapy (SRT)
  agents for, 347
  flavonoids and other mucopolysaccharidoses compounds, 351
  glucose and xylose analogues and rhodamine B, 351
  imino sugars for, 347–350
  morpholinopropanol homologues, 350
  overview, 346
  RNA interference, 351–352
Substrate reduction therapy (SRT), 317–318, 328, 331–332. See also Substrate deprivation therapy
Succinyl-CoA ligase deficiency, 12
Sudden infant death syndrome (SIDS), 73
Susi, A., 3
Sutton, V. R., 3

Taliglucerase alfa, 330
Tandem mass spectroscopy, 3, 6
Tauri disease, 124
Tauroursodeoxycholic acid (TUDCA), for Smith-Lemli-Opitz syndrome, 209
Tay-Sachs disease, 317, 319, 322, 348
3-hydroxy-3-methylglutaryl-CoA lyase deficiency, 29
3-hydroxyacyl-CoA dehydrogenase deficiency, 166
3-Hydroxyisobutyric aciduria, 108–109
3-Hydroxyisobutyryl-CoA hydrolase deficiency, 108
3MCC deficiency, 102

3-Methylglutaconic aciduria (3-MGA), 107–108
3-methylglutaconic aciduria, Type I (3-methylglutaconyl-CoA hydratase deficiency), 30
Threshold effect, in mitochondrial disorders, 183–184
TN (true negatives), in newborn screening, 11
Tolan, D. R., 68
TP (true positives), in newborn screening, 114
TPI (triose phosphate isomerase), 83
Transcription peptide-mediated enzyme replacement therapy, 110
Trifunctional protein and long-chain 3-hydroxyacyl-CoA dehydrogenase deficiency, 165–166
Trifunctional protein deficiency, 23–24
Triose phosphate isomerase (TPI), 83
True negatives (TN), in newborn screening, 11
True positives (TP), in newborn screening, 114
TUDCA (tauroursodeoxycholic acid), for Smith-Lemli-Opitz syndrome, 209
2-methyl-3-hdroxybutyryl-CoA dehydrogenase deficiency, 108
2-methylbutyrylglycinuria (short/branched-chain acyl-CoA dehydrogenase deficiency), 27, 102
2-methyl-3-hydroxybutyric acidemia (2-methyl-3-hydroxybutyryl-CoA dehydrogenase deficiency), 30–31
Tyrosine aminotransferase deficiency (tyrosinemia, type II), 18–19
Tyrosinemia, type I (fumarylacetoacetate hydrolase deficiency), 18, 273
Tyrosinemia, type II (tyrosine aminotransferase deficiency), 18–19
Tyrosinemia, type III (4-hydroxy-phenylpyruvate dioxygenase deficiency), 18–19
Tyrosine synthesis, PET studies of, 252–253

UCDs (urea cycle disorders). See Ureagenesis and non-ureagenic functions
UDP-galactose 4-epimerase deficiency, 31–32
Umaña, L., 225
UOA (urine organic acids) analysis, 12
Urea cycle disorders (UCDs). See Ureagenesis and non-ureagenic functions
Ureagenesis and non-ureagenic functions, 134–151
  arginase 1 deficiency and spastic paraplegia, 143–144
  arginine connection, 140–141
  argininosuccinate lyase and nitric oxide deficiency, 143
  carbamoyl-phosphate synthase 1 and pulmonary hypertension, 142–143
  complex disorders in, 141
  hyperammonemia, 138–139
  liver cell transplantation for, 276–277
  liver transplantation for, 274–275
  regulation of, 137
  treatment, 144–146
Urine acylcarnitines, 3

Urine organic acids (UOAs) analysis, 12
U.S. Centers for Disease Control and Prevention Newborn Screening Quality Assurance Program, 12
U.S. Department of Health and Human Services, 11
U.S. Food and Drug Administration (FDA), 303, 308, 318

Valine. *See* Branched chain amino acid disorders
Velaglucerase, 330
Venditti, C., 92
Very-long-chain acyl-CoA dehydrogenase deficiency, 22, 164–165
Vision screening. *See* Mitochondrial disorders
Visual evoked potential abnormalities, in phenylketonuria, 253–254
Vitamin B12. *See* One-carbon metabolism disorders

Vitamins and minerals, for Smith-Lemli-Opitz syndrome, 209–210
von Gierke disease, 77

Walker Warburg syndrome (WWS), 53
Warburg effect, 130
Wechsler Adult Intelligence Scale, 246
Westbroek, W., 343
White matter disease, phenylketonuria as, 258–259
Wilson's disease, 111, 273
WWS (Walker Warburg syndrome), 53

X-linked multiple congenital anomalies-hypotonia-seizures syndrome 2, 58
Xylose analogues, in substrate deprivation therapy, 351

Zheng, W., 328